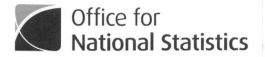
Office for
National Statistics

Annual Abstract
of Statistics

No 146
2010 Edition

Editor: Ian Macrory
Office for National Statistics

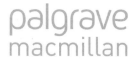
palgrave
macmillan

ISBN 978-0-230-24316-3

ISSN 0072–5730 (print), ISSN 2040–1639 (online)

A National Statistics publication

National Statistics are produced to high professional standards as set out in the Code of Practice for Official Statistics. They are produced free from political influence.

About us

The Office for National Statistics

The Office for National Statistics (ONS) is the executive office of the UK Statistics Authority, a non-ministerial department which reports directly to Parliament. ONS is the UK government's single largest statistical producer. It compiles information about the UK's society and economy, and provides the evidence-base for policy and decision-making, the allocation of resources, and public accountability. The Director-General of ONS reports directly to the National Statistician who is the Authority's Chief Executive and the Head of the Government Statistical Service.

The Government Statistical Service

The Government Statistical Service (GSS) is a network of professional statisticians and their staff operating both within the Office for National Statistics and across more than 30 other government departments and agencies.

Palgrave Macmillan

This publication first published 2010 by Palgrave Macmillan.

Palgrave Macmillan in the UK is an imprint of Macmillan Publishers Limited, registered in England, company number 785998, of Houndmills, Basingstoke, Hampshire RG21 6XS. Palgrave Macmillan in the US is a division of St Martin's Press LLC, 175 Fifth Avenue, New York, NY 10010.

Palgrave Macmillan is the global academic imprint of the above companies and has companies and representatives throughout the world. Palgrave® and Macmillan® are registered trademarks in the United States, the United Kingdom, Europe and other countries. A catalogue record for this book is available from the British Library.

10 9 8 7 6 5 4 3 2 1

19 18 17 16 15 14 13 12 11 10

Contacts

This publication

For information about the content of this publication, contact the ONS Core Table Unit

Tel: 01329 455851

Email: ctu@ons.gsi.gov.uk

Other customer enquiries

ONS Customer Contact Centre

Tel: 0845 601 3034

International: +44 (0)845 601 3034

Minicom: 01633 815044

Email: info@statistics.gsi.gov.uk

Fax: 01633 652747

Post: Room 1.101, Government Buildings, Cardiff Road, Newport, South Wales NP10 8XG

www.ons.gov.uk

Media enquiries

Tel: 0845 604 1858

Email: press.office@ons.gsi.gov.uk

Publication orders

To obtain the print version of this publication, contact Palgrave Macmillan

Tel: 01256 302611

www.palgrave.com/ons

Price: £55.00

Copyright and reproduction

Printing

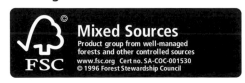

This book is printed on paper suitable for recycling and made from fully managed and sustained forest sources. Logging, pulping and manufacturing processes are expected to conform to the environmental regulations of the country of origin.

Printed and bound in Great Britain by Hobbs the Printer Ltd, Totton, Southampton

Typeset by Kerrypress Ltd, Luton

Contents Whether items are National Statistics, non National Statistics

Contents

Contents

Contents

17: Prices

18: Government finance

Central government

Local authorities

United Kingdom

England and Wales

Contents

		Page	Type*

22: Production

Contents

*   This publication contains a mixture of 'National Statistics' and 'Other Official Statistics'. Statistics accredited as 'National Statistics' (NS) are fully compliant with the Code of Practice for Official Statistics and carry the National Statistics Kitemark. Statistics labelled as 'Other Official Statistics' (Non NS) follow many of the best practice principles set out in the Code but have not been accredited as fully compliant.

Contributors and acknowledgements

The editor would like to thank the following people for their help in producing this book:

Production team: Leah Corten

Tammy Powell

Sue Punt

Dilys Rosen

Karen Whittaker

Andrew White

Contributors
The Editor also wishes to thank all his colleagues in ONS, the rest of the Government Statistical Service and all contributors in other organisations for their generous support and helpful comments, without whose help this publication would not be possible.

Design: ONS Design
Typesetting: Kerrypress Typesetters Ltd
Publishing management: Phil Lewin, Brenda Miles

Units of measurement

Length
1 millimetre (mm)	= 0.03937 inch	
1 centimetre (cm)	= 10 millimetres	= 0.3937 inch
1 metre (m)	= 1,000 millimetres	= 1.094 yards
1 kilometre (km)	= 1,000 metres	= 0.6214 mile
1 inch (in.)		= 25.40 millimetres or 2.540 centimetres
1 foot (ft.)	= 12 inches	= 0.3048 metre
1 yard (yd.)	= 3 feet	= 0.9144 metre
1 mile	= 1,760 yards	= 1.609 kilometres

Area
1 square millimetre (mm2)		= 0.001550 square inch
1 square metre (m2)	= one million square millimetres	= 1.196 square yards
1 hectare (ha)	= 10,000 square metres	= 2.471 acres
1 square kilometre (km2)	= one million square metres	= 247.1 acres
1 square inch (sq. in.)		= 645.2 square millimetres or 6.452 square centimetres
1 square foot (sq. ft.)	= 144 square inches	= 0.09290 square metre or 929.0 square centimetres
1 square yard (sq. yd.)	= 9 square feet	= 0.8361 square metre
1 acre	= 4,840 square yards	= 4,046 square metres or 0.4047 hectare
1 square mile (sq. mile)	= 640 acres	= 2.590 square kilometres or 259.0 hectares

Volume
1 cubic centimetre (cm3)		= 0.06102 cubic inch
1 cubic decimetre (dm3)	= 1,000 cubic centimetres	= 0.03531 cubic foot
1 cubic metre (m3)	= one million cubic centimetres	= 1.308 cubic yards
1 cubic inch (cu.in.)		=16.39 cubic centimetres
1 cubic foot (cu. ft.)	= 1,728 cubic inches	= 0.02832 cubic metre or 28.32 cubic decimetres
1 cubic yard (cu. yd.)	= 27 cubic feet	= 0.7646 cubic metre

Capacity
1 litre (l)	= 1 cubic decimetre	= 0.2200 gallon
1 hectolitre (hl)	= 100 litres	= 22.00 gallons
1 pint		= 0.5682 litre
1 quart	= 2 pints	= 1.137 litres
1 gallon	= 8 pints	= 4.546 litres
1 bulk barrel	= 36 gallons (gal.)	= 1.637 hectolitres

Weight
1 gram (g)		= 0.03527 ounce avoirdupois
1 hectogram (hg)	= 100 grams	= 3.527 ounces or 0.2205 pound
1 kilogram (kg)	= 1,000 grams or 10 hectograms	= 2.205 pounds
1 tonne (t)	= 1,000 kilograms	= 1.102 short tons or 0.9842 long ton
1 ounce avoirdupois (oz.)	= 437.5 grains	= 28.35 grams
1 pound avoirdupois (lb.)	= 16 ounces	= 0.4536 kilogram
1 hundredweight (cwt.)	= 112 pounds	= 50.80 kilograms
1 short ton	= 2,000 pounds	= 907.2 kilograms or 0.9072 tonne
1 long ton (referred to as ton)	= 2,240 pounds	= 1,016 kilograms or 1.016 tonnes
1 ounce troy	= 480 grains	= 31.10 grams

Energy
British thermal unit (Btu)	= 0.2520 kilocalorie (kcal) = 1.055 kilojoule (kj)
Therm	= 105 British thermal units = 25,200 kcal = 105,506 kj
Megawatt hour (MWh)	= 106 watt hours (Wh)
Gigawatt hour (GWh)	= 106 kilowatt hours = 34,121 therms

Food and drink
Butter	23,310 litres milk	= 1 tonne butter (average)
Cheese	10,070 litres milk	= 1 tonne cheese
Condensed milk	2,550 litres milk	= 1 tonne full cream condensed milk
	2,953 litres skimmed milk	= 1 tonne skimmed condensed milk
Milk	1 million litres	= 1,030 tonnes
Milk powder	8,054 litres milk	= 1 tonne full cream milk powder
	10,740 litres skimmed milk	= 1 tonne skimmed milk powder
Eggs	17,126 eggs	= 1 tonne (approximate)
Sugar	100 tonnes sugar beet	= 92 tonnes refined sugar
	100 tonnes cane sugar	= 96 tonnes refined sugar

Shipping

Gross tonnage = The total volume of all the enclosed spaces of a vessel, the unit of measurement being a 'ton' of 100 cubic feet.

Deadweight tonnage = Deadweight tonnage is the total weight in tons of 2,240 lb. that a ship can legally carry, that is the total weight of cargo, bunkers, stores and crew.

Introduction

Introduction

Welcome to the 2010 edition of the *Annual Abstract of Statistics*. This compendium draws together statistics from a wide range of official and other authoritative sources. All contributors' help is gratefully acknowledged.

This will be the last print edition of the *Annual Abstract*. Future web editions will be available free of charge on the Office for National Statistics (ONS) website: www.ons.gov.uk.

Regional information, supplementary to the national figures in *Annual Abstract*, appear in *Regional Trends online*. The latest edition of *Regional Trends* is available electronically on the ONS website free of charge. This can be accessed at: *www.statistics.gov.uk/regionaltrends/data*

Print editions are available from Palgrave Macmillan (see page ii).

Current data for many of the series appearing in this *Annual Abstract* are contained in other ONS publications, such as *Economic & Labour Market Review, Population Trends, Health Statistics Quarterly* and *Financial Statistics*.

Other ONS publications which contain related data are the *Monthly Digest of Statistics* and *Social Trends*. These are also published by Palgrave Macmillan or can be found directly at:

www.statistics.gov.uk/statbase/Product.asp?vlnk=611

www.statistics.gov.uk/socialtrends/

The name (and telephone number, where this is available) of the organisation providing the statistics are shown under each table. In addition, a list of Sources is given at the back of the book, which sets out the official publications or other sources to which further reference can be made.

Identification codes

The four-letter identification code at the top of each data column, or at the side of each row is the ONS reference for this series of data on our database. Please quote the relevant code if you contact us requiring any further information about the data. On some tables it is not possible to include these codes, so please quote the table number in these cases.

Definitions and classification

Time series
So far as possible annual totals are given throughout, but quarterly or monthly figures are given where these are more suitable to the type of series.

Explanatory notes
Most sections are preceded by explanatory notes which should be read in conjunction with the tables. Definitions and explanatory notes for many of the terms occurring in the *Annual Abstract* are also given in the *Annual Supplement to the Monthly Digest of Statistics*, published in the January edition. Detailed notes on items which appear in both the *Annual Abstract and Financial Statistics* are given in an annual supplement to the latter entitled *Financial Statistics Explanatory Handbook*. The original sources listed in the Sources may also be consulted.

Standard Industrial Classification

A Standard Industrial Classification (SIC) was first introduced into the UK in 1948 for use in classifying business establishments and other statistical units by the type of economic activity in which they are engaged. The classification provides a framework for the collection, tabulation, presentation and analysis of data about economic activities. Its use promotes uniformity of data collected by various government departments and agencies.

Since 1948 the classification has been revised in 1958, 1968, 1980, 1992, 2003 and 2007. One of the principal objectives of the 1980 revision was to eliminate differences from the activity classification issued by the Statistical Office of the European Communities (Eurostat) and entitled 'Nomenclature générale des activités économiques dans les Communautés Européennes', usually abbreviated to NACE.

In 1990 the European Communities introduced a new statistical classification of economic activities (NACE Rev 1) by regulation. The regulation made it obligatory for the UK to introduce a new Standard Industrial Classification SIC(92), based on NACE Rev 1. UK SIC(92) was based exactly on NACE Rev 1 but, where it was thought necessary or helpful, a fifth digit was added to form subclasses of the NACE 1 four digit system. Classification systems need to be revised periodically because, over time, new products, processes and industries emerge. In January 2003 a minor revision of NACE Rev 1, known as NACE Rev 1.1, was published in the *Official Journal of the European Communities*.

Introduction

Consequently, the UK was obliged to introduce a new Standard Industrial Classification, SIC(2003) consistent with NACE Rev 1.1. The UK took the opportunity of the 2003 revision also to update the national Subclasses. Full details are available in UK Standard Industrial Classification of Economic Activities 2003 and the Indexes to the UK Standard Industrial Classification of Economic Activities 2003. These are the most recent that are currently used. The most up to date version is the UK Standard Industrial Classification of Economic activities 2007 (SIC2007). It will be implemented in five stages and came into effect on 1 January 2008.

- For reference year 2008, the Annual Business Inquiry (parts 1 & 2) will be based on SIC 2007

- PRODCOM will also be based on SIC 2007 from reference year 2008

- Other annual outputs will be based on SIC 2007 from reference year 2009, unless otherwise determined by regulation

- Quarterly and monthly surveys will be based on SIC 2007 from the first reference period in 2010, unless otherwise determined by regulation

- National Accounts will move to SIC 2007 in September 2011

ONS is currently working on a detailed implementation plan for the introduction of the new classification, covering all of our surveys and outputs. For further information see: www.statistics.gov.uk/statbase/Product.asp?vlnk=14012

Revisions to contents

Some of the figures, particularly for the latest year, are provisional and may be revised in a subsequent issue of the *Annual Abstract*.

Symbols and conventions used

Change of basis
Where consecutive figures have been compiled on different bases and are not strictly comparable, a footnote is added indicating the nature of the difference.

Geographic coverage
Statistics relate mainly to the UK. Where figures relate to other areas, this is indicated on the table.

Units of measurement
The various units of measurement used are listed after the Contents.

Rounding of figures
In tables where figures have been rounded to the nearest final digit, the constituent items may not add up exactly to the total.

Symbols
The following symbols have been used throughout:

- .. = not available or not applicable (also information supressed to avoid disclosure)

- - = nil or less than half the final digit shown

Office for National Statistics online: www.ons.gov.uk

Web-based access to time series, cross-sectional data and metadata from across the Government Statistical Service (GSS), is available using the site search function from the homepage. Download many datasets, in whole or in part, or consult directory information for all GSS statistical resources, including censuses, surveys, periodicals and enquiry services. Information is posted as PDF electronic documents or in XLS and CSV formats, compatible with most spreadsheet packages.

Complete copies of this publication are available to download free of charge at: www.statistics.gov.uk/statbase/product.asp?vlnk=94

Contact point

ONS welcomes any feedback on the content of the *Annual Abstract*, including comments on the format of the data and the selection of topics. Comments and requests for general information should be addressed to:

Core Table Unit
Societal Wellbeing Division
Room 1.059
Office for National Statistics
Government Buildings
Cardiff Road
Newport
South Wales
NP10 8XG

or

Email: info@statistics.gov.uk

July 2010

Area

Chapter 1

Area

The UK comprises Great Britain and Northern Ireland. Great Britain comprises England, Wales and Scotland.

Physical Features

The UK constitutes the greater part of the British Isles. The largest of the islands is Great Britain. The next largest comprises Northern Ireland and the Irish Republic. Western Scotland is fringed by the large island chain known as the Hebrides, and to the north east of the Scottish mainland are the Orkney and Shetland Islands. All these, along with the Isle of Wight, Anglesey and the Isles of Scilly, form part of the UK. The Isle of Man, in the Irish Sea, and the Channel Islands, between Great Britain and France, are largely self-governing and are not part of the UK. The UK is one of the 27 member states of the European Union following the accession of Bulgaria and Romania on 1 January 2007. With an area of about 243,000 sq km (about 94,000 sq miles), the UK is just under 1,000 km (about 600 miles) from the south coast to the extreme north of Scotland and just under 500 km (around 300 miles) across at the widest point.

- Highest mountain: Ben Nevis, in the highlands of Scotland, at 1,343 m (4,406 ft)

- Longest river: the Severn, 354 km (220 miles) long, which rises in central Wales and flows through Shrewsbury, Worcester and Gloucester in England to the Bristol Channel

- Largest lake: Lough Neagh, Northern Ireland, at 396 sqkm (153 sq miles)

- Deepest lake: Loch Morar in the Highlands of Scotland, 310 m (1,017 ft) deep

- Highest waterfall: Eas a'Chual Aluinn, from Glas Bheinn, in the highlands of Scotland, with a drop of 200 m (660 ft)

- Deepest cave: Ogof Ffynnon Ddu, Wales, at 308 m (1,010 ft) deep

- Most northerly point on the British mainland: Dunnet Head, north-east Scotland

- Most southerly point on the British mainland: Lizard Point, Cornwall

- Closest point to mainland continental Europe: Dover, Kent. The Channel Tunnel, which links England and France, is a little over 50 km (31 miles) long, of which nearly 38 km (24 miles) are actually under the Channel.

1.1 Area of the United Kingdom[1,2], 2008

	sq km		sq km
		Shropshire	3 197
United Kingdom	243 122	Staffordshire	2 620
		Warwickshire	1 975
Great Britain	228 972	West Midlands (Met County)	902
		Worcestershire	1 741
England and Wales	151 014		
		East	19 109
		Luton UA	43
England	130 280	Peterborough UA	343
		Southend-on-Sea UA	42
North East	8 573	Thurrock UA	163
Darlington UA	197	Bedfordshire	1 192
Hartlepool UA	94	Cambridgeshire	3 046
Middlesbrough UA	54	Essex	3 465
Redcar and Cleveland UA	245	Hertfordshire	1 643
Stockton-on-Tees UA	204	Norfolk	5 371
		Suffolk	3 800
Durham	2 226		
Northumberland	5 013	**London**	1572
Tyne and Wear (Met County)	540		
		Inner London	319
North West	14 107	Outer London	1 253
Blackburn with Darwen UA	137	**South East**	19 069
Blackpool UA	35		
Halton UA	79	Bracknell Forest UA	109
Warrington UA	181	Brighton and Hove UA	83
		Isle of Wight UA	380
Cheshire	2 083	Medway UA	192
Cumbria	6 767	Milton Keynes UA	309
Greater Manchester (Met County)	1 276	Portsmouth UA	40
Lancashire	2 903	Reading UA	40
Merseyside (Met County)	647	Slough UA	33
		Southampton UA	50
Yorkshire and the Humber	15 408	West Berkshire UA	704
		Windsor and Maidenhead UA	197
East Riding of Yorkshire UA	2 408	Wokingham UA	179
Kingston upon Hull, City of UA	72		
North East Lincolnshire UA	192	Buckinghamshire	1 565
North Lincolnshire UA	846	East Sussex	1 708
York UA	272	Hampshire	3 679
		Kent	3 544
North Yorkshire	8 038	Oxfordshire	2 605
South Yorkshire (Met County)	1 552	Surrey	1 663
West Yorkshire (Met County)	2 029	West Sussex	1 991
East Midlands	15 607	**South West**	23 837
Derby UA	78	Bath and North East Somerset UA	346
Leicester UA	73	Bournemouth UA	46
Nottingham UA	75	Bristol, City of UA	110
Rutland UA	382	North Somerset UA	374
		Plymouth UA	80
Derbyshire	2 547	Poole UA	65
Leicestershire	2 083	South Gloucestershire UA	497
Lincolnshire	5 920	Swindon UA	230
Northamptonshire	2 364	Torbay UA	63
Nottinghamshire	2 085		
		Cornwall and the Isles of Scilly	3 563
West Midlands	12 998	Devon	6 564
		Dorset	2 542
Herefordshire, County of UA	2 180	Gloucestershire	2 653
Stoke-on-Trent UA	93	Somerset	3 451
Telford and Wrekin UA	290	Wiltshire	3 255

1.1 Area of the United Kingdom[1,2], 2008
continued

	sq km		sq km
Wales	20 733	Dumfries and Galloway	6 426
		Dundee City	60
Blaenau Gwent	109	East Ayrshire	1 262
Bridgend	251	East Dunbartonshire	175
Caerphilly	277	East Lothian	679
Cardiff[1]	140		
Carmarthenshire[1]	2 371	East Renfrewshire	174
		Edinburgh, City of	263
Ceredigion[1]	1 785	Eilean Siar (Western Isles)	3 055
Conwy	1 126	Falkirk	297
Denbighshire	837	Fife	1 325
Flintshire	437		
Gwynedd	2 535	Glasgow City	175
		Highland	25 709
Isle of Anglesey	711	Inverclyde	160
Merthyr Tydfil	111	Midlothian	354
Monmouthshire	849	Moray	2 238
Neath Port Talbot	441		
Newport[1]	190	North Ayrshire	885
Pembrokeshire[1]	1 619	North Lanarkshire	470
		Orkney Islands	990
Powys	5 181	Perth and Kinross	5 286
Rhondda, Cynon, Taff	424	Renfrewshire	262
Swansea	378	Scottish Borders	4 732
Torfaen	126		
The Vale of Glamorgan[1]	331	Shetland Islands	1 467
Wrexham	504	South Ayrshire	1 222
		South Lanarkshire	1 772
		Stirling	2 187
Scotland	77 958	West Dunbartonshire	159
		West Lothian	428
Aberdeen City	186		
Aberdeenshire	6 313		
Angus	2 182	**Northern Ireland**	14 150
Argyll and Bute	6 908		
Clackmannanshire	159		

1 On boundaries as at 2001.

Source: Office for National Statistics

Parliamentary elections

Chapter 2

Elections

2.1 Parliamentary elections[1]
United Kingdom

		15 Oct 1964	31 Mar 1966	18 June 1970[1]	28 Feb 1974		10 Oct 1974	3 May 1979	9 June 1983	11 June 1987	9 April 1992	1 May 1997	7 June 2001	5 May 2005
United Kingdom														
Electorate	DZ5P	35 894	35 957	39 615	40 256	DZ6V	40 256	41 573	42 704	43 666	43 719	43 846	44 403	44 246
Average-electors per seat	DZ5T	57.0	57.1	62.9	63.4	DZ6R	63.4	65.5	66.7	67.2	67.2	66.5	67.4	68.5
Valid votes counted	DZ5X	27 657	27 265	28 345	31 340	DZ6N	29 189	31 221	30 671	32 530	33 614	31 286	26 367	27 149
As percentage of electorate	DZ63	77.1	75.8	71.5	77.9	DZ6J	72.5	75.1	71.8	74.5	76.7	71.4	59.4	61.4
England and Wales														
Electorate	DZ5Q	31 610	31 695	34 931	35 509	DZ6W	35 509	36 695	37 708	38 568	38 648	38 719	39 228	39 266
Average-electors per seat	DZ5U	57.8	57.9	63.9	64.3	DZ6S	64.3	66.5	67.2	68.8	68.8	68.0	68.9	69.0
Valid votes counted	DZ5Y	24 384	24 116	24 877	27 735	DZ6O	25 729	27 609	27 082	28 832	29 897	27 679	23 243	24 097
As percentage of electorate	DZ64	77.1	76.1	71.2	78.1	DZ6K	72.5	75.2	71.8	74.8	77.5	71.5	59.3	61.4
Scotland														
Electorate	DZ5R	3 393	3 360	3 659	3 705	DZ6X	3 705	3 837	3 934	3 995	3 929	3 949	3 984	3 840
Average-electors per seat	DZ5V	47.8	47.3	51.5	52.2	DZ6T	52.2	54.0	54.6	55.5	54.6	54.8	55.3	65.1
Valid votes counted	DZ5Z	2 635	2 553	2 688	2 887	DZ6P	2 758	2 917	2 825	2 968	2 931	2 817	2 313	2 334
As percentage of electorate	DZ65	77.6	76.0	73.5	77.9	DZ6L	74.5	76.0	71.8	74.3	74.2	71.3	58.1	60.8
Northern Ireland														
Electorate	DZ5S	891	902	1 025	1 027	DZ6Y	1 037	1 028	1 050	1 090	1 141	1 178	1 191	1 140
Average-electors per seat	DZ5W	74.2	75.2	85.4	85.6	DZ6U	86.4	85.6	61.8	64.1	67.1	65.4	66.2	63.3
Valid votes counted	DZ62	638	596	779	718	DZ6Q	702	696	765	730	785	791	810	718
As percentage of electorate	DZ66	71.7	66.1	76.0	69.9	DZ6M	67.7	67.7	72.9	67.0	68.8	67.1	68.0	62.9
Members of Parliament elected: (numbers)	DZV7	630	630	630	635	DZV8	635	635	650	650	651	659	659	646
Conservative	DZ67	303	253	330	296	DZ6D	276	339	396	375	336	165	166	198
Labour	DZ68	317	363	287	301	DZ6E	319	268	209	229	271	418	412	355
Liberal Democrat[2]	DZ69	9	12	6	14	DZ6F	13	11	23	22	20	46	52	62
Scottish National Party	DZ6A	–	–	1	7	DZ6G	11	2	2	3	3	6	5	6
Plaid Cymru	DZ6B	–	–	–	2	DZ6H	3	2	2	3	4	4	4	3
Other[3]	DZ6C	1	2	6	15	DZ6I	13	13	18	18	17	20	20	22

1 The Representation of the People Act 1969 lowered the minimum voting age from 21 to 18 years with effect from 16 February 1970.
2 Liberal before 1992. The figures for 1983 and 1987 include six and five MPs respectively who were elected for the Social Democratic Party.
3 Including the Speaker.

Sources: British Electoral Facts 1832-2006.; University of Plymouth for the Electoral Commission: 01752 233207

2.2 Parliamentary by-elections
United Kingdom

	May 1997 - June 2001	General[1,2] Election May 1997	June 2001 - November 2004	General[1] Election June 2001	May 2005 - November 2009	General[1,2] Election May 2005
Numbers of by-elections	17		6		14	
Votes recorded						
By party (percentages)						
Conservative	27.0	25.1	17.7	21.2	27.7	25.7
Labour	29.7	40.1	40.8	58.3	29.3	35.7
Liberal Democrat	22.1	14.4	31.3	13.7	20.0	20.6
Scottish National Party	6.0	4.1	-	-	9.5	6.2
Plaid Cymru	2.5	2.3	2.7	2.1	0.4	0.1
Other	12.7	14.1	7.4	4.7	13.0	11.7
Total votes recorded (percentages)	100.0	100.0	100.0	100.0	100.0	100.0
(thousands)	435	723	140	205	436	586

1 Votes recorded in the same seats in the previous General Election.
2 Proportions of 'other' votes inflated by the fact that votes were cast for the retiring Speaker as 'The Speaker seeking re-election' and not as a party candidate.

Source: University of Plymouth for the Electoral Commission: 01752 233207

2.3 Devolved assembly elections
Wales and Scotland

Thousands and percentages

		6 May 1999	1 May 2003	3 May 2007
Welsh Assembly				
Electorate	E28K	2 205	2 230	2 248
Average-electors per seat[1]	E28N	55.1	55.7	56.2
Valid votes counted	E28Q	1 023	850	978
As percentage of electorate	E28T	46.4	38.1	43.5
Members elected:[2] (numbers)	E2XI	60	60	60
Conservative	E2WG	9	11	12
Labour	E2WU	28	30	26
Liberal Democrat	E2WW	6	6	6
Plaid Cymru	E2X3	17	12	15
Other	E2WY	–	1	1
Scottish Parliament				
Electorate	E28L	4 024	3 879	3 899
Average-electors per seat[1]	E28O	55.1	53.1	53.4
Valid votes counted	E28R	2 342	1 916	2 017
As percentage of electorate	E28U	58.2	49.4	51.7
Members elected:[3] (numbers)	E2XJ	129	129	129
Conservative	E2WH	18	18	17
Labour	E2WV	56	50	46
Liberal Democrat	E2WX	17	17	16
Scottish National Party	E2X4	35	27	47
Other	E2WZ	3	17	3

1 This is the average in each first-past-the-post constituency. Additional members are then elected on the basis of a regional 'list' vote.
2 Comprising 40 from constituencies and 20 from the regional 'list'.
3 Comprising 73 from constituencies and 56 from the regional 'list'.

Sources: British Electoral Facts 1832-2006;
University of Plymouth for the Electoral Commission: 01752 233207

2.4 Devolved assembly elections
Northern Ireland

Thousands and percentages

		25 June 1998	26 Nov 2003	8 Mar 2007
Electorate	E28M	1 179	1 098	1 108
Average-electors per seat[1]	E28P	65.5	61.0	61.6
Valid votes counted	E28S	810	702	690
As percentage of electorate	E28V	68.7	64.0	63.0
Members elected: (numbers)	E2XK	108	108	108
Alliance Party	E2X5	6	6	7
SDLP	E2X6	24	18	16
Sinn Fein	E2X7	18	24	28
Democratic Unionist Party	E2X8	20	30	36
UK Unionist Party	E2X9	5	1	–
Ulster Unionist Party	E2XA	28	27	18
Other	E2X2	7	2	3

1 This is the average in each Westminster constituency. Six members are elected by single transferable vote (STV) in each constituency.

Sources: British Electoral Facts 1832-2006;
University of Plymouth for the Electoral Commission: 01752 233207

International development

Chapter 3

International development

Overseas development assistance

(Tables 3.1 and 3.2)

The Department for International Development (DFID) is the UK government department with lead responsibility for overseas development. DFID's aim is to eliminate poverty in poorer countries through achievement of the Millennium Development Goals (MDGs) by 2015. Statistics relating to international development are published on a financial year basis and on a calendar year basis. Statistics on a calendar year basis allow comparisons of aid expenditure with other donor countries. Aid flows can be measured before (gross) or after (net) deductions of repayments of principal on past loans. These tables show only the gross figures.

Aid is provided in two main ways: Bilateral funding is provided directly to partner countries while multilateral funding is provided through international organisations.

Funds can only be classified as multilateral if they are channelled through one of the organisations listed in the OECD Development Assistance Committee (DAC) statistical reporting directives which identifies all multilateral organisations. This list also highlights some bodies that might appear to be multilateral but are actually bilateral (in particular this latter category includes some international non-governmental organisations such as the International Committee of the Red Cross and some public–private partnerships such as the Global Alliance for Vaccines and Immunisation). The DAC list of multilaterals is updated annually based on members nominations. Organisations must be engaged in development work to be classified as multilateral aid channels.[1]

While core funding to multilateral organisations is always classified as multilateral expenditure, additional funding channelled through multilaterals is often classified as bilateral expenditure. This would be the case in circumstances where a DFID country office transfers some money to a multilateral organisation (for example, a UN agency) for a particular programme in that country (or region). That is, where DFID has control over what the money is being spent on and/or where it is being spent. Likewise, if DFID responds to an emergency appeal from an agency for a particular country

or area, the funds will be allocated as bilateral spend to that country or region. As a result, some organisations, such as UN agencies have some of their DFID funding classified as bilateral and some as multilateral.

DFID is planning to introduce a new activity reporting system between 2007/08 and 2009/10. The new system will integrate all DFID's current financial and project management systems. To coincide with the introduction of the new system, DFID is reviewing how it classifies its aid delivery types. The outcome of this review may lead to the introduction of a new set of classifications which may result in changes to the format in future publications.

Table 3.1 shows the main groups of multilateral agencies; the International Development Association being the largest in the World Bank Group.

Bilateral assistance takes various forms:

Financial aid: Poverty Reduction Budget Support (PRBS) – funds provided to developing countries for them to spend in support of their expenditure programmes whose long-term objective is to reduce poverty. Funds are spent using the overseas governments' own financial management, procurement and accountability systems to increase ownership and long-term sustainability. PRBS can take the form of a general contribution to the overall budget – general budget support – or support with a more restricted focus which is earmarked for a specific sector – sector budget support.

Other financial aid – funding of projects and programmes such as sector-wide programmes not classified as PRBS. Financial aid in its broader sense covers all bilateral aid expenditure other than technical cooperation and administrative costs but in *Statistics on International Development* (SID) Humanitarian Assistance, DFID Debt Relief, and 'Other bilateral aid' are separately categorised. Aid and Trade Provision which was previously identified in SID has now been merged into 'Other financial aid' as it is a rapidly declining flow.

Technical co-operation – activities designed to enhance the knowledge, intellectual skills, technical expertise or the productive capability of people in recipient countries. It also covers funding of services which contribute to the design or implementation of development projects and programmes.

This assistance is mainly delivered through research and development, the use of consultants, training (generally overseas partners visiting the UK or elsewhere for a training programme) and employment of 'other personnel' (non-DFID experts on fixed-term contracts). This latter category is growing less significant over time as existing contracted staff reach the end of their assignments.

[1] money may be classified as bilateral while a case is being made for a new multilateral organisation to be recognised.

Other bilateral aid – this category comprises support to the development work of UK and international voluntary organisations, grants to the British Council and for other development work by UK institutions, and non-emergency special appeals through multilateral agencies. The remaining element of 'Other bilateral aid' is made up of a number of categories including, for example, DFID's contributions to two multi-donor trust funds for Sudan, the Development Awareness Fund and the provision of books, equipment and other supplies.

Humanitarian assistance – provides food, aid and other humanitarian assistance including shelter, medical care and advice in emergency situations and their aftermath. Work of the conflict pools is also included.

DFID debt relief – this includes sums for debt relief on DFID aid loans and cancellation of debt under the Commonwealth Debt Initiative (CDI). The non-CDI DFID debt relief is reported on the basis of the 'benefit to the recipient country'. This means that figures shown represent the money available to the country in the year in question that would otherwise have been spent on debt servicing. The CDI debt cancellation is reported on a 'lump sum' basis where all outstanding amounts on a loan are shown at the time the agreement to cancel is made.

CDC investments – CDC Group plc (or CDC) replaced the former Commonwealth Development Corporation in 1999. CDC was founded in 1948 and is now the UK Government's instrument for investing in the private sector in developing economies (it does so through fund management companies, of whom the largest is Actis Capital LLP). CDC has activities in more than 50 developing countries. CDC provides equities an concessional loans to companies in some aid-eligible countries, and these disbursements and repayments are included as UK flows. Although CDC no longer provides loans to governments, it did in the past and these existing loans can become eligible for debt relief.

Non-DFID debt relief – comprises CDC debt and Export Credit Guarantee Department (ECGD) debt. CDC has a portfolio of loans to governments which can become eligible for debt relief under the HIPC (Heavily Indebted Poor Countries) or other debt relief deals. In 2005/06 £90 million of debts owed to CDC were reorganised. ECGD is the UK's official Export Credit Agency which provides insurance for exporters against the main risks in selling overseas and guarantees to banks providing export finance. It also negotiates debt relief arrangements on commercial debt.

Other – This includes contributions from other government departments to civil society organisations, British Council and Global Conflict Pool, and small amounts of drug related assistance funded by the Home Office and the Foreign and Commonwealth Office.

Further details on the UK's development assistance can be found in the Department for International Developments publication *Statistics on International Development* which can be found on the website at: www.dfid.gov.uk/About-DFID/Finance-and-performance/DFID-Expenditure-Statistics/. International Comparisons are available in the OECD Development Assistance Committee's annual report.

3.1 Gross public expenditure on aid (GPEX)[1]
United Kingdom

£ Thousand

		2000 /01	2001 /02	2002 /03	2003 /04	2004 /05	2005 /06	2006 /07	2007 /08	2008 /09
Bilateral Assistance										
Department for International Development										
Poverty Reduction Budget Support (General)	LUJS	239 900	245 500	184 500	288 750	286 500	347 320	297 553	366 453	92 748
Poverty Reduction Budget Support (Sector)	I4UJ	24 098	22 718	23 685	20 724	60 492	128 232	166 064	268 631	255 920
Other Financial Aid	LUJW	206 113	264 905	319 145	389 853	411 018	469 631	454 631	460 554	520 133
Technical Co-operation Projects	LUOS	455 401	473 519	508 574	459 754	462 633	481 053	522 722	474 287	514 235
Other Bilateral Aid	LUOT	370 184	367 736	450 749	480 252	573 382	712 489	810 993	889 723	1 136 074
Humanitarian Assistance	LUOU	222 431	192 446	294 981	311 602	333 318	447 978	383 513	430 773	449 163
DFID Debt Relief	LUOV	20 367	17 682	20 364	59 534	71 485	68 120	147 106	71 386	19 425
CDC Investments	LUOX	201 427	159 352	237 324	350 356	238 279	172 808	278 787	360 821	436 028
Debt Relief	EQ4B	79 850	242 097	399 844	163 059	627 402	1 588 414	1 866 591	3 760	280 337
Other	LUOY	66 978	67 795	79 459	111 197	143 564	153 536	196 122	191 002	329 857
Total	LUOZ	1 918 441	2 081 504	2 540 613	2 635 081	3 208 072	4 569 524	5 124 083	3 517 389	4 333 920
Multilateral Assistance										
European Community[2]	LUPA	723 651	744 141	897 826	1 082 389	1 222 018	1 191 961	1 123 215	1 200 319	1 407 901
World Bank Group	LUPB	342 410	173 722	300 021	150 000	150 000	364 909	493 333	493 387	573 652
IMF Poverty Reduction and Growth Facility	LUPC	–	11 147	11 434	9 417	1 767	23 728	15	..	..
Global Environmental Assistance	EQ4C	21 144	25 337	27 338	61 213	52 445	53 460	50 260	..	..
HIPC Trust Funds	EQ4D	27 518	23 400	17 855	22 910	42 123	11 094	18 666	..	..
UN Agencies	LUPD	122 423	163 645	176 487	196 406	211 638	252 745	245 019	296 940	308 154
Regional Development Banks	LUPE	54 784	75 383	90 648	80 391	82 166	77 759	123 591	..	..
Other[3]	LUPF	134 086	111 076	151 473	155 861	164 750	105 891	360 443	256 348	310 659
Total	LUPG	1 322 571	1 192 584	1 525 807	1 584 656	1 748 406	1 915 506	2 222 010	2 246 995	2 600 365
Administrative costs	LUPH	138 507	132 214	154 127	248 698	227 769	256 451	245 893	262 731	249 000
Total Gross Public Expenditure on Aid	LUPI	3 379 519	3 406 301	4 220 547	4 468 435	5 184 247	6 741 481	7 591 986	6 027 115	7 183 285

1 See chapter text.
2 The institution, not the member states of the European Union.
3 IMF Poverty Reduction and Growth Facility, Global Environmental Assistance, HIPC Trust Funds and Regional Development Banks are now included in Multilateral Assistance Other.

Source: Department for International Development: 01355 843764.

3.2 Total bilateral gross public expenditure on aid (GPEX): by main recipient countries and regions[1]
United Kingdom

£ Thousand

		1999 /00	2000 /01	2001 /02	2002 /03	2003 /04	2004 /05	2005 /06	2006 /07	2007 /08
Main recipients										
Nigeria	C227	14 395	15 940	20 561	29 287	32 630	73 113	1 227 717	1 750 694	157 722
India	LUPJ	104 016	126 700	198 576	182 708	242 736	267 510	270 065	293 706	312 751
Afghanistan	C224	5 452	7 465	50 027	76 018	99 595	98 959	126 949	123 011	146 818
Pakistan	LUPY	23 472	15 890	44 838	46 852	66 299	55 277	97 688	118 150	88 145
Cameroon	I53M	7 005	5 467	3 652	28 971	7 764	16 547	3 170	115 408	2 013
Tanzania	LUPK	74 709	110 590	203 830	102 614	162 372	130 009	114 134	115 023	125 353
Sudan	EU5S	3 189	4 912	5 598	19 222	24 663	83 964	117 114	109 917	138 702
Bangladesh	LUPM	69 670	75 005	60 375	73 246	155 364	149 152	128 258	109 313	129 725
Serbia	I53N	6 393	15 670	11 531	305 036	4 795	4 001	48 971	95 713	3 491
Ethiopia	C225	7 299	16 484	12 088	44 224	43 665	73 044	62 562	90 506	140 011
Malawi	LUPP	49 058	54 648	46 651	49 266	54 437	56 429	68 653	88 686	72 619
Ghana	LUPL	51 887	74 700	54 479	86 294	73 448	145 835	96 315	93 147	93 076
Congo, Dem Rep	C223	2 132	6 752	10 262	15 574	151 657	36 585	58 832	79 283	82 910
Uganda	LUPN	89 978	98 352	68 091	54 041	59 694	62 928	72 064	79 035	77 231
Iraq	C222	6 585	9 545	7 760	18 853	214 313	391 507	426 249	71 829	40 649
Kenya	EU5W	32 665	62 620	34 227	63 404	28 647	37 824	65 486	67 054	52 135
Zambia	LUPO	46 657	93 345	59 203	45 140	32 304	163 537	101 707	63 412	41 942
Indonesia	LUPZ	58 812	28 405	18 232	42 613	17 449	34 526	58 553	62 290	32 715
China	LUPS	26 246	56 740	50 266	44 386	42 406	42 476	36 854	60 086	83 743
Mozambique	LUPV	70 643	43 876	134 133	39 101	36 713	47 941	56 540	56 273	67 799
Total	LUQD	750 261	923 108	1 094 379	1 366 848	1 550 951	1 971 164	3 237 881	3 642 536	1 889 550
Total other countries	LUQE	899 776	837 292	886 021	1 095 698	1 084 130	1 236 908	1 331 643	1 481 547	1 627 839
Regional totals										
Africa	LUQF	628 719	774 692	865 317	891 954	1 058 005	1 282 423	2 425 880	3 071 676	1 552 123
America	LUQG	237 961	180 165	166 949	221 526	103 358	126 278	85 389	119 491	68 545
Asia	LUQH	375 839	413 294	534 954	609 138	969 466	1 243 004	1 356 415	1 091 488	1 116 528
Europe	LUQI	191 697	113 859	97 609	384 240	74 871	62 295	90 086	135 699	39 496
Pacific	LUQJ	7 248	5 029	6 885	5 362	4 484	3 272	3 823	2 670	2 842
World unallocated[2]	LUQK	208 574	273 363	308 686	350 327	451 897	490 800	607 931	703 059	737 855
Total Bilateral GPEX	LUQL	1 650 037	1 760 400	1 980 400	2 462 546	2 635 081	3 208 072	4 569 524	5 124 083	3 517 389

1 See chapter text.
2 Includes grants to VSO, CSOs, Research Institutions and Commonwealth Organisations based in the UK.

Source: Department for International Development: 01355 843764.

Chapter 4

Defence

Defence

This section includes figures on defence expenditure, on the size and role of the Armed Forces and on related support activities.

Much of the material in this section can be found in *UK Defence Statistics 2009*

Defence expenditure

(Table 4.1)

UK Defence Expenditure – the move from cash to resource accounting

Up until financial year 1998/99, government expenditure was accounted for on a cash basis. In April 1999 the introduction of Resource Accounting and Budgeting (RAB) brought in an accruals-based accounting system, although government departments were still controlled on a cash basis. This transitional accounting regime remained for two financial years. Government expenditure has been accounted for on a resource basis only since 2001/02.

The main difference arising from the adoption of RAB is that costs are accounted for as they are incurred (the principle of accruals), rather than when payment is made (the principle of cash). This gives rise to timing differences in accounting between the cash and RAB systems and also to the recognition of depreciation, which expends the cost of an asset over its useful economic life, and the cost of capital charge, equivalent to an interest charge on the net assets held on the balance sheet. At the time that RAB was introduced the cost of capital charge was 6 per cent of the net value of assets; although this was reduced to 3.5 per cent in 2003/04.

The change from cash based accounting to resource (accruals) based accounting, and the two-stage introduction of RAB (outlined below) has affected the time series comparability of the data.

Please refer to UK Defence Statistics 2009 Chapter 1 – Resource Accounting & Budgeting section for a summary of the key events leading to the introduction of RAB. Back copies of this publication are available at www.dasa.mod.uk/applications/newWeb/www/index.php?page=67&pubType=1&thiscontent=10&date=2009-09-30

Control regime

Under resource accounting, government departments are accountable for their spending against Resource and Capital Departmental Expenditure Limits (DELs). Spending against the Resource DEL includes current items, which are explained in the following two paragraphs. The Capital DEL, while part of the overall DEL, reflects investment spending that will appear on the department's balance sheet and be consumed over a number of years, net of the receipts from sale of assets. Departments are also responsible for Annually Managed Expenditure (AME). This spending is demand led (for example, payment of War Pensions) and therefore cannot be controlled by departments in the same way.

In **Stage 1** of RAB, which was introduced at the start of financial year 2001/02, the Resource DEL covered current costs such as in-year personnel costs, equipment, maintenance of land and buildings. Non-cash costs such as depreciation and the cost of capital charge fell within Annually Managed Expenditure (AME) and were not controlled to the same degree as DELs. This allowed departments an interim period to gain experience of managing the new non-cash costs and to review their holdings of stocks and fixed assets, which impact the non-cash costs, prior to the charge impacting on the more tightly controlled DELs.

Stage 2 of RAB was introduced at the start of the financial year 2003/04. This involved the movement of the primary non-cash costs (depreciation and the cost of capital charge) from AME into the Resource DEL, and reduced the cost of capital charge to 3.5 per cent of the net value of assets.

The change in definition of the DELs combined with volatile non-cash costs over the Stage 1 period make time series comparisons over the period 2001/02–2003/04 complex.

From 2006/07, the Ministry of Defence (MOD) has transferred ownership of fixed assets into two TLB's: Defence Estates (DE) for Land and Buildings: and Defence Equipment & Support (DE&S) for Plant and Machinery, Transport, IT and Communications equipment, and Single Use Military Equipment (SUME).

Factors affecting Cash to RAB data consistency

- There are timing differences as to when payments are recognised

- The movement of Non-Cash items of expenditure from AME into the Resource DEL from 2003/04 onwards has the apparent effect of inflating the Resource DEL

- In financial year 2003/04 the rate of interest used to calculate the cost of capital charge was reduced from 6 per cent to 3.5 per cent

- The discount rate for provisions was changed from 3.5 per cent real to 2.2 per cent real with effect from 1 April 2005.

- The discount rate for pension's liabilities was changed from 2.8 per cent real to 1.8 per cent real with effect from 1 April 2007

Table 4.1 provides a breakdown of MOD outturn in terms of resources consumed. This is distributed between the main personnel, fixed assets and other expenditure groups. The table also includes expenditure relating to conflict prevention and operations.

Resource DEL includes expenditure under the following headings:

- Equipment support – internal and contracted out costs for equipment repair and maintenance

- Stock consumption – consumption of armament, medical, dental, veterinary, oil, clothing, and general stores

- Property management – estate and facilities management services and costs for building maintenance

- Movements – cost of transportation of freight and personnel

- Accommodation and utilities – charges include rent, rates, gas, electricity, water and sewerage costs

- Professional fees – fees, such as legal costs paid to professional organisations

- Fuel – relates to fuel consumption by military vehicles, ships and aircraft

- Other Costs – can include grants-in-aid, exchange rate movements, provisions, receipts, welfare, medical and legal costs, research and expensed development, rentals paid under operating leases, fixed assets and stock written off

Expenditure on fixed asset categories in Capital DEL includes:-

- Intangible assets – comprise the development costs of major equipment projects and Intellectual Property Rights

- Single Use Military Equipment (SUME) – are assets which only have a military use, such as tanks and fighter aircrafts. Dual use items, that is those that also have a civilian use, are recorded under the other categories

- Assets under Construction – largely consist of major weapons platforms under construction in the Defence Equipment & Support, and a smaller element of buildings under construction. Once construction is complete, those platforms will transfer to the relevant Top Level Budget holder as Single Use Military Equipment on their balance sheets

- Transport/Capital spares – from 2004/05 transport has been recorded as a separate category and Capital Spares has been removed as a category, with the costs previously recorded here being incorporated into Transport or SUME

- Capital Income – receipts for the sale of fixed assets. Redemption of QinetiQ preference shares refers to the proceeds received from the partial redemption of the redeemable preference shares during 2004/05.

Annual Managed Expenditure includes:

- Other – under Stage 2 of RAB, this category now contains only demand led payments, such as cash release and cost of capital credit on nuclear provisions and QinetiQ loan repayments

In order to give a single measure of spending on public services under full resource budgeting, the Defence Spending line is presented as the sum of the resource and capital budgets, net of depreciation and impairments. This reflects the resources required plus the net investment in them, but avoids double counting the writing down of the existing capital stock and the cash outlay on new assets. Control is exercised separately on gross Capital and Resource DEL.

Service personnel

(Tables 4.2, 4.4, 4.5, 4.8 and 4.10)

The Regular Forces consist entirely of volunteer members serving on a whole-time basis, figures for which include both trained and untrained personnel and exclude Gurkhas, Full Time Reserve Service (FTRS) personnel, the Home Service battalions of the Royal Irish Regiment, mobilised reservists and Naval Activated Reservists.

Locally entered personnel are recruited outside the United Kingdom for whole-time service in special formations with special conditions of service and normally restricted locations. The Brigade of Gurkhas is an example.

The Regular Forces are supported by Reserves and Auxiliary Forces. There are both regular and volunteer Reserves. Regular reserves consist of former service personnel with a reserve liability. Volunteer Reserves are open to both former personnel and civilians. The call-out liabilities of the various reserve forces differ in accordance with their roles.

Defence

All three services run cadet forces for young people and the Combined Cadet Force, which is found in certain schools where education is continued to the age of 17 and over, may operate sections for any or all of the services.

Full Time Reserve Service personnel represent reserves serving full-time in regular posts. This was made possible by the Reserve Forces Act 1996. None existed before 1998. FTRS figures include Full Commitment (FC), Home Commitment (HC) and Limited Commitment (LC) individuals.

Home Service battalions of the Royal Irish Regiment. Up until 1 July 1992, this was the Ulster Defence Regiment. The figures for the Territorial Army include Officer Training Corps and non-regular permanent staff.

The figures for cadet forces for each service include the Combined Cadet Force. Naval Service figures include officers and civilian instructors. The Army and Royal Air Force figures exclude officers and civilian instructors.

Intake of UK regular forces from civilian life: by service

(Table 4.2)

This table shows all intakes to UK Regular Forces including re-enlistments and rejoined reservists.

Formation of the armed forces

(Table 4.3)

This table shows the number of units which comprise the 'teeth' elements of the Armed Forces and excludes supporting units.

Outflow of UK regular forces: by service

(Table 4.4)

This table does not include promotions to officer from other ranks and miscellaneous outflow.

Civilian personnel

(Table 4.6)

In previous years, the MOD civilian workforce definition has reflected the historical requirement to understand the number of civil servants being directly funded. However with changes in employment legislation and the requirement to plan the future of the civilian workforce there was a need to change the definition to a more inclusive one, better reflecting modern human resources methods and policies. In the longer term it will be used for skills planning, ensuring that the MOD has a well-equipped workforce able to provide the best support to the UK Armed Forces.

In summary, the change over previous years is the addition of two further categories of individuals:

Casual personnel – those employed on a short-term casual contract

Those not directly funded – personnel who are employed by the MOD, but whose salaries are paid for by another department/agency etc. This includes personnel on loan to other government departments or working for NATO, as well as those on a career break or long-term sickness absence.

These additions allow two levels of definition to be established:

Definition – Level 1 **includes** permanent and casual personnel, Royal Fleet Auxiliaries, but excludes Trading Funds. This is generally used for internal reporting and planning.

Definition – Level 0 contains all those at Level 1 **plus** Trading Funds and Locally Engaged Civilians. This is used for external reporting, including National Statistics publications CPS1 and UKDS, and Parliamentary business.

For more information on the revised civilian workforce definition, visit: www.dasa.mod.uk/natstats/consultation/consultation.html

From 1 April 2000 a new top-level budget was formed in the Centre called Defence Logistics Organisation, replacing the top-level budgets CinC Fleet Support, Quarter Master General and RAF Logistics Command.

On 1 April 2007, Chief of Defence Logistics and Defence Procurement Agency merged to form Defence Equipment & Support.

The QinetiQ portion of the Defence Evaluation and Research Agency was established as a private company in July 2001. The War Pensions Agency transferred from the Department of Work and Pensions in 2001. The Clyde Dockyards were contractorised in 2002.

Data on manually paid personnel before 1999 is not available, so estimates are used.

Totals and subtotals have been rounded separately and so may not appear to be the sums of their parts.

Family accommodation and defence land holdings

(Table 4.7)

In November 1996 most of the MOD's housing stock in England and Wales was sold to a private company, Annington Homes. The homes retained for use by service families are leased back with the condition that the MOD releases a certain number of houses each year for disposal by Annington. The proceeds of these sales are used to upgrade the housing stock.

The table also presents statistics of land and foreshore in the United Kingdom owned or leased by the MOD or over which it has limited rights under grants or licences. Land declared as surplus to defence requirements is also included.

Deployment of Service personnel

(Table 4.8)

Location data are based on the stationed location of the individual. Personnel deployed on operations to an area away from their stationed location are shown against their most recent stationed location. Naval Service personnel on sea service are included against the local authority containing the home port of their ship.

Prior to 2003, figures for UK distribution and global location are collated from separate sources and comparison is therefore not possible between the two sets of UK personnel figures. From 2001 the grouping of overseas locations has been changed to give a more relevant overview.

UK regular forces – deaths

(Table 4.9)

Rates have been standardised to 2009 Armed Forces population age and gender structure. The data are presented for the Naval Service (Royal Navy and Royal Marines), the Army (including the Gurkhas), the Royal Air Force, and on a Tri-Service basis. Non-regular members of the UK Armed Forces who died whilst deployed on operations are included in the data presented.

Health

(Table 4.10)

The Services operate a number of hospitals in this country and in areas abroad where there is a significant British military presence. These hospitals take as patients, members of all three services and their dependants. In addition, the hospitals in the United Kingdom take civilian patients under arrangements agreed with the National Health Service. Medical support is also supplied by service medical staff at individual units, ships and stations.

Defence services and the civilian community

(Table 4.11)

Search & Rescue (SAR)

This table covers incidents attended by military Search and Rescue units. The Royal Air Force and Royal Navy provide an essential service to the Search and Rescue (SAR) effort around the UK forming part of the national UK SAR coverage throughout the year for air, land and maritime operations. The military SAR teams' primary purpose is to recover aircrew from crashed military aircraft, although each year over 90 per cent of callouts are to civilian incidents. The SAR force currently consists of 6 x RAF and 2 x RN SAR Sea King helicopter units and 4 RAF mountain rescue teams operating from bases around the UK, plus specially equipped RAF Nimrod aircraft based in RAF Kinloss in Scotland.

The table also includes urgent medical incidents in which the military SAR facilities gave assistance (eg inter-hospital transfers).

More than one SAR unit may be called to the same incident; consequently the number of callouts is likely to be greater than the number of incidents.

Persons moved involves moving people from a hostile environment to a safe environment or to a medical facility to receive urgent medical attention. People helped by RAF mountain rescue teams, but subsequently transported from the scene by helicopter, are recorded as having been rescued by the helicopter unit concerned.

Fisheries Protection

The Royal Navy Fishery Protection squadron operates within the British fishery limits under contract to the Department for Environment, Food and Rural Affairs. Boardings carried out by vessels of the Scottish Executive Environment and Rural Affairs Department and the Department of Agriculture for Northern Ireland are not included.

Defence

4.1 United Kingdom defence expenditure[1]

Inclusive of non-recoverable VAT at current prices (£ million)

		2003 /04	2004[2] /05	2005 /06	2006 /07	2007[2] /08	2008 /09
Defence Spending	C228	30 861	32 515	33 164	34 045	37 387	38 579
Departmental Expenditure Limits (DEL)	SNKJ	37 174	38 323	39 751	40 654	43 634	45 473
Resource DEL	E2XV	31 266	31 798	32 911	33 457	35 689	36 715
Expenditure on personnel	SNKK	10 435	10 996	11 255	11 204	11 474	11 723
of which: Armed forces	SNKL	7 974	8 047	8 263	8 423	8 646	8 937
of which: Civilians	SNKM	2 461	2 948	2 992	2 781	2 828	2 786
Depreciation/impairments	SNKN	6 313	5 808	6 587	6 609	6 247	6 894
Cost of capital	SNKO	2 770	3 026	3 106	3 242	3 371	3 626
Equipment support	SNKP	3 804	3 623	3 542	3 793	4 272	4 292
Stock consumption	SNKQ	1 060	1 079	1 039	1 140	1 071	1 181
Property management	SNKR	1 393	1 509	1 367	1 258	1 523	1 508
Movements	SNKS	491	711	729	774	858	975
Accommodation and utilities	SNKT	643	581	735	786	750	866
Professional fees	SNKU	549	565	553	482	471	391
Fuel	SNKV	161	239	369	416	537	695
Hospitality & Entertainment	I4SS	8	6	5	4	4	4
PFI Service Charges	I4ST	..	..	870	1 148	1 276	1 482
IT & Communications	I4SU	738	678	643	719	655	852
Other costs	SNKW	2 900	2 977	2 111	1 882	3 180	2 226
Capital DEL	E2XW	5 908	6 525	6 840	7 197	7 945	8 758
Expenditure on fixed asset categories							
Intangible assets	SNKX	1 665	1 580	1 550	1 744	1 756	1 311
Land and buildings	SNKY	54	388	31	45	126	163
Single Use Military Equipment	SNKZ	90	435	402	404	657	552
Plant, machinery and vehicles	SNLA	78	124	64	32	36	30
IT and communications equipment	SNLB	183	134	180	206	361	336
Assets under construction	SNLC	3 931	4 335	4 879	5 099	5 450	6 515
Transport	E2XX	..	73	13	33	55	239
Capital spares	SNLD	581	..	..	..	..	..
Capital loan repayment	E2XY	−28	−25	−53	−8	−10	−65
Other Costs	E2Y3	−646	−519	−225	−358	−486	−323
Annually Managed Expenditure (AME)	SNLF	1 011	908	890	582	510	214
War pensions	SNLG	1 116	1 110	1 067	1 038	1 014	1 000
Other	SNLH	−105	−202	−177	−456	−504	−785

1 See chapter text. Where rounding has been used, totals and sub-totals have been rounded separately and so may not equal the sums of their rounded parts.

2 Some figures for 2004/05 and 2007/08 have been revised.

Sources: Ministry of Defence/DASA (Defence Expenditure Analysis); 030 6793 4529/30

4.2 Intake of United Kingdom Regular Forces from civilian life: by Service[1]

Numbers

		1998 /99	1999 /00	2000 /01	2001 /02	2002 /03	2003 /04	2004 /05	2005 /06	2006[2] /07	2007[2] /08	2008[2] /09
All Services:												
Male	KCJB	22 560	22 390	20 410	20 950	23 040	20 760	15 660	16 410	17 830	19 230	20 690
Female	KCJC	3 440	3 160	2 610	2 700	3 240	2 710	1 900	1 740	1 960	2 090	2 080
Total	KCJA	26 000	25 550	23 020	23 650	26 280	23 470	17 560	18 150	19 790	21 330	22 770
Naval Service:												
Male	KCJE	4 110	4 250	3 990	4 270	4 420	3 530	3 240	3 480	3 300	3 400	3 590
Female	KCJF	660	700	630	740	800	580	460	460	460	470	410
Total	KCJD	4 770	4 950	4 620	5 010	5 220	4 120	3 690	3 940	3 770	3 860	4 000
Army:												
Male	KCJJ	15 010	14 750	13 450	13 620	15 060	13 930	10 780	11 740	13 160	13 390	13 500
Female	KCJK	1 980	1 750	1 320	1 240	1 550	1 260	910	990	1 140	1 150	1 020
Total	KCJI	16 990	16 500	14 770	14 850	16 610	15 190	11 690	12 730	14 300	14 540	14 510
Royal Air Force:												
Male	KCJM	3 450	3 380	2 980	3 070	3 550	3 290	1 640	1 190	1 370	2 450	3 600
Female	KCJN	800	710	660	720	890	870	530	290	360	480	660
Total	KCJL	4 250	4 100	3 630	3 780	4 450	4 160	2 180	1 480	1 720	2 930	4 260

1 See chapter text.
2 Due to ongoing validation of data from the new Personnel Administration System, Naval Service statistics from 1 October 2006, Army statistics from 1 April 2007 and RAF statistics from 1 May 2007 are provisional and subject to review.

Source: Ministry of Defence/DASA (Quad-Service): 0207 8078896

4.3 Formation of the United Kingdom armed forces[1]
As at 1 April

Numbers

				1999	2000	2001	2002	2003	2004	2005	2006	2007	2008	2009
			Front Line Units											
Royal Navy[2]														
Submarines	KCGA		Vessels	15	16	16	16	16	15	15	14[3]	13[4]	13	12[5]
Carriers and assault ships	KCGB		"	6	6	6	4	4	5	6	5[6]	5	5	5
Destroyers and frigates	KCGC		"	35	32	32	32	31	31	28	25[7]	25	25	24[8]
Mine counter-measure	KCGE		"	20	21	23	22	22	19	16	16	16	16	16
Patrol ships and craft	KCGF		"	24	23	23	23	22	26	26	22[9]	22	22[10]	22
Fixed wing aircraft[11]	KCGG		Squadrons	3	1	1	1	1	1	1	1	1	1	1
Helicopters[12]	KCGH		"	12	9	9	8	8	5	6	6	7	7	7
Royal Marines	KCGI		Commandos	3	3	3	3	3	3	3	3	3	3	3
Regular Army														
Royal Armoured Corps[13]	KCGJ		Regiments	11	10	10	10	10	10	10	10	10	10	10
Royal Artillery	KCGK		"	15	15	15	15	15	14	14	14	14	14	14
Royal Engineers[14]	KCGL		"	10	11	11	11	11	11	11	11	11	11	11
Infantry	KCGM		Battalions	40	40	40	40	40	40	40	36	36	36	36
Special Air Service	KCGN		Regiments	1	..	..	..	..	..	..	..	..	..	..
Army Air Corps[12]	KCGO		"	5	..	..	..	..	..	..	..	..	..	..
Royal Air Force														
Strike/attack	KCGP		Squadrons	5	5	5	5	5	5	5)				
Offensive support[11]	KCGQ	ZIZM	"	5	2	2	2	2	2	1)	13[15]	13	11[16]	11
Reconnaissance	KCGT		"	5	5	5	5	5	5	5)				
Air defence	KCGR		"	5	5	5	5	4	4	4)	..	..	..	..
Maritime patrol	KCGS		"	3	3	3	3	3	3	3	2	2	2	2
Airborne early warning & ISTAR[17]	KCGU		"	2	2	2	2	2	2	2	3	3	4[18]	4
Air transport and tankers and helicopters[12]	KCGV		"	14	8	9	9	9	9	9	8	8	8	8
Search and rescue	KCGX		"	2	2	2	2	2	2	2	2	2	2	2
RAF FP Wg	GHN7		HQs	..	..	4	4	4	4	4	6	6	7	7
RAF Ground based air defence[19,20]	GHN8		Squadrons	..	..	4	4	4	4	4	3	2	–	–
RAF Regiment Field[20]	GJ2F		"	..	..	6	6	6	6	6	6	6	7	7
RAF Regt (Jt CBRN)	I63Y		"	..	..	..	..	..	..	..	..	1	1	1
Tactical Provost Wg	GJ2G		HQs	–	–	–	–	–	–	–	1	1	1	1
Tactical Provost	GJ2H		Squadrons	–	–	–	–	–	–	–	2	1	1	1
Joint Helicopter Command														
Royal Navy Helicopter	JUAT		"	..	4	4	4	4	4	4	4	4	4	4
Army Aviation	JUAU		Regiments	..	5	5	5	5	5	5	5	5	5	5
Royal Air Force Helicopter	JUAV		Squadrons	..	6	6	6	6	6	6	6	5	6[21]	6
Joint Force Harrier														
Royal Navy	JUAW		"	..	3	3	3	3	2	1	1	2[22]	2	2
Royal Air Force	JUAX		"	..	3	3	3	3	3	3	2	2	2	2

1 See chapter text.
2 Only active vessels are shown.
3 HMS Spartan was withdrawn from service during the year.
4 HMS Sovereign was withdrawn from the service during the year.
5 HMS Superb was withdrawn from the service during the year.
6 HMS Invincible went into Extended Readiness in late 2005.
7 HMS Cardiff, HMS Marlborough and HMS Grafton were withdrawn from service during the year.
8 HMS Southampton was withdrawn from the service during the year.
9 HMS Leeds Castle and the NI Squadron, consisting of HMS Brecon, HMS Cottesmore and HMS Dulverton, were withdrawn from service during the year.
10 This figure has been revised due to a compiling error last year.
11 From 2000 excludes aircraft transferred to the Joint Force Harrier squadron.
12 From 2000 excludes helicopters transferred to the Joint Helicopter command.
13 From 2000 includes one Armoured Regiment which is committed to the new Joint Nuclear Biological and Chemical Regiment.
14 Figure for 2000 includes an additional Close Support Regiment formed as a result of the Stategic Defence Review.

15 From 2006, 4 Air Defence squadrons amalgamated with Strike/Attack, Offensive support and Reconnaissance to form multi-roled squadrons. One squadron moved from reconnaissance to ISTAR, and one squadron was disbanded.
16 6 Sqn (Jag) was disbanded 30 April 2007, 25 Sqn was disbanded 1 April 2008. 43 Squadron also cover the role of the OCU since the disbandment of 56 Sqn, however this is not their only role.
17 Figure for 2001 includes an embedded Operational Conversion Unit at the Sentry Operation Establishments.
18 39 Sqn was re-formed on 23 January 2008
19 Delivery of Ground Based Air Defence is now vested with the Army. The remaining 2 Squadrons were reroled on 1 April 2008 to increase the numbers of FP Wgs and field Regts.
20 In UKDS editions 2003 and 2004, Ground Based Air Defence and Field Squadrons for years 2001 to 2004 were also included under Regular Air Force.
21 Reflects the standing up of 78 Sqn RAF to accommodate the endorsed increase in Merlin Mk3 crews and aircraft.
22 The Fleet Air Arm Strike wing, the equivalent to an RAF Squadron, comprises 800 and 801 Naval Air Squadrons.

Source: MOD/DASA: 020 7218 0390

Defence

4.4 Outflow of United Kingdom Regular Forces: by Service[1]

Numbers

		1998 /99	1999 /00	2000 /01	2001 /02	2002 /03	2003 /04	2004 /05	2005 /06	2006[2] /07	2007[2] /08	2008[2] /09
All Services:												
Male	KDNA	24 500	23 870	22 520	22 360	21 770	21 200	21 330	21 290	23 000	22 510	19 940
Female	KDNB	2 970	2 750	2 430	2 350	2 340	2 200	2 100	1 980	2 160	2 170	1 940
Total	KDNC	27 470	26 620	24 950	24 710	24 100	23 400	23 430	23 260	25 160	24 690	21 880
Naval Service:												
Male	KDND	4 920	5 160	4 480	5 110	4 680	4 230	4 150	4 000	3 830	3 870	3 970
Female	KDNE	610	630	550	690	620	540	490	480	490	470	460
Total	KDNF	5 530	5 800	5 040	5 800	5 300	4 770	4 630	4 490	4 320	4 340	4 430
Army:												
Male	KDNI	15 320	14 620	13 900	13 290	13 420	13 500	13 990	13 240	14 660	14 230	12 210
Female	KDNJ	1 730	1 580	1 330	1 090	1 140	1 090	1 080	950	1 110	1 100	930
Total	KDNK	17 050	16 200	15 230	14 380	14 560	14 600	15 070	14 190	15 770	15 330	13 140
Royal Air Force:												
Male	KDNL	4 250	4 080	4 140	3 960	3 670	3 470	3 200	4 050	4 500	4 420	3 770
Female	KDNM	640	540	540	570	580	570	530	540	560	610	550
Total	KDNN	4 890	4 620	4 680	4 530	4 250	4 040	3 730	4 590	5 070	5 020	4 320

1 See chapter text. Comprises all those who left the Regular Forces and includes deaths.
2 Due to ongoing validation of data from the new Personnel Administration System, Naval Service statistics from 1 October 2006, Army statistics from 1 April 2007 and RAF statistics from 1 May 2007 are provisional and subject to review.

Source: Ministry of Defence/DASA (Quad-Service): 0207 8078896

4.5 United Kingdom Defence: Service manpower strengths[1]
As at 1 April

Thousands

		1999	2000	2001	2002	2003	2004	2005	2006	2007	2008	2009
UK Service personnel												
Full-time trained strength	ZBTR	191.1	190.3	189.1	187.1	188.5	190.2	188.1	183.2	177.8	174.0	173.9
Trained Naval Service	ZBTS	39.3	38.9	38.5	37.5	37.6	37.5	36.4	35.6	34.9	35.1	35.0
UK regulars	ZBTT	39.1	38.5	38.0	36.8	36.6	36.4	35.5	34.9	34.3	34.5	34.4
Full-time Reserve Service	ZBTU	0.3	0.3	0.5	0.7	1.0	1.1	0.9	0.7	0.6	0.5	0.6
Trained Army	ZBTV	99.8	100.2	100.4	100.4	102.0	103.6	102.4	100.6	99.3	98.3	99.3
UK regulars	ZBTW	96.3	96.5	96.3	96.0	97.6	99.4	98.5	96.8	95.4	93.8	94.6
Full-time Reserve Service	ZBTX	0.2	0.5	0.7	0.9	1.0	0.7	0.4	0.5	0.7	0.9	1.1
Gurkhas	ZBTY	3.4	3.4	3.5	3.4	3.4	3.4	3.5	3.3	3.3	3.6	3.6
Trained Royal Air Force	ZBTZ	51.9	51.2	50.1	49.2	48.9	49.1	49.2	46.9	43.6	40.6	39.7
UK regulars	ZBUA	51.8	51.0	49.8	48.9	48.5	48.7	48.8	46.6	43.2	40.3	39.3
Full-time Reserve Service	ZBUB	0.1	0.2	0.3	0.3	0.4	0.4	0.4	0.3	0.3	0.4	0.4
Untrained UK regulars	ZBUC	21.5	21.6	21.5	23.0	24.2	22.5	18.3	17.5	17.5	18.4	20.1
Naval Service	ZBUD	4.6	4.3	4.4	4.9	5.0	4.5	4.4	4.5	4.5	4.0	3.9
Army	ZBUE	13.4	13.6	13.2	14.0	14.5	13.3	10.8	10.9	10.8	11.3	11.9
Royal Air Force	ZBUF	3.5	3.7	3.9	4.1	4.7	4.7	3.0	2.1	2.2	3.1	4.3
Locally Entered Personnel[2] (excluding Gurkhas)	ZBUG	0.4	0.4	0.3	0.4	0.4	0.4	0.4	0.4	0.4	0.4	0.4
Royal Irish Regiment[3] Home Service batallions	ZBUH	4.4	4.2	3.8	3.6	3.5	3.4	3.2	3.1	2.1	–	–
Reserve personnel	ZBUI	307.0	294.8	284.2	273.4	259.7	246.7	235.6	..	..	..	..
Regular Reserves	ZBUJ	247.6	241.6	234.9	224.9	212.6	201.4	191.5	..	..	..	..
Naval Services	ZBUK	24.7	24.2	23.5	23.5	23.2	22.8	22.2	..	..	19.6	..
Army[4]	ZBUL	180.5	175.5	169.8	161.1	151.5	141.9	134.2	127.6	121.8	..	..
of which mobilised:	SNEO	0.1	0.3	0.2	0.3	0.4	0.1	0.2	0.3	0.1	–	–
Royal Air Force	ZBUM	42.4	41.9	41.5	40.2	37.7	36.4	35.0	34.4	33.4	..	..
of which mobilised:	SNEP	–	–	–	–	–	–	..	–	–	–	–
Volunteer Reserves	ZBUN	59.4	53.2	47.3	46.3	44.9	43.4	42.3	..	42.7	39.2	41.5
Royal Naval Reserve and Royal Marine Reserve	ZBUO	4.5	4.8	4.8	5.0	4.9	4.5	4.4	..	3.0	2.9	3.0
of which mobilised:	SNEQ	..	..	..	..	0.4	0.1	..	..	0.1	0.2	0.2
Territorial Army[4]	ZBUP	52.3	45.6	41.7	40.7	39.3	38.1	37.3	38.5	36.8	35.0	35.3
of which mobilised:	SNER	0.5	0.8	0.4	0.5	4.1	2.9	1.5	1.1	1.0	1.4	1.4
Royal Auxilliary Air Force	ZBUQ	2.6	2.7	1.6	1.5	1.5	1.4	1.4	1.4	1.3	1.3	1.4
of which mobilised:	SNES	–	–	–	0.1	0.8	–	..	0.1	0.2	0.1	0.2
Cadet Forces	ZBUR	151.0	154.5	151.0	152.3	155.6	155.6	153.1	..	150.5	150.4	153.8
Naval Service	ZBUS	24.5	24.1	23.8	23.8	23.2	22.6	21.9	..	18.2	18.6	19.0
Army[4]	ZBUT	74.6	77.4	75.4	75.8	78.7	80.5	80.9	81.7	81.9	82.7	84.9
Royal Air Force	ZBUU	51.9	53.0	51.8	52.7	53.7	52.5	50.3	51.0	50.4	49.5	50.1

1 See chapter text.
2 Locally Entered Personnel includes Gibraltar Volunteer Reserves and Gibraltar Permanent Cadre.
3 The Royal Irish Regiment disbanded on 31 March 2008.
4 2008 Army Reserves data are as at 1 June. 2007 Army Reserves data are as at 1 March.

Source: Ministry of Defence/DASA (Quad-Service): 0207 8078896

4.6 United Kingdom defence: civilian manpower strengths[1]
As at 1 April

Thousands: Full-time Equivalent

		1999	2000	2001	2002	2003	2004	2005	2006	2007	2008	2009
Ministry of Defence civilians												
MOD Head Office, HQ and centrally managed expenditure[2,3]												
Non-industrial	KDQE	21.5	19.7	19.1	20.0	21.2	22.7	24.0	24.6	19.8	19.6	19.3
Industrial	KDQF	1.0	0.9	0.9	0.8	0.7	0.6	0.7	0.8	0.8	0.7	0.7
Defence Logistics Organisation[3]												
Non-industrial	ZBTJ	..	19.7	17.8	17.3	16.4	16.5	16.5	14.1	..	..	..
Industrial	ZBTK	..	11.5	8.4	6.3	4.4	4.3	4.1	3.9	..	..	..
Defence Equipment & Support[3]												
Non-industrial	I6P5	..	..	..	..	..	..	..	..	17.3	15.2	14.3
Industrial	I6P6	..	..	..	..	..	..	..	..	3.6	2.8	2.4
Naval Service												
Non-industrial	KYCW	11.3	3.0	3.0	2.9	2.7	2.9	2.6	2.3	2.3	1.8	1.8
Industrial	KYCX	5.3	1.0	0.9	0.8	0.8	0.8	0.7	0.6	0.6	0.5	0.5
Royal Fleet Auxiliary	EQS9	2.4	2.4	2.4	2.4	2.5	2.3	2.3	2.3	2.4	2.3	2.3
Army												
Non-industrial	KDQK	21.6	16.3	16.4	16.0	16.0	14.7	14.5	13.4	12.7	12.2	11.9
Industrial	KDQL	10.6	5.8	5.7	5.5	5.4	5.6	5.5	5.2	5.3	5.0	4.6
Royal Air Force												
Non-industrial	KDQM	12.2	7.1	7.0	7.1	7.0	7.3	7.0	6.7	6.0	5.7	5.7
Industrial	KDQN	7.1	4.5	4.4	4.3	4.4	4.4	4.0	4.0	3.0	3.0	2.8
Level 1 Total	C7PE	94.1	91.9	86.0	83.6	81.5	82.2	82.0	78.1	73.8	69.1	66.4
Non-industrial	C7PF	66.6	65.8	63.4	63.4	63.3	64.1	64.7	61.3	58.1	54.7	53.0
Industrial	C7PG	25.1	23.7	20.2	17.8	15.7	15.7	15.0	14.5	13.3	12.1	11.1
Royal Fleet Auxiliary	EQT2	2.4	2.4	2.4	2.4	2.5	2.3	2.3	2.3	2.4	2.3	2.3
Locally engaged overseas	KDQA	14.9	14.8	13.3	14.1	13.8	15.4	15.7	15.1	14.2	11.2	10.5
Non-industrial	KDQT	6.7	6.7	6.3	6.5	6.5	7.3	..	..	..	..	..
Industrial	KDQU	8.1	8.2	7.0	7.6	7.4	8.1	..	..	..	..	..
Trading funds	GQHI	14.0	14.5	18.8	12.4	12.2	11.4	10.8	10.7	10.1	9.2	9.6
Level 0 Total	C7PH	123.0	121.3	118.2	110.1	107.6	109.0	108.5	103.9	98.0	89.5	86.6

1 See chapter text. Individuals on temporary and geographic (T&G) promotion are classed as non-industrial. From 2004, personnel who cannot be correctly allocated to Top Level Budgets (TLBs) are included with the Centre figures (numbering approx 200 in 2006).
2 The MOD Head Office, HQ and centrally managed expenditure budgetary area was formerly referred to as Centre.
3 At 1 April 2007, the Defence Logistics Organisation and the Defence Procurement Agency (formerly part of the MOD Head Office, HQ and centrally managed expenditure budgetary area) merged to form Defence Equipment & Support.

Source: Ministry of Defence/DASA (SMG): 01225 467144

4.7 Family accommodation and defence land holdings[1]
As at 1 April

Thousands and thousand hectares

		1999	2000	2001	2002	2003	2004	2005	2006	2007	2008	2009
Family accommodation (thousands)												
United Kingdom: Total	KDPA	65.5	64.8	59.2	55.8	53.8	52.8	51.9	51.8	51.1	51.2	49.9
Land holdings												
United Kingdom												
Land[2]	KDPF	220.2	219.9	224.3	222.4	221.4	221.3	222.1	222.0	222.0	221.7	221.0
Foreshore[2]	KDPH	18.6	18.6	18.6	18.6	18.6	18.6	18.6	18.6	18.6	18.6	18.0
Rights held	KDPJ	124.8	124.8	124.8	124.9	131.1	131.1	124.9	124.9	124.9	133.1	133.0

1 See chapter text.
2 Freehold and leasehold.

Sources: Ministry of Defence/Defence Estates Directorate of Operations;
Housing : 01480 52151;
Ministry of Defence/Defence Estates: 0121 311 2140

Defence

4.8 Location of United Kingdom service personnel[1]
As at 1 April

Thousands

		1999	2000	2001	2002	2003	2004	2005	2006	2007	2008[13]	2009[13]
UK Service personnel, Regular Forces:												
UK distribution[2,3]												
In United Kingdom[4]	KDOB	171.7	170.3	172.0	..	..	..	169.7	167.3	161.4	158.7	162.7
England	KDOC	144.3	143.0	144.1	..	..	..	145.0	142.1	141.4	140.3	143.6
Wales	KDOD	3.3	3.2	2.6	..	..	..	2.9	3.3	2.6	2.6	2.7
Scotland	KDOE	14.9	15.1	14.5	..	..	..	13.2	13.5	12.6	12.0	12.0
Northern Ireland	KDOF	9.0	8.4	9.4	..	..	..	7.0	6.8	4.8	3.7	4.4
Global location[2,3]												
United Kingdom	MKCN	161.0	163.1	162.8	..	..	..	169.7	167.3	161.4	158.7	162.7
Overseas	KDOG	47.1	43.0	40.9	..	..	..	29.2	28.5	28.0	27.6	25.4
Mainland European States[4,5]	KDOI	15.2	8.2	8.6	..	..	..	27.0	26.6	26.2	26.0	23.4
Germany[6]	KDOH	18.0	19.5	17.3	..	..	..	22.2	22.0	21.7	21.7	19.1
Balkans	MKCO	..	..	..	..	..	..	0.1	–	0.1	–	–
Mediterranean[7,8]	KDOM	1.3	1.1	2.3	..	..	..	..	..	..	..	..
Gibraltar	KDOJ	0.6	0.6	0.5	..	..	..	0.4	0.3	0.3	0.3	0.3
Cyprus	KDOL	3.6	3.5	3.5	..	..	..	3.2	3.0	3.0	2.8	2.9
Far East/Asia[9]	MKCT	0.3	1.0	0.3	..	..	..	0.3	0.3	0.2	0.3	0.3
Africa[10]	MKCP	..	..	–	..	..	..	0.6	0.6	0.5	0.5	0.5
North America	MKCQ	..	..	2.5	..	..	..	0.7	0.7	0.7	0.7	0.8
Central/South America	MKCR	..	..	–	..	..	..	0.1	0.1	0.1	0.1	0.1
Falkland Islands	MKCS	..	..	0.8	..	..	..	0.3	0.3	0.3	0.1	0.3
Other locations, including unallocated	KDOQ	8.2	9.1	5.1	..	..	..	1.1	1.0	1.1	1.2	0.3
Locally entered service personnel:[11]												
United Kingdom	KDOS	2.0	2.1	2.3	2.6	2.6	2.6	2.5[12]	2.6[12]	2.8[12]	3.0[12]	3.2
Gibraltar	KDOT	0.4	0.3	0.4	0.4	0.4	0.4	0.4	0.4	0.4	0.4	0.4
Hong Kong	KDOV	–	–	–	–	–	–	–	–	–	–	–
Brunei	KDOW	0.8	0.8	0.8	0.8	0.8	0.7	0.8	0.8	0.8	0.8	0.7
India/Nepal	KDOX	0.5	0.5	0.4	0.3	0.4	0.4	0.4[12]	0.3	0.1	–	–
Total	KDOK	3.7	3.7	3.9	4.2	4.1	4.1	4.1[12]	4.0[12]	4.1[12]	4.2[12]	4.3

1 See chapter text.
2 Prior to 2003, figures for UK distribution and global location are collated from seperate sources. Comparison is therefore not possible between the two sets of UK personnel figures.
3 Includes personnel within the UK whose location is unknown.
4 Includes the Balkans until 2002.
5 Post 2002 Mainland European States figure includes Germany, Balkans, Mediterranean, Gibraltar and Cyprus.
6 Prior to 1996, figures for the Federal Republic of Germany and Mainland European States were combined.
7 Includes Med Near East and Middle East until 2002.
8 Post 2002 Mediterranean figure is not shown separately but is included in Mainland European States figure.
9 Prior to 1997, figures include personnel serving in Hong Kong.
10 Post 2002, the Africa figure includes Middle East.
11 Up to 2001 includes trained Gurkhas. Post 2001 includes trained and untrained Gurkhas.
12 Revised to make data consistent with UK Defence Statistics.
13 All data for 2008 and 2009 are provisional.

Source: Ministry of Defence/DASA (Quad-Service): 02072 180 390

4.9 United Kingdom regular forces: deaths[1]

Numbers and rates per hundred thousand

		2000	2001	2002	2003	2004	2005	2006	2007	2008	2009
Deaths											
Total	SNIA	147	142	147	177	170	160	191	204	137	205
Male	SNIB	143	139	138	170	164	152	184	195	129	202
Female	SNIC	4	3	9	7	6	8	7	9	8	3
Rates per 100,000 strength[2]											
All	SNIH	72	70	74	83	81	81	98	106	72	106
Navy	SNII	63	80	72	89	92	70	86	71	109	55
Army	SNIJ	80	72	85	83	76	86	95	129	72	134
RAF	SNIK	64	51	53	72	63	72	86	70	34	51

1 Gurkhas and non-regular Service personnel who died whilst on Operations are included in the numbers and rates presented in Table 4.9.
2 Rates have been age and gender standardised to the 2009 Armed Forces population.

Source: Ministry of Defence/DASA (Health Information): 01225 467538

4.10 Strength of uniformed United Kingdom medical staff[1]
As at 1 April

Numbers

		1998	1999	2000	2001	2002	2003	2004	2005	2006	2007[8]	2008[9]
Qualified doctors:[2]												
Naval Service	KDMA	210	210	210	220	220	230	240	260	260	290	283
Army[3]	KDMB	440	450	460	470	490	550	600	610	650	550	598
Royal Air Force	KDMC	210	200	180	180	180	190	200	220	230	220	229
All Services	KDMD	850	860	860	870	890	970	1 040	1 090	1 140	1 060	1 110
Qualified dentists:[2]												
Naval Service	KDME	60	60	60	60	60	60	60	60	60	50	55
Army[3]	KDMF	140	140	140	150	140	150	150	150	140	130	132
Royal Air Force	KDMG	80	80	80	80	70	70	80	70	70	60	63
All Services	KDMH	280	290	280	290	280	270	290	280	270	240	250
Support staff:[4]												
Naval Service[5]	KDMI	990	970	1 000	1 030	1 010	1 060	1 110	1 110	1 120	1 130	1 278
Nursing services[5]	ZBTL	..	200	210	210	220	250	280	290	300	300	295
Support[5]	ZBTM	..	770	790	820	790	810	840	820	820	830	983
Army[3]	KDMJ	3 090	3 120	3 210	3 260	3 320	3 410	3 560	..	..	3 000	4 071
Nursing services[3,4,6]	ZBTN	..	520	570	610	650	710	770	770	800	790	962
Support[3]	ZBTO	..	2 600	2 640	2 650	2 670	2 700	2 800	..	..	2 210	3 109
Royal Air Force	KDMK	1 190	1 360	1 460	1 480	1 500	1 600	1 680	1 660	1 550	1 340	1 375
Nursing services[7]	ZBTP	..	330	400	420	450	470	480	510	480	490	437
Support	ZBTQ	..	1 030	1 060	1 070	1 050	1 130	1 200	1 160	1 070	850	938
All Services	KDML	5 230	5 540	5 760	5 800	5 930	6 180	6 440	..	..	..	..

1 See chapter text. Includes staff employed at units (including ships) and in hospitals.

2 The Medical and Dental Officers are trained only and exclude Late Entry Personnel. For 2007 includes all those individuals who hold a basic registrable qualification but may not necessarily be fully trained in their speciality. "Qualified" Doctors and Dentists refers to personnel who hold a basic registrable qualification, but may not necessarily have completed their career directed professional training, and as such may not necessarily be fully trained in their speciality.

3 Due to a change in source data, Army figures prior to 2005 cannot be verified.

4 Includes all members of the Nursing Services/Nursing Corps. From 1999, figures for support staff have been split so that nurses are separate from other support staff. From 2007, includes all medical support staff which the Defence Medical Services Department collects in its tri-service return.

5 From 2007, includes trained and untrained.

6 The 2006 Nursing Services figure is trained and untrained Soldiers with Nursing trades in the QARANC and all trained Officers in QARANC. From 2007, includes trained and untrained.

7 From 2007, includes trained and untrained.

8 Figures from 2007 provided by DMSD.

9 2008 support figures include all support staff both trained and untrained.

Source: DASA DMSD: 0207 2181429

Defence

4.11 United Kingdom defence services and the civilian community[1]

		1999	2000	2001	2002	2003	2004	2005	2006	2007	2008	2009
Military Search and rescue operations at home												
Call outs: total	GPYC	1 912	1 941	1 763	1 684	1 714	1 638	1 702	1 875	1 973	2 083	2 337
Royal Navy helicopters	GPXO	499	499	502	436	424	453	478	497	592	586	758
Royal Air Force helicopters	GPXP	1 235	1 278	1 115	1 122	1 173	1 079	1 114	1 258	1 258	1 377	1 479
Contractorised and other helicopters	GPXQ	–	–	–	–	–	–	–	1	–	–	–
Royal Air Force Nimrod aircraft	GPXR	65	71	54	46	37	37	37	32	21	29	13
Other fixed wing aircraft[2]	GPXS	–	1	1	1	–	2	–	1	–	–	1
HM ships and auxilliary vessels[2]	KCMG	–	–	–	–	–	–	–	–	–	–	–
Royal Air Force mountain rescue teams	KCMH	113	92	91	79	80	67	73	86	102	91	86
Persons moved: total	KCMI	1 204	1 316	1 182	1 224	1 273	1 412	1 384	1 463	1 767	1 607	1 810
Persons moved by rescue service												
Royal Navy helicopters	GPXT	355	360	386	314	320	416	380	479	507	516	656
Royal Air Force helicopters	GPXU	832	934	781	900	922	978	907	968	1 219	1 062	1 135
Royal Air Force mountain rescue teams	GPXV	17	22	15	10	31	17	97	16	41	29	19
Other	GPXW	–	–	–	–	–	1	–	–	–	–	–
Persons moved by type of assistance												
Rescue[3]	GPXX	307	276	281	343	280	494	408	384	582	450	445
Medrescue[4]	GPXY	640	713	629	654	779	672	778	830	946	869	1 064
Medtransfer[5]	GPXZ	216	241	228	201	174	195	143	175	198	219	224
Recovery[6]	GPYA	32	29	36	21	25	33	31	43	24	40	44
Transfer[7]	GPYB	9	57	8	5	15	18	24	31	17	29	33
Search and rescue incidents: total	KCMM	1 714	1 781	1 608	1 544	1 600	1 504	1 584	1 703	1 803	1 941	2 191

Source: Ministry of Defence/DASA (Statistical Methodology Group): 01225 468701

		1999 /00	2000 /01	2001 /02	2002 /03	2003 /04	2004 /05	2005 /06	2006 /07	2007 /08	2008 /09
Fishery protection											
Vessels boarded	KCMO	1 716	1 603	1 464	1 375	1 709	1 747	1 371	1 335	1 309	1 102

Source: Fisheries Protection - Ministry of Defence

1 See chapter text.
2 Not permanently on stand-by.
3 Rescue: Moving an uninjured person from a hostile to a benign environment.
4 Medrescue: Moving an injured casualty from a hostile environment to a medical facility.
5 Medtransfer (formerly Medevac): Moving a sick person between medical facilities such as a hospital or occasionally to move transplant organs.
6 Recovery: Moving people declared dead on scene or confirmed dead on arrival by a qualified doctor.
7 Transfer (formerly Airlift): Moving military personnel, or their families, on compassionate grounds.

Population and vital statistics

Chapter 5

Population and vital statistics

This section begins with a summary of population figures for the UK and constituent countries for 1851 to 2031 and for Great Britain from 1801 (Table 5.1). Table 5.2 analyses the components of population change. Table 5.3 gives details of the national sex and age structures for years up to the present date, with projected figures up to the year 2026. Legal marital condition of the population is shown in Table 5.4. The distribution of population at regional and local levels is summarised in Table 5.5.

In the main, historical series relate to census information, while mid-year estimates, which make allowance for under-enumeration in the census, are given for the recent past and the present (from 1961 onwards).

Population

(Tables 5.1 – 5.3)

Figures shown in these tables relate to the population enumerated at successive censuses (up to 1951), mid-year estimates (from 1961 to 2008) and population projections (up to 2031). Further information can be found on the Office for National Statistics (ONS) website at: www.statistics.gov.uk/popest

Population projections are 2008-based and were published by ONS on 21 October 2009. Further information can be found at: www.statistics.gov.uk/StatBase/Product.asp?vlnk=8519.

Definition of resident population

The estimated resident population of an area includes all the people who usually live there, whatever their nationality. Members of HM and US Armed Forces in England and Wales are included on a residential basis wherever possible. HM Forces stationed outside England and Wales are not included. Students are taken to be resident at their term-time address.

The projections of the resident population of the UK and constituent countries were prepared by the National Statistics Centre for Demography within ONS, in consultation with the Registrars General, as a common framework for use in national planning in a number of different fields. New projections are made every second year on assumptions regarding future fertility, mortality and migration which seem most appropriate on the basis of the statistical evidence available at the time. The population projections in

Tables 5.1 – 5.3 are based on the estimates of the population of the UK at mid-2008 made by the Registrars General.

Marital condition (de jure): estimated population

(Table 5.4)

This table shows population estimates by marital status.

Geographical distribution of the population

(Table 5.5)

The population enumerated in the censuses for 1911–1951 and the mid-year population estimates for later years are provided for standard regions of the UK, for metropolitan areas, for broad groupings of local authority districts by type within England and Wales and for some of the larger cities. Projections of future sub-national population levels are prepared from time to time by the Registrar General, but are not shown in this publication.

Migration into and out of the UK

(Tables 5.7, 5.9)

A migrant is defined as a person who changes his or her country of usual residence for a period of at least a year so that the country of destination effectively becomes the country of usual residence.

The main source of international migration data is the International Passenger Survey (IPS). This is a continuous voluntary sample survey that provides information on passengers entering and leaving the UK by the principal air, sea and tunnel routes. Being a sample survey, the IPS is subject to some uncertainty; therefore, it should be noted that international migration estimates, in particular the difference between inflow and outflow, may be subject to large sampling errors. The IPS excludes routes between the Channel Islands and Isle of Man and the rest of the world.

The IPS data are supplemented with three types of additional information in order to provide a full picture of total international migration:

1. The IPS is based on intentions to migrate and intentions are liable to change. Adjustments are made for visitor switchers (those who intend to stay in the UK or abroad for less than one year but subsequently stay for longer and become migrants) and for migrant switchers (those who intend to stay in the UK or abroad for one year or more but then return earlier so are no longer migrants). These adjustments are primarily based on IPS data but

for years prior to 2001 Home Office data on short-term visitors who were subsequently granted an extension of stay for a year or longer for other reasons have been incorporated.

2. Home Office data on applications for asylum and dependants of asylum seekers entering the UK are used to estimate inflows of asylum seekers and dependants not already captured by the IPS. In addition, Home Office data on removals and refusals are used to estimate outflows of failed asylum seekers not identified by the IPS.

3. Migration flows between the UK and the Irish Republic are added to these data as the IPS did not cover this route until recently and the quality of these data are still being assessed. Migration flows are obtained mainly from the Quarterly National Household Survey and are agreed between the Irish Central Statistics Office and ONS.

The international migration estimates in Table 5.7 are derived from all these sources and represent total international migration. The estimates in Tables 5.8 and 5.9 are based on the IPS only (without the three adjustments outlined above).

Grants for settlement in the UK

(Table 5.10)

This table presents, in geographic regions, the statistics of individual countries of nationality, arranged alphabetically within each region. The figures are on a different basis from those derived from IPS (Tables 5.8 and 5.9) and relate only to people subject to immigration control. Persons granted settlement are allowed to stay indefinitely in the UK. They exclude temporary migrants such as students and generally relate only to non-EEA nationals. Settlement can occur several years after entry to the country.

Applications received for asylum in the United Kingdom, excluding dependants

(Table 5.11)

This table shows statistics of applications for asylum in the UK. Figures are shown for the main applicant nationalities by geographic region. The basis of assessing asylum applications, and hence of deciding whether to grant asylum in the UK, is the 1951 United Nations Convention on Refugees.

Marriages

(Table 5.12)

The figures in this table relate to marriages solemnised in the constituent countries of the UK. They take no account of the growing trend towards marrying abroad.

Divorces

(Tables 5.13 and 5.14)

A marriage may be either **dissolved**, following a petition for divorce and the granting of a decree absolute, or **annulled**, following a petition for nullity and the awarding of a decree of nullity. The first group of decrees are known as dissolutions of marriage and the second as annulments of marriage. In Table 5.13 the term 'divorce' includes both types of decrees.

Births

(Tables 5.15 – 5.17)

For Scotland and Northern Ireland the number of births relate to those **registered** during the year. For England and Wales the figures up to and including the period from 1930 to 1932 are for those registered, while later figures relate to births **occurring** in each year.

All data for England and Wales and for Scotland include births occurring in those countries to mothers not usually resident in them. Data for Northern Ireland, and hence the UK, prior to 1981 include births occurring in Northern Ireland to non-resident mothers; from 1981 such births are excluded.

Deaths

(Tables 5.19 and 5.21)

The figures relate to the number of deaths registered during each calendar year.

Infant and maternal mortality

(Table 5.20)

On 1 October 1992 the legal definition of a stillbirth was altered from a baby born dead after 28 completed weeks gestation or more to one born after 24 completed weeks of gestation or more. The 258 stillbirths of 24 to 27 weeks gestation that occurred between 1 October and 31 December 1992 are excluded from this table.

Population and vital statistics

Life tables

(Table 5.22)

The current set of interim life tables are constructed from the estimated population in the period from 2004 to 2006 and corresponding data on births, infant deaths and deaths by individual age occurring in those years.

The estimates used in these interim life tables are the estimates, or revised estimates, issued on the following dates:

Mid-year population estimates	England	Wales	Scotland	Northern Ireland
2004	August 2007	August 2007	July 2007	July 2005
2005	August 2007	August 2007	July 2007	October 2006
2006	August 2007	August 2007	July 2007	July 2007
2007	August 2008	August 2008	July 2008	July 2008

Adoptions

(Tables 5.23)

The figures shown within these tables relate to the date the adoption was entered in the Adopted Children Register. Figures based on the date of the court order are available for England and Wales in the volume *Marriage, divorce and adoption statistics 2007* (no. 35 in the FM2 series) available on the ONS website at: www.ons.gov.uk or from the enquiry point in the ONS shown at the foot of the tables.

5.1 Population summary: by country and sex

Thousands

	United Kingdom			England and Wales			Wales	Scotland			Northern Ireland		
	Persons	Males	Females	Persons	Males	Females	Persons	Persons	Males	Females	Persons	Males	Females
Enumerated population: Census figures													
1801	..	..	..	8 893	4 255	4 638	587	1 608	739	869	..	..	..
1851	22 259	10 855	11 404	17 928	8 781	9 146	1 163	2 889	1 376	1 513	1 442	698	745
1901	38 237	18 492	19 745	32 528	15 729	16 799	2 013	4 472	2 174	2 298	1 237	590	647
1911	42 082	20 357	21 725	36 070	17 446	18 625	2 421	4 761	2 309	2 452	1 251	603	648
1921[1]	44 027	21 033	22 994	37 887	18 075	19 811	2 656	4 882	2 348	2 535	1 258	610	648
1931[1]	46 038	22 060	23 978	39 952	19 133	20 819	2 593	4 843	2 326	2 517	1 243	601	642
1951	50 225	24 118	26 107	43 758	21 016	22 742	2 599	5 096	2 434	2 662	1 371	668	703
1961	52 709	25 481	27 228	46 105	22 304	23 801	2 644	5 179	2 483	2 697	1 425	694	731
Resident population: mid-year estimates													
	DYAY	BBAB	BBAC	BBAD	BBAE	BBAF	KGJM	BBAG	BBAH	BBAI	BBAJ	BBAK	BBAL
1973	56 223	27 332	28 891	49 459	24 061	25 399	2 773	5 234	2 515	2 719	1 530	756	774
1974	56 236	27 349	28 887	49 468	24 075	25 393	2 785	5 241	2 519	2 722	1 527	755	772
1975	56 226	27 361	28 865	49 470	24 091	25 378	2 795	5 232	2 516	2 716	1 524	753	770
1976	56 216	27 360	28 856	49 459	24 089	25 370	2 799	5 233	2 517	2 716	1 524	754	770
1977	56 190	27 345	28 845	49 440	24 076	25 364	2 801	5 226	2 515	2 711	1 523	754	769
1978	56 178	27 330	28 849	49 443	24 067	25 375	2 804	5 212	2 509	2 704	1 523	754	770
1979	56 240	27 373	28 867	49 508	24 113	25 395	2 810	5 204	2 505	2 699	1 528	755	773
1980	56 330	27 411	28 919	49 603	24 156	25 448	2 816	5 194	2 501	2 693	1 533	755	778
1981	56 357	27 412	28 946	49 634	24 160	25 474	2 813	5 180	2 495	2 685	1 543	757	786
1982	56 291	27 364	28 927	49 582	24 119	25 462	2 804	5 165	2 487	2 677	1 545	757	788
1983	56 316	27 371	28 944	49 617	24 133	25 484	2 803	5 148	2 479	2 669	1 551	759	792
1984	56 409	27 421	28 989	49 713	24 185	25 528	2 801	5 139	2 475	2 664	1 557	761	796
1985	56 554	27 489	29 065	49 861	24 254	25 606	2 803	5 128	2 470	2 658	1 565	765	800
1986	56 684	27 542	29 142	49 999	24 311	25 687	2 811	5 112	2 462	2 649	1 574	768	805
1987	56 804	27 599	29 205	50 123	24 371	25 752	2 823	5 099	2 455	2 644	1 582	773	809
1988	56 916	27 652	29 265	50 254	24 434	25 820	2 841	5 077	2 444	2 633	1 585	774	812
1989	57 076	27 729	29 348	50 408	24 510	25 898	2 855	5 078	2 443	2 635	1 590	776	814
1990	57 237	27 819	29 419	50 561	24 597	25 964	2 862	5 081	2 444	2 637	1 596	778	818
1991	57 439	27 909	29 530	50 748	24 681	26 067	2 873	5 083	2 445	2 639	1 607	783	824
1992	57 585	27 977	29 608	50 876	24 739	26 136	2 878	5 086	2 445	2 640	1 623	792	831
1993	57 714	28 039	29 675	50 986	24 793	26 193	2 884	5 092	2 448	2 644	1 636	798	837
1994	57 862	28 108	29 754	51 116	24 853	26 263	2 887	5 102	2 453	2 649	1 644	802	842
1995	58 025	28 204	29 821	51 272	24 946	26 326	2 889	5 104	2 453	2 650	1 649	804	845
1996	58 164	28 287	29 877	51 410	25 030	26 381	2 891	5 092	2 447	2 645	1 662	810	851
1997	58 314	28 371	29 943	51 560	25 113	26 446	2 895	5 083	2 442	2 641	1 671	816	856
1998	58 475	28 458	30 017	51 720	25 201	26 519	2 900	5 077	2 439	2 638	1 678	819	859
1999	58 684	28 578	30 106	51 933	25 323	26 610	2 901	5 072	2 437	2 635	1 679	818	861
2000	58 886	28 690	30 196	52 140	25 438	26 702	2 907	5 063	2 432	2 631	1 683	820	862
2001	59 113	28 832	30 281	52 360	25 574	26 786	2 910	5 064	2 434	2 630	1 689	824	865
2002	59 323	28 964	30 359	52 572	25 704	26 868	2 920	5 055	2 432	2 623	1 697	829	868
2003	59 557	29 109	30 449	52 797	25 841	26 956	2 931	5 057	2 435	2 623	1 703	833	870
2004	59 846	29 278	30 568	53 057	25 995	27 062	2 946	5 078	2 446	2 632	1 710	836	874
2005	60 238	29 497	30 741	53 419	26 197	27 223	2 954	5 095	2 456	2 639	1 724	844	880
2006	60 587	29 694	30 893	53 729	26 371	27 358	2 966	5 117	2 469	2 647	1 742	853	888
2007	60 975	29 916	31 059	54 072	26 569	27 503	2 980	5 144	2 486	2 659	1 759	862	897
2008	61 383	30 151	31 232	54 440	26 780	27 659	2 993	5 169	2 500	2 668	1 775	871	904
Resident population: projections (mid-year)[2]													
	C59J	C59K	C59L	C59M	C59N	C59O	C59P	C59Q	C59R	C59S	C59T	C59U	C59V
2011	62 649	30 842	31 807	55 601	27 412	28 189	3 024	5 233	2 537	2 695	1 815	892	923
2016	64 773	31 986	32 787	57 576	28 474	29 102	3 104	5 324	2 589	2 736	1 874	924	950
2021	66 958	33 134	33 824	59 620	29 547	30 073	3 187	5 411	2 635	2 776	1 927	952	975
2026	69 051	34 210	34 841	61 597	30 563	31 035	3 263	5 483	2 672	2 811	1 971	975	996
2031	70 933	35 162	35 772	63 397	31 473	31 924	3 326	5 532	2 696	2 835	2 005	992	1 012

1 Figures for Northern Ireland are estimated. The population at the Census of 1926 was 1 257 thousand (608 thousand males and 649 thousand females).

2 These projections are 2008-based. See chapter text for more detail.

Sources: Office for National Statistics: 01329 444661;
General Register Office for Scotland;
Northern Ireland Statistics and Research Agency

5.2 Population changes: by country

Thousands

	Population[1] at start of period	Average annual change				
		Overall annual change	Births	Deaths[2]	Natural change	Net migration and other changes
United Kingdom						
1901 - 1911	38 237	385	1 091	624	467	-82
1911 - 1921	42 082	195	975	689	286	-92
1921 - 1931	44 027	201	824	555	268	-67
1931 - 1951	46 038	213	793	603	190	22
1951 - 1961	50 225	258	839	593	246	12
1961 - 1971	52 807	312	962	638	324	-12
1971 - 1981	55 928	42	736	666	69	-27
1981 - 1991	56 357	108	757	655	103	5
1991 - 2001	57 439	161	731	631	100	61
2001 - 2007	59 113	310	710	591	119	191
2001 - 2008	59 113	324	722	588	134	191
2011 - 2021	62 649	431	791	544	248	183
England and Wales						
1901 - 1911	32 528	354	929	525	404	-50
1911 - 1921	36 070	182	828	584	244	-62
1921 - 1931	37 887	207	693	469	224	-17
1931 - 1951	39 952	193	673	518	155	38
1951 - 1961	43 758	244	714	516	197	47
1961 - 1971	46 196	296	832	560	272	23
1971 - 1981	49 152	48	638	585	53	-5
1981 - 1991	49 634	111	664	576	89	23
1991 - 2001	50 748	155	647	556	92	63
2001 - 2007	52 360	285	634	520	114	171
2001 - 2008	52 360	297	644	517	127	170
2011 - 2021	55 601	402	709	477	232	170
Scotland						
1901 - 1911	4 472	29	131	76	54	-25
1911 - 1921	4 761	12	118	82	36	-24
1921 - 1931	4 882	-4	100	65	35	-39
1931 - 1951	4 843	13	92	67	25	-12
1951 - 1961	5 096	9	95	62	34	-25
1961 - 1971	5 184	5	97	63	34	-30
1971 - 1981	5 236	-6	70	64	6	-11
1981 - 1991	5 180	-7	66	63	3	-10
1991 - 2001	5 083	-2	60	60	-1	-1
2001 - 2007	5 064	13	54	57	-3	16
2001 - 2008	5 064	15	55	57	-2	17
2011 - 2021	5 233	18	58	52	5	12
Northern Ireland						
1901 - 1911	1 237	1	31	23	8	-6
1911 - 1921	1 251	1	29	22	7	-6
1921 - 1931	1 258	-2	30	21	9	-11
1931 - 1951	1 243	6	28	18	10	-4
1951 - 1961	1 371	6	30	15	15	-9
1961 - 1971	1 427	11	33	16	17	-6
1971 - 1981	1 540	-	28	17	11	-11
1981 - 1991	1 543	6	27	16	12	-5
1991 - 2001	1 607	8	24	15	9	-
2001 - 2008	1 689	11	23	14	8	4
2011 - 2021	1 815	11	25	14	11	1

1 Census enumerated population up to 1951; mid-year estimates of resident population from 1961 to 2008 and mid-2008-based projections of resident population thereafter.

2 Including deaths of non-civilians and merchant seamen who died outside the country. These numbered 577 000 in 1911-1921 and 240 000 in 1931-1951 for England and Wales; 74 000 in 1911-1921 and 34 000 in 1931-1951 for Scotland; and 10 000 in 1911-1926 for Northern Ireland.

Sources: Office for National Statistics: 01329 444661;
General Register Office for Scotland;
Northern Ireland Statistics and Research Agency

5.3 Age distribution of the resident population: by sex and country

Thousands

| | | United Kingdom | | | | | | | | | | | | | | |
| | | Population enumerated in Census | | | Estimated mid-year resident population | | | | | | | | Projected mid-year resident population[1] | | | |
		1901	1931	1951	1981	1991[2]	2001[3]	2003	2004	2005	2006	2007	2008	2011	2016	2021	2026
Persons: All ages	KGUA	38 237	46 038	50 225	56 357	57 439	59 114	59 557	59 846	60 238	60 587	60 975	61 383	62 649	64 773	66 958	69 051
Under 1	KGUK	938	712	773	730	790	663	680	705	716	732	756	788	775	787	801	795
1 - 4	KABA	3 443	2 818	3 553	2 726	3 077	2 819	2 706	2 686	2 713	2 765	2 837	2 912	3 108	3 111	3 190	3 199
5 - 9	KGUN	4 106	3 897	3 689	3 677	3 657	3 735	3 650	3 608	3 554	3 490	3 424	3 395	3 508	3 892	3 906	3 999
10 - 14	KGUO	3 934	3 746	3 310	4 470	3 485	3 890	3 896	3 867	3 819	3 751	3 704	3 659	3 500	3 515	3 898	3 912
15 - 19	KGUP	3 826	3 989	3 175	4 735	3 719	3 678	3 856	3 921	3 957	3 996	4 016	3 988	3 832	3 571	3 585	3 968
20 - 29	KABB	6 982	7 865	7 154	8 113	9 138	7 499	7 400	7 496	7 691	7 880	8 107	8 302	8 758	8 920	8 471	8 223
30 - 44	KABC	7 493	9 717	11 125	10 956	12 125	13 405	13 506	13 460	13 419	13 302	13 141	12 978	12 646	12 600	13 408	14 085
45 - 59	KABD	4 639	7 979	9 558	9 540	9 500	11 168	11 412	11 507	11 616	11 744	11 728	11 792	12 288	13 080	12 951	12 323
60 - 64	KGUY	1 067	1 897	2 422	2 935	2 888	2 884	2 949	3 027	3 114	3 240	3 483	3 639	3 746	3 442	3 840	4 300
65 - 74	KBCP	1 278	2 461	3 689	5 195	5 067	4 947	5 001	5 028	5 046	5 029	5 058	5 155	5 501	6 344	6 551	6 703
75 - 84	KBCU	470	844	1 555	2 677	3 119	3 296	3 398	3 431	3 420	3 416	3 424	3 440	3 540	3 829	4 360	5 130
85 and over	KGVD	61	113	224	603	873	1 130	1 104	1 111	1 174	1 243	1 298	1 335	1 447	1 682	1 995	2 413
School ages (5-15)	KBWU	..	13 120	7 649	9 086	7 818	8 381	8 334	8 254	8 159	8 041	7 917	7 817	7 739	8 077	8 543	8 692
Under 18	KGUD	..	10 557	13 248	14 472	13 120	13 357	13 259	13 219	13 176	13 120	13 111	13 121	13 120	13 375	13 978	14 269
Pensionable ages[5]	KFIA	2 387	4 421	6 828	10 035	10 557	10 845	11 012	11 117	11 232	11 344	11 562	11 791	12 178	12 493	12 906	13 457
Males: All ages	KGWA	18 492	22 060	24 118	27 412	27 909	28 832	29 109	29 278	29 497	29 694	29 916	30 151	30 842	31 986	33 134	34 210
Under 1	KGWK	471	361	397	374	403	338	349	362	367	374	387	404	397	403	410	407
1 - 4	KBCV	1 719	1 423	1 818	1 400	1 572	1 445	1 384	1 376	1 389	1 416	1 453	1 492	1 591	1 592	1 632	1 637
5 - 9	KGWN	2 052	1 967	1 885	1 889	1 871	1 913	1 870	1 847	1 819	1 785	1 750	1 737	1 795	1 989	1 995	2 043
10 - 14	KGWO	1 972	1 892	1 681	2 295	1 784	1 993	1 998	1 985	1 962	1 924	1 898	1 873	1 791	1 802	1 995	2 002
15 - 19	KGWP	1 898	1 987	1 564	2 424	1 905	1 879	1 989	2 018	2 030	2 060	2 069	2 049	1 966	1 831	1 841	2 034
20 - 29	KBCW	3 293	3 818	3 509	4 103	4 578	3 744	3 709	3 773	3 878	3 978	4 116	4 235	4 479	4 555	4 318	4 193
30 - 44	KBCX	3 597	4 495	5 461	5 513	6 045	6 645	6 695	6 669	6 655	6 597	6 522	6 449	6 311	6 353	6 812	7 180
45 - 59	KBUU	2 215	3 753	4 493	4 711	4 732	5 534	5 646	5 691	5 745	5 804	5 786	5 815	6 048	6 431	6 373	6 099
60 - 64	KGWY	490	894	1 061	1 376	1 390	1 412	1 440	1 479	1 522	1 584	1 701	1 778	1 824	1 673	1 864	2 078
65 - 74	KBWL	565	1 099	1 560	2 264	2 272	2 308	2 347	2 365	2 380	2 379	2 398	2 447	2 623	3 032	3 127	3 201
75 - 84	KBWM	196	335	617	922	1 146	1 308	1 369	1 392	1 400	1 413	1 432	1 452	1 535	1 716	1 988	2 355
85 and over	KGXD	23	36	70	141	212	312	312	321	350	379	403	422	482	610	778	982
School ages (5-15)	KBWV	..	6 711	3 895	4 666	4 001	4 294	4 273	4 233	4 185	4 122	4 054	4 002	3 961	4 134	4 369	4 445
Under 18	KGWD	..	3 630	6 753	7 430	6 711	6 845	6 799	6 780	6 756	6 727	6 721	6 723	6 719	6 848	7 154	7 301
Pensionable ages[5]	KFIB	785	1 471	2 247	3 327	3 630	3 928	4 028	4 078	4 130	4 171	4 233	4 321	4 639	5 358	5 893	6 158
Females: All ages	KGYA	19 745	23 978	26 107	28 946	29 530	30 281	30 449	30 568	30 741	30 893	31 059	31 232	31 807	32 787	33 824	34 841
Under 1	KGYK	466	351	376	356	387	324	331	343	349	357	368	385	378	384	391	388
1 - 4	KBWN	1 724	1 397	1 735	1 327	1 505	1 375	1 322	1 310	1 324	1 349	1 383	1 420	1 517	1 519	1 558	1 562
5 - 9	KGYN	2 054	1 930	1 804	1 788	1 786	1 822	1 781	1 761	1 735	1 705	1 674	1 658	1 713	1 903	1 911	1 956
10 - 14	KGYO	1 962	1 854	1 629	2 175	1 701	1 897	1 897	1 882	1 857	1 827	1 806	1 785	1 709	1 714	1 903	1 911
15 - 19	KGYP	1 928	2 002	1 611	2 311	1 815	1 799	1 867	1 903	1 927	1 936	1 947	1 939	1 866	1 740	1 745	1 934
20 - 29	KBWO	3 690	4 047	3 644	4 009	4 560	3 755	3 691	3 723	3 813	3 902	3 990	4 067	4 278	4 366	4 153	4 031
30 - 44	KBWP	3 895	5 222	5 663	5 442	6 080	6 760	6 811	6 792	6 764	6 706	6 620	6 529	6 335	6 247	6 596	6 905
45 - 59	KBWR	2 424	4 226	5 065	4 829	4 769	5 634	5 766	5 816	5 871	5 940	5 942	5 978	6 240	6 649	6 579	6 223
60 - 64	KGYY	577	1 003	1 361	1 559	1 498	1 473	1 509	1 548	1 591	1 656	1 782	1 861	1 923	1 769	1 976	2 223
65 - 74	KBWS	713	1 361	2 127	2 931	2 795	2 640	2 654	2 662	2 666	2 650	2 660	2 708	2 878	3 312	3 424	3 503
75 - 84	KBWT	274	509	937	1 756	1 972	1 987	2 029	2 040	2 020	2 002	1 992	1 988	2 005	2 113	2 371	2 775
85 and over	KGZD	38	77	154	462	661	817	792	789	825	864	895	914	965	1 072	1 218	1 431
School ages (5-15)	KBWW	..	6 409	3 753	4 421	3 817	4 087	4 061	4 022	3 974	3 919	3 863	3 815	3 778	3 943	4 174	4 247
Under 18	KGYD	..	6 927	6 495	7 042	6 409	6 512	6 460	6 439	6 419	6 393	6 390	6 398	6 402	6 527	6 824	6 969
Pensionable ages[5]	KFIC	1 601	2 950	4 580	6 708	6 927	6 917	6 984	7 039	7 102	7 172	7 329	7 471	7 539	7 135	7 013	7 299

Population and vital statistics

5.3 Age distribution of the resident population: by sex and country
continued

Thousands

		England										Wales								
		Estimated mid-year resident population							Projected population[1]			Estimated mid-year resident population							Projected population[1]	
		1991[2]	2002[4]	2003[4]	2004[4]	2005[4]	2006	2008	2011	2026		1991[2]	2002[4]	2003[4]	2004[4]	2005[4]	2006	2008	2011	2026
Persons: All ages	KCCI	47 875	49 652	49 866	50 111	50 466	50 763	51 446	52 577	58 334	KERY	2 873	2 920	2 931	2 946	2 954	2 966	2 993	3 024	3 263
Under 1	KCCJ	660	559	576	597	606	620	668	657	682	KFAC	38	30	31	32	32	33	35	35	35
1 - 4	KCCK	2 560	2 313	2 275	2 262	2 289	2 335	2 462	2 632	2 735	KFBX	153	132	129	127	126	127	133	140	143
5 - 9	KCCL	3 019	3 084	3 055	3 020	2 976	2 922	2 849	2 959	3 402	KFCA	186	183	180	178	175	172	163	163	183
10 - 14	KCCM	2 865	3 264	3 250	3 225	3 185	3 130	3 055	2 926	3 313	KFCB	177	197	197	195	193	189	183	174	182
15 - 19	KCCN	3 067	3 115	3 203	3 261	3 297	3 334	3 331	3 199	3 354	KFCC	187	190	196	199	200	202	203	194	186
20 - 29	KCEG	7 651	6 244	6 232	6 315	6 483	6 633	6 974	7 385	7 009	KFCD	415	333	334	340	348	359	384	401	366
30 - 44	KCEH	10 147	11 347	11 369	11 337	11 318	11 230	10 975	10 711	12 003	KFCE	583	610	608	606	599	590	567	544	619
45 - 59	KCEQ	7 920	9 439	9 522	9 591	9 675	9 777	9 809	10 235	10 392	KFCF	486	578	582	586	589	592	589	602	565
60 - 64	KCEW	2 399	2 399	2 445	2 509	2 586	2 697	3 039	3 118	3 583	KFCG	154	156	161	166	171	177	197	203	216
65 - 74	KCGD	4 222	4 129	4 155	4 175	4 189	4 171	4 274	4 572	5 541	KFCH	284	265	268	270	271	273	282	303	357
75 - 84	KCJG	2 626	2 803	2 850	2 875	2 865	2 860	2 877	2 958	4 288	KFCI	164	185	187	188	186	186	185	188	283
85 and over	KCKJ	739	956	936	942	996	1 055	1 135	1 226	2 032	KFCK	45	59	59	60	63	67	72	79	128
School ages (5-15)	KCWX	6 439	6 984	6 960	6 895	6 817	6 719	6 540	6 495	7 375	KFCL	397	419	417	413	407	401	385	373	402
Under 18	KCWY	10 840	11 119	11 089	11 064	11 036	10 997	11 008	11 035	12 130	KFCM	662	659	654	651	646	641	634	623	653
Pensionable ages[5]	KEAA	8 827	9 111	9 188	9 273	9 370	9 462	9 839	10 164	11 207	KFEB	573	589	595	602	608	615	639	661	728
Males: All ages	KEAB	23 291	24 290	24 419	24 563	24 758	24 926	25 319	25 932	28 952	KFEI	1 391	1 414	1 423	1 432	1 439	1 445	1 461	1 480	1 610
Under 1	KEAC	336	286	296	306	310	317	342	337	349	KFEJ	20	16	16	16	17	17	18	18	18
1 - 4	KEAD	1 307	1 182	1 163	1 159	1 172	1 196	1 260	1 347	1 400	KFEK	78	68	66	65	65	65	68	72	73
5 - 9	KEAE	1 545	1 581	1 564	1 546	1 522	1 493	1 457	1 513	1 738	KFEL	95	94	92	91	90	88	84	84	94
10 - 14	KEAF	1 467	1 672	1 667	1 657	1 638	1 606	1 564	1 497	1 695	KFFA	91	101	101	100	99	97	94	89	93
15 - 19	KECA	1 572	1 607	1 654	1 679	1 691	1 720	1 712	1 642	1 720	KFFN	95	97	100	102	103	104	104	99	95
20 - 29	KECB	3 835	3 130	3 126	3 182	3 270	3 349	3 561	3 780	3 569	KFHA	207	164	166	170	176	181	195	205	188
30 - 44	KECC	5 064	5 644	5 658	5 639	5 637	5 591	5 475	5 363	6 126	KFHB	289	297	296	295	292	287	276	266	315
45 - 59	KECD	3 957	4 673	4 715	4 748	4 791	4 839	4 845	5 051	5 166	KFHW	242	285	287	288	290	291	288	293	275
60 - 64	KECE	1 159	1 176	1 197	1 228	1 267	1 320	1 485	1 518	1 738	KFQO	74	77	79	82	84	87	97	100	104
65 - 74	KECF	1 900	1 942	1 958	1 972	1 984	1 981	2 035	2 183	2 650	KFQV	128	125	127	128	129	130	135	146	171
75 - 84	KECG	970	1 128	1 154	1 172	1 179	1 190	1 222	1 290	1 970	KFUK	60	74	75	76	77	77	78	82	132
85 and over	KECH	181	269	267	274	298	324	361	411	832	KFUL	11	16	16	17	19	20	23	26	53
School ages (5-15)	KECI	3 295	3 580	3 569	3 536	3 497	3 444	3 348	3 323	3 771	KFUV	204	215	214	212	209	206	198	192	206
Under 18	KECJ	5 545	5 699	5 686	5 675	5 658	5 638	5 640	5 650	6 207	KFVE	339	338	336	335	332	329	326	320	334
Pensionable ages[5]	KECK	3 050	3 339	3 379	3 419	3 461	3 494	3 617	3 885	5 137	KFVF	198	215	218	221	224	227	236	254	336
Females: All ages	KEJV	24 584	25 362	25 448	25 548	25 708	25 837	26 127	26 645	29 382	KFVL	1 482	1 506	1 508	1 514	1 515	1 521	1 532	1 545	1 653
Under 1	KEJW	324	273	280	291	296	303	326	321	333	KFYW	19	15	15	15	16	16	17	17	17
1 - 4	KEJX	1 253	1 131	1 112	1 103	1 117	1 139	1 201	1 285	1 336	KFZJ	75	65	63	62	61	62	65	68	70
5 - 9	KEKP	1 474	1 503	1 490	1 474	1 454	1 428	1 392	1 445	1 664	KGCK	91	89	88	87	85	84	79	79	90
10 - 14	KEKQ	1 399	1 591	1 583	1 569	1 547	1 523	1 491	1 429	1 617	KGCM	86	96	95	95	94	92	89	84	89
15 - 19	KEKR	1 495	1 508	1 549	1 582	1 606	1 615	1 619	1 557	1 634	KGCN	91	93	95	97	97	98	99	95	91
20 - 29	KEKS	3 816	3 114	3 106	3 133	3 213	3 284	3 414	3 606	3 440	KGCO	208	168	167	170	172	178	189	196	177
30 - 44	KENR	5 083	5 703	5 711	5 699	5 682	5 638	5 499	5 348	5 877	KGCP	294	313	312	311	307	303	291	278	304
45 - 59	KEOQ	3 964	4 767	4 808	4 843	4 885	4 938	4 963	5 184	5 226	KGGZ	244	293	295	298	299	301	301	308	290
60 - 64	KEOZ	1 239	1 223	1 248	1 280	1 319	1 377	1 554	1 600	1 846	KGIY	80	80	82	84	87	90	100	104	112
65 - 74	KEQJ	2 323	2 187	2 197	2 203	2 206	2 190	2 239	2 388	2 891	KGKR	156	140	141	142	142	143	147	157	186
75 - 84	KEQK	1 656	1 676	1 696	1 703	1 686	1 670	1 655	1 668	2 318	KGTQ	104	111	112	112	110	108	107	106	151
85 and over	KEQL	558	687	669	667	697	731	774	815	1 200	KGTZ	34	43	42	42	44	47	50	52	76
School ages (5-15)	KEQM	3 143	3 404	3 392	3 359	3 320	3 275	3 192	3 172	3 603	KGVG	194	204	203	201	198	195	187	181	196
Under 18	KEQN	5 295	5 419	5 403	5 389	5 377	5 358	5 368	5 385	5 924	KGVH	323	321	318	317	314	311	309	303	319
Pensionable ages[5]	KEQO	5 777	5 772	5 809	5 854	5 908	5 968	6 222	6 279	6 070	KGVK	375	374	377	380	383	387	403	407	392

5.3 Age distribution of the resident population: by sex and country
continued

Thousands

		Scotland										Northern Ireland								
		Estimated mid-year resident population							Projected population[1]			Estimated mid-year resident population							Projected population[1]	
		2001[3]	2003	2004	2005	2006	2007	2008	2011	2026		2001[3]	2003	2004	2005	2006	2007	2008	2011	2026
Persons: All ages	KGVP	5 064	5 057	5 078	5 095	5 117	5 144	5 169	5 233	5 483	KIOY	1 689	1 703	1 710	1 724	1 742	1 759	1 775	1 815	1 971
Under 1	KHAQ	52	52	54	54	55	57	60	58	55	KIOZ	22	21	22	23	23	24	26	25	23
1 - 4	KHCT	224	212	210	211	213	218	223	235	226	KIPA	93	89	87	88	89	91	94	101	94
5 - 9	KHDN	306	294	290	285	279	273	269	273	291	KIPN	123	121	120	119	117	115	113	114	123
10 - 14	KHDQ	323	320	319	315	308	303	298	282	292	KIPP	132	129	128	126	125	124	123	119	126
15 - 19	KHDT	318	324	328	327	328	330	327	316	303	KIPQ	130	133	133	132	131	128	127	124	125
20 - 29	KHDU	630	614	617	630	649	671	689	709	624	KIPR	225	221	224	230	239	249	255	263	225
30 - 44	KHDV	1 163	1 150	1 140	1 124	1 107	1 086	1 065	1 027	1 068	KIPS	376	378	378	377	375	374	371	364	394
45 - 59	KHFK	979	1 008	1 025	1 042	1 058	1 060	1 068	1 106	1 010	KIPT	290	301	305	310	316	321	327	345	355
60 - 64	KHOZ	262	265	270	273	280	301	312	331	380	KIPU	74	78	81	84	87	90	91	94	121
65 - 74	KHTU	447	452	455	457	456	457	463	480	614	KIPV	123	126	127	128	130	132	136	146	192
75 - 84	KHUO	272	281	286	286	287	290	293	305	426	KIPW	77	81	82	83	83	84	85	89	132
85 and over	KHUQ	89	86	85	91	95	98	100	110	193	KIPX	23	24	24	25	26	27	28	32	60
School ages (5-15)	KHVV	694	679	672	664	653	642	631	614	642	KIPY	282	278	274	271	268	265	262	257	274
Under 18	KIMT	1 098	1 074	1 067	1 059	1 050	1 047	1 046	1 029	1 044	KIQL	451	443	437	435	432	432	433	433	442
Pensionable ages[5]	KIMU	944	958	968	975	983	1 001	1 017	1 045	1 161	KIQM	262	271	275	280	284	290	296	309	361
Males: All ages	KIMV	2 434	2 435	2 446	2 456	2 469	2 486	2 500	2 537	2 672	KIQN	824	833	836	844	853	862	871	892	975
Under 1	KIMW	26	26	28	28	28	29	30	30	28	KIQO	11	11	11	12	12	13	13	13	12
1 - 4	KIMX	115	108	107	107	109	112	115	120	116	KIQP	48	46	45	45	46	47	48	52	48
5 - 9	KIMY	156	151	149	146	143	140	138	139	148	KIQQ	63	62	62	61	60	59	58	58	63
10 - 14	KIMZ	166	164	163	161	157	155	152	145	149	KIQR	68	66	65	64	64	63	63	61	64
15 - 19	KINA	161	166	168	168	169	169	168	161	155	KIQS	66	68	68	68	67	66	65	64	65
20 - 29	KINB	311	306	309	317	328	339	350	361	318	KIQT	113	111	112	116	121	126	129	134	118
30 - 44	KINC	563	556	550	542	534	524	515	502	540	KIQU	185	186	185	185	184	183	183	180	199
45 - 59	KIND	483	496	503	511	517	517	520	534	486	KIQV	144	149	151	153	156	158	161	170	173
60 - 64	KINE	125	126	129	131	135	146	152	161	178	KIQW	35	38	39	41	42	44	44	45	58
65 - 74	KINR	200	204	207	208	209	210	213	224	288	KIRJ	56	57	58	59	60	61	63	69	92
75 - 84	KINS	103	108	111	112	113	116	118	126	193	KIRK	30	31	32	32	33	33	34	37	60
85 and over	KINT	23	23	23	25	27	29	30	35	74	KIRL	6	7	7	7	8	8	8	10	23
School ages (5-15)	KINU	356	348	344	340	334	328	322	314	328	KIRM	145	142	141	139	138	136	134	132	140
Under 18	KINV	562	550	546	543	538	536	535	527	533	KIRN	231	227	225	223	222	222	222	222	226
Pensionable ages[5]	KINW	327	336	341	345	349	354	361	385	520	KIRO	92	95	97	99	101	103	106	116	165
Females: All ages	KINX	2 630	2 623	2 632	2 639	2 648	2 659	2 668	2 695	2 811	KIRP	865	870	874	880	888	897	904	923	996
Under 1	KINY	26	25	26	26	27	28	29	28	27	KIRQ	10	10	11	11	11	12	12	12	11
1 - 4	KINZ	109	104	103	103	104	106	109	115	111	KIRR	45	43	42	43	43	44	46	49	46
5 - 9	KIOA	149	143	141	139	136	134	132	133	142	KIRS	60	59	58	58	57	56	55	56	60
10 - 14	KIOB	157	156	156	154	151	148	145	137	143	KIRT	65	63	62	62	61	60	60	58	61
15 - 19	KIOC	156	158	160	159	160	160	160	155	148	KIRU	64	65	65	64	64	62	62	60	61
20 - 29	KIOO	319	307	308	314	321	332	339	348	306	KISH	113	110	111	114	118	123	126	129	108
30 - 44	KIOP	600	595	590	583	573	562	550	526	529	KISI	191	193	192	192	191	190	188	184	195
45 - 59	KIOQ	496	512	521	531	541	542	548	572	525	KISJ	146	152	154	157	160	163	165	176	182
60 - 64	KIOR	137	139	141	142	145	155	160	171	202	KISK	38	40	42	43	45	46	47	48	63
65 - 74	KIOS	246	248	248	249	248	247	250	256	326	KISL	68	68	69	69	69	70	72	77	100
75 - 84	KIOT	169	173	175	174	174	174	175	179	234	KISM	47	49	50	50	51	51	51	52	72
85 and over	KIOU	66	63	62	65	68	70	71	76	119	KISN	17	17	17	18	18	19	20	22	36
School ages (5-15)	KIOV	339	331	328	324	319	314	308	299	314	KISO	138	135	134	132	130	129	127	125	134
Under 18	KIOW	536	524	520	516	512	511	510	502	510	KISP	220	215	213	212	210	210	211	211	216
Pensionable ages[5]	KIOX	617	622	627	630	634	646	656	660	641	KISQ	170	175	178	181	183	187	190	193	197

1 2008-based national population projections . See explanatory notes at beginning of chapter for further details.

2 Data for mid 1991 for UK, England and Wales and Scotland are revised in light of the results of the 2001 Census.

3 Data for mid-2001 were revised as a result of local authority population studies.

4 England & Wales population estimates for mid-2003 to mid-2005 were revised in August 2007 to take account of improved estimates of international migration.

5 The pensionable age population is that over state retirement age. The 2011 figures take account of planned changes in retirement age from 65 for men and 60 for women at present to 65 for both sexes. This change will be phased in between April 2010 and March 2020.

Sources: Office for National Statistics: 01329 444661; General Register Office for Scotland; General Register Office for Northern Ireland

Population and vital statistics

5.4 Marital condition (*de jure*): estimated population: by age and sex
England and Wales

Thousands

		Males									Females							
		2001	2002[1]	2003[1]	2004[1]	2005[1]	2006[1]	2007[1]	2008[1]		2001	2002[1]	2003[1]	2004[1]	2005[1]	2006[1]	2007[1]	2008[1]
All ages:																		
Single	KRPL	12 270	12 408	12 550	12 714	12 893	13 078	13 279	13 472	KUBS	10 917	11 035	11 167	11 310	11 494	11 673	11 853	12 045
Married	KRPM	11 090	11 043	10 995	10 941	10 923	10 881	10 851	10 849	KVCC	11 150	11 094	11 033	10 980	10 943	10 893	10 851	10 812
Widowed	KRPN	733	730	726	722	719	716	715	713	KVCD	2 745	2 709	2 669	2 628	2 588	2 548	2 511	2 477
Divorced	KRPO	1 482	1 524	1 571	1 617	1 662	1 696	1 724	1 746	KVCE	1 975	2 031	2 087	2 144	2 198	2 244	2 289	2 326
Age groups:																		
0 - 14: Single	KRPP	5 036	4 999	4 967	4 941	4 912	4 880	4 872	4 888	KVCF	4 796	4 763	4 726	4 696	4 670	4 648	4 644	4 660
15 - 19: Single	KRPQ	1 645	1 698	1 749	1 778	1 792	1 822	1 832	1 814	KVCG	1 560	1 587	1 631	1 667	1 693	1 706	1 718	1 711
Married	KRPR	5	5	4	3	2	2	2	2	KVCH	16	13	12	11	10	7	7	7
Widowed	KRPS	1	1	1	–	–	–	–	–	KVCI	1	1	1	–	–	–	–	–
Divorced	KRPT	1	1	1	–	–	–	–	–	KVCJ	1	1	–	–	–	–	–	–
20 - 24: Single	KRPU	1 501	1 530	1 568	1 632	1 693	1 741	1 813	1 855	KVCK	1 390	1 427	1 459	1 491	1 539	1 591	1 637	1 689
Married	KRPV	74	73	74	75	73	67	64	61	KVCL	178	170	166	163	157	146	136	126
Widowed	KRPW	1	1	1	1	1	1	1	1	KVCM	1	1	1	2	2	1	1	1
Divorced	KRPX	3	3	3	3	3	3	3	2	KVCN	8	8	8	8	8	7	6	6
25 - 34: Single	KRPY	2 227	2 229	2 230	2 245	2 292	2 343	2 383	2 452	KVCO	1 770	1 788	1 811	1 846	1 906	1 961	2 000	2 046
Married	KRPZ	1 391	1 311	1 237	1 173	1 125	1 068	1 027	1 006	KVCP	1 768	1 671	1 584	1 506	1 452	1 386	1 326	1 281
Widowed	KRQA	3	3	3	3	3	2	2	3	KVCQ	10	9	8	7	7	7	7	6
Divorced	KRQB	136	129	124	118	111	103	96	90	KVCR	231	217	206	193	182	169	158	147
35 - 44: Single	KRQC	963	1 027	1 080	1 126	1 173	1 219	1 259	1 289	KVEH	692	749	801	853	903	955	1 004	1 044
Married	KRQD	2 494	2 499	2 488	2 466	2 452	2 419	2 385	2 333	KVEI	2 649	2 653	2 638	2 623	2 597	2 564	2 525	2 463
Widowed	KRQE	12	12	12	11	11	11	10	10	KVEJ	36	35	33	32	31	30	29	27
Divorced	KRQF	411	420	427	433	436	431	422	407	KVEK	558	570	579	588	590	585	574	555
45 - 54: Single	KRQG	419	432	450	473	499	530	563	601	KVEL	256	271	288	310	334	363	397	436
Married	KUAR	2 511	2 432	2 383	2 356	2 348	2 355	2 365	2 390	KVEM	2 548	2 477	2 428	2 401	2 391	2 398	2 413	2 437
Widowed	KUBA	37	35	34	32	31	30	29	29	KVEN	111	105	99	96	92	90	87	85
Divorced	KUBB	448	451	461	474	489	504	518	532	KVEO	557	565	576	591	609	630	654	676
55 - 59: Single	KUBC	128	141	150	158	164	170	170	171	KVEP	74	81	86	91	96	102	104	108
Married	KUBD	1 156	1 238	1 278	1 288	1 285	1 271	1 201	1 148	KVEQ	1 125	1 212	1 256	1 271	1 271	1 260	1 197	1 145
Widowed	KUBE	34	36	36	37	37	36	34	32	KVER	112	115	114	111	109	106	98	91
Divorced	KUBF	174	194	208	219	228	234	231	230	KVES	210	235	255	269	281	290	288	287
60 - 64: Single	KUBG	97	97	100	104	108	114	124	134	KVET	62	61	62	63	65	69	75	80
Married	KUBH	980	977	991	1 013	1 039	1 077	1 150	1 196	KVEU	906	910	932	958	988	1 029	1 110	1 158
Widowed	KUBI	50	49	48	47	47	48	51	52	KVEV	178	172	167	163	160	159	162	162
Divorced	KUBJ	125	131	138	147	156	168	186	200	KVEW	151	158	169	180	193	210	234	254
65 - 74: Single	KUBK	155	154	153	152	151	149	150	152	KMGN	130	126	123	120	117	113	111	111
Married	KUBL	1 569	1 581	1 595	1 606	1 614	1 610	1 620	1 649	KMGO	1 322	1 336	1 356	1 373	1 389	1 393	1 410	1 449
Widowed	KUBM	188	183	178	174	170	165	162	160	KMGP	697	675	655	633	611	584	563	550
Divorced	KUBN	139	148	158	168	178	186	196	208	KMGQ	177	190	204	218	232	243	257	275
75 and over: Single	KUBO	99	101	103	106	109	111	114	116	KMGR	188	182	177	173	169	166	163	160
Married	KUBP	909	928	944	962	984	1 011	1 038	1 064	KMGS	639	651	661	673	689	709	728	746
Widowed	KUBQ	407	411	414	417	419	422	425	427	KMGT	1 598	1 597	1 590	1 583	1 576	1 571	1 564	1 553
Divorced	KUBR	44	48	51	56	61	66	71	77	KMGU	81	86	90	96	103	110	118	126

1 Mid-2002 to Mid-2008 are revised to include marriages abroad.

Source: Office for National Statistics: 01329 444661

5.5 Geographical distribution of the population

Thousands

		Population enumerated in Census			Mid-year population estimates[1]									
		1911	1931	1951	1971	1991	2001	2002	2003	2004	2005	2006	2007	2008
United Kingdom	KIUR	42 082	46 074	50 225	55 928	57 439	59 113	59 323	59 557	59 846	60 238	60 587	60 975	61 383
Great Britain	KISR	40 831	44 795	48 854	54 388	55 831	57 424	57 627	57 855	58 136	58 514	58 846	59 216	59 608
England	KKOJ	33 650	37 359	41 159	46 412	47 875	49 450	49 652	49 866	50 111	50 466	50 763	51 092	51 446
Standard Regions														
North	KKNA	2 729	2 938	3 009	3 152	3 073	3 028	3 029	3 033	3 037	3 045	3 052	3 061	3 072
Yorkshire and Humberside	KKNB	3 896	4 319	4 567	4 902	4 936	4 977	5 002	5 028	5 064	5 108	5 142	5 177	5 213
East Midlands	KKNC	2 467	2 732	3 118	3 652	4 011	4 190	4 222	4 254	4 291	4 328	4 364	4 400	4 433
East Anglia	KKND	1 191	1 231	1 381	1 688	2 068	2 181	2 195	2 220	2 242	2 268	2 287	2 311	2 335
South East	KKNE	11 613	13 349	14 877	17 125	17 511	18 566	18 646	18 706	18 783	18 936	19 069	19 216	19 393
South West	KKNF	2 818	2 984	3 479	4 112	4 688	4 943	4 973	5 005	5 042	5 087	5 124	5 178	5 209
West Midlands	KKNG	3 277	3 743	4 423	5 146	5 230	5 281	5 295	5 312	5 327	5 351	5 367	5 382	5 411
North West	KKNH	5 659	6 062	6 305	6 634	6 357	6 285	6 290	6 309	6 325	6 344	6 357	6 367	6 379
Government Office Regions														
North East	JZBU	..	..	..	2 679	2 587	2 540	2 541	2 541	2 542	2 550	2 556	2 564	2 575
North West (including Merseyside)	JZBV	..	..	..	7 108	6 843	6 773	6 778	6 800	6 820	6 840	6 853	6 864	6 876
Yorkshire and The Humber	JZBX	..	..	..	4 902	4 936	4 977	5 002	5 028	5 064	5 108	5 142	5 177	5 213
East Midlands	JZBY	..	..	..	3 652	4 011	4 190	4 222	4 254	4 291	4 328	4 364	4 400	4 433
West Midlands	JZBZ	..	..	..	5 146	5 230	5 281	5 295	5 312	5 327	5 351	5 367	5 382	5 411
South West	JZCA	..	..	..	4 112	4 688	4 943	4 973	5 005	5 042	5 087	5 124	5 178	5 209
East of England	JZCB	..	..	..	4 454	5 121	5 400	5 433	5 475	5 511	5 563	5 607	5 661	5 729
London	JZCC	..	..	..	7 529	6 829	7 322	7 362	7 364	7 389	7 456	7 512	7 557	7 620
South East	JZCD	..	..	..	6 830	7 629	8 023	8 047	8 087	8 125	8 185	8 238	8 309	8 380
Wales	KKNI	2 421	2 593	2 599	2 740	2 873	2 910	2 920	2 931	2 946	2 954	2 966	2 980	2 993
Scotland	KGJB	4 761	4 843	5 096	5 236	5 083	5 064	5 055	5 057	5 078	5 095	5 117	5 144	5 169
Northern Ireland[4]	KGJC	1 251	1 280	1 371	1 540	1 607	1 689	1 697	1 703	1 710	1 724	1 742	1 759	1 775
Greater London	KKNJ	7 161	8 110	8 197	7 529	6 829	7 322	7 362	7 364	7 389	7 456	7 512	7 557	7 620
Inner London[2]	KISS	4 998	4 893	3 679	3 060	2 599	2 859	2 886	2 891	2 907	2 944	2 973	3 000	3 030
Outer London[2]	KITF	2 162	3 217	4 518	4 470	4 230	4 463	4 475	4 473	4 482	4 512	4 539	4 557	4 590
Metropolitan areas of England and Wales	KITG	9 716	10 770	11 365	11 862	11 085	10 888	10 907	10 930	10 956	11 010	11 049	11 086	11 141
Tyne and Wear	KGJN	1 105	1 201	1 201	1 218	1 124	1 087	1 087	1 085	1 083	1 086	1 088	1 089	1 093
West Yorkshire	KGJP	1 852	1 939	1 985	2 090	2 062	2 083	2 094	2 103	2 119	2 142	2 161	2 181	2 201
South Yorkshire	KGJO	963	1 173	1 253	1 331	1 289	1 266	1 270	1 273	1 279	1 288	1 293	1 299	1 306
West Midlands	KGJQ	1 780	2 143	2 547	2 811	2 619	2 568	2 574	2 578	2 582	2 594	2 600	2 604	2 620
Greater Manchester	KGJR	2 638	2 727	2 716	2 750	2 554	2 516	2 518	2 528	2 534	2 543	2 554	2 562	2 573
Merseyside	KGJS	1 378	1 587	1 663	1 662	1 438	1 368	1 364	1 362	1 359	1 357	1 354	1 350	1 348
Principal Metropolitan Cities[2]	KITH	3 154	3 906	3 915	3 910	3 415	3 344	3 356	3 364	3 382	3 417	3 441	3 467	3 495
Newcastle	KGJT	267	286	292	312	275	266	267	267	267	270	270	272	274
Leeds	KGJX	446	483	505	749	707	716	720	723	729	741	750	761	771
Sheffield	KGJV	455	512	513	579	520	513	514	513	517	522	526	530	534
Birmingham	KGKF	526	1 003	1 113	1 107	1 005	985	989	992	996	1 003	1 007	1 010	1 017
Manchester	KGKJ	714	766	703	554	433	423	426	431	436	445	452	458	464
Liverpool	KGKM	746	856	789	610	476	442	441	439	437	437	436	435	435
Other metropolitan districts[2]	KITI	6 562	6 864	7 450	7 952	7 670	7 544	7 551	7 565	7 574	7 593	7 608	7 619	7 646
Non-metropolitan districts of England and Wales	KITJ	19 194	21 072	24 196	29 761	32 834	31 239	31 383	31 572	31 766	32 000	32 201	32 449	32 685
Non-metropolitan cities[2,3]	KITK	..	–	–	4 715	..	–	–	–	–	–	–	..	..
Incl. Kingston-upon-Hull	KKNZ	278	314	299	288	263	250	250	251	253	255	256	257	259
Leicester	KKOA	227	239	285	285	281	283	282	282	283	286	290	293	295
Nottingham	KKNX	260	269	308	302	279	269	272	275	279	283	286	289	292
Bristol	KKNV	357	397	443	433	392	390	391	394	397	406	410	416	421
Plymouth	KITL	207	215	225	249	251	241	242	242	244	246	248	251	253
Stoke-on-Trent	KKOD	235	277	275	265	249	240	239	239	239	239	240	239	240
Cardiff	KKOB	182	224	244	291	297	310	311	310	312	314	318	321	325
Newport	IFX3	84	89	106	132	135	138	139	139	139	140	140	140	141
Industrial districts[2,3]	KITM	..	–	–	6 486	..	–	–	–	–	–	–	..	..
New Towns[2,3]	KITN	..	–	–	1 895	..	–	–	–	–	–	–	..	..
Resort, port and retirement districts[2,3]	KITO	..	–	–	3 184	–	–	–	–	–	–	–	–	..
Urban and mixed urban/rural districts[2,3]	KITP	..	–	–	8 821	–	–	–	–	–	–	–	–	..
Remoter, mainly rural districts[2,3]	KITQ	..	–	–	4 661	–	–	–	–	–	–	–	–	..
City of Edinburgh local government district	KGKU	320	439	467	478	436	449	448	448	455	458	464	468	472
City of Glasgow local government district	KGKT	784	1 088	1 090	983	629	579	577	577	578	579	581	582	584
Belfast[4]	KGKV	387	438	444	–	293	277	274	272	269	268	267	268	268

1 Mid-2002 to mid-2005 population estimates for the UK and England &
Wales have been updated to include the latest revised estimates that take
into account improved estimates of international migration.

2 Details of the classification by broad area type are given in recent issues of
the ONS annual reference volume *Key Population and Vital Statistics; local
and health authority areas* (Series VS). The ten broad area types include all
local authorities in England and Wales.

3 The breakdown of non-metropolitan districts by area type has not been provided from mid-2001 onwards. This is because the effect of boundary
changes due to the major local government reorganisation on 1 April 1995
and 1 April 1996 (particularly in Wales) make the comparison of 2001 data
with data for earlier years invalid.

4 1931 figures shown for Northern Ireland and the City of Belfast relate to the
1937 Census.

*Sources: Office for National Statistics: 01329 813318;
General Register Office for Scotland;
Northern Ireland Statistics and Research Agency*

5.6 Population: by ethnic group and age, January - December 2007
United Kingdom

Percentages and thousands

	0 to 4	5 to 9	10 to 14	15 to 19	20 to 24	25 to 29	30 to 34	35 to 44	45 to 59	60 to 74	75 and over	All ages (=100%) (thousands)
White[1]												
British	6	5	6	6	6	6	6	15	20	16	8	49 139
Other	5	4	4	4	9	13	11	17	17	12	6	3 188
Mixed												
White and Black Caribbean	21	16	16	14	9	6	4	8	4	1	1	241
White and Black African	24	16	11	9	9	5	5	10	8	2	0	98
White and Asian	22	17	11	13	8	7	5	8	5	2	1	187
Other Mixed	15	12	10	11	9	10	8	13	7	3	1	151
Asian												
Indian	7	6	6	7	8	11	11	15	18	9	3	1 245
Pakistani	13	11	9	9	9	10	9	15	10	4	1	995
Bangladeshi	14	10	10	7	10	11	12	13	8	4	1	364
Other Asian	8	7	6	7	8	11	12	19	15	5	2	501
Black												
Black Caribbean	6	7	6	7	7	5	6	20	20	10	5	618
Black African	13	10	9	9	7	9	10	19	11	3	0	829
Black Other	15	9	11	8	9	8	5	18	10	6	1	83
Chinese	4	4	3	7	16	14	11	16	19	4	2	255
Other	8	6	6	7	10	12	11	19	14	5	2	903
All[2]	6	6	6	6	7	7	6	15	19	14	7	60 554

1 Respondents in Northern Ireland who state that their ethnicity is white are not asked this question.

2 Includes those who did not state their ethnic origin and those in Northern Ireland who stated that their ethnicity was white.

Source: Office for National Statistics, Annual Population Survey

5.7 Total international migration estimates: citizenship[1,2]
United Kingdom

Citizenship by country of next or last residence

Thousands[3]

					Commonwealth		
	All citizenships	British	Non-British	European Union[4]	Old	New[5]	Other foreign[6]
Inflow							
	C58E	C58H	C58K	C58N	C58Q	C58T	C58W
2000	479	99	379	63	56	91	169
2001	479	110	370	57	65	84	164
2002	513	97	416	59	63	92	201
2003	508	99	409	64	62	105	177
2004	586	88	498	128	73	141	155
2005	563	96	466	149	62	117	137
2006	591	81	510	167	62	139	142
2007	577	75	502	197	45	130	131
Outflow							
	C58F	C58I	C58L	C58O	C58R	C58U	C58X
2000	321	161	160	57	32	15	55
2001	306	158	149	49	32	19	49
2002	358	185	174	52	42	16	64
2003	361	191	171	50	42	17	62
2004	342	195	147	42	33	19	52
2005	359	185	174	54	37	23	59
2006	400	207	194	66	42	24	61
2007	340	171	169	68	31	26	43
Balance							
	C58G	C58J	C58M	C58P	C58S	C58V	C58Y
2000	158	−62	220	6	24	76	114
2001	173	−48	221	8	33	65	115
2002	154	−87	242	7	21	77	137
2003	147	−91	238	14	20	88	115
2004	244	−107	351	85	40	122	104
2005	204	−89	293	95	25	94	78
2006	191	−126	316	100	20	115	81
2007	237	−96	333	128	13	103	88

1 The1998-2005 were revised, following changes to the weightings used to gross up the IPS data, in November 2007. Therefore they may not agree with previously published estimates.

2 Based mainly on data from the IPS. Includes adjustments for (1) those whose intended length of stay changes so that their migrant status changes; (2) asylum seekers and their dependants not identified by the IPS; and (3) flows between the UK and the Republic of Ireland.

3 Estimates of international migration flows are shown rounded to the nearest thousand, rather than nearest hundred, as they are considered less reliable at the more detailed level.

4 European Union estimates are for the EU15 (Austria, Belgium, Denmark, Finland, France, Germany, Greece, Republic of Ireland, Italy, Luxembourg, Netherlands, Portugal, Spain and Sweden) from 1998- 2003, EU25 (EU15 and Czech Republic, Estonia, Hungary, Latvia, Lithuania, Malta, Poland,Cyprus, Slovakia and Slovenia). from 2004-2006, and for the EU27 (EU25 plus Bulgaria and Romania) from 2007. British citizens are excluded from all EU citizenship groupings and are shown separately.

5 For 2004 onwards, the New Commonwealth excludes Malta and Cyprus.

6 For 2004 onwards, Other foreign excludes the eight Central and Eastern European member states that joined the EU in May 2004. For 2007 other foreign excludes Bulgaria and Romania which joined the EU in January 2007.

Source: Office for National Statistics: 01329 444645

5.8 Estimates of migration into and out of the United Kingdom by usual occupation[1,2] and sex

Thousands

	Total			Professional and managerial			Manual and clerical			Not gainfully employed[3]		
	Persons	Males	Females	Persons	Males	Females	Persons	Males	Females	Persons	Males	Females
Inflow												
	KGOA	KGOB	KGOC	KGOD	KGOE	KGOF	KGOG	KGOH	KGOI	KGOJ	KGOK	KGOL
1991	255	117	138	76	47	28	53	22	31	127	48	79
1992	207	95	112	59	37	22	42	16	26	106	42	65
1993	204	97	108	63	40	23	41	20	21	100	37	63
1994	243	121	121	79	47	32	54	30	24	110	44	65
1995	235	125	111	83	55	28	44	19	25	108	51	57
1996	261	124	137	86	51	35	55	24	31	120	50	71
1997	273	137	136	89	57	33	42	23	19	141	57	84
1998	318	160	158	112	65	47	71	35	35	136	60	76
1999	354	181	173	131	77	54	75	40	35	148	63	84
2000	359	188	171	162	98	64	64	33	31	133	57	76
2001	372	187	185	138	77	62	77	39	38	157	72	85
2002	386	200	186	139	78	62	83	45	38	163	77	87
2003	427	211	215	146	76	71	92	46	46	189	90	99
2004	518	261	257	175	102	73	132	66	65	212	92	119
2005	496	273	223	168	97	71	145	90	55	184	86	98
2006	529	280	249	154	82	72	136	79	57	239	120	119
2007	527	286	241	168	99	69	136	79	57	223	108	115
Outflow												
	KGPA	KGPB	KGPC	KGPD	KGPE	KGPF	KGPG	KGPH	KGPI	KGPJ	KGPK	KGPL
1991	247	124	123	87	50	37	51	29	21	110	46	64
1992	235	117	118	85	51	33	49	24	25	101	41	60
1993	223	117	106	73	39	33	46	25	21	105	53	52
1994	197	96	102	57	33	24	50	24	26	90	38	52
1995	198	105	93	64	43	21	43	23	20	91	39	52
1996	223	109	114	87	54	32	48	23	24	89	31	58
1997	232	125	107	88	59	29	50	23	26	94	43	51
1998	206	103	103	82	48	34	42	22	21	82	33	48
1999	245	132	114	97	60	38	69	32	37	79	41	39
2000	278	154	124	128	80	48	59	36	23	90	37	53
2001	250	135	115	102	66	36	60	30	30	88	39	49
2002	305	161	144	123	79	45	80	40	40	102	42	59
2003	314	165	149	108	60	49	103	59	44	102	46	57
2004	310	152	158	114	65	49	73	40	33	123	47	76
2005	328	187	141	137	88	50	83	47	37	108	53	55
2006	369	208	162	125	77	48	119	73	46	126	58	68
2007	318	178	139	112	65	48	101	60	42	104	54	50
Balance												
	KGRA	KGRB	KGRC	KGRD	KGRE	KGRF	KGRG	KGRH	KGRI	KGRJ	KGRK	KGRL
1991	8	−7	16	−11	−3	−8	2	−8	10	17	3	14
1992	−28	−22	−6	−26	−14	−12	−7	−8	1	5	–	5
1993	−19	−20	2	−9	–	−10	−5	−5	–	−4	−15	11
1994	45	26	20	22	14	8	4	6	−2	20	6	13
1995	37	19	18	18	11	7	1	−4	6	17	12	5
1996	37	15	22	−1	−3	2	7	–	7	31	18	13
1997	40	12	29	1	−2	3	−7	−1	−7	47	14	33
1998	113	57	55	30	17	13	28	13	15	54	27	27
1999	109	49	60	34	18	16	6	8	−2	69	23	46
2000	82	35	47	34	18	16	5	−3	8	43	20	23
2001	122	52	70	36	11	25	17	9	8	70	33	36
2002	81	39	42	16	−1	17	3	5	−2	62	34	27
2003	113	47	67	38	16	22	−11	−13	2	86	44	42
2004	208	109	99	61	37	24	58	26	32	89	45	43
2005	168	86	82	31	9	21	61	43	18	76	34	43
2006	160	72	87	29	5	24	17	6	11	113	62	51
2007	209	108	101	55	34	21	34	19	15	119	54	65

1 See chapter text.
2 The 1991-2005 estimates were revised, following changes to the weightings used to gross up the IPS data, in November 2007. Therefore the above figures may not agree with estimates published before then.
3 Includes housewives, students, children and retired persons.

Source: Office for National Statistics: 01329 444645

Population and vital statistics

5.9 Estimates of migration into and out of the United Kingdom[1] by citizenship and country of last or next residence

Thousands

	All citizens	British citizens						European Union citizens[1] (excluding British)			
	All residences Total	Total	European Union[1]	Old Common-wealth	New Common-wealth[2]	United States of America	Other countries[3]	Total	European Union[1]	Other Europe[3]	Other countries[4]

Inflow

	KEZR	KGLA	KGLB	KGLC	KGLD	KGLE	KGLF	KGLG	KGLH	KGLI	KGLJ
1991	255	110	38	27	19	9	16	33	30	–	3
1992	207	94	46	19	10	8	11	25	23	–	2
1993	204	86	31	21	13	9	12	26	23	–	2
1994	243	111	44	20	14	15	18	31	28	1	3
1995	235	86	31	15	12	12	16	42	37	–	5
1996	261	97	32	19	16	13	18	55	50	1	4
1997	273	90	34	20	11	7	18	62	57	–	4
1998	318	104	28	29	15	16	17	70	64	–	5
1999	354	115	30	37	15	13	20	59	54	–	5
2000	359	99	28	29	14	8	20	59	52	–	6
2001	372	110	26	34	18	10	22	53	50	–	3
2002	386	97	30	23	10	9	25	55	50	2	3
2003	427	99	37	25	11	10	15	61	54	1	6
2004	518	84	21	23	15	9	16	106	99	–	6
2005	496	91	35	24	14	8	11	118	110	2	7
2006	529	77	32	16	7	4	18	136	129	1	7
2007	527	71	25	18	9	5	15	172	161	4	6

Outflow

	KEZS	KGMA	KGMB	KGMC	KGMD	KGME	KGMF	KGMG	KGMH	KGMI	KGMJ
1991	247	141	47	43	16	13	22	32	23	2.0	6
1992	235	137	45	35	13	17	27	17	14	–	3
1993	223	130	45	35	12	17	21	24	21	–	3
1994	197	111	35	29	11	15	21	23	19	–	4
1995	198	122	39	35	10	18	20	20	16	–	4
1996	223	143	53	38	16	16	20	24	18	–	6
1997	232	135	41	38	13	16	27	32	27	1.0	4
1998	206	114	37	36	8	15	19	26	21	1.0	4
1999	245	115	37	41	8	14	14	47	41	–	6
2000	278	141	41	48	9	19	24	46	39	1.0	6
2001	250	133	41	47	7	15	22	40	34	1.0	5
2002	305	164	68	44	10	18	24	42	38	–	4
2003	314	170	71	55	9	13	22	42	33	3.0	5
2004	310	184	68	62	12	16	27	34	30	1.0	3
2005	328	174	74	62	6	10	22	47	42	1.0	4
2006	369	196	71	69	10	16	30	59	52	–	7
2007	318	159	54	60	7	12	27	65	57	2.0	5

Balance

	KEZT	KGNA	KGNB	KGNC	KGND	KGNE	KGNF	KGNG	KGNH	KGNI	KGNJ
1991	8	–30	–8	–16	3	–3	–5	–	6	–2	–3
1992	–28	–43	1	–16	–3	–9	–16	8	10	–	–1
1993	–19	–44	–14	–14	1	–8	–9	2	3	–	–
1994	45	–	10	–10	2	–	–3	8	10	1	–2
1995	37	–36	–8	–21	2	–6	–4	22	22	–	1
1996	37	–46	–21	–20	–	–3	–3	31	32	1	–1
1997	40	–45	–7	–18	–2	–9	–9	30	30	–1	1
1998	113	–10	–10	–6	7	1	–2	44	43	–1	1
1999	109	–	–8	–4	7	–2	6	12	13	–	–1
2000	82	–42	–14	–19	6	–11	–3	13	14	–1	–
2001	122	–23	–15	–13	11	–5	–	13	16	–1	–2
2002	81	–66	–37	–21	–	–9	1	13	11	2	–1
2003	113	–70	–34	–29	2	–2	–7	19	21	–3	1
2004	208	–100	–47	–39	3	–7	–11	72	69	–1	3
2005	168	–83	–39	–38	8	–2	–12	72	67	1	3
2006	160	–119	–39	–53	–3	–12	–12	78	78	1	–
2007	209	–88	–29	–42	2	–7	–12	107	104	2	1

The 1991-2005 estimates were revised following changes to the weightings used to gross up the IPS data, in November 2007. Therefore the above figures may not agree with previous estimates published before then.

1 EU estimates are for the EU15 (Austria, Belgium, Denmark, Finland, France, Germany, Greece, the Irish Republic, Italy, Luxembourg, Netherlands, Portugal, Spain and Sweden) from 1991-2003, EU25 (EU15 and A8 groupings plus Malta and Cyprus) form 2004 -2006 and for the EU27 (EU25 plus Bulgaria and Romania) from 2007.

2 From 2004 onwards, the New Commonwealth excludes Malta and Cyprus.

3 From 2004 onwards these categories exclude the A8 Central and Eastern countries that joined the EU in 2004. From 2007 these categories exclude the A2 countries (Bulgaria and Romania) that joined the EU in 2007.

4 From 2004 onwards Other countries excludes Malta and cyprus.

5.9 Estimates of migration into and out of the United Kingdom[1] by citizenship and country of last or next residence

continued

Thousands

	Commonwealth[1] citizens								Other foreign citizens[3]				
	Total	Australia	Canada	New Zealand	South Africa	Indian[2] sub-continent	Other African Commonwealth	Other countries	Total	European Union[4]	Other Europe[5]	United States of America	Other countries
Inflow													
	KGLK	KGLL	KGLM	KGLN	KTDK	IBH3	KGLQ	IBH4	KGLU	KGLV	KGLW	KGLX	KGLY
1991	61	11	4	6	1	16	8	15	51	6	7	14	26
1992	47	9	2	6	–	12	6	13	41	2	7	9	23
1993	48	10	3	5	2	13	5	10	44	2	11	11	19
1994	48	9	2	6	1	10	8	13	52	5	14	11	22
1995	56	12	5	6	2	11	4	16	52	2	10	11	29
1996	59	14	3	7	4	15	6	11	49	–	7	15	27
1997	75	14	5	7	5	20	6	20	45	–	7	11	27
1998	88	24	5	13	11	13	10	12	56	4	7	18	27
1999	101	27	2	12	12	22	14	12	79	3	18	15	43
2000	113	22	6	11	13	30	13	18	89	2	11	13	63
2001	120	30	4	9	13	31	17	17	89	1	13	12	63
2002	121	20	4	9	20	33	22	11	113	2	11	16	84
2003	142	21	5	7	20	46	24	18	124	2	22	17	84
2004	204	24	5	8	30	77	38	21	125	1	12	14	98
2005	172	22	4	11	23	74	24	13	115	3	13	14	85
2006	193	29	6	8	16	95	17	21	122	9	13	15	86
2007	169	16	4	8	13	89	17	21	115	5	11	15	84
Outflow													
	KGMK	KGML	KGMM	KGMN	KTDL	IBH5	KGMQ	IBH7	KGMU	KGMV	KGMW	KGMX	KGMY
1991	33	7	4	5	–	4	3	10	41	2	3	17	20
1992	28	6	2	5	1	3	3	8	53	1	12	20	21
1993	32	8	2	4	1	4	4	8	38	2	3	17	16
1994	28	6	2	4	1	4	2	9	35	1	10	8	16
1995	27	6	1	4	2	2	2	10	30	–	5	9	16
1996	29	8	2	3	2	3	2	10	27	1	7	5	14
1997	36	7	1	5	5	4	2	13	29	3	5	9	13
1998	30	9	1	3	4	3	2	7	35	2	7	9	18
1999	38	11	2	6	4	2	1	11	45	–	9	14	21
2000	43	12	3	8	5	3	2	10	48	3	11	9	24
2001	44	15	3	6	5	4	2	9	33	1	9	7	16
2002	52	18	6	9	5	5	2	7	47	2	12	16	18
2003	53	19	2	8	9	5	2	8	48	2	12	8	26
2004	50	17	4	5	7	4	3	12	42	5	2	8	28
2005	59	15	4	8	9	13	2	7	49	1	7	14	28
2006	65	17	5	7	13	11	3	8	50	3	7	11	29
2007	56	17	2	5	9	15	3	6	37	4	5	6	23
Balance													
	KGNK	KGNL	KGNM	KGNN	KTDM	IBH6	KGNQ	IBH8	KGNU	KGNV	KGNW	KGNX	KGNY
1991	28	5	–	2	1	12	5	5	10	4	4	–3	6
1992	19	3	–	1	–1	9	3	4	–13	1	–5	–11	2
1993	16	2	1	1	1	8	2	2	7	–	9	–5	3
1994	20	3	1	2	–	5	6	3	17	4	4	3	7
1995	29	5	4	2	–	9	2	6	22	2	5	2	13
1996	30	7	1	4	2	12	4	1	22	–1	–	10	13
1997	39	7	4	2	1	16	4	7	16	–2	2	3	14
1998	59	15	3	10	7	10	8	6	21	2	1	9	9
1999	63	16	–	5	8	20	13	1	34	3	8	2	21
2000	70	10	4	2	9	26	10	8	41	–1	–	4	38
2001	76	15	1	3	8	27	14	8	56	–	3	6	47
2002	69	2	–1	–	15	29	21	4	66	–	–1	–	66
2003	89	2	3	–1	11	41	23	10	76	–1	10	9	57
2004	153	7	1	3	23	74	35	10	83	–4	10	7	71
2005	113	7	1	3	14	61	22	7	66	2	7	1	57
2006	128	13	2	1	3	84	14	12	72	5	6	4	57
2007	112	–	2	4	4	74	14	15	78	1	6	10	61

The 1991 - 2005 estimates were revised following changes to the weightings used to gross up the IPS data, in November 2007. Therefore the above data may not agree with previous estimates published before then.

1 From 2004 onwards, the Commonwealth excludes Malta and Cyprus.

2 Indian sub-contitent consists of Bangladesh, India, Sir Lanka and Pakistan.

3 From 2004 onwards Other foreign citizens excludes the A8 Central and Eastern European countries (Czech Republic, Estonia, Hungary, Latvia, Lithuania, Poland, Slovakia and Slovenia) that joined the EU in 2004. From 2007 Other foreign citizens exlcudes the A2 countries (Bulagria and Romania) that joined the EU in 2007.

4 European Union estimates are for the EU15 (Austria, Belgium, Denmark, Finland, France, Germany, Greece, the Irish Republic, Italy, Luxembourg, Netherlands, Portugal, Spain and Sweden) from 1991-2003, EU25 (EU15 and A8 groupings plus Malta and Cyprus) from 2004-2006 and for the EU27 (EU25 plus Bulgaria and Romania) from 2007.

5 From 2004 onwards Other Europe excludes the 8 Central and Eastern European countries that joined the EU in 2004. From 2007 these categories exclude the A2 countries that joined the EU in 2007.

Source: Office for National Statistics: 01329 444645

5.10 Grants of settlement by country of nationality[1,2]
United Kingdom

Number of persons

Geographical region and country of nationality		2006	2007[7]	2008[8]
Grand Total	KGFA	134 445	124 855	148 740
Europe[1]				
Accession States				
Bulgaria	KGFW	4 250	..	..
Romania	KGGB	1 610	..	..
Total Accession States	EL2O	5 860	..	..
Remainder of Europe				
Albania	I4UK	1 185	1 220	1 250
Croatia	LQMA	180	175	175
Russia	LQLX	1 375	1 310	1 255
Serbia & Montenegro[3]	LQMC	2 070	1 400	1 520
Turkey	KGFT	3 040	2 545	3 670
Ukraine	LQLY	850	865	845
Other former USSR	LQLZ	630	855	935
Other former Yugoslavia	LQMD	290	225	270
Other Europe	KOSO	110	65	35
Total Remainder of Europe	EL2P	9 715	8 660	9 955
Total Europe[1]	KOSP	15 580	8 660	9 955
Americas				
Argentina	KGGF	125	155	170
Barbados	KGGG	130	80	95
Brazil	KGGH	850	865	940
Canada	KGGI	1 125	1 015	1 190
Chile	KGGJ	105	80	65
Colombia	KGGK	855	590	655
Guyana	KGGM	165	140	350
Jamaica	KGGN	2 900	2 440	2 750
Mexico	KGGO	220	185	240
Peru	KGGP	200	145	150
Trinidad and Tobago	KGGQ	375	405	505
USA	KGGR	3 845	3 310	3 335
Venezuela	KGGT	145	150	140
Other Americas	KOSR	1 055	885	995
Total Americas	KGGU	12 085	10 435	11 585
Africa				
Algeria	KGGV	735	750	905
Angola	KOSS	965	1 590	640
Congo (Dem. Rep.)[4]	KOST	1 345	2 055	1 845
Egypt	KGGW	510	485	630
Ethiopia	KGGX	505	635	640
Ghana	KGGY	2 870	2 560	3 885
Kenya	KGHA	1 670	1 575	1 890
Libya	KGHB	260	185	305
Mauritius	KGHC	675	715	1 035
Morocco	KGHD	390	360	420
Nigeria	KGHE	4 440	3 965	5 145
Sierra Leone	KGHF	1 145	725	905
Somalia	KGHG	2 125	2 845	2 425
South Africa	KGHH	5 665	5 805	6 955
Sudan	KGHI	400	365	425
Tanzania	KGHJ	480	360	495
Tunisia	KGHK	195	175	220

Geographical region and country of nationality		2006	2007[7]	2008[8]
Africa (continued)				
Uganda	KGHL	670	530	665
Zambia	KGHM	460	495	1 000
Zimbabwe	KGHN	3 415	4 280	6 330
Other Africa	KOSU	3 320	3 595	3 630
Total Africa	KGHO	32 240	34 050	40 395
Asia				
Indian sub-continent				
Bangladesh	KGHP	2 850	3 330	4 325
India	KGHQ	11 190	14 865	22 880
Pakistan	KGHR	10 960	10 825	12 595
Total Indian sub-continent	KGHS	25 005	29 020	39 800
Middle East				
Iran	KGHT	1 035	1 755	1 470
Iraq	KGHU	7 285	7 020	4 170
Israel	KGHV	340	370	420
Jordan	KGHW	150	150	205
Kuwait	KGHX	20	20	15
Lebanon	KGHY	265	450	380
Saudi Arabia	KGHZ	60	30	40
Syria	KGIA	220	200	325
Yemen	KOSV	315	325	305
Other Middle East	KOSW	110	330	370
Total Middle East	KGIB	9 795	10 655	7 700
Remainder of Asia				
Afghanistan	I4UL	7 395	3 165	2 915
China[5]	KGIC	3 320	3 440	6 890
Hong Kong[6]	KOSX	1 060	785	1 040
Indonesia	KGID	250	225	230
Japan	KGIE	1 255	925	915
Malaysia	KGIF	1 785	1 635	2 190
Nepal	I4UM	6 940	4 155	2 920
Philippines	KGIG	6 315	8 485	11 290
Singapore	KGIH	205	240	240
South Korea	KOTE	620	565	740
Sri Lanka	KGII	3 080	2 440	3 315
Thailand	KGIJ	2 425	1 605	1 740
Other Asia	KOSZ	600	625	675
Total Remainder of Asia	KGIL	35 245	28 280	35 100
Total Asia	KGIM	70 045	67 955	82 605
Oceania				
Australia	KGIN	2 645	2 215	2 620
New Zealand	KGIO	1 405	1 280	1 335
Other Oceania	KOTA	165	125	80
Total Oceania	KGIP	4 215	3 615	4 040
British Overseas citizens	KGIQ	60	35	25
Nationality unknown	KGIS	220	100	135
Grand Total	KGFA	134 445	124 855	148 740

1 Members of the European Economic Area prior to 2005 and Swiss nationals are excluded throughout the period covered.
2 Data also excludes dependants of EEA and Swiss nationals in confirmed relationships granted permanent residence.
3 Serbia and Montenegro continue to be counted together due to the use of a single (Federal Republic of Yugoslavia) passport.
4 Formerly known as Zaire.
5 Includes Taiwan.
6 Hong Kong (Special Administrative Region of China) includes British overseas territories citizens and stateless persons from Hong Kong and British Nationals (overseas).
7 Excludes nationals of Bulgaria and Romania from 1 January 2007.
8 Provisional.

Source: Home Office: 020 8760 8291

5.11 Applications[1] received for asylum in the United Kingdom, excluding dependants, by country of nationality - 2000 to 2008

Number of principal applicants

		2000[2]	2001	2002	2003	2004	2005	2006	2007	2008[5]
Europe										
Albania	LQME	1 490	1 065	1 150	595	295	175	155	165	160
Macedonia	PTDW	65	755	310	60	15	5	–	25	–
Moldova	VQHP	235	425	820	380	170	115	45	30	20
Russia	ZAEQ	1 000	450	295	280	190	130	115	80	50
Serbia & Montenegro[3]	ZAFA	6 070	3 230	2 265	815	290	155	70	..	..
Turkey	KEAW	3 990	3 695	2 835	2 390	1 230	755	425	210	195
Ukraine	ZAER	770	445	365	300	120	55	50	40	30
E U Accession States[4]	GH5T	5 985	3 455	4 455	875	370	130	95	25	5
Other Former USSR	ZAES	1 050	485	615	520	315	265	220	155	180
Other Europe	ZAEU	2 230	210	130	70	35	30	35	95	95
Total Europe	KEAZ	22 880	14 215	13 235	6 295	3 025	1 810	1 210	825	740
Americas										
Colombia	KEBZ	505	365	420	220	120	70	60	30	25
Ecuador	KYDB	445	255	315	150	35	10	15	10	15
Jamaica	PTDX	310	525	1 310	965	455	325	215	240	240
Other Americas	PTDY	155	170	240	230	130	100	95	115	130
Total Americas	KECT	1 420	1 315	2 290	1 560	740	505	385	390	405
Africa										
Algeria	KOTB	1 635	1 140	1 060	550	490	255	225	260	345
Angola	KECU	800	1 015	1 420	850	400	145	95	95	80
Burundi	PTDZ	620	610	700	650	265	90	35	25	15
Cameroon	VQHU	355	380	615	505	360	290	260	160	115
Congo	PTEA	485	540	600	320	150	65	45	25	25
Dem. Rep. Congo	KEEH	1 030	1 370	2 215	1 540	1 475	1 080	570	370	335
Eritrea	PTEC	505	620	1 180	950	1 105	1 760	2 585	1 810	2 255
Ethiopia	KECW	415	610	700	640	540	385	200	90	130
Gambia	DMMA	50	65	130	95	100	90	110	100	125
Ghana	KECX	285	190	275	325	355	230	130	120	140
Ivory Coast	DMLZ	445	275	315	390	280	210	170	100	70
Kenya	KOTC	455	305	350	220	145	100	95	115	150
Liberia	C53K	55	115	450	740	405	175	50	40	20
Libya	GH5U	155	140	200	145	160	125	90	45	45
Nigeria	KECY	835	810	1 125	1 010	1 090	1 025	790	780	820
Rwanda	ZAEV	760	530	655	260	75	40	20	15	20
Sierra Leone	KOTD	1 330	1 940	1 155	380	230	135	125	85	55
Somalia	KECZ	5 020	6 420	6 540	5 090	2 585	1 760	1 845	1 615	1 345
Sudan	KEEE	415	390	655	930	1 305	885	670	330	265
Tanzania	DMMC	60	80	40	30	20	20	15	20	25
Uganda	KEEG	740	480	715	705	405	205	165	130	130
Zimbabwe	GRFS	1 010	2 140	7 655	3 295	2 065	1 075	1 650	1 800	3 165
Africa	PTEB	720	665	970	985	1 050	735	555	510	600
Total Africa	KEEJ	18 185	20 840	29 710	20 605	15 045	10 885	10 500	8 630	10 270
Middle East										
Iran	KEEK	5 610	3 420	2 630	2 875	3 455	3 150	2 375	2 210	2 270
Iraq	KEEL	7 475	6 680	14 570	4 015	1 695	1 415	945	1 825	1 850
Syria	GH5V	140	110	70	110	350	330	160	155	155
Other Middle East	ZAEX	930	810	725	735	730	595	660	755	620
Total Middle East	KEGY	14 150	11 020	17 990	7 740	6 225	5 490	4 140	4 940	4 895
Asia & Oceania										
Afghanistan	DMLY	5 555	8 920	7 205	2 280	1 395	1 580	2 400	2 500	3 505
Bangladesh	ZAEY	795	510	720	735	510	425	440	540	455
China (exc Taiwan)	KEGZ	4 000	2 390	3 675	3 450	2 365	1 730	1 945	2 100	1 400
India	KEIL	2 120	1 850	1 865	2 290	1 405	940	680	510	715
Pakistan	KEIM	3 165	2 860	2 405	1 915	1 710	1 145	965	1 030	1 230
Sri Lanka	KEIN	6 395	5 510	3 130	705	330	395	525	990	1 475
Vietnam	VQIB	180	400	840	1 125	755	380	90	165	230
Other Asia & Oceania	PTEE	1 025	1 040	910	650	375	320	275	740	535
Total Asia & Oceania	KEJO	23 230	23 480	20 755	13 150	8 850	6 915	7 315	8 570	9 550
Other and Nationality not known	KEJP	450	160	150	55	70	105	55	75	75
Grand Total	KEJQ	80 315	71 025	84 130	49 405	33 960	25 710	23 610	23 430	25 930

1 Figures rounded to the nearest 5 (- =0,1 or 2, .. = not available/ applicable).
2 May exclude some cases lodged at Local Enforcement Offices between January 1999 and March 2000.
3 Serbia (Inc Kosovo) and Montenegro counted separately under 'Other Europe' from 2007.
4 EU Accession States: Bulgaria, Cyprus, Czech Republic, Estonia, Hungary, Latvia, Lithuania, Malta, Poland, Romania, Slovakia and Slovenia. Figures between 1998 and 2000 exclude Malta but include Cyprus (Northerm part of).
5 Provisional figures.

Sources: Home Office: 020 7035 4848;
Migrationstatsenquiries@homeoffice.gsi.gov.uk

5.12 Marriages: by previous marital status, sex, age and country

Numbers

		1997	1998	1999	2000	2001	2002	2003	2004	2005	2006	2007
United Kingdom												
Marriages	KKAA	310 218	304 797	301 083	305 912	286 129	293 021	308 623	313 551	286 826	277 611	273 920
Persons marrying per 1,000 resident population	KKAB	10.6	10.4	10.3	10.4	9.7	9.9	10.4	10.5	9.5	9.2	9.0
Previous marital status												
Single men[1]	KKAC	216 237	214 005	211 820	213 777	202 690	206 196	217 534	221 477	201 791	197 137	196 800
Divorced men	KKAD	85 625	82 977	81 750	84 771	76 852	80 040	84 011	85 210	78 537	74 262	71 101
Widowers	KKAE	8 356	7 815	7 513	7 364	6 587	6 785	7 078	6 864	6 498	6 212	6 019
Single women[1]	KKAF	216 776	215 399	213 246	215 865	205 048	208 385	219 828	224 344	205 569	201 384	200 518
Divorced women	KKAG	85 648	82 016	80 816	83 166	74 807	78 182	82 181	82 559	75 120	70 256	67 676
Widows	KKAH	7 794	7 382	7 021	6 881	6 274	6 454	6 614	6 648	6 137	5 971	5 726
First marriage for both partners	KMGH	181 135	180 404	178 759	180 020	171 912	174 374	184 661	188 517	173 123	170 410	171 085
First marriage for one partner	KMGI	70 743	68 596	67 548	69 602	63 914	65 833	68 040	68 787	61 114	57 701	55 148
Remarriage for both partners	KMGJ	58 340	55 797	54 776	56 290	50 303	52 814	55 922	56 247	52 589	49 500	47 687
Males												
Under 21 years	KKAI	5 126	5 173	5 234	5 019	4 625	4 396	4 340	4 233	3 262	2 821	2 611
21-24	KKAJ	36 875	32 723	29 390	28 467	25 840	26 293	27 155	27 223	22 355	20 768	20 057
25-29	KKAK	97 345	94 696	90 412	85 870	78 687	74 858	75 580	74 873	67 943	66 234	66 979
30-34	KKAL	70 904	71 096	72 129	73 809	70 657	72 592	75 892	75 705	68 453	64 688	62 287
35-44	KKAM	58 292	59 838	62 114	68 019	65 242	69 747	75 695	79 510	74 343	72 416	71 196
45-54	KKAN	26 472	26 118	26 581	28 791	26 122	27 801	30 387	31 851	30 737	30 800	30 751
55 and over	KKAO	15 204	15 153	15 223	15 937	14 956	17 334	19 574	20 156	19 733	19 884	20 039
Females												
Under 21 years	KKAP	17 254	16 793	16 082	15 938	13 874	13 194	13 510	12 878	9 113	8 110	7 454
21-24	KKAQ	59 549	54 645	50 350	48 578	45 687	45 789	47 400	46 891	39 482	36 955	35 751
25-29	KKAR	97 932	97 181	94 703	92 753	85 647	82 892	84 066	84 714	79 579	78 478	79 731
30-34	KKAS	58 589	59 349	60 446	62 478	59 859	62 279	65 979	66 508	61 047	57 899	55 793
35-44	KKAT	47 267	47 721	50 136	54 697	52 209	56 997	61 682	65 007	60 969	59 248	57 930
45-54	KKAU	21 038	20 708	20 822	22 621	20 459	22 187	24 721	25 846	24 982	25 041	25 349
55 and over	KKAV	8 589	8 400	8 544	8 847	8 394	9 683	11 265	11 707	11 654	11 880	11 912
England and Wales												
Marriages	KKBA	272 536	267 303	263 515	267 961	249 227	255 596	270 109	273 069	247 805	239 454	235 367
Persons marrying per 1,000 resident population	KKBB	10.6	10.3	10.1	10.3	9.5	9.7	10.2	10.3	9.3	8.9	8.7
Previous marital status												
Single men[1]	KKBC	188 268	186 329	184 266	186 113	175 721	179 121	189 470	191 956	173 413	169 248	168 570
Divorced men	KKBD	76 839	74 029	72 617	75 378	67 678	70 506	74 397	75 129	68 672	64 777	61 533
Widowers	KKBE	7 429	6 945	6 632	6 470	5 828	5 969	6 242	5 984	5 720	5 429	5 264
Single women[1]	KKBF	188 457	187 391	185 328	187 717	177 506	180 675	191 170	194 348	176 505	172 803	171 531
Divorced women	KKBG	77 098	73 330	71 971	74 092	66 120	69 234	73 071	72 875	65 915	61 435	58 800
Widows	KKBH	6 981	6 582	6 216	6 152	5 601	5 687	5 868	5 846	5 385	5 216	5 036
First marriage for both partners	KMGK	156 907	156 539	155 027	156 140	148 642	151 014	160 283	163 007	148 405	145 995	146 216
First marriage for one partner	KMGL	62 911	60 642	59 540	61 550	55 943	57 768	60 074	60 290	53 108	50 061	47 669
Remarriage for both partners	KMGM	52 718	50 122	48 948	50 271	44 642	46 814	49 752	49 772	46 292	43 398	41 482
Males												
Under 21 years	KKBI	4 574	4 608	4 629	4 536	4 160	3 952	3 885	3 803	2 883	2 521	2 345
21-24	KKBJ	31 907	28 389	25 424	24 764	22 436	22 961	23 802	23 873	19 430	18 002	17 486
25-29	KKBK	84 644	82 135	78 364	74 367	67 934	64 619	65 568	64 701	58 066	56 607	57 116
30-34	KKBL	62 265	62 323	63 212	64 611	61 409	62 998	66 060	65 510	58 830	55 595	53 221
35-44	KKBM	51 654	52 812	54 528	59 834	56 872	61 196	66 364	69 364	64 394	62 539	61 023
45-54	KKBN	23 688	23 385	23 676	25 470	22 949	24 336	26 785	27 830	26 679	26 508	26 404
55 and over	KKBO	13 804	13 651	13 682	14 379	13 467	15 534	17 645	17 988	17 523	17 682	17 772
Females												
Under 21 years	KKBP	15 439	15 065	14 379	14 421	12 467	11 916	12 270	11 667	8 182	7 286	6 741
21-24	KKBQ	51 766	47 446	43 691	42 265	39 746	39 968	41 567	40 962	34 185	32 082	30 970
25-29	KKBR	85 352	84 399	82 250	80 312	73 799	71 540	72 790	73 072	68 062	67 090	67 844
30-34	KKBS	51 405	51 982	52 721	54 649	51 865	53 970	57 348	57 592	52 369	49 617	47 653
35-44	KKBT	41 838	42 245	44 199	48 245	45 672	49 984	54 103	56 660	52 758	51 032	49 595
45-54	KKBU	18 938	18 575	18 572	20 083	18 071	19 535	21 858	22 648	21 811	21 688	21 902
55 and over	KKBV	7 798	7 591	7 703	7 986	7 607	8 683	10 173	10 468	10 438	10 659	10 662

5.12 Marriages: by previous marital status, sex, age and country
continued

Numbers

		1997	1998	1999	2000	2001	2002	2003	2004	2005	2006	2007
Scotland												
Marriages	KKCA	29 611	29 668	29 940	30 367	29 621	29 826	30 757	32 154	30 881	29 898	29 866
Persons marrying per 1,000 resident population	KKCB	11.7	11.7	11.8	12.0	11.7	11.8	12.2	12.7	12.1	11.7	11.6
Previous marital status												
Single men[1]	KKCC	20 994	20 987	21 052	21 201	20 737	20 671	21 477	22 526	21 421	20 912	20 851
Divorced men	KKCD	7 845	7 934	8 142	8 427	8 238	8 475	8 574	8 930	8 796	8 330	8 361
Widowers	KKCE	772	747	746	739	646	680	706	698	664	656	654
Single women[1]	KKCF	21 303	21 241	21 308	21 608	21 223	21 180	21 974	22 884	21 991	21 460	21 482
Divorced women	KKCG	7 621	7 754	7 949	8 141	7 825	8 008	8 157	8 622	8 244	7 802	7 793
Widows	KKCH	687	673	683	618	573	638	626	648	646	636	591
First marriage for both partners	KEZV	17 751	17 677	17 680	17 864	17 468	17 426	18 232	19 039	18 221	17 922	18 005
First marriage for one partner	KEZW	6 795	6 874	7 000	7 081	7 024	6 999	6 987	7 332	6 970	6 528	6 323
Remarriage for both partners	KEZX	5 065	5 117	5 260	5 422	5 129	5 401	5 538	5 783	5 690	5 448	5 538
Males												
Under 21 years	KKCI	406	421	490	364	371	367	361	336	304	228	211
21-24	KKCJ	3 494	3 147	2 853	2 720	2 489	2 395	2 507	2 501	2 120	2 012	1 840
25-29	KKCK	9 495	9 439	9 031	8 536	7 949	7 468	7 219	7 365	6 981	6 795	6 902
30-34	KKCL	6 911	6 988	7 179	7 419	7 464	7 692	7 752	7 992	7 516	6 935	6 744
35-44	KKCM	5 649	5 945	6 470	7 018	7 215	7 328	8 007	8 553	8 390	8 234	8 357
45-54	KKCN	2 459	2 412	2 575	2 960	2 816	3 033	3 213	3 503	3 588	3 772	3 805
55 and over	KKCO	1 197	1 316	1 342	1 350	1 317	1 543	1 698	1 904	1 982	1 922	2 007
Females												
Under 21 years	KKCP	1 302	1 289	1 322	1 171	1 111	996	1 007	954	724	635	554
21-24	KKCQ	5 568	5 248	4 778	4 581	4 343	4 171	4 199	4 358	3 772	3 473	3 325
25-29	KKCR	9 574	9 764	9 539	9 495	8 994	8 520	8 321	8 528	8 339	8 230	8 500
30-34	KKCS	5 927	6 036	6 433	6 463	6 618	6 832	7 110	7 235	7 016	6 511	6 289
35-44	KKCT	4 722	4 726	5 150	5 633	5 712	6 115	6 583	7 163	7 083	7 003	7 063
45-54	KKCU	1 844	1 900	1 994	2 279	2 147	2 322	2 589	2 821	2 862	2 975	3 016
55 and over	KKCV	674	705	724	745	696	870	948	1 095	1 085	1 071	1 119
Northern Ireland												
Marriages	KKDA	8 071	7 826	7 628	7 584	7 281	7 599	7 757	8 328	8 140	8 259	8 687
Persons marrying per 1,000 resident population	KKDB	9.7	9.3	9.1	9.0	8.6	9.0	9.1	9.7	9.4	8.0	9.9
Previous marital status												
Single men[1]	KKDC	6 975	6 689	6 502	6 463	6 232	6 404	6 587	6 995	6 957	6 977	7 379
Divorced men	KKDD	941	1 014	991	966	936	1 059	1 040	1 151	1 069	1 155	1 207
Widowers	KKDE	155	123	135	155	113	136	130	182	114	127	101
Single women[1]	KKDF	7 016	6 767	6 610	6 540	6 319	6 530	6 684	7 112	7 073	7 121	7 505
Divorced women	KKDG	929	932	896	933	862	940	953	1 062	961	1 019	1 083
Widows	KKDH	126	127	122	111	100	129	120	154	106	119	99
First marriage for both partners	KEZY	6 477	6 188	6 052	6 016	5 802	5 934	6 146	6 471	6 497	6 493	6 864
First marriage for one partner	KEZZ	1 037	1 080	1 008	971	947	1 066	979	1 165	1 036	1 112	1 156
Remarriage for both partners	KFBI	557	558	568	597	532	599	632	692	607	654	667
Males												
Under 21 years	KKDI	146	144	115	119	94	77	94	94	75	72	55
21-24	KKDJ	1 474	1 187	1 113	983	915	937	846	849	805	754	731
25-29	KKDK	3 206	3 122	3 017	2 967	2 804	2 771	2 793	2 807	2 896	2 832	2 961
30-34	KKDL	1 728	1 785	1 738	1 779	1 784	1 902	2 080	2 203	2 107	2 158	2 322
35-44	KKDM	989	1 081	1 116	1 167	1 155	1 223	1 324	1 593	1 559	1 643	1 816
45-54	KKDN	325	321	330	361	357	432	389	518	470	520	542
55 and over	KKDO	203	186	199	208	172	257	231	264	228	280	260
Females												
Under 21 years	KKDP	513	439	381	346	296	282	233	257	207	189	159
21-24	KKDQ	2 215	1 951	1 881	1 732	1 598	1 650	1 634	1 571	1 525	1 400	1 456
25-29	KKDR	3 006	3 018	2 914	2 946	2 854	2 832	2 955	3 114	3 178	3 158	3 387
30-34	KKDS	1 257	1 331	1 292	1 366	1 376	1 477	1 521	1 681	1 662	1 771	1 851
35-44	KKDT	707	750	787	819	825	898	996	1 184	1 128	1 213	1 272
45-54	KKDU	256	233	256	259	241	330	274	377	309	378	431
55 and over	KKDV	117	104	117	116	91	130	144	144	131	150	131

1 Single men and single women are those who have never been married.

Sources: Office for National Statistics: 01329 444110;
General Register Office for Scotland;
Northern Ireland Statistics and Research Agency

5.13 Divorce: by duration of marriage, age of wife and country

Numbers

		1997	1998	1999	2000	2001	2002	2003	2004	2005	2006	2007
United Kingdom												
Decrees absolute granted[1,2,5]												
Number	ZBRL	161 087	160 057	158 746	154 628	156 814	160 726	166 737	167 138	155 052	148 141	144 220
Duration of marriage												
0-4 years	ZBRM	33 719	33 087	31 047	28 933	28 306	28 591	28 781	28 746	26 549	25 005	24 704
5-9 years	ZBRN	45 040	44 243	43 357	41 621	42 360	42 924	43 558	42 855	39 070	37 116	35 772
10-14 years	ZBRO	29 085	29 706	30 270	30 166	30 849	31 257	32 564	31 775	29 007	27 647	26 446
15-19 years	ZBRP	20 211	20 078	20 147	19 902	20 568	21 881	23 119	23 898	22 593	21 244	20 894
20 years and over	ZBRQ	33 020	32 935	33 916	34 000	34 729	36 073	38 713	39 844	37 824	37 116	36 397
Not stated	ZBRR	12	8	9	6	2	..	2	20	9	13	7
Age of wife at marriage												
16-19 years	ZBRS	28 987	27 627	25 440	23 505	22 558	22 107	22 367	20 948	18 507	16 707	15 430
20-24 years	ZBRT	72 971	71 416	69 509	66 215	66 282	66 264	67 070	65 671	58 829	55 085	52 438
25-29 years	ZBRU	33 452	34 195	35 585	36 009	37 418	39 116	41 464	42 544	40 143	38 812	38 315
30-34 years	ZBRV	12 968	13 719	14 420	14 892	15 842	17 374	18 658	19 729	19 366	19 419	19 294
35-39 years	ZBRW	6 155	6 571	6 848	6 993	7 417	8 070	8 742	9 456	9 275	9 261	9 663
40-44 years	ZBRX	3 375	3 360	3 557	3 568	3 778	4 104	4 404	4 550	4 703	4 677	4 784
45 years and over	ZBRY	3 094	3 086	3 291	3 352	3 429	3 572	3 917	4 093	4 042	3 985	4 081
Not stated	ZBRZ	85	83	96	94	90	119	115	147	187	195	215
Age of wife at divorce												
16-24 years	ZBSA	7 371	6 758	5 671	5 115	4 874	4 998	5 092	4 885	4 388	3 739	3 492
25-29 years	ZBSB	28 814	26 968	24 120	21 280	19 635	18 340	17 633	16 972	14 870	14 216	13 772
30-34 years	ZBSC	37 257	36 795	36 052	34 356	34 194	33 555	32 774	30 754	26 431	23 641	21 911
35-39 years	ZBSD	30 641	31 688	32 605	32 588	33 997	35 050	36 465	35 894	32 722	30 567	28 765
40-44 years	ZBSE	22 246	22 810	23 614	23 879	25 579	27 564	30 154	31 372	30 359	29 412	28 990
45 years and over	ZBSF	34 662	34 947	36 578	37 311	38 442	41 102	44 498	47 108	46 085	46 352	47 071
Not stated	ZBSG	96	91	106	99	93	117	121	153	197	214	219
Divorces in which there were[3,4]												
No children aged under 16	ZBSH	..	..	..	..	..	..	..	..	..	..	..
One or more children aged under 16	ZBSI	..	..	..	..	..	..	..	..	..	..	..
England and Wales												
Decrees absolute granted[1,2]												
Number	KKEA	146 689	145 214	144 556	141 135	143 818	147 735	153 490	153 399	141 750	132 562	128 534
Rate per 1,000 married couples	KKEB	13.0	12.9	12.9	12.7	12.9	13.4	14.0	14.1	13.0	12.2	12.0
Duration of marriage												
0-4 years	KKEC	31 767	31 136	29 307	27 474	26 987	27 344	27 511	27 389	25 345	23 427	23 039
5-9 years	KKED	41 260	40 239	39 676	38 206	39 079	39 730	40 599	39 779	36 161	33 864	32 522
10-14 years	KKEE	26 215	26 698	27 384	27 459	28 176	28 592	29 831	29 086	26 394	24 680	23 496
15-19 years	KKEF	18 027	17 934	18 072	17 870	18 603	19 784	20 923	21 591	20 363	18 792	18 266
20 years and over	KKEG	29 408	29 199	30 108	30 120	30 971	32 285	34 624	35 554	33 478	31 786	31 204
Not stated	KKEH	12	8	9	6	2	–	2	–	9	13	7
Age of wife at marriage												
16-19 years	KKEI	25 579	24 276	22 486	20 930	20 218	19 828	20 063	18 709	16 519	14 478	13 273
20-24 years	KKEJ	66 167	64 453	62 853	59 874	60 211	60 353	61 057	59 548	53 041	48 550	45 929
25-29 years	KKEK	31 022	31 533	32 867	33 282	34 759	36 387	38 722	39 575	37 103	35 177	34 675
30-34 years	KKEL	12 094	12 788	13 507	13 972	14 890	16 339	17 567	18 545	18 118	17 834	17 637
35-39 years	KKEM	5 767	6 153	6 432	6 562	6 956	7 623	8 249	8 912	8 755	8 560	8 880
40-44 years	KKEN	3 156	3 135	3 331	3 378	3 559	3 841	4 154	4 274	4 421	4 318	4 393
45 years and over	KKEO	2 904	2 876	3 080	3 137	3 225	3 364	3 678	3 836	3 773	3 645	3 747
Age of wife at divorce												
16-24 years	KKEP	6 871	6 298	5 318	4 839	4 643	4 808	4 867	4 658	4 216	3 525	3 273
25-29 years	KKEQ	26 435	24 586	22 173	19 650	18 231	17 227	16 539	15 867	13 905	13 182	12 653
30-34 years	KKER	33 967	33 446	32 837	31 420	31 489	30 982	30 345	28 368	24 381	21 409	19 865
35-39 years	KKES	27 715	28 605	29 663	29 820	31 164	32 282	33 519	33 013	29 864	27 479	25 665
40-44 years	KKET	20 125	20 521	21 325	21 469	23 190	25 017	27 610	28 558	27 570	26 128	25 548
45 years and over	KKEU	31 564	31 750	33 231	33 931	35 099	37 419	40 608	42 935	41 805	40 826	41 523
Not stated	KKEV	12	8	9	6	2	–	2	–	9	13	7
Divorces in which there were[3]												
No children aged under 16	ZBSJ	66 019	64 738	65 258	64 359	64 541	66 738	69 681	71 382	88 349	62 667	62 497
One or more children aged under 16	ZBSK	80 670	80 476	79 298	76 776	79 277	80 997	83 809	82 017	75 340	69 895	66 037

5.13 Divorce: by duration of marriage, age of wife and country

continued

Numbers

		1997	1998	1999	2000	2001	2002	2003	2004	2005	2006	2007
Scotland												
Decrees absolute granted[2]												
Number	KKFA	12 222	12 384	11 864	11 143	10 631	10 826	10 928	11 227	10 940	13 014	12 773
Rate per 1,000 married couples	KKFB	11.0	11.3	10.9	10.3	9.7	10.0	10.2	10.5	10.3	12.3	12.2
Duration of marriage												
0-4 years	KKFC	1 793	1 766	1 588	1 304	1 159	1 128	1 141	1 204	1 089	1 444	1 526
5-9 years	KKFD	3 224	3 360	3 095	2 890	2 721	2 689	2 450	2 536	2 403	2 759	2 659
10-14 years	KKFE	2 385	2 456	2 368	2 168	2 163	2 183	2 222	2 173	2 113	2 418	2 345
15-19 years	KKFF	1 804	1 729	1 686	1 622	1 562	1 705	1 773	1 810	1 789	2 033	2 100
20 years and over	KKFG	3 016	3 073	3 127	3 159	3 026	3 121	3 342	3 504	3 546	4 360	4 143
Not stated	ZBSL	–	–	–	–	·	–	–	–	–	–	–
Age of wife at marriage												
16-19 years	ZBSM	2 749	2 654	2 374	2 043	1 839	1 845	1 816	1 753	1 557	1 764	1 700
20-24 years	ZBSN	5 714	5 744	5 453	5 142	4 873	4 823	4 869	4 892	4 721	5 373	5 141
25-29 years	KKFJ	2 151	2 314	2 333	2 318	2 233	2 316	2 307	2 462	2 515	3 075	2 999
30-34 years	KKFK	791	824	829	805	827	895	958	1 025	1 065	1 387	1 404
35-39 years	KKFL	360	382	379	378	401	407	432	489	455	619	699
40-44 years	KKFM	199	198	208	170	193	235	219	252	252	325	336
45 years and over	KKFN	173	185	192	193	175	186	212	221	232	312	298
Not stated	KKFO	85	83	96	94	90	119	115	133	143	159	196
Age of wife at divorce												
16-24 years	KKFP	426	377	301	232	182	180	191	192	148	190	199
25-29 years	KKFQ	2 021	1 957	1 597	1 330	1 109	974	884	869	777	877	938
30-34 years	KKFR	2 736	2 767	2 642	2 381	2 215	2 174	1 943	1 918	1 641	1 837	1 655
35-39 years	KKFS	2 469	2 562	2 450	2 298	2 311	2 281	2 388	2 278	2 304	2 544	2 445
40-44 years	KKFT	1 819	1 951	1 929	1 999	1 963	2 110	2 106	2 341	2 330	2 751	2 801
45 years and over	KKFU	2 667	2 687	2 848	2 810	2 760	2 990	3 297	3 496	3 596	4 650	4 542
Not stated	KKFV	84	83	97	93	91	117	119	133	144	165	193
Divorces in which there were[3,4]												
No children aged under 16	KKFW	..	..	..	..	..	..	..	..	..	..	..
One or more children under 16	KKFX	..	..	..	..	..	..	..	..	..	..	..
Northern Ireland												
Decrees absolute granted:[2,5]												
Number	ZBSO	2 176	2 459	2 326	2 350	2 365	2 165	2 319	2 512	2 362	2 565	2 913
Duration of marriage												
0-4 years	ZBSP	159	185	152	155	160	119	129	153	115	134	139
5-9 years	ZBSQ	556	644	586	525	560	505	509	540	506	493	591
10-14 years	ZBSR	485	552	518	539	510	482	511	516	500	549	605
15-19 years	ZBSS	380	415	389	410	403	392	423	497	441	419	528
20 years and over	ZBST	596	663	681	721	732	667	747	786	800	970	1 050
Not stated[5]	EK8B	–	–	–	–	–	–	–	20	–	..	..
Age of wife at marriage												
16-19 years	ZBSU	659	697	580	532	501	434	488	486	431	465	457
20-24 years	ZBSV	1 090	1 219	1 203	1 199	1 198	1 088	1 144	1 231	1 067	1 162	1 368
25-29 years	ZBSW	279	348	385	409	426	413	435	507	525	560	641
30-34 years	ZBSX	83	107	84	115	125	140	133	159	163	198	253
35-39 years	ZBSY	28	36	37	53	60	40	61	55	65	82	84
40-44 years	ZBSZ	20	27	18	20	26	28	31	24	30	34	55
45 years and over	ZBTA	17	25	19	22	29	22	27	36	37	28	36
Not stated[6]	EK8C	–	–	–	–	–	–	–	14	44	36	19
Age of wife at divorce												
16-24 years	ZBTB	74	83	52	44	49	10	34	35	24	24	20
25-29 years	ZBTC	358	425	350	300	295	139	210	236	188	157	181
30-34 years	ZBTD	554	582	573	555	490	399	486	468	409	395	391
35-39 years	ZBTE	457	521	492	470	522	487	558	603	554	544	655
40-44 years	ZBTF	302	338	360	411	426	437	438	473	459	533	641
45 years and over	ZBTG	431	510	499	570	583	693	593	677	684	876	1 006
Not stated[6]	EK8D	–	–	–	–	–	–	–	20	44	36	19
Divorces in which there were[3]												
No children aged under 16	ZBTH	1 573	1 807	1 649	1 051	1 054	972	1 050	1 218	982	662	1 372
One or more children aged under 16	ZBTI	603	652	677	1 299	1 311	1 193	1 269	1 282	1 380	1 903	1 541
Not stated[6]	EK8E	–	–	–	–	–	–	–	12	–	..	..

1 Data for 2007 are provisional.
2 Includes decrees of nullities.
3 Children of the family as defined by the Matrimonial Causes Act 1973.
4 Data not available in Scotland.
5 Marital estimates are not available for Northern Ireland - no divorce rate for UK/Northern Ireland.
6 Due to some incomplete records.

Sources: Office for National Statistics: 01329 444410;
General Register Office for Scotland;
Northern Ireland Statistics and Research Agency

5.14 Divorce proceedings: by country

Numbers

		1997	1998	1999	2000	2001	2002	2003	2004	2005	2006	2007
United Kingdom												
Dissolution of marriage[1,4]												
Decree absolute/decree granted	ZBXR	160 733	159 688	158 418	154 273	156 562	160 528	166 536	166 937	154 879	147 989	144 071
On grounds of:												
Adultery	ZBXS	38 652	37 302	35 545	34 082	33 452	33 389	33 844	32 586	28 411	25 293	23 355
Behaviour	ZBXT	68 546	68 685	67 851	65 687	66 818	68 499	70 866	70 879	66 824	63 782	62 238
Desertion	ZBXU	956	828	748	722	718	727	697	675	612	516	461
Separation (2 years and consent)	ZBXV	39 398	39 627	40 368	39 763	40 699	42 579	44 012	44 819	41 433	36 917	33 612
Separation(5 years)	ZBXW	12 552	12 697	13 389	13 653	14 575	15 076	16 831	17 714	17 101	15 297	13 192
Combination of more than one ground and other	ZBXX	629	549	517	366	300	258	286	264	498	601	325
Separation[2]												
1 year and consent	IE9T	..	..	..	..	..	..	..	..	..	1 456	3 003
2 years	IE9U	..	..	..	..	..	..	..	..	..	4 127	4 127
Decree absolute/decree granted to:												
the wife	ZBXY	111 910	111 555	109 824	106 957	107 345	108 104	114 664	113 970	105 008	100 003	96 749
the husband	ZBXZ	48 393	47 764	48 236	47 069	49 015	52 251	51 691	52 793	49 725	47 847	47 205
both	ZBYA	430	369	358	247	202	173	181	174	146	139	119
Nullity of marriage												
Decree absolute/decree granted	ZBYB	354	369	328	355	252	198	201	201	173	152	149
England and Wales												
Dissolution of marriage[4]												
Petitions filed[3]	KKGA	163 769	165 870	162 137	157 809	172 341	177 224	173 265	167 340	151 824	148 564	137 465
Decree nisi granted[3]	KKGM	148 310	144 231	143 446	143 729	163 146	170 980	168 037	166 334	150 917	145 242	143 153
Decree absolute granted	KKGN	146 339	144 851	144 233	140 783	143 568	147 538	153 294	153 199	141 583	132 418	128 393
On grounds of:												
Adultery	KKGB	37 592	36 319	34 584	33 310	32 839	32 829	33 331	32 035	27 992	24 936	23 125
Behaviour	KKGC	65 047	65 257	64 816	63 182	64 768	66 480	68 944	68 859	65 169	62 234	61 004
Desertion	KKGD	912	790	713	680	689	681	665	654	593	499	451
Separation (2 years and consent)	KKGE	32 638	32 394	33 482	32 820	33 703	35 476	36 931	37 543	34 388	31 794	31 268
Separation(5 years)	KKGF	9 592	9 616	10 193	10 498	11 355	11 896	13 239	13 933	13 196	12 628	12 220
Combination of more than one ground and other	ZBYC	558	475	445	293	214	176	184	175	245	327	325
Decree absolute granted to:												
the wife	ZBYD	102 173	101 583	100 469	98 227	98 992	102 676	106 208	105 381	96 855	90 587	87 362
the husband	ZBYE	43 739	42 902	43 413	42 311	44 378	44 694	46 915	47 651	44 583	41 702	40 928
both	ZBYF	427	366	351	245	198	168	171	167	145	129	103
Nullity of marriage												
Petitions filed[3]	KKGO	485	505	549	452	492	443	463	495	440	406	352
Decree nisi granted[3]	KKGR	248	281	495	274	160	216	204	308	260	240	190
Decree absolute granted	KKGS	350	363	323	352	250	197	196	200	167	144	141
Judicial separation												
Petitions filed[4]	KKGT	1 078	916	882	650	1 078	1 001	826	745	697	613	502
Decrees granted[4]	KKGW	589	519	696	540	925	560	467	419	387	353	329

5.14 Divorce proceedings: by country
continued

Numbers

		1997	1998	1999	2000	2001	2002	2003	2004	2005	2006	2007
Scotland												
Dissolution of marriage[1]												
Decree granted	ZBYG	12 220	12 383	11 860	11 142	10 631	10 825	10 927	11 226	10 939	13 013	12 771
On grounds of:												
Adultery	ZBYH	909	832	770	610	473	428	401	413	327	263	131
Behaviour	ZBYI	3 081	3 005	2 611	2 099	1 639	1 656	1 537	1 546	1 344	1 215	875
Desertion	ZBYJ	33	28	18	34	24	42	23	15	17	15	7
Separation (2 years and consent)	ZBYK	5 773	6 121	5 908	5 878	5 943	6 101	6 016	6 122	5 989	4 014	971
Separation(5 years)	ZBYL	2 424	2 397	2 553	2 521	2 552	2 598	2 950	3 130	3 262	1 923	182
Separation[2]												
1 year and consent	IE9T	..	..	..	..	..	..	..	..	..	1 456	3 003
2 years	IE9U	..	..	..	..	..	..	..	..	..	4 127	4 127
Decree granted to[2]												
the wife	ZBYM	8 266	8 328	7 770	7 190	6 775	6 800	6 926	6 938	6 653	7 750	7 528
the husband	ZBYN	3 954	4 055	4 090	3 952	3 856	4 025	4 001	4 288	4 286	5 263	5 245
Nullity of marriage												
Decree granted	ZBYO	2	1	4	1	–	1	1	1	1	1	2
Northern Ireland												
Dissolution of marriage												
Petitions filed	ZBYP	2 808	2 760	2 414	3 005	2 869	2 929	3 192	2 808	3 299	3 098	3 010
Decree nisi granted	ZBYQ	2 532	2 904	2 393	2 456	2 615	2 454	2 616	2 697	2 594	2 607	2 985
Decree absolute granted	ZBYR	2 174	2 454	2 325	2 348	2 363	2 165	2 315	2 512	2 357	2 558	2 907
On grounds of:												
Adultery	ZBYS	151	151	191	162	140	132	112	138	92	94	99
Behaviour	ZBYT	418	423	424	406	411	363	385	474	311	333	359
Desertion	ZBYU	11	10	17	8	5	3	9	6	2	2	3
Separation (2 years and consent)	ZBYV	991	1 112	978	1 065	1 053	1 002	1 065	1 154	1 056	1 109	1 373
Separation(5 years)	ZBYW	536	684	643	634	668	582	642	651	643	746	790
Combination of more than one ground and other	ZBYX	67	74	72	73	86	83	102	89	253	274	283
Decree absolute granted to:												
the wife	ZBYY	1 473	1 644	1 585	1 540	1 578	1 405	1 530	1 651	1 500	1 666	1 859
the husband	ZBYZ	698	807	733	806	781	755	775	854	856	882	1 032
both	ZBZA	3	3	7	2	4	5	10	7	1	10	16
Nullity of marriage												
Petitions filed	ZBZB	7	5	1	2	1	5	4	8	9	–	5
Decree nisi granted	ZBZC	2	6	2	5	2	2	5	3	3	3	4
Decree absolute granted	ZBZD	2	5	1	2	2	–	4	–	5	7	6
Judicial separation												
Petitions filed	ZBZE	70	64	50	54	40	27	35	18	3	7	2
Decrees granted	ZBZF	34	40	31	23	25	15	22	12	4	8	12

1 The terms petition filed, decree nisi granted, decree absolute and judicial separation are not used in Scotland. Decree absolute granted to 'both' and 'Combination of more than one ground and other' are not procedures used in Scotland.

2 New categories introduced with effect from 4 May 2006 by the Family Law (Scotland) Act 2006. These replace the two 'non-cohabitation' categories (non-cohabiation is a category that is used in Scotland only) of 2 years with consent and 5 years.

3 Data supplied by Ministry of Justice (12 February 2008) see Judicial and Court Statistics.

4 2007 data are provisional.

Sources: Office for National Statistics: 01329 444410;
General Register Office for Scotland;
Northern Ireland Statistics and Research Agency;
Ministry of Justice (England & Wales);
Scottish Courts Administration;
Northern Ireland Courts Administration

5.15 Births:[1] by country and sex

Thousands

| | Live births | | | | Rates | | | | |
	Total	Male	Female	Sex ratio[2]	Crude birth rate[3]	General fertility rate[4]	TFR[5]	Still-births[6]	Still-birth rate[6]
United Kingdom[7]									
1900 - 02	1 095	558	537	1 037	28.6	115.1	..	..	..
1910 - 12	1 037	528	508	1 039	24.6	99.4	..	..	..
1920 - 22	1 018	522	496	1 052	23.1	93.0	..	..	..
1930 - 32	750	383	367	1 046	16.3	66.5	..	..	..
1940 - 42	723	372	351	1 062	15.0	..	1.89	..	..
1950 - 52	803	413	390	1 061	16.0	73.7	2.21	..	..
1960 - 62	946	487	459	1 063	17.9	90.3	2.80	18.6	19.2
1970 - 72	880	453	427	1 064	15.8	82.5	2.36	11.3	12.7
1980 - 82	735	377	358	1 053	13.0	62.5	1.83	5.0	6.8
1990 - 92	790	405	385	1 051	13.8	63.7	1.81	3.6	4.6
2000 - 02	672	345	328	1 052	11.4	54.7	1.64	3.6	5.4
	BBCA	KBCZ	KBCY	KMFW	KBCT	KBCS	KBCR	KBCQ	KMFX
1998	716.9	367	350	1 052	12.3	58.8	1.71	3.9	5.4
1999	700.0	359	341	1 056	11.9	57.3	1.68	3.7	5.3
2000	679.0	348	331	1 051	11.5	55.4	1.64	3.6	5.3
2001	669.1	343	326	1 050	11.3	54.3	1.63	3.6	5.3
2002	668.8	343	326	1 054	11.3	54.2	1.64	3.8	5.6
2003	695.6	357	339	1 052	11.7	56.2	1.71	4.0	5.7
2004	716.0	368	348	1 055	12.0	57.7	1.77	4.0	5.7
2005	722.5	370	353	1 050	12.0	57.8	1.78	4.0	5.3
2006	748.6	383	366	1 047	12.4	59.7	1.84	4.0	5.3
2007	772.2	397	376	1 056	12.7	61.5	1.90	4.0	5.2
2008	794.4	407	388	1 049	12.9	63.4	1.96	4.0	5.1
England and Wales									
1900 - 02	932	475	458	1 037	28.6	114.7	..	..	..
1910 - 12	884	450	433	1 040	24.5	98.6	..	..	..
1920 - 22	862	442	420	1 051	22.8	91.1	..	..	..
1930 - 32	632	323	309	1 047	15.8	64.4	..	27.0	..
1940 - 42	607	312	295	1 057	15.6	61.3	1.81	22.0	..
1950 - 52	683	351	332	1 058	15.6	72.1	2.16	16.0	..
1960 - 62	812	418	394	1 061	17.6	88.9	2.77	15.6	18.9
1970 - 72	764	394	371	1 061	15.6	81.4	2.31	9.7	12.5
1980 - 82	639	328	311	1 053	12.9	61.8	1.81	4.3	6.7
1990 - 92	698	358	340	1 051	13.8	63.8	1.82	3.2	4.5
2000 - 02	598	307	292	1 052	11.4	55.2	1.65	3.2	5.4
	BBCB	KMFY	KMFZ	KMGA	KMGB	KMGC	KMGD	KMGE	KMGF
1998	635.9	326	310	1 051	12.3	59.2	1.72	3.4	5.3
1999	621.9	319	303	1 055	12.0	57.8	1.70	3.3	5.3
2000	604.4	310	295	1 050	11.6	55.9	1.65	3.2	5.3
2001	594.6	305	290	1 050	11.4	54.7	1.63	3.2	5.3
2002	596.1	306	290	1 055	11.3	54.7	1.65	3.4	5.6
2003	621.5	318	303	1 051	11.8	56.8	1.73	3.6	5.8
2004	639.7	328	311	1 054	12.1	58.2	1.78	3.7	5.7
2005	645.8	331	315	1 049	12.1	58.4	1.80	3.5	5.4
2006	669.6	342	327	1 047	12.5	60.2	1.86	3.6	5.4
2007	690.0	354	336	1 057	12.8	62.0	1.92	3.6	5.2
2008	708.7	363	346	1 050	13.0	63.8	1.97	3.6	5.1

5.15 Births:[1] by country and sex
continued

Thousands

	Live births				Rates				
	Total	Male	Female	Sex ratio[2]	Crude birth rate[3]	General fertility rate[4]	TFR[5]	Still-births[6]	Still-birth rate[6]
Scotland									
1900 - 02	132	67	65	1 046	29.5	120.6	..	..	..
1910 - 12	123	63	60	1 044	25.9	107.4	..	..	..
1920 - 22	125	64	61	1 046	25.6	105.9	..	..	..
1930 - 32	93	47	45	1 040	19.1	78.8	..	..	..
1940 - 42	89	46	43	1 051	18.5	73.7	..	4.0	..
1950 - 52	91	47	44	1 060	17.9	81.4	2.41	2.0	..
1960 - 62	102	53	50	1 060	19.7	97.8	2.98	2.2	20.8
1970 - 72	84	43	41	1 057	16.1	83.3	2.46	1.1	13.5
1980 - 82	68	35	33	1 051	13.1	62.2	1.80	0.4	6.3
1990 - 92	66	34	32	1 052	13.0	59.2	1.68	0.4	5.7
2000 - 02	52	27	26	1 046	10.3	48.6	1.48	0.3	5.6
	BBCD	KMEU	KMEV	KMEW	KMEX	KMEY	KMEZ	KMFM	KMFN
1998	57.3	29	28	1 060	11.3	52.7	1.55	0.4	6.1
1999	55.1	28	27	1 050	10.9	50.9	1.51	0.3	5.2
2000	53.1	27	26	1 051	10.5	49.2	1.48	0.3	5.6
2001	52.5	27	26	1 041	10.4	48.8	1.49	0.3	5.7
2002	51.3	26	25	1 047	10.1	48.1	1.48	0.3	5.4
2003	52.4	27	26	1 054	10.4	49.4	1.54	0.3	5.6
2004	54.0	28	26	1 060	10.6	51.0	1.60	0.3	5.8
2005	54.4	28	26	1 068	10.7	51.5	1.62	0.3	5.3
2006	55.7	28	27	1 046	10.9	52.8	1.67	0.3	5.3
2007	57.8	30	28	1 057	11.2	54.8	1.73	0.3	5.6
2008	60.0	31	29	1 037	11.6	57.2	1.80	0.3	5.4
Northern Ireland[7]									
1900 - 02	..	..	..	..	..	..	..	..	..
1910 - 12	..	..	..	..	..	..	..	..	..
1920 - 22	31	16	15	1 048	24.2	105.9	..	..	..
1930 - 32	26	13	12	1 047	20.5	78.8	..	..	..
1940 - 42	27	14	13	1 078	20.8	73.7	..	..	..
1950 - 52	29	15	14	1 066	20.9	81.4	..	..	..
1960 - 62	31	16	15	1 068	22.5	111.5	3.47	0.7	22.0
1970 - 72	31	16	15	1 074	20.4	105.7	3.13	0.5	14.3
1980 - 82	28	14	13	1 048	18.0	87.5	2.59	0.2	8.4
1990 - 92	26	13	13	1 051	16.1	74.8	2.15	0.1	4.6
2000 - 02	22	11	11	1 054	12.8	58.8	1.78	0.1	5.0
	BBCE	KMFO	KMFP	KMFQ	KMFR	KMFS	KMFT	KMFU	KMFV
1998	23.7	12	12	1 039	14.1	65.0	1.90	0.1	5.1
1999	23.0	12	11	1 084	13.7	62.9	1.86	0.1	5.7
2000	21.5	11	10	1 070	12.8	58.7	1.75	0.1	4.3
2001	22.0	11	11	1 058	13.0	59.7	1.80	0.1	5.1
2002	21.4	11	11	1 035	12.6	58.1	1.77	0.1	5.7
2003	21.6	11	10	1 081	12.7	59.0	1.81	0.1	5.0
2004	22.3	11	11	1 059	13.0	60.6	1.87	0.1	5.0
2005	22.3	11	11	1 032	12.9	60.4	1.87	0.1	4.0
2006	23.3	12	11	1 066	14.0	62.5	1.94	0.1	3.8
2007	24.5	13	12	1 049	13.9	65.1	2.02	0.1	4.2
2008	25.6	13	12	1 063	14.4	68.2	2.11	0.1	4.5

1 See chapter text.
2 Males per 1,000 females (calculated using whole numbers).
3 Rate per 1,000 population (calculated using whole numbers).
4 Rate per 1,000 women aged 15 - 44.
5 Total fertility rate is the average number of children which would be born to a woman if she experienced the age-specific fertility rates of the period in question throughout her child-bearing life span. UK figures for the years 1970-72 and earlier are estimates.
6 On 1 October 1992 the legal definition of a stillbirth was changed from a baby born dead after 28 completed weeks gestation or more to one born

dead after 24 completed weeks gestation or more. Between 1 October and 31 December 1992 in the UK there were 258 babies born dead between 24 and 27 completed weeks gestation (216 in England and Wales, 35 in Scotland and 7 in Northern Ireland). If these babies were included in the stillbirth figures given, the stillbirth rate would be 4.7 for the UK and England and Wales, while Scotland and Northern Ireland stillbirth rate would remain as stated.
7 From 1981, data for the United Kingdom and Northern Ireland have been revised to exclude births in Northern Ireland to non-residents of Northern Ireland.

Sources: Office for National Statistics: 01329 444410;
General Register Office for Scotland;
Northern Ireland Statistics and Research Agency

49

5.16 Birth occurrence inside and outside marriage by age of mother

Thousands

	Inside marriage						Outside marriage					
	All ages	Under 20	20 - 24	25 - 29	Over 30	Mean[1] age (Years)	All ages	Under 20	20 - 24	25 - 29	Over 30	Mean[1] age (Years)
United Kingdom[2]												
	KKEY	KKEZ	KKFY	KKFZ	KKGX	KKGY	KKGZ	KKIC	KKID	KKIE	KKIF	KKIG
1961	890	55	273	280	282	27.7	54	13	17	10	13	25.5
1971	828	70	301	271	185	26.4	74	24	25	13	12	23.8
1981	640	36	193	231	180	27.3	91	30	33	16	13	23.4
1988	589	16	144	234	195	28.2	198	51	76	42	29	24.1
1989	570	14	130	228	198	28.4	207	49	79	46	32	24.3
1990	576	13	121	233	209	28.6	223	51	83	53	37	24.5
1991	556	10	109	224	213	28.9	236	50	87	58	41	24.8
1992	540	9	98	216	218	29.1	241	46	86	62	46	25.1
1993	520	8	87	204	221	29.3	242	44	84	64	50	25.4
1994	510	7	78	194	231	29.6	240	41	80	65	55	25.7
1995	486	6	69	180	232	29.8	246	42	79	66	60	25.9
1996	473	6	61	170	237	30.1	260	45	80	69	66	26.0
1997	460	6	55	159	240	30.3	267	47	79	71	71	26.1
1998	447	6	51	149	243	30.5	270	49	77	70	74	26.2
1999	428	6	47	136	239	30.7	272	49	77	68	77	26.3
2000	411	5	44	126	237	30.9	268	47	77	66	78	26.4
2001	401	5	44	116	236	30.9	268	45	77	64	82	26.7
2002	397	5	44	109	239	31.1	272	44	80	62	85	26.7
2003	407	5	44	110	249	31.2	289	45	86	65	92	26.8
2004	413	4	44	110	255	31.3	303	47	90	69	97	26.9
2005	412	4	43	111	254	31.4	310	47	93	72	98	26.9
2006	422	3	43	115	260	31.4	327	48	99	78	102	26.9
2007	429	3	42	119	265	31.5	343	47	104	85	106	27.1
2008	434	3	41	123	266	31.5	361	48	110	93	110	27.0
Great Britain												
	KKIH	KKII	KKIJ	KKIK	KKIL	KKIM	KKIN	KKIO	KKIP	KKIQ	KKIR	KKIS
1961	859	53	264	270	272	27.7	53	13	17	10	13	25.5
1971	797	68	293	261	176	26.4	73	24	25	13	12	23.8
1981	614	34	186	223	171	27.2	89	29	32	16	13	23.3
1988	566	16	138	226	186	28.2	194	49	74	42	29	23.6
1989	549	13	125	220	190	28.4	202	48	77	45	32	24.2
1990	554	12	116	225	201	28.6	218	49	81	52	36	24.6
1991	535	10	105	216	205	28.9	231	48	85	57	41	24.8
1992	520	9	94	208	210	29.1	235	45	84	61	46	25.1
1993	500	7	84	196	213	29.3	236	42	82	62	49	25.4
1994	492	7	75	188	222	29.6	235	41	78	63	53	25.7
1995	468	6	66	173	223	29.8	240	40	77	65	59	25.9
1996	455	6	59	163	227	30.1	254	44	78	68	65	26.0
1997	442	6	53	152	231	30.3	261	46	76	69	69	26.2
1998	430	6	49	143	233	30.5	263	48	74	68	73	26.3
1999	412	6	46	131	230	30.7	265	48	74	67	76	26.4
2000	396	5	43	121	228	30.9	261	46	74	65	77	26.5
2001	386	5	43	112	227	30.9	261	44	75	62	80	26.6
2002	383	5	43	105	230	31.1	265	43	77	61	84	26.7
2003	393	4	43	106	239	31.2	281	44	83	64	90	26.9
2004	399	4	43	106	245	31.3	295	45	88	67	95	26.9
2005	398	4	42	107	245	31.4	302	45	90	70	97	26.9
2006	407	3	42	111	251	31.4	318	46	96	76	100	26.9
2007	414	3	41	114	255	31.5	334	46	101	83	104	27.1
2008	418	3	41	119	256	31.5	351	46	107	90	107	27.0

1 The mean ages presented in this table are unstandardised and therefore take no account of the age structure of the population.
2 From 1981, data for the United Kingdom have been revised to exclude births in Northern Ireland to non-residents of Northern Ireland.

Sources: Office for National Statistics: 01329 444410; General Register Office for Scotland; Northern Ireland Statistics and Research Agency

5.17 Live births: by age of mother and country

Numbers

	All ages	Under 20	20 - 24	25 - 29	30 - 34	35 - 39	40 - 44	45 and over

United Kingdom

All live births[1,2]

	KMBZ	KMDV	KMDW	KMDX	KMDY	KMDZ	KMES	KMET
1998	716 888	54 822	127 230	218 072	212 876	88 729	14 453	640
1999	699 976	54 921	124 036	204 808	208 986	91 272	15 210	695
2000	679 029	52 059	120 305	191 583	202 893	95 400	16 032	708
2001	669 123	50 157	121 664	179 776	202 017	97 379	17 271	831
2002	668 777	49 165	123 844	171 852	203 261	101 379	18 273	968
2003	695 549	49 874	129 867	175 473	210 071	109 038	20 233	933
2004	715 996	50 752	134 614	179 050	213 620	114 852	22 107	975
2005	722 549	50 396	135 891	183 513	211 076	116 902	23 518	1 176
2006	748 563	51 066	142 171	192 800	212 333	123 867	24 999	1 288
2007	772 245	50 515	145 725	204 276	214 020	129 599	26 633	1 420
2008	794 383	50 396	151 608	216 466	215 964	130 520	27 845	1 558

Age-specific fertility rates[3]

	KMBY	KMBR	KMBS	KMBT	KMBU	KMBV	KMBW	KMBX
1998	58.8	30.8	73.6	101.4	90.4	40.0	7.4	0.3
1999	57.3	30.7	71.8	98.0	89.4	40.2	7.6	0.4
2000	55.4	29.2	68.7	93.9	87.7	41.0	7.8	0.4
2001	54.3	27.9	68.0	91.5	88.0	41.3	8.2	0.4
2002	54.2	27.0	68.0	91.3	89.7	42.6	8.4	0.5
2003	56.2	26.7	70.2	95.4	94.6	45.9	9.1	0.5
2004	57.7	26.7	71.5	97.3	99.2	48.6	9.7	0.5
2005	57.8	26.2	70.4	97.4	100.5	50.0	10.6	0.6
2006	59.7	26.4	72.0	100.1	104.6	53.4	10.6	0.6
2007	61.5	25.9	72.3	103.5	109.8	56.6	11.2	0.7
2008	63.4	26.0	73.5	107.9	113.1	58.2	12.4	0.7

England and Wales

All live births

	KGSH	KGSA	KGSB	KGSC	KGSD	KGSE	KGSF	KGSG
1998	635 901	48 285	113 537	193 144	188 499	78 881	12 980	575
1999	621 872	48 375	110 722	181 931	185 311	81 281	13 617	635
2000	604 441	45 846	107 741	170 701	180 113	84 974	14 403	663
2001	594 634	44 189	108 844	159 926	178 920	86 495	15 499	761
2002	596 122	43 467	110 959	153 379	180 532	90 449	16 441	895
2003	621 469	44 236	116 622	156 931	187 214	97 386	18 205	875
2004	639 721	45 094	121 072	159 984	190 550	102 228	19 884	909
2005	645 835	44 830	122 145	164 348	188 153	104 113	21 155	1 091
2006	669 601	45 509	127 828	172 642	189 407	110 509	22 512	1 194
2007	690 013	44 805	130 784	182 570	191 124	115 380	24 041	1 309
2008	708 711	44 691	135 971	192 960	192 450	116 220	24 991	1 428

Age-specific fertility rates[3]

	KGSP	KGSI	KGSJ	KGSK	KGSL	KGSM	KGSN	KGSO
1998	59.2	30.9	74.9	101.5	90.6	40.4	7.5	0.3
1999	57.8	30.9	73.0	98.3	89.6	40.6	7.7	0.4
2000	55.9	29.3	70.0	94.3	87.9	41.4	8.0	0.4
2001	54.7	28.0	69.0	91.7	88.0	41.5	8.4	0.5
2002	54.7	27.0	69.1	91.5	89.9	43.0	8.6	0.5
2003	56.8	26.9	71.1	95.8	94.9	46.4	9.3	0.5
2004	58.2	26.9	72.8	97.6	99.6	48.8	9.9	0.5
2005	58.3	26.3	71.6	97.9	100.7	50.3	10.8	0.6
2006	60.2	26.6	73.2	100.6	104.8	53.8	10.8	0.6
2007	62.0	26.0	73.5	104.0	110.2	56.9	11.4	0.7
2008	63.8	26.0	74.6	108.4	113.1	58.4	12.6	0.7

5.17 Live births: by age of mother and country
continued

Numbers

	All ages	Under 20	20 - 24	25 - 29	30 - 34	35 - 39	40 - 44	45 and over
Scotland								
All live births[1]								
	KGTH	KGTA	KGTB	KGTC	KGTD	KGTE	KGTF	KGTG
1998	57 319	4 802	9 804	17 477	17 207	6 893	1 027	43
1999	55 147	4 755	9 440	16 011	16 722	7 034	1 096	41
2000	53 076	4 599	8 962	14 676	16 233	7 395	1 133	29
2001	52 527	4 444	9 121	13 763	16 206	7 701	1 224	40
2002	51 270	4 195	9 267	12 694	16 038	7 727	1 267	47
2003	52 432	4 155	9 626	12 725	16 085	8 310	1 432	39
2004	53 957	4 172	9 950	13 131	16 085	8 912	1 631	50
2005	54 386	4 171	10 008	13 229	15 962	9 179	1 694	66
2006	55 690	4 130	10 399	13 876	15 878	9 535	1 775	58
2007	57 781	4 305	10 913	14 917	15 622	10 035	1 849	83
2008	60 041	4 279	11 373	16 171	16 028	10 025	2 044	95
Age-specific fertility rates[3]								
	KGTP	KGTI	KGTJ	KGTK	KGTL	KGTM	KGTN	KGTO
1998	52.7	30.6	62.8	94.3	83.2	34.1	5.7	0.3
1999	50.9	30.3	61.0	90.4	82.0	34.3	5.9	0.2
2000	49.2	29.3	57.6	86.5	81.3	35.6	6.0	0.2
2001	48.8	28.4	57.8	85.1	82.2	36.9	6.3	0.2
2002	48.1	26.8	58.3	83.3	83.6	37.1	6.4	0.3
2003	49.4	26.3	60.1	86.5	86.8	40.0	7.1	0.2
2004	51.0	26.1	61.8	89.4	90.3	43.3	7.9	0.3
2005	51.5	26.2	60.9	88.6	93.2	45.4	8.1	0.3
2006	52.8	25.8	61.9	90.2	97.1	47.8	8.4	0.3
2007	54.8	26.9	63.6	93.1	100.1	51.3	8.8	0.4
2008	57.2	26.8	65.3	98.1	105.4	53.1	10.2	0.5
Northern Ireland								
All live births[2]								
	KMDM	KMDF	KMDG	KMDH	KMDI	KMDJ	KMDK	KMDL
1998	23 668	1 735	3 889	7 451	7 170	2 955	446	22
1999	22 957	1 791	3 874	6 866	6 953	2 957	497	19
2000	21 512	1 614	3 602	6 206	6 547	3 031	496	16
2001	21 962	1 524	3 699	6 087	6 891	3 183	548	30
2002	21 385	1 502	3 619	5 779	6 691	3 203	565	26
2003	21 648	1 483	3 619	5 817	6 772	3 342	596	19
2004	22 318	1 486	3 592	5 935	6 985	3 712	592	16
2005	22 328	1 395	3 738	5 936	6 961	3 610	669	19
2006	23 272	1 427	3 944	6 282	7 048	3 823	712	36
2007	24 451	1 405	4 028	6 789	7 274	4 184	741	30
2008	25 631	1 426	4 264	7 335	7 486	4 275	810	35
Age-specific fertility rates[2,3]								
	KMDU	KMDN	KMDO	KMDP	KMDQ	KMDR	KMDS	KMDT
1998	65.0	27.8	69.6	119.0	108.4	47.2	8.2	0.4
1999	62.9	28.6	70.6	112.3	105.6	46.1	8.9	0.4
2000	58.7	25.6	66.0	103.9	100.4	46.2	8.5	0.3
2001	59.7	23.9	67.5	105.1	106.0	48.0	9.1	0.6
2002	58.1	23.3	66.0	102.9	104.2	48.2	9.2	0.5
2003	59.0	22.9	65.5	106.8	107.0	50.2	9.8	0.3
2004	60.6	23.0	62.8	109.8	112.6	56.1	9.5	0.3
2005	60.4	21.7	63.2	108.6	114.8	55.0	10.2	0.3
2006	62.5	22.5	63.6	112.0	119.2	58.2	10.8	0.6
2007	65.1	22.5	62.6	116.1	124.6	64.2	11.1	0.5
2008	68.2	23.0	65.6	120.5	131.1	67.0	12.6	0.6

1 The 'All ages' figure for Scotland includes births to mothers whose age was not known. There were 66 such births in 1998, 48 in 1999, 49 in 2000, 28 in 2001, 35 in 2002, 60 in 2003, 26 in 2004, 77 in 2005, 39 in 2006, 57 in 2007 and 26 in 2008.

2 From 1981 data for the United Kingdom and Northern Ireland have been revised to exclude births in Northern Ireland to non residents in Northern Ireland.

3 The rates for women of all ages, under 20, and 45 and over are based upon the populations of women aged 15-44, 15-19 and 45 respectively.

Sources: Office for National Statistics: 01329 444410;
General Register Office for Scotland;
Northern Ireland Statistics and Research Agency

5.18 Legal abortions[1]: by age for residents

Numbers

	All ages	Under 15	15	16 - 19	20 - 24	25 - 29	30 - 34	35 - 39	40 - 44	45 and over	Not stated
England and Wales											
	C53Z	C542	C543	C544	C545	C546	C547	C548	C549	C54A	C54B
1987	156 191	907	2 858	35 167	49 256	31 243	18 960	12 639	4 757	390	14
1988	168 298	859	2 709	37 928	54 067	34 584	20 000	12 681	5 047	412	11
1989	170 463	803	2 580	36 182	54 880	36 604	21 284	12 713	5 020	388	9
1990	173 900	873	2 549	35 520	55 281	38 770	22 431	12 956	5 104	404	12
1991	167 376	886	2 272	31 130	52 678	38 611	23 445	13 035	4 901	408	10
1992	160 501	905	2 095	27 589	49 052	38 430	23 870	13 252	4 844	452	12
1993	157 846	964	2 119	25 806	46 846	38 139	24 690	13 885	4 889	494	14
1994	156 539	1 080	2 166	25 223	44 871	38 081	25 507	14 156	5 008	440	7
1995	154 315	946	2 324	24 945	43 394	37 254	25 759	14 352	4 868	457	16
1996	167 916	1 098	2 547	28 790	46 356	39 311	28 228	16 118	5 027	428	13
1997	170 145	1 020	2 414	29 947	44 960	40 159	28 892	16 858	5 413	482	..
1998	177 871	1 103	2 656	33 236	45 766	40 366	30 449	18 174	5 576	511	34
1999	173 701	1 066	2 537	32 807	45 004	38 492	29 139	18 341	5 755	502	58
2000	175 542	1 048	2 700	33 218	47 099	37 852	28 735	18 589	5 794	459	48
2001	176 364	1 066	2 592	33 431	48 267	36 506	28 782	19 146	6 094	456	24
2002	175 932	1 075	2 658	32 985	48 359	35 795	28 503	19 450	6 531	457	119
2003	181 582	1 171	2 796	34 247	51 201[2]	36 018	28 749	19 868	7 032	500	–
2004	185 415	1 034	2 722	35 386	52 701[2]	37 759	28 064	19 820	7 422	507	–
2005	186 416	1 083	2 703	35 313	53 342	38 330	27 836	19 782	7 459	568	–
2006	193 737	1 042	2 948	37 296	55 340	40 396	28 153	20 074	7 825	663	–
2007	198 499	1 171	3 205	39 579	56 963	41 704	27 257	19 976	7 915	729	–
2008	195 296	1 097	3 016	38 577	56 171	41 896	26 985	19 228	7 663	663	–
Scotland											
	C54C	C54D	C54E	C54F	C54G	C54H	C54I	C54J	C54K	C54L	EVH4
1987	9 449	70	210	2 415	2 991	1 728	1 082	695	241	17	–
1988	10 111	65	217	2 526	3 299	1 965	1 105	662	257	15	–
1989	10 191	53	209	2 554	3 199	1 967	1 225	704	266	14	–
1990	10 198	54	185	2 536	3 235	2 061	1 157	698	253	19	–
1991	11 046	77	203	2 567	3 479	2 247	1 443	740	262	28	–
1992	10 791	73	173	2 368	3 383	2 283	1 444	798	252	17	–
1993	11 059	92	193	2 297	3 365	2 443	1 489	889	262	29	–
1994	11 371	78	214	2 311	3 480	2 427	1 640	876	315	30	–
1995	11 131	79	233	2 168	3 395	2 437	1 606	885	295	33	–
1996	11 957	87	234	2 360	3 569	2 595	1 798	957	330	27	–
1997	12 087	85	204	2 429	3 438	2 644	1 849	1 091	322	25	–
1998	12 458	73	213	2 703	3 419	2 740	1 801	1 148	339	22	–
1999	12 140	69	182	2 628	3 349	2 546	1 807	1 178	358	23	–
2000	11 976	93	181	2 606	3 348	2 400	1 765	1 174	381	28	–
2001	12 108	66	210	2 717	3 459	2 315	1 815	1 126	377	23	–
2002	11 840	80	194	2 646	3 447	2 165	1 731	1 166	382	29	–
2003	12 267	71	242	2 781	3 673	2 224	1 725	1 112	411	28	–
2004	12 419	104	207	2 901	3 689	2 261	1 660	1 182	383	32	–
2005	12 605	94	248	2 966	3 765	2 334	1 682	1 094	397	25	–
2006	13 109	91	273	3 085	3 967	2 433	1 614	1 205	413	28	–
2007	13 672	98	275	3 170	4 108	2 722	1 636	1 219	407	37	–
2008[3]	13 762	94	247	3 125	4 259	2 736	1 641	1 204	427	29	–

1 Refers to therapeutic abortions notified in accordance with the Abortion Act 1967.
2 Records with missing ages were assigned to the 20 - 24 age group.
3 Provisional.

Sources: Department of Health;
Notifications (to the Chief Medical Officer for Scotland) of abortions performed;
under the Abortion Act 1967: ISD Scotland

5.19 Deaths: by sex and age[1]

Numbers

	All ages[2]	Under 1 year	1-4	5-9	10-14	15-19	20-24	25-34	35-44	45-54	55-64	65-74	75-84	85 and over
United Kingdom														
Males														
1900 - 02	340 664	87 242	37 834	8 429	4 696	7 047	8 766	19 154	24 739	30 488	37 610	39 765	28 320	6 563
1910 - 12	303 703	63 885	29 452	7 091	4 095	5 873	6 817	16 141	21 813	28 981	37 721	45 140	29 397	7 283
1920 - 22	284 876	48 044	19 008	6 052	3 953	5 906	6 572	13 663	19 702	29 256	40 583	49 398	34 937	7 801
1930 - 32	284 249	28 840	11 276	4 580	2 890	5 076	6 495	12 327	16 326	29 376	47 989	63 804	45 247	10 022
1940 - 42	314 643	24 624	6 949	3 400	2 474	4 653	4 246	11 506	17 296	30 082	57 076	79 652	59 733	12 900
1950 - 52	307 312	14 105	2 585	1 317	919	1 498	2 289	5 862	11 074	27 637	53 691	86 435	79 768	20 131
1960 - 62	318 850	12 234	1 733	971	871	1 718	1 857	3 842	8 753	26 422	63 009	87 542	83 291	26 605
1970 - 72	335 166	9 158	1 485	1 019	802	1 778	2 104	3 590	7 733	24 608	64 898	105 058	82 905	30 027
1980 - 82	330 495	4 829	774	527	652	1 999	1 943	3 736	6 568	19 728	54 159	105 155	98 488	31 936
1990 - 92	312 521	3 315	623	372	396	1 349	2 059	4 334	6 979	15 412	40 424	87 849	106 376	43 032
2000 - 02	288 261	2 065	365	233	326	1 032	1 502	4 270	7 181	15 370	32 328	66 808	98 363	58 419
	KHUA	KHUB	KHUC	KHUD	KHUE	KHUF	KHUG	KHUH	KHUI	KHUJ	KHUK	KHUL	KHUM	KHUN
1997	301 713	2 414	465	301	366	1 134	1 738	4 558	6 678	15 770	33 910	78 121	101 817	54 441
1998	299 655	2 315	465	297	361	1 145	1 651	4 782	6 893	15 836	33 673	75 608	101 066	55 563
1999	299 235	2 323	459	260	333	1 088	1 548	4 647	6 930	15 862	33 181	73 457	101 327	57 820
2000	291 337	2 136	390	263	305	1 068	1 595	4 491	7 168	15 458	32 661	69 707	98 398	57 697
2001	287 942	2 052	358	230	369	1 106	1 518	4 459	7 275	15 668	32 135	66 257	98 041	58 474
2002	289 083	2 050	382	224	327	1 071	1 575	4 345	7 362	15 222	32 509	65 140	99 387	59 489
2003	289 185	2 047	356	228	308	1 013	1 586	4 041	7 530	14 692	32 895	63 520	100 900	60 069
2004	278 918	2 033	345	206	282	975	1 484	3 831	7 454	14 510	31 660	60 760	98 466	56 912
2005	277 349	2 117	339	194	312	1 022	1 449	3 660	7 454	14 241	31 645	58 828	95 641	60 447
2006	274 201	2 078	328	213	299	1 008	1 482	3 712	7 485	14 406	32 012	56 319	92 532	62 327
2007	274 883	2 106	379	200	270	979	1 491	3 711	7 423	14 045	31 994	55 338	91 488	65 459
2008	276 745	2 123	319	211	218	955	1 487	3 718	7 519	14 420	31 406	55 445	90 367	68 557
Females														
1900 - 02	322 058	68 770	36 164	8 757	5 034	6 818	8 264	18 702	21 887	25 679	34 521	42 456	34 907	10 099
1910 - 12	289 608	49 865	27 817	7 113	4 355	5 683	6 531	15 676	19 647	24 481	32 813	46 453	37 353	11 828
1920 - 22	274 772	35 356	17 323	5 808	4 133	5 729	6 753	14 878	18 121	24 347	34 026	48 573	45 521	14 203
1930 - 32	275 336	21 072	9 995	3 990	2 734	4 721	5 931	12 699	15 373	24 695	39 471	59 520	56 250	18 886
1940 - 42	296 646	17 936	5 952	2 743	2 068	4 180	5 028	11 261	14 255	23 629	42 651	70 907	71 377	24 658
1950 - 52	291 597	10 293	2 098	880	625	1 115	1 717	5 018	8 989	18 875	37 075	75 220	92 848	36 844
1960 - 62	304 871	8 887	1 334	627	522	684	811	2 504	6 513	16 720	36 078	73 118	105 956	51 117
1970 - 72	322 968	6 666	1 183	654	459	718	900	2 110	5 345	15 594	36 177	75 599	109 539	68 024
1980 - 82	330 269	3 561	585	355	425	733	772	2 099	4 360	12 206	32 052	72 618	117 760	82 743
1990 - 92	328 218	2 431	485	259	255	520	714	1 989	4 340	9 707	25 105	61 951	115 467	104 994
2000 - 02	317 356	1 586	283	188	208	446	536	1 877	4 426	10 270	20 549	47 324	101 650	128 012
	KIUA	KIUB	KIUC	KIUD	KIUE	KIUF	KIUG	KIUH	KIUI	KIUJ	KIUK	KIUL	KIUM	KIUN
1997	330 804	1 863	336	221	236	489	587	1 953	4 320	10 451	21 103	55 947	108 777	124 521
1998	327 937	1 744	339	221	233	511	554	2 015	4 316	10 441	20 819	54 048	106 703	125 993
1999	330 241	1 736	346	195	244	487	567	1 963	4 359	10 400	20 963	52 098	106 323	130 560
2000	319 242	1 677	288	181	215	468	573	1 975	4 488	10 477	20 620	49 138	102 052	127 090
2001	316 451	1 639	299	218	200	447	557	1 895	4 475	10 354	20 479	47 138	101 135	127 615
2002	318 962	1 488	280	181	229	456	556	1 838	4 380	10 080	20 707	46 094	102 503	130 170
2003	322 900	1 639	309	182	237	441	563	1 869	4 506	9 870	20 974	45 374	105 182	131 754
2004	305 873	1 626	279	160	201	480	572	1 765	4 486	9 463	20 500	43 118	100 775	122 448
2005	305 615	1 555	256	153	216	450	557	1 684	4 432	9 492	20 655	41 839	98 338	125 988
2006	298 023	1 659	303	151	201	437	520	1 604	4 434	9 474	20 855	40 290	92 877	125 218
2007	299 797	1 627	266	137	212	423	522	1 575	4 398	9 487	21 026	39 685	90 822	129 617
2008	302 952	1 622	296	158	161	430	544	1 667	4 446	9 680	21 060	39 496	89 459	133 933

5.19 Deaths: by sex and age[1]
continued

Numbers

	All ages[2]	Under 1 year	1-4	5-9	10-14	15-19	20-24	25-34	35-44	45-54	55-64	65-74	75-84	85 and over
England and Wales														
Males														
1900 - 02	288 886	76 095	32 051	7 066	3 818	5 611	7 028	15 869	21 135	26 065	31 600	33 568	23 835	5 144
1910 - 12	257 253	54 678	24 676	5 907	3 348	4 765	5 596	13 603	18 665	24 820	32 217	38 016	24 928	6 036
1920 - 22	240 605	39 796	15 565	5 151	3 314	4 901	5 447	11 551	17 004	25 073	34 639	42 025	29 685	6 455
1930 - 32	243 147	23 331	9 099	3 844	2 435	4 354	5 580	10 600	14 041	25 657	41 581	54 910	39 091	8 624
1940 - 42	268 876	19 393	5 616	2 834	2 051	3 832	3 156	9 484	14 744	25 983	50 058	68 791	51 779	11 158
1950 - 52	266 879	11 498	2 131	1 087	778	1 248	1 947	4 990	9 489	23 815	46 948	75 774	69 496	17 677
1960 - 62	278 369	10 157	1 444	812	742	1 523	1 624	3 278	7 524	22 813	54 908	77 000	73 180	23 364
1970 - 72	293 934	7 818	1 259	860	677	1 524	1 788	3 079	6 637	21 348	56 667	92 389	73 365	26 522
1980 - 82	290 352	4 168	657	452	555	1 716	1 619	3 169	5 590	16 909	47 144	92 485	87 338	28 551
1990 - 92	275 550	2 926	545	325	338	1 157	1 757	3 717	6 057	13 258	34 977	77 063	94 672	38 757
2000 - 02	253 706	1 836	323	200	282	862	1 244	3 619	6 104	13 184	27 696	58 114	87 481	52 761
	KHVA	KHVB	KHVC	KHVD	KHVE	KHVF	KHVG	KHVH	KHVI	KHVJ	KHVK	KHVL	KHVM	KHVN
1997	266 164	2 160	421	268	327	970	1 468	3 915	5 718	13 565	29 110	68 275	90 659	49 308
1998	264 202	2 058	415	254	309	962	1 404	4 111	5 886	13 606	28 947	65 989	90 048	50 213
1999	263 166	2 080	408	221	289	905	1 265	3 978	5 918	13 633	28 532	64 017	89 963	51 957
2000	256 698	1 902	345	227	263	898	1 328	3 849	6 135	13 355	28 003	60 801	87 449	52 143
2001	253 608	1 818	329	192	320	927	1 276	3 830	6 184	13 424	27 599	57 638	87 238	52 833
2002	254 390	1 831	329	198	286	912	1 310	3 665	6 255	13 011	27 807	56 584	88 493	53 709
2003	254 433	1 827	310	203	263	852	1 348	3 478	6 440	12 697	28 291	55 064	89 596	54 064
2004	245 208	1 809	303	174	252	833	1 257	3 281	6 360	12 417	27 117	52 709	87 367	51 329
2005	243 870	1 877	297	166	272	856	1 217	3 146	6 362	12 158	27 292	51 019	84 661	54 547
2006	240 888	1 863	292	187	261	844	1 212	3 132	6 315	12 256	27 551	48 881	81 912	56 182
2007	240 780	1 882	339	182	226	797	1 218	3 138	6 264	11 893	27 508	47 830	80 573	58 930
2008	243 014	1 920	284	180	190	779	1 255	3 088	6 419	12 269	27 093	47 862	79 799	61 876
Females														
1900 - 02	269 432	60 090	30 674	7 278	4 010	5 265	6 497	15 065	18 253	21 474	28 424	35 307	29 118	7 977
1910 - 12	242 079	42 642	23 335	5 883	3 519	4 522	5 256	12 742	16 363	20 611	27 571	38 489	31 363	9 782
1920 - 22	229 908	29 178	14 174	4 928	3 456	4 719	5 533	12 244	15 142	20 580	28 633	41 010	38 439	11 871
1930 - 32	233 915	16 929	8 013	3 338	2 293	3 969	5 039	10 716	13 022	21 190	33 798	50 844	48 531	16 234
1940 - 42	253 702	14 174	4 726	2 265	1 695	3 426	4 198	9 470	12 093	20 413	36 814	60 987	61 891	21 550
1950 - 52	252 176	8 367	1 727	732	520	893	1 365	4 131	7 586	16 161	31 875	65 087	81 154	32 579
1960 - 62	266 849	7 409	1 103	527	444	591	700	2 147	5 576	14 389	31 083	63 543	93 548	45 789
1970 - 72	284 181	5 677	1 020	562	396	620	806	1 814	4 585	13 417	31 222	65 817	96 952	61 293
1980 - 82	290 026	3 064	511	301	365	635	670	1 821	3 740	10 420	27 606	63 023	103 676	74 194
1990 - 92	288 851	2 161	420	227	217	455	625	1 718	3 765	8 347	21 466	53 783	101 752	93 914
2000 - 02	279 482	1 412	251	168	182	382	455	1 629	3 805	8 893	17 659	40 734	89 387	114 525
	KIVA	KIVB	KIVC	KIVD	KIVE	KIVF	KIVG	KIVH	KIVI	KIVJ	KIVK	KIVL	KIVM	KIVN
1997	291 888	1 664	300	183	206	428	503	1 711	3 734	9 055	18 053	48 553	96 009	111 489
1998	289 233	1 547	301	185	207	432	466	1 768	3 705	9 077	17 872	46 742	94 281	112 650
1999	290 366	1 555	308	168	219	399	484	1 707	3 773	8 999	17 949	44 958	93 360	116 487
2000	281 179	1 497	257	160	191	403	504	1 702	3 853	9 108	17 722	42 318	89 651	113 813
2001	278 890	1 449	272	198	171	386	472	1 665	3 858	8 984	17 608	40 639	89 036	114 152
2002	280 966	1 337	240	160	204	391	467	1 597	3 767	8 689	17 807	39 645	90 213	116 449
2003	284 718	1 479	278	159	209	370	485	1 636	3 884	8 554	18 001	39 001	92 694	117 968
2004	269 042	1 462	251	140	173	410	494	1 536	3 855	8 139	17 649	37 041	88 404	109 488
2005	269 123	1 371	222	134	189	379	478	1 481	3 805	8 175	17 797	35 913	86 309	112 870
2006	261 711	1 505	267	135	169	381	444	1 382	3 802	8 098	17 948	34 502	81 210	111 868
2007	263 265	1 456	235	121	192	357	453	1 360	3 787	8 072	18 166	33 903	79 411	115 752
2008	266 076	1 449	270	137	140	351	458	1 445	3 811	8 291	18 187	33 883	77 827	119 827

Population and vital statistics

5.19 Deaths: by sex and age[1]
continued

Numbers

	All ages[2]	Under 1 year	1-4	5-9	10-14	15-19	20-24	25-34	35-44	45-54	55-64	65-74	75-84	85 and over
Scotland														
Males														
1900 - 02	40 224	9 189	4 798	1 083	672	1 069	1 292	2 506	2 935	3 591	4 597	4 531	3 117	834
1910 - 12	35 981	7 510	3 935	962	595	826	910	1 969	2 469	3 325	4 356	5 113	3 182	813
1920 - 22	34 649	6 757	2 847	710	489	747	791	1 616	2 128	3 314	4 785	5 624	3 928	911
1930 - 32	32 476	4 426	1 771	610	365	568	706	1 352	1 848	2 979	5 095	6 906	4 839	1 010
1940 - 42	36 384	3 973	1 011	449	321	668	888	1 643	2 090	3 348	5 728	8 556	6 317	1 337
1950 - 52	32 236	1 949	349	175	105	200	265	693	1 267	3 151	5 574	8 544	8 094	1 871
1960 - 62	32 401	1 578	222	121	102	146	185	456	1 013	2 986	6 682	8 505	7 980	2 425
1970 - 72	32 446	944	168	119	93	178	233	396	875	2 617	6 641	10 176	7 383	2 624
1980 - 82	31 723	451	80	56	71	206	233	423	776	2 280	5 601	10 152	8 804	2 591
1990 - 92	29 421	287	57	34	40	137	230	485	744	1 730	4 402	8 611	9 311	3 353
2000 - 02	27 526	165	30	23	30	119	196	523	882	1 775	3 781	7 038	8 535	4 430
	KHWA	KHWB	KHWC	KHWD	KHWE	KHWF	KHWG	KHWH	KHWI	KHWJ	KHWK	KHWL	KHWM	KHWN
1997	28 305	186	32	22	27	114	208	521	788	1 794	3 876	7 909	8 791	4 037
1998	28 132	183	37	34	39	134	200	524	843	1 796	3 828	7 746	8 585	4 183
1999	28 605	161	31	23	33	138	215	545	818	1 820	3 773	7 569	8 908	4 571
2000	27 511	173	33	24	28	115	198	512	842	1 716	3 789	7 224	8 523	4 334
2001	27 324	155	22	27	35	131	179	510	902	1 820	3 751	6 950	8 433	4 409
2002	27 743	167	34	17	27	111	211	546	901	1 789	3 804	6 940	8 648	4 548
2003	27 832	146	35	15	31	122	186	469	893	1 634	3 787	6 797	8 994	4 723
2004	26 775	160	29	21	23	105	181	449	889	1 676	3 629	6 507	8 733	4 373
2005	26 522	159	33	19	30	106	150	385	882	1 654	3 478	6 352	8 691	4 583
2006	26 251	145	21	18	21	112	206	461	938	1 697	3 567	5 966	8 353	4 746
2007	26 895	154	25	13	31	127	207	461	908	1 685	3 572	6 082	8 547	5 083
2008	26 504	140	22	19	16	106	174	503	868	1 715	3 481	6 052	8 290	5 118
Females														
1900 - 02	39 891	7 143	4 477	1 162	747	1 058	1 246	2 625	2 732	3 130	4 485	5 273	4 305	1 508
1910 - 12	36 132	5 854	3 674	981	618	836	910	2 149	2 473	2 909	3 960	5 636	4 588	1 552
1920 - 22	34 449	5 029	2 602	687	489	711	889	1 947	2 266	2 828	4 157	5 587	5 443	1 814
1930 - 32	32 377	3 319	1 602	527	339	568	666	1 508	1 812	2 731	4 380	6 630	6 178	2 117
1940 - 42	33 715	2 852	921	373	283	595	656	1 382	1 672	2 528	4 630	7 674	7 613	2 536
1950 - 52	31 525	1 432	284	115	84	185	293	714	1 127	2 188	4 204	8 157	9 310	3 431
1960 - 62	30 559	1 107	170	80	63	72	87	287	762	1 897	4 115	7 752	9 991	4 177
1970 - 72	30 978	694	118	69	46	73	74	231	608	1 769	4 036	7 823	10 112	5 324
1980 - 82	32 326	337	49	37	44	74	73	213	493	1 456	3 565	7 781	11 333	6 871
1990 - 92	31 747	190	45	20	29	49	72	218	458	1 093	2 966	6 630	11 079	8 898
2000 - 02	30 235	123	24	14	21	50	64	199	493	1 110	2 341	5 326	9 785	10 685
	KIWA	KIWB	KIWC	KIWD	KIWE	KIWF	KIWG	KIWH	KIWI	KIWJ	KIWK	KIWL	KIWM	KIWN
1997	31 189	130	23	28	21	43	71	199	496	1 128	2 480	5 985	10 164	10 421
1998	31 032	137	26	28	19	55	68	198	485	1 106	2 416	5 955	9 913	10 626
1999	31 676	115	26	20	17	65	58	201	467	1 128	2 431	5 837	10 198	11 113
2000	30 288	132	20	10	21	46	56	222	510	1 086	2 324	5 512	9 875	10 474
2001	30 058	135	20	16	21	47	71	189	480	1 111	2 361	5 235	9 695	10 677
2002	30 360	103	32	15	20	58	65	185	489	1 134	2 339	5 232	9 784	10 904
2003	30 640	119	24	18	20	57	64	181	489	1 062	2 446	5 194	9 977	10 989
2004	29 412	106	19	15	22	52	62	179	492	1 065	2 291	4 924	9 924	10 261
2005	29 225	125	27	11	18	55	58	163	506	1 073	2 316	4 841	9 620	10 412
2006	28 842	103	26	11	17	40	58	170	497	1 090	2 351	4 722	9 303	10 454
2007	29 091	118	26	11	14	50	52	166	490	1 124	2 311	4 732	9 083	10 914
2008	29 196	113	17	11	18	55	68	172	497	1 083	2 315	4 560	9 299	10 988

5.19 Deaths: by sex and age[1]

continued

Numbers

	All ages[2]	Under 1 year	1-4	5-9	10-14	15-19	20-24	25-34	35-44	45-54	55-64	65-74	75-84	85 and over
Northern Ireland														
Males														
1900 - 02	11 554	1 958	985	280	206	367	446	779	669	832	1 413	1 666	1 368	585
1910 - 12	10 469	1 697	841	222	152	282	311	569	679	836	1 148	2 011	1 287	434
1920 - 22	9 622	1 491	596	191	150	258	334	496	570	869	1 159	1 749	1 324	435
1930 - 32	8 626	1 083	406	126	90	154	209	375	437	740	1 313	1 988	1 317	388
1940 - 42	9 383	1 258	322	117	102	153	202	379	462	751	1 290	2 305	1 637	405
1950 - 52	8 197	658	105	55	36	50	77	179	318	671	1 169	2 117	2 178	583
1960 - 62	8 080	499	67	38	27	49	48	108	216	623	1 419	2 037	2 131	816
1970 - 72	8 786	396	58	40	32	76	83	115	221	643	1 590	2 493	2 157	881
1980 - 82	8 420	211	37	20	26	77	92	144	202	539	1 414	2 518	2 346	795
1990 - 92	7 550	102	21	13	18	55	73	132	178	423	1 044	2 175	2 393	922
2000 - 02	7 029	64	13	11	14	50	62	128	195	411	851	1 656	2 347	1228
	KHXA	KHXB	KHXC	KHXD	KHXE	KHXF	KHXG	KHXH	KHXI	KHXJ	KHXK	KHXL	KHXM	KHXN
1997	7 244	68	12.0	11	12	50	62	122	172	411	924	1 937	2 367	1 096
1998	7 321	74	13.0	9	13	49	47	147	164	434	898	1 873	2 433	1 167
1999	7 464	82	20.0	16	11	45	68	124	194	409	876	1 871	2 456	1 292
2000	7 128	61	12.0	12	14	55	69	130	191	387	869	1 682	2 426	1 220
2001	7 007	79	7.0	11	14	48	63	119	189	423	785	1 669	2 370	1 231
2002	6 948	52	19.0	9	14	48	54	134	206	421	898	1 616	2 245	1 232
2003	6 920	74	11.0	10	14	39	52	94	197	361	817	1 659	2 310	1 282
2004	6 935	64	13.0	11	7	37	46	101	205	417	914	1 544	2 366	1 210
2005	6 957	81	9.0	9	10	60	82	129	210	429	875	1 457	2 289	1 317
2006	7 062	70	15.0	8	17	52	64	119	232	453	894	1 472	2 267	1 399
2007	7 208	70	15.0	5	13	55	66	112	251	467	914	1 426	2 368	1 446
2008	7 227	63	13.0	12	12	70	58	127	232	436	832	1 531	2 278	1 563
Females														
1900 - 02	12 735	1 537	1 013	317	277	495	521	1 012	902	1 075	1 612	1 876	1 484	614
1910 - 12	11 397	1 369	808	249	218	325	365	785	811	961	1 282	2 328	1 402	494
1920 - 22	10 415	1 149	547	193	188	299	331	687	713	939	1 236	1 976	1 639	518
1930 - 32	9 044	824	380	125	102	184	226	475	539	774	1 293	2 046	1 541	535
1940 - 42	9 229	910	305	105	90	159	174	409	490	688	1 207	2 246	1 873	572
1950 - 52	7 896	494	87	33	21	37	59	173	276	526	996	1 976	2 384	834
1960 - 62	7 463	371	61	20	15	21	24	70	175	434	880	1 823	2 417	1 151
1970 - 72	7 809	295	45	23	17	25	20	65	152	408	919	1 959	2 475	1 407
1980 - 82	7 917	160	26	17	17	23	29	65	127	329	881	1 813	2 752	1 678
1990 - 92	7 620	80	20	12	9	16	17	53	117	267	672	1 538	2 636	2 182
2000 - 02	7 638	50	9	7	5	13	17	49	129	266	548	1 263	2 479	2 802
	KIXA	KIXB	KIXC	KIXD	KIXE	KIXF	KIXG	KIXH	KIXI	KIXJ	KIXK	KIXL	KIXM	KIXN
1997	7 727	69	13	10	9	18	13	43	90	268	570	1 409	2 604	2 611
1998	7 672	60	12	8	7	24	20	49	126	258	531	1 351	2 509	2 717
1999	8 199	66	12	7	8	23	25	55	119	273	583	1 303	2 765	2 960
2000	7 775	48	11	11	3	19	13	51	125	283	574	1 308	2 526	2 803
2001	7 506	55	7	4	8	14	14	41	137	260	510	1 265	2 404	2 787
2002	7 638	48	8	6	5	7	24	56	124	258	561	1 217	2 507	2 817
2003	7 542	41	7	5	8	14	14	52	133	254	527	1 179	2 511	2 797
2004	7 419	58	9	5	6	18	16	50	139	259	560	1 153	2 447	2 699
2005	7 267	59	7	8	9	16	21	40	121	244	542	1 085	2 409	2 706
2006	7 470	51	10	5	15	16	18	52	135	286	556	1 066	2 364	2 896
2007	7 441	53	5	5	6	16	17	49	121	291	549	1 050	2 328	2 951
2008	7 680	60	9	10	3	24	18	50	138	306	558	1 053	2 333	3 118

1 See chapter text.
2 In some years the totals include a small number of persons whose age was not stated.

Sources: Office for National Statistics: 01329 444410;
General Register Office for Scotland;
Northern Ireland Statistics and Research Agency

Population and vital statistics

5.20 Infant and maternal mortality[1]
(i) - By country. (ii) - Infant mortality by country, type of death and sex

| | Deaths of Infants under 1 year of age per thousand live births | | | | | | | | | | | | Maternal deaths per thousand live births[3] | | | |
| | United Kingdom | | | England and Wales[2] | | | Scotland | | | Northern Ireland | | | United Kingdom | England and Wales | Scotland | Northern Ireland |
	Total	Males	Females	Total	Males	Females	Total	Males	Females	Total	Males	Females				
1900 - 02	142	156	128	146	160	131	124	136	111	113	123	103	4.71	4.67	4.74	6.03
1910 - 12	110	121	98	110	121	98	109	120	97	101	110	92	3.95	3.67	5.65	5.28
1920 - 22	82	92	71	80	90	69	94	106	82	86	95	77	4.37	4.03	6.36	5.62
1930 - 32	67	75	58	64	72	55	84	94	73	75	83	66	4.54	4.24	6.40	5.24
1940 - 42	59	66	51	55	62	48	77	87	66	80	89	70	3.29	2.74	4.50	3.79
1950 - 52	30	34	26	29	33	25	37	42	32	40	45	36	0.88	0.79	1.09	1.09
1960 - 62	22	25	19	22	24	19	26	30	22	27	30	24	0.36	0.36	0.37	0.43
1970 - 72	18	20	16	18	20	15	19	22	17	22	24	20	0.17	0.17	0.17	0.12
1980 - 82	12	13	10	11	13	10	12	13	10	13	15	12	0.09	0.09	0.14	0.06
1990 - 92	7	8	6	7	8	6	7	8	6	7	8	6	0.07	0.07	0.10	-
2000 - 02	5	6	5	5	6	5	5	6	5	5	6	5	0.07	0.06	0.12	0.05
	KKAW	KKAX	KKAY	KKAZ	KKBW	KKBX	KKBY	KKBZ	KKCW	KKCX	KKCY	KKCZ	KKDW	KKDX	KKDY	KKDZ
1997	5.8	6.4	5.3	5.9	6.5	5.3	5.3	6.1	4.5	5.6	5.5	5.8	0.06	0.06	0.07	–
1998	5.7	6.3	5.0	5.7	6.4	5.0	5.6	6.2	4.9	5.6	6.1	5.1	0.07	0.07	0.09	0.04
1999	5.8	6.4	5.1	5.8	6.5	5.1	5.0	5.7	4.3	6.4	6.8	5.9	0.05	0.05	0.13	–
2000	5.6	6.1	5.0	5.6	6.1	5.1	5.7	6.4	5.1	5.0	5.4	4.6	0.07	0.06	0.15	–
2001	5.5	6.0	5.0	5.4	5.9	4.9	5.5	5.8	5.2	6.0	6.9	5.1	0.07	0.07	0.11	0.09
2002	5.2	5.9	4.5	5.2	5.9	4.5	5.3	6.4	4.1	4.6	4.7	4.5	0.06	0.06	0.10	0.05
2003	5.3	5.7	4.9	5.3	5.7	4.9	5.1	5.4	4.7	5.2	6.5	3.9	0.10	0.07	0.10	0.14
2004	5.0	5.5	4.6	5.0	5.5	4.6	4.9	5.8	4.0	5.3	5.4	5.2	0.07	0.07	0.11	0.04
2005	5.1	5.7	4.5	5.0	5.7	4.4	5.2	5.7	4.8	6.1	7.0	5.3	0.06	0.06	0.07	0.04
2006	5.0	5.4	4.5	5.0	5.4	4.6	4.5	5.1	3.8	5.1	5.7	4.4	0.07	0.06	0.13	0.13
2007	4.8	5.3	4.3	4.8	5.3	4.3	4.7	5.2	4.2	4.9	5.5	4.4	0.07	0.07	0.14	–
2008	4.7	5.2	4.2	4.8	5.3	4.2	4.2	4.6	3.8	4.7	4.7	4.7	0.06	0.06	0.08	–

5.20
continued

Infant and maternal mortality[1]
(i) - By country. (ii) - Infant mortality by country, type of death and sex

Deaths per thousand live births

		1998	1999	2000	2001	2002	2003	2004	2005	2006	2007	2008
Total												
United Kingdom:												
Stillbirths[4]	KHNQ	5.4	5.3	5.3	5.3	5.6	5.7	5.7	5.3	5.3	5.2	5.1
Perinatal[4]	KHNR	8.3	8.2	8.1	8.0	8.3	8.5	8.3	8.0	7.9	7.7	7.5
Neonatal	KHNS	3.8	3.9	3.9	3.6	3.5	3.6	3.4	3.5	3.5	3.3	3.2
Post neonatal	KHNT	1.9	1.9	1.7	1.8	1.7	1.7	1.6	1.6	1.5	1.5	1.5
England and Wales:												
Stillbirths[4]	KHNU	5.3	5.3	5.3	5.3	5.6	5.7	5.7	5.4	5.4	5.2	5.1
Perinatal[4]	KHNV	8.2	8.2	8.2	8.0	8.3	8.5	8.4	8.0	8.0	7.7	7.6
Neonatal	KHNW	3.8	3.9	3.9	3.6	3.6	3.6	3.5	3.4	3.5	3.3	3.2
Post neonatal	KHNX	1.9	1.9	1.7	1.9	1.7	1.7	1.6	1.6	1.5	1.5	1.5
Scotland:												
Stillbirths[4]	KHNY	6.1	5.2	5.6	5.7	5.4	5.6	5.8	5.3	5.3	5.6	5.4
Perinatal[4]	KHNZ	8.7	7.6	8.4	8.5	7.6	8.0	8.1	7.7	7.4	7.8	7.4
Neonatal	KHOA	3.6	3.3	4.0	3.8	3.2	3.4	3.1	3.5	3.5	3.3	2.8
Post neonatal	KHOB	2.0	1.7	1.8	1.7	2.1	1.7	1.9	1.7	1.5	1.5	1.4
Northern Ireland:												
Stillbirths[4]	KHOC	5.1	5.7	4.3	5.1	5.7	5.0	5.0	4.0	3.8	4.2	4.5
Perinatal[4]	KHOD	8.1	10.0	7.2	8.4	8.7	8.0	8.0	8.1	6.9	6.9	7.4
Neonatal	KHOE	3.9	4.8	3.8	4.4	3.4	3.9	3.6	4.9	3.8	3.2	3.6
Post neonatal	KHOF	1.7	1.6	1.2	1.6	1.2	1.3	1.7	1.3	1.3	1.7	1.1
Males												
United Kingdom:												
Perinatal[4]	KHOG	8.8	8.7	8.7	8.6	8.9	8.8	8.8	8.3	8.3	8.1	7.9
Neonatal	KHOH	4.2	4.3	4.2	4.0	4.0	3.9	3.8	3.9	3.9	3.6	3.6
Infant mortality	KHOI	6.3	6.4	6.1	6.0	5.9	5.7	5.5	5.7	5.5	5.3	5.2
England and Wales:												
Perinatal[4]	KHOK	8.8	8.6	8.7	8.5	8.9	8.9	8.8	8.4	8.3	8.1	7.9
Neonatal	KHOL	4.3	4.3	4.2	3.9	4.0	3.8	3.8	3.8	3.8	3.6	3.6
Infant mortality	KHOM	6.4	6.5	6.1	5.9	5.9	5.7	5.5	5.7	5.4	5.3	5.3
Scotland:												
Perinatal[4]	KHOO	9.6	8.4	9.5	9.2	7.9	8.4	8.8	7.6	7.7	8.4	8.1
Neonatal	KHOP	4.0	3.8	4.5	4.0	3.7	3.6	3.6	3.8	4.0	3.5	3.0
Infant mortality	KHOQ	6.2	5.7	6.4	5.8	6.4	5.4	5.8	5.7	5.6	5.2	4.6
Northern Ireland:												
Perinatal[4]	KHOS	8.9	10.5	7.9	9.6	9.8	8.1	8.2	9.2	7.3	7.3	7.6
Neonatal	KHOT	4.4	5.5	4.2	5.2	3.7	4.6	3.7	5.5	4.6	3.4	3.7
Infant mortality	KHOU	6.1	6.8	5.4	6.9	4.7	6.5	5.4	7.0	5.7	5.5	4.7
Females												
United Kingdom:												
Perinatal[4]	KHOW	7.7	7.8	7.5	7.4	7.7	8.2	7.9	7.6	7.5	7.3	7.1
Neonatal	KHOX	3.3	3.4	3.5	3.3	3.1	3.4	3.1	3.1	3.2	3.0	2.9
Infant mortality	KHOY	5.0	5.1	5.0	5.0	4.5	4.9	4.6	4.5	4.5	4.3	4.2
England and Wales:												
Perinatal[4]	KHPA	7.7	7.8	7.6	7.3	7.7	8.2	8.0	7.6	7.6	7.4	7.2
Neonatal	KHPB	3.3	3.5	3.5	3.2	3.1	3.4	3.1	3.0	3.2	3.0	2.9
Infant mortality	KHPC	5.0	5.1	5.1	4.9	4.5	4.9	4.6	4.4	4.6	4.3	4.2
Scotland:												
Perinatal[4]	KHPE	7.9	6.7	7.2	7.8	7.2	7.7	7.3	7.9	7.1	7.3	6.7
Neonatal	KHPF	3.2	2.8	3.5	3.5	2.6	3.1	2.5	3.2	2.9	3.0	2.6
Infant mortality	KHPG	4.9	4.3	5.1	5.2	4.1	4.7	4.0	4.8	3.8	4.2	3.8
Northern Ireland:												
Perinatal[4]	KHPI	7.3	9.5	6.4	6.9	7.6	7.8	7.8	6.9	6.5	6.5	7.0
Neonatal	KHPJ	3.4	4.1	3.3	3.5	3.0	3.2	3.5	4.2	2.9	3.0	3.5
Infant mortality	KHPK	5.1	5.9	4.6	5.1	4.5	3.9	5.2	5.3	4.4	4.4	4.7

1 See chapter text.
2 From 1937 to 1956 death rates are based on the births to which they relate in the current and preceding years.
3 Deaths in pregnancy and childbirth.
4 Deaths per 1,000 live and stillbirths. See chapter introduction.

Sources: Office for National Statistics;
General Register Office for Scotland;
General Register Office (Northern Ireland)

5.21 Death rates by sex and age[1]
United Kingdom

Rates per 1,000 population

	All ages	0-4	5-9	10-14	15-19	20-24	25-34	35-44	45-54	55-64	65-74	75-84	85 and over
Males													
1900 - 02	18.4	57.0	4.1	2.4	3.7	5.0	6.6	11.0	18.6	35.0	69.9	143.6	289.6
1910 - 12	14.9	40.5	3.3	2.0	3.0	3.9	5.0	8.0	14.9	29.8	62.1	133.8	261.5
1920 - 22	13.5	33.4	2.9	1.8	2.9	3.9	4.5	6.9	11.9	25.3	57.8	131.8	259.1
1930 - 32	12.9	22.3	2.3	1.5	2.6	3.3	3.5	5.7	11.3	23.7	57.9	134.2	277.0
1940 - 42	..	..	..	..	..	..	..	..	..	..	..	..	..
1950 - 52	12.6	7.7	0.7	0.5	0.9	1.4	1.6	3.0	8.5	23.2	55.2	127.6	272.0
1960 - 62	12.5	6.4	0.5	0.4	0.9	1.1	1.1	2.5	7.4	22.2	54.4	123.4	251.0
1970 - 72	12.4	4.6	0.4	0.4	0.9	1.0	1.0	2.4	7.3	20.9	52.9	116.3	246.1
1980 - 82	12.1	3.2	0.3	0.3	0.8	0.9	0.9	1.9	6.3	18.2	46.7	107.1	224.9
1990 - 92	11.2	2.0	0.2	0.2	0.7	0.9	1.0	1.8	4.6	14.2	38.6	93.0	201.4
2000 - 02	10.0	1.4	0.1	0.2	0.5	0.8	1.0	1.6	4.0	10.4	28.9	75.2	187.7
	KHZA	KHZB	KHZC	KHZD	KHZE	KHZF	KHZG	KHZH	KHZJ	KHZK	KHZL	KHZM	KHZN
1997	10.6	1.5	0.2	0.2	0.6	1.0	1.0	1.7	4.1	11.8	33.9	83.2	196.7
1998	10.5	1.5	0.1	0.2	0.6	0.9	1.1	1.7	4.1	11.6	33.0	81.8	193.6
1999	10.5	1.5	0.1	0.2	0.6	0.9	1.0	1.7	4.1	11.2	32.2	80.9	195.7
2000	10.1	1.4	0.1	0.2	0.6	0.8	1.0	1.6	4.0	10.7	30.3	76.8	187.9
2001	9.9	1.3	0.1	0.2	0.6	0.8	1.0	1.6	4.0	10.4	28.6	74.8	186.9
2002	9.9	1.4	0.1	0.2	0.5	0.8	1.0	1.6	4.0	10.1	27.8	74.1	188.2
2003	9.9	1.4	0.1	0.1	0.5	0.8	1.0	1.6	3.9	9.9	27.0	73.6	191.7
2004	9.5	1.4	0.1	0.1	0.5	0.7	0.9	1.6	3.8	9.3	25.5	70.6	176.3
2005	9.5	1.4	0.1	0.1	0.5	0.7	0.9	1.6	3.7	9.3	24.8	68.7	187.8
2006	9.2	1.3	0.1	0.2	0.5	0.7	0.9	1.6	3.7	9.1	23.7	65.5	164.5
2007	9.2	1.3	0.1	0.1	0.5	0.7	0.9	1.6	3.6	9.0	23.1	63.9	162.5
2008	9.2	1.3	0.1	0.1	0.5	0.7	0.9	1.7	3.6	8.8	22.7	62.2	162.6
Females													
1900 - 02	16.3	47.9	4.3	2.6	3.5	4.3	5.8	9.0	14.4	27.9	59.3	127.0	262.6
1910 - 12	13.3	34.0	3.3	2.1	2.9	3.4	4.4	6.7	11.5	23.1	50.7	113.7	234.0
1920 - 22	11.9	26.9	2.8	1.9	2.8	3.4	4.1	5.6	9.3	19.2	45.6	111.5	232.4
1930 - 32	11.5	17.7	2.1	1.5	2.4	2.9	3.3	4.6	8.3	17.6	43.7	110.1	246.3
1940 - 42	..	..	..	..	..	..	..	..	..	..	..	..	..
1950 - 52	11.2	6.0	0.5	0.4	0.7	1.0	1.4	2.3	5.3	12.9	35.5	98.4	228.8
1960 - 62	11.2	4.9	0.3	0.3	0.4	0.5	0.8	1.8	4.5	11.0	30.8	87.3	218.5
1970 - 72	11.3	3.6	0.3	0.2	0.4	0.4	0.6	1.6	4.5	10.5	27.5	76.7	196.1
1980 - 82	11.4	2.3	0.2	0.2	0.3	0.4	0.5	1.3	3.9	9.9	24.8	67.2	179.5
1990 - 92	11.1	1.5	0.1	0.2	0.3	0.3	0.4	1.1	2.9	8.4	22.1	58.7	157.2
2000 - 02	10.5	1.1	0.1	0.1	0.2	0.3	0.4	1.0	2.6	6.4	17.9	51.1	157.3
	KHZO	KHZP	KHZQ	KHZR	KHZS	KHZT	KHZU	KHZV	KHZW	KHZX	KHZY	KHZZ	KHZI
1997	11.0	1.2	0.1	0.1	0.3	0.3	0.4	1.1	2.7	7.1	20.5	55.2	160.3
1998	11.0	1.2	0.1	0.1	0.3	0.3	0.4	1.0	2.7	7.0	20.2	54.4	159.8
1999	11.0	1.2	0.1	0.1	0.3	0.3	0.4	1.0	2.7	6.9	19.6	54.2	163.7
2000	10.5	1.1	0.1	0.1	0.3	0.3	0.5	1.0	2.7	6.6	18.5	51.6	155.8
2001	10.4	1.1	0.1	0.1	0.2	0.3	0.4	1.0	2.6	6.4	17.8	50.8	155.8
2002	10.5	1.0	0.1	0.1	0.2	0.3	0.4	1.0	2.6	6.2	17.4	51.0	160.3
2003	10.6	1.2	0.1	0.1	0.2	0.3	0.4	1.0	2.6	6.1	17.1	51.8	166.4
2004	10.0	1.1	0.1	0.1	0.2	0.3	0.4	1.0	2.4	5.8	16.2	49.3	155.2
2005	10.0	1.1	0.1	0.1	0.2	0.3	0.4	0.9	2.5	5.9	15.8	48.2	160.1
2006	9.6	1.1	0.1	0.1	0.2	0.3	0.4	0.9	2.4	5.7	15.2	46.4	144.9
2007	9.7	1.1	0.1	0.1	0.2	0.3	0.4	0.9	2.3	5.7	14.9	45.6	144.8
2008	9.7	1.1	0.1	0.1	0.2	0.3	0.4	1.0	2.3	5.7	14.6	45.0	146.6

1 See chapter text.

Sources: Office for National Statistics;
General Register Office for Scotland;
Northern Ireland Statistics and Research Agency

5.22 Interim life tables, 2006-08

Age(x)	United Kingdom Males l_x	Males e^0_x	Females l_x	Females e^0_x	England and Wales Males l_x	Males e^0_x	Females l_x	Females e^0_x
0 years	100 000	77.4	100 000	81.6	100 000	77.7	100 000	81.8
5 years	99 373	72.9	99 481	77.1	99 370	73.2	99 479	77.3
10 years	99 314	67.9	99 437	72.1	99 312	68.2	99 435	72.3
15 years	99 246	63.0	99 385	67.1	99 246	63.3	99 383	67.3
20 years	99 011	58.1	99 275	62.2	99 027	58.4	99 278	62.4
25 years	98 663	53.3	99 145	57.3	98 703	53.6	99 153	57.5
30 years	98 262	48.5	98 979	52.4	98 324	48.8	98 991	52.6
35 years	97 740	43.8	98 739	47.5	97 833	44.0	98 759	47.7
40 years	97 069	39.1	98 378	42.7	97 196	39.3	98 412	42.8
45 years	96 157	34.4	97 810	37.9	96 325	34.6	97 856	38.1
50 years	94 797	29.9	96 911	33.2	95 016	30.1	96 985	33.4
55 years	92 677	25.5	95 484	28.7	92 962	25.7	95 596	28.8
60 years	89 489	21.3	93 373	24.3	89 852	21.5	93 537	24.4
65 years	84 583	17.4	90 117	20.0	85 077	17.5	90 362	20.2
70 years	77 232	13.8	85 149	16.1	77 865	13.9	85 532	16.2
75 years	66 692	10.5	77 413	12.4	66 477	10.6	77 951	12.5
80 years	51 826	7.8	65 356	9.2	52 668	7.9	65 040	9.2
85 years	32 514	5.7	47 007	6.6	34 258	5.7	48 733	6.6
90 years	16 658	4.0	27 849	4.5	17 169	4.0	28 475	4.5

Age(x)	Scotland Males l_x	Males e^0_x	Females l_x	Females e^0_x	Northern Ireland Males l_x	Males e^0_x	Females l_x	Females e^0_x
0 years	100 000	75.0	100 000	79.9	100 000	76.3	100 000	81.2
5 years	99 423	70.4	99 519	75.3	99 338	71.8	99 466	76.6
10 years	99 364	65.4	99 478	70.3	99 268	66.9	99 407	71.7
15 years	99 292	60.5	99 423	65.3	99 159	62.0	99 341	66.7
20 years	98 955	55.7	99 273	60.4	98 715	57.2	99 193	61.8
25 years	98 403	51.0	99 101	55.5	98 254	52.5	99 056	56.9
30 years	97 799	46.3	98 893	50.6	97 740	47.7	98 890	52.0
35 years	96 910	41.7	98 572	45.8	97 239	43.0	98 631	47.1
40 years	95 889	37.1	98 081	41.0	96 496	38.3	98 225	42.3
45 years	94 608	32.6	97 385	36.3	95 430	33.7	97 654	37.5
50 years	92 821	28.1	96 256	31.7	93 817	29.2	96 662	32.9
55 years	90 118	23.9	94 513	27.2	91 575	24.9	95 102	28.4
60 years	86 187	19.9	91 933	22.9	88 394	20.7	92 859	24.0
65 years	80 137	16.2	87 839	18.8	82 994	16.8	89 669	19.8
70 years	71 517	12.8	81 603	15.1	75 558	13.2	84 762	15.7
75 years	59 691	9.8	72 542	11.6	64 767	10.0	76 934	12.1
80 years	43 431	7.3	59 215	8.6	49 454	7.3	64 738	8.9
85 years	27 194	5.4	41 475	6.2	30 645	5.2	47 390	6.1
90 years	12 522	3.9	22 504	4.4	13 759	3.7	25 924	4.1

Note Column l_x shows the number who would survive to exact **age**(x), out of 100,000 born, who were subject throughout their lives to the death rates experienced in the three-year period indicated. Column e^0_x is 'the expectation of life', that is, the average future lifetime which would be lived by a person aged exactly x if likewise subject to the death rates experienced in the three-year period indicated. See introductory notes.

Source: Office for National Statistics: 01329 444681

Population and vital statistics

5.23 Adoptions by date of entry in Adopted Children Register: by sex, age and country

Numbers and Percentages

	All ages		Under 1		1-4		5-9		10-14		15-17	
	Numbers	Percentages	Numbers	Percentages	Numbers	Percentages	Numbers	Percentages	Numbers	Percentages	Numbers	Percentages
United Kingdom **Persons**												
	VOXI	VOXJ	VOXK	VOXL	VOXM	VOXN	VOXO	VOXP	VOXQ	VOXR	VOXS	VOXT
2002	6 239	100	313	5	2 737	44	1 937	31	999	16	253	4
2003	5 426	100	212	4	2 481	46	1 716	32	789	15	228	4
2004	6 116	100	274	5	2 843	46	1 856	30	847	14	269	4
2005	6 151	100	242	4	3 127	51	1 757	29	798	13	228	4
2006	5 539	100	216	4	2 788	50	1 608	29	696	13	226	4
2007	5 224	100	163	3	2 761	53	1 400	27	672	13	205	4
Males												
	VOXU	VOXV	VOXW	VOXX	VOXY	VOXZ	VOYA	VOYB	VOYC	VOYD	VOYE	VOYF
2002	3 140	100	176	6	1 425	45	935	30	488	16	116	4
2003	2 634	100	104	4	1 224	46	844	32	351	13	111	4
2004	3 051	100	145	5	1 426	47	936	31	418	14	126	4
2005	3 072	100	121	4	1 566	51	910	30	370	12	105	3
2006	2 708	100	97	4	1 377	51	806	30	314	12	113	4
2007	2 614	100	83	3	1 392	53	714	27	314	12	103	4
Females												
	VOYG	VOYH	VOYI	VOYJ	VOYK	VOYL	VOYM	VOYN	VOYO	VOYP	VOYQ	VOYR
2002	3 099	100	137	4	1 312	42	1 002	32	511	16	137	4
2003	2 792	100	108	4	1 257	45	872	31	438	16	117	4
2004	3 065	100	129	4	1 417	46	920	30	456	15	143	5
2005	3 079	100	121	4	1 561	51	847	28	428	14	122	4
2006	2 831	100	119	4	1 411	50	802	28	382	13	113	4
2007	2 610	100	80	3	1 369	52	686	26	358	14	102	4
England and Wales[1] **Persons**												
	GQTP	GQTQ	GQTR	GQTS	GQTT	GQTU	GQTV	GQTW	GQTX	GQTY	GQTZ	GQUA
2002	5 680	100	287	5	2 532	45	1 748	31	900	16	213	4
2003	4 818	100	183	4	2 260	47	1 503	31	683	14	189	4
2004	5 562	100	253	5	2 627	47	1 651	30	786	14	245	4
2005	5 565	100	222	4	2 906	52	1 555	28	683	12	199	4
2006	4 980	100	197	4	2 592	52	1 406	28	585	12	195	4
2007	4 637	100	151	3	2 510	54	1 206	26	576	12	171	4
Males												
	GQUB	GQUC	GQUD	GQUE	GQUF	GQUG	GQUH	GQUI	GQUJ	GQUK	GQUL	GQUM
2002	2 871	100	160	6	1 324	46	846	29	443	15	98	3
2003	2 339	100	91	4	1 115	48	737	32	301	13	95	4
2004	2 777	100	132	5	1 327	48	831	30	373	13	114	4
2005	2 791	100	112	4	1 461	52	808	29	320	11	90	3
2006	2 446	100	95	4	1 282	52	707	29	267	11	94	4
2007	2 315	100	77	3	1 253	54	618	27	270	12	89	4
Females												
	GQUN	GQUO	GQUP	GQUQ	GQUR	GQUS	GQUT	GQUU	GQUV	GQUW	GQUX	GQUY
2002	2 809	100	127	5	1 208	43	902	32	457	16	115	4
2003	2 479	100	92	4	1 145	46	766	31	382	15	94	4
2004	2 785	100	121	4	1 300	47	820	29	413	15	131	5
2005	2 774	100	110	4	1 445	52	747	27	363	13	109	4
2006	2 534	100	102	4	1 310	52	699	28	318	13	101	4
2007	2 322	100	74	3	1 257	54	588	25	306	13	82	4

5.23 Adoptions by date of entry in Adopted Children Register: by sex, age and country
continued

Numbers and Percentages

	All ages		Under 1		1-4		5-9		10-14		15-17	
	Numbers	Percentages	Numbers	Percentages	Numbers	Percentages	Numbers	Percentages	Numbers	Percentages	Numbers	Percentages

Scotland[1]
Persons

	GQUZ	GQVA	GQVB	GQVC	GQVD	GQVE	GQVF	GQVG	GQVH	GQVI	GQVJ	GQVK
2002	385	100	13	3	143	37	130	34	73	19	26	7
2003	468	100	25	5	153	33	170	36	88	19	32	7
2004	393	100	21	5	144	37	143	36	67	17	18	5
2005	439	100	18	4	162	37	155	35	81	18	23	5
2006	418	100	16	4	153	37	150	36	73	17	26	6
2007	440	100	9	2	198	45	141	32	65	15	27	6

Males

	GQVL	GQVM	GQVN	GQVO	GQVP	GQVQ	GQVR	GQVS	GQVT	GQVU	GQVV	GQVW
2002	193	100	8	4	75	39	60	31	37	19	13	7
2003	228	100	11	5	78	34	85	37	43	19	11	5
2004	200	100	13	7	67	34	77	39	34	17	9	5
2005	217	100	9	4	80	37	79	36	36	17	13	6
2006	194	100	2	1	72	37	78	40	25	13	17	9
2007	229	100	4	2	115	50	70	31	30	13	10	4

Females

	GQVX	GQVY	GQVZ	GQWA	GRFK	GRFL	GRFM	GRFN	GRFO	GRFP	GRFQ	GRFR
2002	192	100	5	3	68	35	70	36	36	19	13	7
2003	240	100	14	6	75	31	85	35	45	19	21	9
2004	193	100	8	4	77	40	66	34	33	17	9	5
2005	222	100	9	4	82	37	76	34	45	20	10	5
2006	224	100	14	6	81	36	72	32	48	22	9	4
2007	211	100	5	2	83	39	71	34	35	17	17	8

Northern Ireland[1]
Persons

	VOYS	VOYT	VOYU	VOYV	VOYW	VOYX	VOYY	VOYZ	VOZA	VOZB	VOZC	VOZD
2003	140	100	4	3	68	49	43	31	18	13	7	5
2004	161	100	4	2	70	43	61	38	20	12	6	4
2005	140	100	6	4	53	38	45	32	30	21	6	4
2006	141	100	3	2	44	31	51	36	38	27	5	4
2007	147	100	3	2	53	36	53	36	31	21	7	5
2008	97	100	–	–	48	49	30	31	13	13	6	6

Males

	VOZE	VOZF	VOZG	VOZH	VOZI	VOZJ	VOZK	VOZL	VOZM	VOZN	VOZO	VOZP
2003	67	100	2	3	31	46	22	33	7	10	5	7
2004	74	100	1	1	32	43	28	38	10	14	3	4
2005	61	100	2	3	23	38	21	34	12	20	3	5
2006	68	100	–	–	24	35	20	29	22	32	2	3
2007	70	100	2	3	24	34	26	37	14	20	4	6
2008	48	100	–	–	20	42	17	35	6	13	5	10

Females

	VOZQ	VOZR	VOZS	VOZT	VOZU	VOZV	VOZW	VOZX	VOZY	VOZZ	VPAA	VPVD
2003	73	100	2	3	37	51	21	29	11	15	2	3
2004	87	100	3	3	38	44	33	38	10	11	3	3
2005	79	100	4	5	30	38	24	30	18	23	3	4
2006	73	100	3	4	20	27	31	42	16	22	3	4
2007	77	100	1	1	29	38	27	35	17	22	3	4
2008	49	100	–	–	28	57	13	27	7	14	1	2

1 England & Wales: number of persons aged over 17 (counted into 'All ages')

Year	Persons	Male	Female
2006	5	1	4
2007	23	8	15

Scotland: number of persons aged over 17 (counted into 15-17 age group)

Year	Persons	Male	Female
2002	4	1	3
2003	4	3	1
2004	3	-	3
2006	5	5	-

Northern Ireland: number of persons aged over 17 (counted into 15-17 age group)

Year	Persons	Male	Female
2007	1	1	

Sources: Office for National Statistics: 01329 444410;
General Register Office for Scotland;
Northern Ireland Statistics and Research Agency

Education

Chapter 6

Education

Educational establishments in the UK are administered and financed in several ways. Most schools are controlled by local authorities, which are part of the structure of local government, but some are 'assisted', receiving grants direct from central government sources and being controlled by governing bodies which have a substantial degree of autonomy. Completely outside the public sector are non maintained schools run by individuals, companies or charitable institutions.

For the purposes of UK education statistics, schools fall under the following broad categories:

Mainstream state schools
(In Northern Ireland, grant-aided mainstream schools)

These schools work in partnership with other schools and local authorities and they receive funding from local authorities. Since 1 September 1999, the categories (typically in England) are:

Community – schools formerly known as 'county' plus some former grant-maintained (GM) schools

Foundation – most former GM schools

Voluntary Aided – schools formerly known as 'aided' and some former GM schools

Voluntary Controlled – schools formerly known as 'controlled'

Non-maintained mainstream schools

These consist of:

(a) Independent schools

Schools which charge fees and may also be financed by individuals, companies or charitable institutions. These include Direct Grant schools, where the governing bodies are assisted by departmental grants and a proportion of the pupils attending them do so free or under an arrangement by which local authorities meet tuition fees. City Technology Colleges (CTCs) and Academies (applicable in England only) are also included as independent schools..

(b) Non-maintained schools

Run by voluntary bodies who may receive some grant from central government for capital work and for equipment, but their current expenditure is met primarily from the fees charged to the local authorities for pupils placed in schools.

Special schools

Special schools provide education for children with Special Educational Needs (SEN) (In Scotland, Record of Needs or a Co-ordinated Support Plan), who cannot be educated satisfactorily in an ordinary school. Maintained special schools are run by local authorities, while non-maintained special schools are financed as described at (b) above.

Pupil Referral Units

Pupil Referral Units (PRUs) operate in England and Wales and provide education outside of a mainstream or special school setting, to meet the needs of difficult or disruptive children.

Schools in Scotland are categorised as Education Authority, Grant-aided, Opted-out/Self-governing (these three being grouped together as 'Publicly funded' schools), Independent schools and Partnership schools.

The home government departments dealing with education statistics are:

Department for Education (DE)

Department for Business, Innovation and Skills (BIS)

Welsh Assembly Government (WAG)

Scottish Government (SG)

Northern Ireland Department of Education (DENI)

Northern Ireland Department for Employment and Learning (DELNI)

Each of the home education departments in Great Britain, along with the Northern Ireland Department of Education, have overall responsibility for funding the schools sectors in their own country.

Up to March 2001, further education (FE) courses in FE sector colleges in England and in Wales were largely funded through grants from the respective FE funding councils. In April 2001 however, the Learning and Skills Council (LSC) took over the responsibility for funding the FE sector in England, and the National Council for Education and Training for Wales (part of Education and Learning Wales – ELWa) did so for Wales.

The LSC in England is also responsible for funding provision for FE and some non-prescribed higher education in FE sector colleges; it also funds some FE provided by local authority maintained and other institutions referred to as 'external institutions'. In Wales, the National Council – ELWa, funds FE provision made by FE institutions via a third party or sponsored arrangements. The Scottish Further Education Funding Council (SFEFC) funds FE colleges in Scotland, while the Department for Employment and Learning funds FE colleges in Northern Ireland.

Higher education (HE) courses in higher education establishments are largely publicly funded through block grants from the HE funding councils in England and Scotland, the Higher Education Council – ELWa in Wales, and the Department for Employment and Learning in Northern Ireland. In addition, some designated HE (mainly HND/HNC Diplomas and Certificates of HE) is also funded by these sources. The FE sources mentioned above fund the remainder.

Statistics for the separate systems obtained in England, Wales, Scotland and Northern Ireland are collected and processed separately in accordance with the particular needs of the responsible departments. Since 1994/95 the Higher Education Statistics Agency (HESA) has undertaken the data collection for all higher education institutions (HEIs) in the UK. This includes the former Universities Funding Council (UFC) funded UK universities, previously collected by the Universities Statistical Record. There are some structural differences in the information collected for schools, FE and HE in each of the four home countries and in some tables the GB/UK data presented are amalgamations from sources that are not entirely comparable.

Stages of education

There are five stages of education: early years, primary, secondary, FE and HE, and education is compulsory for all children between the ages of 5 (4 in Northern Ireland) and 16. The non-compulsory fourth stage, FE, covers non-advanced education, which can be taken at further (including tertiary) education colleges, HE institutions (HEIs) and increasingly in secondary schools. The fifth stage, HE, is study beyond GCE A levels and their equivalent which, for most full-time students, takes place in universities and other HEIs.

Early years education

Children under 5 attend a variety of settings including state nursery schools, nursery classes within primary schools and, in England and Wales, reception classes within primary schools, as well as settings outside the state sector such as voluntary pre-schools or privately run nurseries. In recent years there has been a major expansion of early years education, and the *Education Act 2002* extended the National Curriculum for England to include the foundation stage. The foundation stage was introduced in September 2000, and covered children's education from the age of 3 to the end of the reception year, when most are just 5 and some almost 6 years old. The Early Years Foundation Stage (EYFS), came into force in September 2008, and is a single regulatory and quality framework for the provision of learning, development and care for children in all registered early years settings between birth and the academic year in which they turn 5.

Children born in Scotland between March and December are eligible for early years education at the time the Pre-School Education and Day Care Census is carried out. In Scotland, early years education is called ante-pre-school education for those aged 3 to 4 years old, and pre-school education for those aged 4.

Primary education

The primary stage covers three age ranges: nursery (under 5), infant (5 to 7 or 8) and junior (up to 11 or 12) but in Scotland and Northern Ireland there is generally no distinction between infant and junior schools. Most public sector primary schools take both boys and girls in mixed classes. It is usual to transfer straight to secondary school at age 11 (in England, Wales and Northern Ireland) or 12 (in Scotland), but in England some children make the transition via middle schools catering for various age ranges between 8 and 14. Depending on their individual age ranges middle schools are classified as either primary or secondary.

Secondary education

Public provision of secondary education in an area may consist of a combination of different types of school, the pattern reflecting historical circumstance and the policy adopted by the local authority. Comprehensive schools largely admit pupils without reference to ability or aptitude and cater for all the children in a neighbourhood, but in some areas they co-exist with grammar, secondary modern or technical schools. In 2005/06, 88 per cent of secondary pupils in England attended comprehensive schools while all secondary schools in Wales are comprehensive schools. The majority of education authority secondary schools in Scotland are comprehensive in character and offer six years of secondary education; however in remote areas there are several two-year and four-year secondary schools. In Northern Ireland, post-primary education is provided by grammar schools and non-selective secondary schools. In England, the Specialist Schools Programme helps schools, in partnership with private sector sponsors and supported by additional government funding, to establish distinctive identities through their chosen specialisms and achieve their targets to raise standards. Specialist schools have a special focus on their chosen subject area but must meet the National Curriculum requirements and deliver a broad and balanced education to all pupils. Any maintained secondary school in England can apply to be designated as a specialist school in one of ten specialist areas: arts, business and enterprise, engineering, humanities, languages, mathematics and computing, music, science, sports and technology. Schools can also combine any two specialisms.

Academies, operating in England, are publicly funded independent local schools that provide free education. They are all ability schools established by sponsors from business, faith or voluntary groups working with partners from the local community. The Secretary of State for the former Department for Children, Schools and Families announced in July 2007, that all new academies (that is, not including those with a signed agreement although they could if they wished), would be required to follow the National Curriculum programmes of study in English, mathematics, science and information and communication technology (ICT). This is different to the previous model whereby academies had to teach English, mathematics, science and ICT to all pupils and the curriculum had to be broad and balanced.

Special schools

Special schools (day or boarding) provide education for children who require specialist support to complete their education, for example because they have physical or other difficulties. Many pupils with special educational needs are educated in mainstream schools. All children attending special schools are offered a curriculum designed to overcome their learning difficulties and to enable them to become self-reliant. Since December 2005, special schools have also been able to apply for the Special Educational Needs (SEN) specialism, under the Specialist Schools Programme. They can apply for a curriculum specialism, but not for both the SEN and a curriculum specialism.

Further education

The term further education may be used in a general sense to cover all non-advanced courses taken after the period of compulsory education, but more commonly it excludes those staying on at secondary school and those in higher education, that is courses in universities and colleges leading to qualifications above GCE A Level, Scottish

Certificate of Education (SCE) Higher Grade, GNVQ/NVQ level 3, and their equivalents. Since 1 April 1993, sixth form colleges in England and Wales have been included in the further education sector.

Higher education

Higher education is defined as courses that are of a standard that is higher than GCE A level, the Higher Grade of the SCE/National Qualification, GNVQ/NVQ level 3 or the Edexcel (formerly BTEC) or SQA National Certificate/Diploma. There are three main levels of HE course:

(i)   Postgraduate courses leading to higher degrees, diplomas and certificates (including postgraduate certificates of education (PGCE) and professional qualifications) which usually require a first degree as entry qualification.

(ii) Undergraduate courses which includes first degrees, first degrees with qualified teacher status, enhanced first degrees, first degrees obtained concurrently with a diploma, and intercalated first degrees (where first degree students, usually in medicine, dentistry or veterinary medicine, interrupt their studies to complete a one-year course of advanced studies in a related topic).

(iii) Other undergraduate courses which includes all other higher education courses, for example HNDs and Diplomas in HE.

As a result of the *Further and Higher Education Act 1992*, former polytechnics and some other HEIs were designated as universities in 1992/93. Students normally attend HE courses at HEIs, but some attend at FE colleges. Some also attend institutions which do not receive public grant (such as the University of Buckingham) and these numbers are excluded from the tables, however, the University of Buckingham is included in Table 6.10.

6.1 Number of schools by type and establishments of further and higher education
Academic years

Numbers

		1995[1]/96	2003[1]/04	2004[1]/05	2005[1]/06	2006[1]/07	2007/08	2008/09
United Kingdom:								
Public sector mainstream								
Nursery[2,3]	KBFK	1 486	3 438	3 425	3 349	3 326	3 273	3 209
Primary[4]	KBFA	23 441	22 509	22 343	22 156	21 968	21 768	21 568
Secondary[5,6,7]	KBFF	4 478	4 281	4 261	4 244	4 232	4 209	4 183
of which 6th form colleges	KPGM	..	..	..	..	..	..	..
Non-maintained mainstream[8]	KBFU	2 485	2 498	2 445	2 455	2 486	2 527	2 547
Special - all	KBFP	1 560	1 465	1 436	1 416	1 391	1 378	1 378
maintained	KPVX	1 456	1 362	1 329	1 311	1 285	1 264	1 264
non maintained	KPGO	104	103	107	105	106	114	114
Pupil referral units	KXEP	315	457	478	481	489	506	511
Universities (including Open University)[9,10,11]	KAHG	114	112	117	119	120	120	127
All other further and higher education institutions	KJPQ	611	522	530	523	507	489	..
Higher education institutions	KPVY	68	57	50	47	48	45	37
Further education institutions	KSNY	543	465	480	476	459	444	..
of which 6th form colleges	KPGP	110	102	102	102	96	95	..
England:								
Public sector mainstream								
Nursery	KBAK	547	468	456	453	446	445	438
Primary	KBAA	18 480	17 762	17 642	17 504	17 361	17 205	17 064
Secondary[5,6,7]	KBAF	3 609	3 435	3 416	3 405	3 399	3 383	3 361
of which 6th form colleges	KPGS	..	..	..	..	..	..	..
Non-maintained maintream[8]	KBAU	2 251	2 304	2 252	2 263	2 286	2 329	2 358
Special - all	KBAP	1 263	1 148	1 122	1 105	1 078	1 065	1 058
maintained	KPGT	1 191	1 078	1 049	1 033	1 006	993	985
non maintained	KPGU	72	70	73	72	72	72	73
Pupil referral units	KXEQ	291	426	447	449	448	455	458
Universities (including Open University)[9,10]	KAHM	92	89	95	96	98	98	103
All other further and higher education institutions	KJPR	503	423	431	425	411	406	..
Higher education institutions	KPXA	50	43	36	34	34	33	27
Further education institutions	KPWC	453	380	395	391	377	373	..
of which 6th form colleges	KPGV	110	102	102	102	96	95	..
Wales:								
Public sector mainstream								
Nursery	KBBK	52	34	34	33	31	28	28
Primary	KBBA	1 681	1 588	1 572	1 555	1 527	1 509	1 478
Secondary[6]	KBBF	228	227	227	224	224	222	223
of which 6th form colleges	KPGY	..	..	..	..	..	..	..
Non-maintained	KBBU	62	60	58	56	66	66	60
Special (Maintained)	KBBP	54	43	43	43	44	44	44
Pupil referral units	KZBF	24	31	31	32	41	51	53
Universities[9,11]	KAHS	7	8	7	7	7	7	9
All other further and higher education institutions	KJQP	33	28	28	28	28	26	..
Higher education institutions	KSNZ	7	5	5	5	5	4	2
Further education institutions	KPGZ	26	23	23	23	23	22	..
Scotland:								
Public sector mainstream								
Nursery[2]	KBDK	796	2 836	2 836	2 763	2 750	2 702	2 645
Primary	KBDA	2 332	2 248	2 217	2 194	2 184	2 169	2 153
Secondary	KBDF	405	386	386	385	381	378	376
Non-maintained	KBDU	151	117	118	117	116	115	113
Special - all	KBDP	196	227	226	223	224	226	234
maintained	KYCZ	164	194	192	190	190	184	193
non-maintained	KYDA	32	33	34	33	34	42	41
Universities[9]	KAHX	13	13	13	14	13	13	13
All other further and higher education institutions	KJRA	56	53	53	52	50	49	..
Higher education institutions	KPWE	9	7	7	6	7	6	6
Further education institutions	KPHB	47	46	46	46	43	43	..
Northern Ireland:								
Grant aided mainstream								
Nursery[3]	KBEK	91	100	99	100	99	98	98
Primary[4]	KBEA	948	911	912	903	896	885	873
Secondary	KBEF	236	233	232	230	228	226	223
Non-maintained	KBEU	21	17	17	19	18	17	16
Special (Maintained)	KBEP	47	47	45	45	45	43	42
Universities	KIAD	2	2	2	2	2	2	2
Colleges of education	KIAE	2	2	2	2	2	2	2
Further education colleges	KIAG	17	16	16	16	16	6	..

1 Includes revised data.

2 Nursery schools figures for Scotland prior to 1998/99 only include data for Local Authority pre-schools. Data thereafter include partnership pre-schools. From 2005/06, figures exclude pre-school education centres not in partnership with the Local Authority.

3 Excludes voluntary and private pre-school education centres in Northern Ireland (366 in total in 2007/08).

4 From 1995/96, includes Preparatory Departments in Northern Ireland Grammar Schools (17 in total in 2007/08).

5 Time series revised to show State-funded secondary schools (i.e. including City Technology Colleges (CTCs) and Academies in England, previously included in the 'Non-maintained' category). In 2007/08, there were 5 CTCs and 83 Academies in England.

6 Excludes sixth form colleges in England and Wales which were reclassified as further education colleges on 1 April 1993.

7 Includes Specialist schools in England, operational from September of the first year shown (2,799 in total in 2007/08).

8 Revised to exclude CTCs and Academies - see footnote 5.

9 Includes former polytechnics and colleges which became universities as a result of the Further and Higher Education Act 1992.

10 Includes the members of the University of London separately.

11 Includes the members of the University of Wales separately.

Sources: Department for Education;
Department for Children, Schools and Families;
Welsh Assembly Government;
Scottish Government;
Northern Ireland Department of Education;
Northern Ireland Department for Employment and Learning;
01325 391266

6.2 Full-time and part-time pupils in school[1] by age and sex[2]
United Kingdom
All schools at January[3]

Thousands

		1999	2000	2001	2002	2003	2004	2005	2006	2007[4]	2008[5]	2009
Age at previous 31 August[6]												
Number (thousands)												
England[7]	KBIA	8 310	8 346	8 374	8 369	8 367	8 335	8 274	8 216	8 149	8 102	8 071
Wales	KBIB	513	512	512	511	509	506	501	495	490	485	479
Scotland	KBIC	844	874	882	876	874	866	851	850	845	829	818
Northern Ireland[2]	KBID	352	349	348	346	345	341	337	333	329	326	323
United Kingdom	KBIE	10 020	10 081	10 116	10 102	10 095	10 048	9 963	9 893	9 813	9 742	9 691
Boys and girls												
2 - 4[8]	KBIF	1 154	1 184	1 187	1 180	1 189	1 145	1 138	1 130	1 139	1 160	1 181
5[9] - 10	KBIG	4 661	4 629	4 597	4 537	4 489	4 403	4 378	4 321	4 264	4 212	4 163
11	KBIH	762	783	771	783	791	784	758	756	739	730	744
12 - 14	KBII	2 211	2 256	2 297	2 320	2 343	2 355	2 369	2 344	2 309	2 265	2 236
15	KBIK	706	705	732	737	751	775	764	777	786	783	757
16	KBIL	283	285	287	298	290	314	304	304	314	320	329
17	KBIM	218	213	219	223	217	238	226	235	234	242	249
18 and over	KBIN	25	27	27	23	24	32	27	26	28	30	32
Boys												
14	KBIO	367	381	384	391	401	394	402	407	404	391	389
15	KBIP	361	359	374	377	384	394	390	397	401	401	387
16	KBIQ	137	138	139	145	140	150	146	146	150	154	160
17	KBIR	104	101	105	107	104	112	107	111	110	114	119
18 and over	KBIS	13	14	15	13	13	17	14	15	15	16	17
Girls												
14	KBIT	352	364	365	373	384	378	384	388	385	373	372
15	KBIU	345	346	358	360	368	379	375	380	385	382	370
16	KBIV	146	147	148	153	150	161	159	159	164	165	169
17	KBIW	114	111	114	116	113	124	119	123	124	128	131
18 and over	KBIX	11	13	12	11	11	15	12	12	13	14	15

1 From 1 April 1993 excludes 6th form colleges in England and Wales which were reclassified as further education colleges.
2 In Northern Ireland, a gender split is not collected by age but is available by year group and so this is used as a proxy.
3 In Scotland, as at the previous September.
4 Includes revised figures.
5 Provisional.
6 1 July for Northern Ireland and 31 December for non-maintained primary and secondary schools pupils in Scotland and age at census date in January for pre-school education in Scotland.
7 From 1992, figures for independent schools in England include pupils aged less than 2.
8 Includes the so-called "rising 5s" (i.e. those pupils who become 5 during the autumn term).
9 In Scotland, includes some 4-year-olds.

Sources: Department for Education;
Department for Business, Innovation and Skills;
Welsh Assembly Government;
Scottish Government;
Northern Ireland Department of Education;
Northern Ireland Department for Employment and Learning;
01325 391266

6.3 Number of pupils and teachers, and pupil:teacher ratios:[1] by school type
United Kingdom

At January[2]

Numbers

		2004	2005[3]	2006[3]	2007[3,4]	2008[3,5]	2009[3]
All schools or departments							
Total							
Pupils (thousands)							
Full-time and full-time							
equivalent of part-time	KBCA	9 812.6	9 686.7	9 613.9	9 527.6	9 459.8	9 412.1
Teachers[6] (thousands)	KBCB	561.4	562.6	568.6	570.1	575.8	579.7
Pupils per teacher[6]:							
United Kingdom	KBCC	17.6	17.3	17.0	16.8	16.5	16.4
England	KBCD	17.8	17.5	17.2	17.1	16.8	16.5
Wales	KBCE	18.0	18.0	17.6	17.6	17.5	17.5
Scotland	KBCF	15.0	14.3	13.8	13.1	12.8	12.9
Northern Ireland	KBCG	16.5	16.5	16.7	16.8	16.7	16.6
Public sector mainstream schools or departments							
Nursery							
Pupils (thousands)							
Full-time and full-time							
equivalent of part-time	KBFM	83.9	29.1	29.1	29.4	29.0	28.9
Teachers[6] (thousands)	KBFN	3.5	1.7	1.7	1.7	1.7	1.6
Pupils per teacher[6]	KBFO	23.7	17.6	17.3	17.7	17.3	17.5
Primary[7]							
Pupils (thousands)							
Full-time and full-time							
equivalent of part-time	KBFB	4 953.9	4 896.6	4 831.9	4 778.8	4 747.6	4 725.1
Teachers[6] (thousands)	KBFD	224.9	224.2	226.6	226.3	227.5	228.3
Pupils per teacher[6]	KBFE	22.0	21.8	21.3	21.1	20.9	20.7
Secondary[8,9]							
Pupils (thousands)							
Full-time and full-time							
equivalent of part-time	KBFG	4 014.1	4 001.9	3 987.1	3 941.3	3 872.8	3 803.3
Teachers[6] (thousands)	KBFH	243.8	246.6	248.5	247.6	248.0	246.5
Pupils per teacher[6]	KBFI	16.5	16.2	16.0	15.9	15.6	15.4
Special schools							
Pupils (thousands)							
Full-time and full-time							
equivalent of part-time	KPGE	102.2	100.4	99.5	99.4	99.3	100.1
Teachers[6] (thousands)	KPGG	16.9	16.8	17.0	17.0	17.1	17.2
Pupils per teacher[6]	KPGI	6.1	6.0	5.9	5.9	5.8	5.8

1 'All schools' pupil: teacher ratios exclude Pupil Referral Units and non-maintained special schools.
2 In Scotland, as at the previous September.
3 Excluding nursery school figures for Scotland as FTE pupils numbers are not available.
4 Includes revised figures.
5 Provisional.
6 Figures of teachers and of pupil/teacher ratios take account of the full-time equivalent of part-time teachers.

7 Includes preparatory departments attached to grammar schools in Northern Ireland.
8 Includes voluntary grammar schools in Northern Ireland.
9 For 2007/08, State-funded secondary schools (i.e. including City Technology Colleges (CTCs) and Academies in England, which were previously included under 'Non-maintained').

Sources: Department for Education;
Department for Business, Innovation and Skills;
Welsh Assembly Government;
Scottish Government;
Northern Ireland Department of Education;
Northern Ireland Department for Employment and Learning;
01325 391266

6.4 Full-time and part-time pupils with special educational needs (SEN) or nearest equivalent)[1], 2008/09[2] United Kingdom

By type of school

Thousands and percentages

	United Kingdom	England[2]	Wales	Scotland	Northern Ireland
All schools					
Total pupils	9 692.1	8 071.0	479.4	817.7	324.0
SEN pupils with statements	258.2	221.7	14.5	8.8	13.3
Incidence (%)[3]	2.7	2.7	3.0	1.1	4.1
State-funded schools[4]					
Nursery[5]					
Total pupils[6]	150.3	37.2	1.8	105.4	5.9
SEN pupils[7] with statements[9]	0.9	0.3	-	0.6	0.1
Incidence (%)[3]	0.6	0.8	0.8	0.5	0.9
Placement (%)[8]	0.4	0.1	0.1	6.4	0.4
Primary[10]					
Total pupils	4 868.8	4 074.9	258.3	370.8	164.8
SEN pupils without statements[10]	836.4	743.1	49.9	15.6	27.8
SEN pupils with statements	69.1	57.9	4.6	2.0	4.5
SEN Pupils with statements-incidence (%)[3]	1.4	1.4	1.8	0.5	2.8
SEN Pupils with statements-placement (%)[8]	26.7	26.1	31.5	23.2	34.2
Secondary[11]					
Total pupils	3 928.5	3 271.1	205.4	304.0	148.0
SEN pupils without statements[10]	685.2	622.9	32.7	11.9	17.6
SEN pupils with statements	77.6	65.2	5.6	2.4	4.4
SEN Pupils with statements - incidence (%)[3]	2.0	2.0	2.7	0.8	3.0
SEN Pupils with statements - placement (%)[8]	30.1	29.4	38.3	27.5	33.5
Special[12,13]					
Total pupils	100.9	85.5	4.1	6.8	4.6
SEN pupils with statements	94.8	83.1	4.0	3.5	4.2
Incidence (%)[3]	93.9	97.3	96.6	51.8	91.8
Placement (%)[8]	36.7	37.5	27.4	39.9	31.8
Pupil referral units[12]					
Total pupils	15.7	15.2	0.5	..	..
SEN pupils[4] with statements	2.1	2.0	0.1	..	..
Incidence (%)[3]	13.4	13.2	19.7	..	..
Placement (%)[8]	0.8	0.9	0.7	..	..
Other schools					
Independent[11]					
Total pupils	622.2	582.5	9.3	29.7	..
SEN pupils[4] with statements	9.0	8.7	0.3	-	..
Incidence (%)[3]	1.5	1.5	3.3	0.1	..
Placement (%)[8]	3.5	3.9	2.1	0.4	..
Non-maintained special[12]					
Total pupils	5.7	4.6	..	1.0	..
SEN pupils with statements	4.7	4.5	..	0.2	..
Incidence (%)[3]	83.3	96.7	..	22.6	..
Placement (%)[8]	1.8	2.0	..	2.6	..

1 Scotland no longer has Special Educational Needs as the Education (Additional Support for Learning) (Scotland) Act 2004 (the Act) replaces the system for assessment and recording of children and young people with special educational needs. Nursery schools include the number of children registered for pre-school education with Additional Support Needs with a Coordinated Support Plan. Primary and secondary schools include pupils with a Record of Needs or a Coordinated Support Plan, including some who also had an individualised educational Programme (IEP).

2 Includes new codes for recording SEN status following the introduction of a new SEN Code of Practice from January 2002.

3 Incident of pupils - the number of pupils with statements within each school type expressed as a proportion of the total number of pupils on roll in each school type.

4 Grant-Aided schools in Northern Ireland.

5 Includes 6,629 pupils in Voluntary and Private Pre-School Centres in Northern Ireland funded under the Pre-School Expansion Programme which began in 1998/99.

6 In Scotland, pre-school registrations for places funded by the local authority, in centres providing pre-school education as a local authority centre or in partnership with the local authority only. Children are counted once for each centre they are registered with. Figures are not directly comparable with previous years.

7 For Scotland, number of children registered for pre-school education and Additional Support Needs with a Coordinated Support Plan are likely to be an undercount as only centres that returned the full census form were asked about Coordinated Support Plans, and of those who were asked, not all completed them. Out of 2,702 centres, 713 did not provide this information.

8 Placement of pupils - the number of pupils with statements within each school type expressed as a proportion of the number of pupils with statements in all schools.

9 Includes nursery classes (except for Scotland, where they are included with Nursery schools) and reception classes in Primary schools.

10 For Scotland, those with IEP only used for the 'without statement' category.

11 City Technology Colleges (CTCs) and Acadamies in England, previously included with Independent schools are included with State-funded secondary schools, therefore figures are not directly comparable with previous years.

12 England and Wales figures exclude dually registered pupils, where applicable.

13 Including general and hospital special schools.

Sources: Department for Education;
Department for Business, Innovation and Skills;
Welsh Assembly Government;
Scottish Government;
Northern Ireland Department of Education;
Northern Ireland Department for Employment and Learning;
01325 391266

6.5 GCE, GCSE and SCE/NQ[1] and vocational qualifications obtained by pupils and students

United Kingdom

Percentages and thousands

| | Pupils in their last year of compulsory education[2] | | | | | Pupils/students in education[3] | |
| | | | | | | % achieving GCE A Levels and equivalent[4,5,6] | |
	5 or more grades A*-C[6]	1-4 grades A*-C	Grades D-G[7] only	No graded results	Total (=100%) (Thousands)	2 or more passes [8]	Population aged 17 (thousands)
2000/01							
All	51.0	24.1	19.4	5.5	729.7	37.4	717.9
Males	45.7	24.6	23.1	6.5	372.1	33.4	366.6
Females	56.5	23.6	15.5	4.4	357.6	41.6	351.3
2001/02							
All	52.5	23.7	18.4	5.4	732.5	37.4	739.0
Males	47.2	24.3	22.0	6.4	374.0	33.0	379.8
Females	58.0	23.1	14.6	4.3	358.5	42.0	359.2
2002/03							
All	53.5	23.1	18.2	5.2	750.2	38.4	771.2
Males	48.3	23.6	21.8	6.3	382.7	33.9	397.2
Females	58.8	22.7	14.4	4.1	367.6	43.2	374.0
2003/04							
All	54.2	22.7	18.8	4.4	772.0	39.2	769.5
Males	49.2	23.1	22.4	5.3	392.6	34.7	395.8
Females	59.3	22.2	15.0	3.4	379.4	44.0	373.7
2004/05							
All	57.0	22.1	17.9	3.0	759.1	38.3	788.5
Males	52.1	22.8	21.4	3.7	385.5	33.8	405.2
Females	62.1	21.4	14.2	2.3	373.5	43.1	383.4
2005/06							
All	59.0	21.4	16.9	2.7	773.8	37.3	807.3
Males	54.3	22.1	20.3	3.3	394.2	32.7	415.5
Females	63.9	20.6	13.5	2.1	379.6	42.1	391.8
2006/07							
All	61.3	20.1	17.0	1.6	778.2	45.2	791.6
Males	56.9	20.6	20.5	2.1	395.8	39.5	407.8
Females	65.8	19.5	13.4	1.2	382.4	51.2	383.8
2007/08[9]							
All	64.4	-	-	-	-	46.3	806.1
Males	60.0	-	-	-	-	41.2	415.7
Females	69.0	-	-	-	-	51.9	390.4

1 From 1999/00, National Qualifications (NQ) were introduced in Scotland but are not all shown until 2000/01. NQs include Standard Grades, Intermediate 1 & 2 and Higher Grades. The figures for Higher Grades combine the new NQ Higher and the old SCE Higher and include Advanced Highers.

2 Pupils aged 15 at the start of the acadamic year, pupils in Year S4 in Scotland. From 2004/05, pupils at the end of Key Stage 4 in England.

3 Pupils in schools and students in further education institutions generally aged 16-18 at the start of the academic year in England, Wales and Northern Ireland as a percentage of the 17 year old population. Data from 2002/03 for Wales and Northern Ireland however, relate to schools only. Pupils in Scotland generally sit Highers one year earlier than those sitting A levels in the rest of the UK, and the figures relate to the results of the pupils in Year S5/S6.

4 Figures, other than for Scotland, include Vocational Certificates of Education (VCE) and, previously, Advanced level GNVQ which is equivalent to 2 GCE A level or AS equivalents.

5 2 AS levels or 2 Highers/1Adavanced Higher or 1 each in Scotland, count as 1 A level pass.

6 Standard Grades 1-3/Intermediate 2 A-C/Intermediate 1 A in Scotland, count as 1 A level pass.

7 Grades D-G at GCSE and Scottish Standard Grades 4-6/Intermediate 1 B and C/Access 3 (pass).

8 3 or more SCE/NQ Higher Grades/2 or more Advanced Highers/1 Advanced Higher with 2 or more Higher Passes in Scotland.

9 Provisional.

Sources: Department for Education;
Department for Business, Innovation and Skills;
Welsh Assembly Government;
Scottish Government;
Northern Ireland Department of Education;
Northern Ireland Department for Employment and Learning;
01325 391266

Education

6.6 Students in further[1] education: by country, mode of study,[2] sex and age,[3] during 2007/08

United Kingdom (home and overseas students)

Thousands

	United Kingdom		England[4]		Wales		Scotland[5]		Northern Ireland	
	Full-time	Part-time	Full-time	Part-time	Full-time	Part-time	Full-time	Part-time	Full-time	Part-time
All										
Age under 16	5.1	89.8	3.7	9.0	0.3	4.0	1.0	66.7	-	10.1
16	327.4	70.8	298.0	35.8	14.3	2.9	7.7	16.3	7.5	15.8
17	284.6	71.1	255.6	40.9	12.0	3.6	9.1	17.5	8.0	9.1
18	135.5	72.5	117.5	49.5	6.1	4.0	7.2	13.0	4.7	5.9
19	53.9	65.8	45.7	46.9	2.6	4.3	3.6	10.7	2.0	3.8
20	27.5	59.3	23.1	44.0	1.3	3.9	2.2	8.5	0.9	2.9
21	18.8	57.7	15.9	44.5	0.9	3.7	1.5	7.0	0.5	2.6
22	15.2	59.0	13.0	46.4	0.7	3.8	1.2	6.3	0.3	2.4
23	12.6	58.7	10.9	46.6	0.5	3.6	0.9	6.1	0.2	2.3
24	11.2	59.8	9.8	48.0	0.5	3.7	0.8	5.8	0.2	2.4
25	10.0	60.6	8.9	48.7	0.3	3.8	0.7	5.8	0.1	2.3
26	9.3	60.6	8.2	49.0	0.3	3.7	0.7	5.8	0.1	2.1
27	9.0	60.7	8.1	49.1	0.3	3.6	0.6	5.8	0.1	2.1
28	7.9	57.5	7.1	46.8	0.3	3.5	0.5	5.3	0.1	1.9
29	7.1	51.8	6.4	42.1	0.2	3.1	0.4	5.0	0.1	1.6
30+	114.0	1 343.1	108.2	1 129.9	0.1	16.3	5.1	157.8	0.6	39.1
Unknown	0.8	10.7	0.8	8.9	-	1.9	-	-	-	-
All ages	1 053.3	2 415.7	940.9	1 786.1	43.9	179.6	43.2	343.4	25.3	106.5
Males										
Age under 16	2.9	47.8	2.1	5.3	0.2	2.2	0.5	33.7	-	6.7
16	162.9	37.7	147.4	19.2	7.2	1.4	4.0	7.9	4.4	9.1
17	139.4	37.8	124.5	22.0	5.9	1.9	4.3	9.2	4.7	4.7
18	67.8	38.6	58.8	25.3	3.0	2.2	3.2	8.0	2.7	3.1
19	28.7	35.2	24.5	24.2	1.3	2.3	1.6	6.8	1.3	2.0
20	14.9	29.7	12.7	21.4	0.7	1.8	1.0	5.1	0.6	1.4
21	9.8	26.9	8.4	20.3	0.5	1.7	0.6	3.8	0.3	1.1
22	7.8	25.8	6.8	20.2	0.3	1.7	0.5	3.0	0.2	0.9
23	6.2	24.9	5.4	19.8	0.2	1.5	0.4	2.7	0.1	0.9
24	5.4	24.8	4.8	19.9	0.2	1.5	0.3	2.5	0.1	0.9
25	4.8	25.1	4.3	20.3	0.1	1.5	0.3	2.4	0.1	0.9
26	4.3	24.6	3.9	20.0	0.1	1.5	0.3	2.3	-	0.8
27	4.1	25.0	3.8	20.3	0.1	1.5	0.2	2.3	-	0.8
28	3.7	23.5	3.4	19.2	0.1	1.4	0.2	2.2	-	0.7
29	3.2	20.9	3.0	16.9	0.1	1.2	0.1	2.1	-	0.6
30+	51.9	490.0	50.2	411.6	-	5.2	1.5	59.0	0.2	14.2
Unknown	0.7	6.0	0.7	5.2	-	0.8	-	-	-	-
All Ages	519.7	983.6	465.0	711.0	21.0	70.9	19.0	153.1	14.7	48.7
Females										
Age under 16	2.2	42.0	1.6	3.7	0.1	1.9	0.5	33.0	-	3.4
16	164.5	33.1	150.6	16.6	7.1	1.5	3.6	8.4	3.1	6.7
17	145.2	33.3	131.1	18.8	6.1	1.7	4.8	8.4	3.3	4.4
18	67.8	33.9	58.7	24.2	3.1	1.8	4.0	5.0	2.0	2.9
19	25.2	30.6	21.1	22.7	1.3	2.1	2.0	4.0	0.8	1.8
20	12.5	29.6	10.4	22.6	0.7	2.0	1.2	3.4	0.3	1.5
21	9.0	30.8	7.5	24.2	0.4	2.0	0.8	3.2	0.2	1.5
22	7.4	33.1	6.2	26.2	0.4	2.1	0.7	3.3	0.2	1.5
23	6.5	33.8	5.5	26.8	0.3	2.1	0.5	3.4	0.1	1.5
24	5.8	35.1	5.0	28.0	0.3	2.2	0.5	3.3	0.1	1.5
25	5.2	35.6	4.5	28.5	0.2	2.2	0.4	3.5	-	1.4
26	4.9	36.0	4.3	29.0	0.2	2.2	0.4	3.4	-	1.3
27	4.8	35.7	4.3	28.9	0.2	2.1	0.4	3.4	-	1.3
28	4.3	34.0	3.7	27.6	0.2	2.1	0.3	3.1	-	1.2
29	3.9	30.9	3.4	25.1	0.1	1.9	0.3	2.9	-	1.0
30+	62.1	853.0	58.0	718.3	0.1	11.1	3.6	98.8	0.4	24.9
Unkown	0.1	4.7	0.1	3.7	-	1.1	-	-	-	-
All ages	533.6	1 432.1	475.9	1 075.1	22.9	108.8	24.2	190.4	10.7	57.9

1 Further education (FE) institution figures are whole year counts. Higher education (HE) institution figures are based on the HESA 'standard registration' count.

2 Full-time includes sandwich. Part-time comprises both day and evening, including block release and open/distance learning.

3 Ages as at 31 August 2007 (1 July in Northern Ireland and 31 December in Scotland).

4 FE institution figures for England include LSC funded students only.

5 Figures for Scotland FE colleges are vocational course enrolments rather than headcounts.

Sources: Department for Education;
Department for Business, Innovation and Skills;
Welsh Assembly Government;
Scottish Government;
Northern Ireland Department of Education;
Northern Ireland Department for Employment and Learning;
01325 391266

6.7 Students in further education:[1] by country, mode of study,[2] sex and area[3] 2007/08

United Kingdom - Home and overseas students

Thousands

	United Kingdom		England[4]		Wales		Scotland[5]		Northern Ireland	
	Full-time	Part-time	Full-time	Part-time	Full-time	Part-time	Full-time	Part-time	Full-time	Part-time
All persons										
Health, Public Services and Care	110.0	330.0	100.5	265.4	-	-	6.4	56.3	3.1	8.4
Science and Mathematics	62.9	42.3	59.7	27.3	-	-	1.5	6.4	1.8	8.6
Agriculture, Horticulture and Animal Care	24.6	35.8	23.2	25.8	-	-	1.2	9.4	0.2	0.6
Engineering and Manufacturing Technologies	56.4	111.5	48.9	76.9	-	0.1	4.7	28.1	2.7	6.5
Construction, Planning and the Built Environment	58.0	76.8	48.9	52.8	-	-	3.4	17.9	5.7	6.0
Information & Communication Technology	54.7	285.1	50.6	225.3	-	-	2.5	49.4	1.6	10.4
Retail and Commercial Enterprise	72.3	78.9	69.1	68.3	-	-	0.1	1.3	3.0	9.3
Leisure,Travel and Tourism	66.1	79.8	61.7	53.7	-	-	2.5	24.4	2.0	1.7
Arts, Media and Publishing	119.3	109.4	115.5	96.7	-	-	1.4	8.8	2.4	3.9
History, Philosophy and Theology	14.9	19.6	14.3	18.3	-	-	0.5	0.8	0.1	0.5
Social Sciences	20.4	9.8	19.0	4.6	-	-	1.2	2.9	0.2	2.2
Languages, Literature and Culture	30.0	148.4	28.3	102.2	-	13.0	1.6	20.2	0.1	13.0
Education and Training	7.3	108.4	5.3	83.3	1.0	1.9	0.7	5.7	0.3	17.6
Preparation for Life and Work	174.4	570.2	165.5	507.2	-	-	8.4	53.8	0.5	9.3
Business Adiminstration & Law	66.5	158.1	62.6	135.5	-	-	2.2	14.0	1.7	8.5
Other subjects[6] / Unknown	115.6	251.6	67.8	42.8	42.9	164.7	4.9	44.1	-	-
All subjects	1 053.3	2 415.7	940.9	1 786.1	43.9	179.6	43.2	343.4	25.3	106.5
Males										
Health, Public Services and Care	28.0	74.8	27.3	57.5	-	-	0.5	15.8	0.2	1.5
Science and Mathematics	29.0	14.4	27.7	8.3	-	-	0.5	2.7	0.8	3.3
Agriculture, Horticulture and Animal Care	11.1	17.5	10.3	11.4	-	-	0.7	5.9	0.1	0.2
Engineering and Manufacturing Technologies	52.4	97.2	45.4	68.3	-	0.1	4.4	23.1	2.6	5.7
Construction, Planning and the Built Environment	55.6	72.2	46.9	49.6	-	-	3.2	16.9	5.6	5.7
Information & Communication Technology	41.1	111.4	38.1	88.9	-	-	1.8	18.4	1.3	4.1
Retail and Commercial Enterprise	11.1	20.8	10.6	18.4	-	-	-	0.5	0.4	1.9
Leisure, Travel and Tourism	38.5	43.3	36.4	34.1	-	-	1.1	8.4	1.1	0.9
Arts Media and Publishing	55.0	32.8	53.0	28.0	-	-	0.7	3.8	1.3	1.1
History, Philosophy and Theology	6.2	6.4	6.0	5.9	-	-	0.2	0.2	-	0.2
Social Sciences	8.2	3.1	7.7	1.4	-	-	0.3	0.9	0.1	0.9
Languages, Literature and Culture	10.4	50.9	9.8	33.9	-	4.0	0.6	7.4	0.1	5.6
Education and Training	2.6	36.9	1.9	24.9	0.5	0.7	0.1	1.7	0.2	9.7
Preparation for Life and Work	84.7	241.0	82.7	216.0	-	-	1.7	19.3	0.3	5.7
Business Administration & Law	31.9	54.2	30.8	47.4	-	-	0.6	4.6	0.6	2.1
Other Subjects[6]/Unknown	53.7	106.7	30.5	17.1	20.6	66.1	2.7	23.5	-	-
All subjects	519.7	983.6	465.0	711.0	21.0	70.9	19.0	153.1	14.7	48.7
Females										
Health, Public Services and Care	82.0	255.3	73.3	207.9	-	-	5.8	40.5	2.9	6.9
Science and Mathematics	34.0	27.9	32.0	19.0	-	-	0.9	3.7	1.1	5.2
Agriculture, Horticulture and Animal Care	13.5	18.4	12.8	14.5	-	-	0.5	3.5	0.1	0.4
Engineering and Manufacturing Technologies	4.0	14.3	3.6	8.6	-	-	0.3	4.9	0.1	0.9
Construction, Planning and the Built Environment	2.3	4.6	2.0	3.2	-	-	0.2	1.0	0.1	0.3
Information & Communication Technology	13.6	173.8	12.6	136.4	-	-	0.8	31.0	0.3	6.3
Retail and Commercial Enterprise	61.2	58.1	58.5	49.9	-	-	0.1	0.8	2.6	7.4
Leisure, Travel and Tourism	27.6	36.4	25.3	19.6	-	-	1.4	16.0	0.9	0.8
Arts, Media and Publishing	64.3	76.6	62.5	68.8	-	-	0.6	5.0	1.1	2.8
History, Philosophy and Theology	8.7	13.2	8.3	12.4	-	-	0.4	0.5	-	0.3
Social Sciences	12.2	6.7	11.3	3.2	-	-	0.8	2.0	0.1	1.4
Language, Literature and Culture	19.6	97.5	18.5	68.2	-	9.0	1.0	12.9	0.1	7.4
Education and Training	4.6	71.5	3.4	58.4	0.5	1.2	0.6	4.0	0.1	7.9
Preparation for Life and Work	89.7	329.2	82.8	291.2	-	-	6.7	34.5	0.2	3.6
Business Administration & Law	34.6	103.9	31.8	88.1	-	-	1.6	9.4	1.1	6.4
Other subjects[6]/Unknown	61.9	144.9	37.3	25.7	22.3	98.6	2.3	20.6	-	-
All subjects	533.6	1 432.1	475.9	1 075.1	22.9	108.8	24.2	190.4	10.7	57.9

1 Further education (FE) institution figures are whole year counts. Higher education (HE) institution figures are based on the HESA 'standard registration' count.

2 Full-time includes sandwich. Part-time comprises both day and evening including block release and open/distance learning.

3 Data are shown by sector subject area and are not directly comparable with previous years prior to 2005/06.

4 FE institution figures for England include LSC funded students only.

5 Figures for Scotland FE colleges are vocational course enrolments rather than headcounts.

6 For UK HE institutions, includes the previous subject groups not allocated to specific sector subject areas, i e. medicine & dentistry, subjects allied to medicine, biological, veterinary, physical, mathematical and computer sciences and creative arts & design.

Sources: Department for Education;
Department for Business, Innovation and Skills;
Welsh Assembly Government;
Scottish Government;
Northern Ireland Department of Education;
Northern Ireland Department for Employment and Learning;
01325 391266

6.8 Students in higher[1] education by level, mode of study,[2] sex and age,[3] 2007/08[4],[5]
United Kingdom (home and overseas students)

Thousands

	Postgraduate level						First degree		Other undergraduate		Total higher education[6]	
	PhD and equivalent		Masters and others		Total Postgraduate							
	Full-time	Part-time	Full-time	Part-time	Full-time	Part-time	Full-time	Part-time	Full-time	Part-time	Full-time	Part-time
All												
Age under 16	-	-	-	-	-	-	-	-	-	0.4	0.1	0.5
16	-	-	-	-	-	-	0.3	0.1	0.5	4.8	0.8	4.8
17	-	-	0.1	-	0.1	-	9.9	0.2	4.1	3.0	14.0	3.2
18	-	-	0.1	-	0.1	-	180.1	1.7	20.1	7.7	200.4	9.4
19	-	-	0.2	0.1	0.2	0.1	248.2	5.0	25.1	11.8	273.6	17.0
20	0.1	-	2.0	0.4	2.1	0.4	251.0	7.8	18.6	13.3	271.8	21.7
21	0.7	-	17.9	1.9	18.6	1.9	161.2	9.7	13.4	13.1	193.3	24.8
22	3.0	0.1	29.1	4.7	32.1	4.8	77.9	9.4	10.3	13.3	120.3	27.7
23	5.3	0.2	27.7	7.2	33.0	7.3	40.0	8.3	8.2	13.7	81.2	29.5
24	6.7	0.3	22.0	9.0	28.7	9.3	24.6	7.7	6.8	14.1	60.0	31.2
25	6.4	0.4	16.3	9.9	22.7	10.3	17.7	7.2	5.6	14.2	46.0	31.8
26	5.7	0.6	12.5	10.4	18.2	11.0	13.5	7.1	4.9	14.8	36.6	32.9
27	4.7	0.7	9.8	10.5	14.5	11.2	10.8	7.0	4.3	14.4	29.6	32.7
28	3.8	0.8	7.9	10.3	11.7	11.1	8.6	6.4	4.0	13.9	24.3	31.5
29	3.0	0.8	6.4	9.3	9.4	10.1	6.8	5.9	3.3	12.7	19.5	28.8
30+	18.8	18.9	39.0	161.4	57.8	180.3	66.5	121.3	43.8	303.7	168.3	606.0
Unknown	-	-	0.1	0.9	0.1	0.9	0.1	0.1	0.1	2.6	0.2	3.6
All ages	58.2	22.8	191.0	236.1	249.2	258.9	1 117.1	205.0	173.1	471.7	1 539.9	936.9
Males												
Age under 16	-	-	-	-	-	-	-	-	-	0.2	-	0.2
16	-	-	-	-	-	-	0.1	-	0.3	2.0	0.4	2.0
17	-	-	-	-	-	-	4.3	0.1	1.7	1.3	6.1	1.4
18	-	-	0.1	-	0.1	-	79.6	0.7	8.9	4.3	88.6	5.0
19	-	-	0.1	-	0.1	-	111.8	2.6	11.2	6.6	123.2	9.2
20	-	-	1.0	0.1	1.0	0.1	113.7	4.0	8.0	7.0	122.7	11.1
21	0.3	-	7.8	0.7	8.1	0.7	77.8	4.9	5.6	6.3	91.6	11.9
22	1.7	-	12.9	1.7	14.6	1.8	39.5	4.7	4.2	5.9	58.3	12.3
23	2.9	0.1	12.6	2.6	15.6	2.7	20.3	3.9	3.3	5.4	39.2	12.0
24	3.8	0.1	10.4	3.3	14.2	3.5	12.1	3.4	2.7	5.3	28.9	12.2
25	3.4	0.2	8.1	3.6	11.5	3.8	8.5	3.1	2.0	5.1	22.0	12.0
26	3.0	0.3	6.2	4.0	9.2	4.3	6.1	2.8	1.8	5.2	17.1	12.3
27	2.4	0.3	5.0	4.0	7.5	4.4	4.8	2.7	1.6	5.2	13.8	12.3
28	2.0	0.4	4.2	4.1	6.1	4.5	3.8	2.5	1.5	5.0	11.4	12.0
29	1.6	0.4	3.4	3.9	5.0	4.3	2.9	2.3	1.2	4.6	9.1	11.2
30+	10.7	9.6	20.6	69.5	31.3	79.1	21.8	44.6	12.3	102.4	65.5	226.4
Unknown	-	-	-	0.3	-	0.3	-	-	-	0.9	0.1	1.2
All ages	31.9	11.5	92.3	97.9	124.2	109.4	507.2	82.3	66.4	172.5	698.1	364.8
Females												
Age under 16	-	-	-	-	-	-	-	-	-	0.2	-	0.2
16	-	-	-	-	-	-	0.2	-	0.3	2.8	0.4	2.8
17	-	-	-	-	-	-	5.5	0.1	2.3	1.6	7.9	1.8
18	-	-	0.1	-	0.1	-	100.4	0.9	11.2	3.4	111.7	4.4
19	-	-	0.1	-	0.1	-	136.4	2.5	13.8	5.2	150.4	7.8
20	-	-	1.1	0.3	1.1	0.3	137.3	3.9	10.6	6.3	149.1	10.6
21	0.3	-	10.2	1.2	10.5	1.2	83.4	4.9	7.8	6.8	101.7	13.0
22	1.2	-	16.2	3.0	17.5	3.0	38.5	4.8	6.0	7.5	62.0	15.3
23	2.3	0.1	15.1	4.6	17.4	4.7	19.7	4.4	4.9	8.4	42.0	17.5
24	2.9	0.2	11.6	5.7	14.5	5.9	12.5	4.3	4.1	8.8	31.0	19.0
25	3.0	0.2	8.2	6.3	11.3	6.5	9.1	4.1	3.6	9.2	24.0	19.8
26	2.7	0.3	6.3	6.4	9.0	6.7	7.3	4.2	3.1	9.6	19.4	20.6
27	2.2	0.3	4.8	6.5	7.0	6.9	6.0	4.3	2.7	9.3	15.7	20.5
28	1.9	0.4	3.7	6.2	5.6	6.6	4.9	3.9	2.5	8.9	12.9	19.5
29	1.4	0.4	3.0	5.4	4.4	5.8	3.9	3.6	2.1	8.2	10.4	17.6
30+	8.1	9.3	18.3	91.9	26.5	101.2	44.8	76.7	31.5	201.3	102.9	379.5
Unknown	-	-	-	0.6	0.1	0.6	-	0.1	-	1.7	0.1	2.3
All ages	26.3	11.3	98.7	138.3	124.9	149.5	609.9	122.7	106.7	299.2	841.8	572.1

1 Includes Open University students. Part-time figures include dormant modes, those writing up at home and on sabbaticals.
2 Full-time includes sandwich. Part-time comprises both day and evening, including block release and open/distance learning.
3 Ages as at 31 August 2007 (1 July in Northern Ireland and 31 December in Scotland).
4 Figures for higher education (HE) institutions are based on the HESA 'standard registration' count. Figure for further education (FE) institutions are whole year enrolments.

5 FE institution figures for England include Learning and Skills Council (LSC) funded students only.
6 Includes data for HE students in FE institutions in Wales which cannot be split by level.

Sources: Department for Education;
Department for Business, Innovation and Skills;
Welsh Assembly Government;
Scottish Government;
Northern Ireland Department of Education;
Northern Ireland Department for Employment and Learning;
01325 391266

6.9 Students in higher[1] education by level, mode of study[2], sex and subject group[3], 2007/08[3,4]

United Kingdom - Home and overseas students

Thousands

	Postgraduate level						First degree		Other undergraduate		Total higher education[5]	
	PhD and equivalent		Masters and others		Total Postgraduate							
	Full-time	Part-time	Full-time	Part-time	Full-time	Part-time	Full-time	Part-time	Full-time	Part-time	Full-time	Part-time
All persons												
Medicine & Dentistry	4.5	2.5	3.2	7.6	7.7	10.2	43.4	0.1	0.4	0.1	51.5	10.4
Subjects Allied to Medicine	2.7	2.0	8.9	33.2	11.7	35.2	86.6	27.5	58.4	69.4	156.7	132.0
Biological Sciences	8.9	2.1	7.8	7.8	16.6	9.9	107.9	17.3	4.1	6.0	128.6	33.3
Vet. Science, Agriculture & related	0.8	0.1	1.4	1.1	2.1	1.2	11.2	0.5	3.4	4.7	16.8	6.4
Physical Sciences	8.6	0.7	5.3	3.2	13.9	3.9	51.5	6.5	1.3	5.2	66.7	15.6
Mathematical and Computing Sciences	4.7	1.0	12.3	7.0	17.0	8.0	73.2	13.1	8.1	13.8	98.3	34.9
Engineering & Technology	8.5	1.5	15.3	10.3	23.9	11.8	74.2	11.2	8.7	15.3	106.7	38.3
Architecture, Building & Planning	0.8	0.4	5.1	8.7	5.9	9.1	27.8	8.6	4.5	9.2	38.2	26.9
Social Sciences (inc Law)	6.3	2.2	31.1	21.7	37.4	23.9	158.4	28.9	10.5	37.0	206.3	89.8
Business & Administrative Studies	2.5	2.0	45.0	49.2	47.5	51.1	145.7	18.2	17.4	43.6	210.5	112.9
Mass Communication & Documentation	0.4	0.2	5.3	3.2	5.7	3.5	34.2	1.5	1.7	1.6	41.7	6.6
Languages	3.3	1.1	6.6	4.1	9.9	5.2	75.7	9.6	2.3	33.5	87.9	48.3
Historical and Philosophical Studies	3.3	1.8	5.0	5.9	8.3	7.7	52.1	12.8	0.4	15.2	60.9	35.7
Creative Arts & Design	1.4	1.0	9.4	5.5	10.8	6.6	119.7	5.2	16.9	7.4	147.4	19.1
Education[6]	1.3	3.9	28.5	59.4	29.8	63.3	42.8	9.8	9.2	48.4	81.9	121.4
Other subjects[7]	-	0.1	0.1	2.3	0.1	2.3	5.0	28.5	3.8	81.5	8.9	112.3
Unknown[5,8]	-	-	0.8	6.0	0.8	6.0	7.8	5.8	21.8	79.9	30.9	93.0
All subjects	58.2	22.8	191.0	236.2	249.2	259.0	1 117.2	205.0	173.2	471.7	1 540.0	936.9
of which overseas students	28.3	5.7	-	28.8	133.1	34.6	134.4	10.0	14.7	20.5	282.2	65.1
Males												
Medicine and Dentistry	1.8	1.3	1.3	3.5	3.1	4.8	18.0	0.1	0.1	0.1	21.2	4.9
Subjects Allied to Medicine	1.2	0.7	3.0	9.0	4.2	9.7	18.9	4.4	7.0	9.8	30.1	23.9
Biological Sciences	3.3	0.8	2.8	2.4	6.0	3.2	40.6	4.7	2.3	1.9	48.9	9.8
Vet. Science, Agriculture & related	0.3	0.1	0.7	0.6	1.0	0.6	3.3	0.1	1.5	2.2	5.7	3.0
Physical Sciences	5.4	0.4	3.0	1.9	8.4	2.3	30.2	3.8	0.7	2.7	39.3	8.8
Mathematical and Computing Sciences	3.6	0.8	9.5	5.4	13.1	6.2	55.9	9.8	6.7	9.0	75.7	24.9
Engineering & Technology	6.7	1.2	12.2	8.2	18.9	9.3	62.0	10.0	7.5	13.8	88.4	33.1
Architecture, Building & Planning	0.5	0.2	3.1	5.3	3.6	5.6	19.2	6.8	3.4	6.9	26.2	19.2
Social Sciences (inc Law)	3.1	1.1	13.4	8.7	16.6	9.8	62.5	9.9	3.3	10.0	82.4	29.7
Business & Administrative Studies	1.5	1.3	24.6	26.0	26.1	27.3	75.8	8.4	8.0	18.9	109.8	54.5
Mass Communication & Documentation	0.2	0.1	1.8	1.0	2.0	1.2	15.2	0.6	1.0	0.7	18.2	2.4
Languages	1.4	0.5	2.1	1.3	3.5	1.8	22.6	2.6	1.2	13.1	27.3	17.5
Historical and Philosophical Studies	1.9	1.0	2.5	3.0	4.3	4.0	25.1	5.2	0.2	5.3	29.6	14.5
Creative Arts & Design	0.7	0.5	3.6	2.2	4.3	2.7	46.9	1.8	7.3	2.3	58.4	6.7
Education[6]	0.4	1.5	8.4	16.6	8.8	18.1	6.5	1.2	2.3	12.2	17.6	31.5
Other subjects[7]	-	-	0.1	1.0	0.1	1.1	2.0	11.0	2.1	30.8	4.2	42.9
Unknown[5,8]	-	-	0.2	1.8	0.2	1.8	2.7	2.1	12.0	33.0	15.2	37.4
All subjects	31.9	11.5	92.3	97.9	124.2	109.4	507.2	82.3	66.4	172.5	698.1	364.7
of which overseas students	16.4	3.3	56.2	16.1	72.7	19.4	67.5	5.6	8.2	9.2	148.4	34.2
Females												
Medicine & Dentistry	2.7	1.3	1.9	4.1	4.6	5.4	25.4	-	0.4	0.1	30.4	5.5
Subjects Allied to Medicine	1.6	1.3	6.0	24.2	7.5	25.5	67.7	23.0	51.4	59.6	126.6	108.1
Biological Sciences	5.6	1.4	5.0	5.4	10.6	6.8	67.3	12.6	1.8	4.1	79.7	23.59
Vet. Science, Agriculture & related	0.4	0.1	0.7	0.5	1.2	0.6	8.0	0.3	2.0	2.4	11.1	3.4
Physical Sciences	3.2	0.3	2.3	1.3	5.5	1.6	21.2	2.7	0.7	2.5	27.4	6.8
Mathematical and Computing Sciences	1.2	0.2	2.7	1.6	3.9	1.9	17.3	3.3	1.4	4.8	22.6	10.1
Engineering & Technology	1.9	0.3	3.1	2.2	5.0	2.5	12.2	1.2	1.1	1.5	18.3	5.2
Architecture, Building & Planning	0.3	0.1	1.9	3.4	2.3	3.5	8.6	1.8	1.1	2.3	12.0	7.6
Social Sciences (inc Law)	3.2	1.1	17.7	13.0	20.9	14.1	95.9	19.0	7.2	27.0	123.9	60.1
Business & Administrative Studies	1.0	0.7	20.3	23.1	21.4	23.8	69.9	9.8	9.4	24.7	100.7	58.3
Mass Communication & Documentation	0.2	0.1	3.5	2.2	3.7	2.3	19.0	0.9	0.7	0.9	23.4	4.1
Languages	1.9	0.7	4.5	2.7	6.4	3.4	53.1	7.0	1.1	20.4	60.7	30.8
Historical and Philosophical Studies	1.5	0.8	2.5	2.9	4.0	3.7	27.0	7.6	0.2	9.9	31.3	21.2
Creative Arts & Design	0.7	0.5	5.8	3.4	6.5	3.9	72.8	3.4	9.7	5.2	89.0	12.4
Education[6]	0.8	2.4	20.1	42.8	21.0	45.1	36.3	8.6	7.0	36.2	64.2	89.9
Other subjects[7]	-	-	0.1	1.2	0.1	1.3	3.0	17.6	1.6	50.6	4.7	69.4
Unknown[5,8]	-	-	0.5	4.3	0.5	4.3	5.1	3.8	9.9	46.9	15.7	55.6
All subjects	26.3	11.3	98.7	138.3	124.9	149.5	609.9	122.7	106.7	299.2	841.8	572.1
of which overseas students	11.8	2.5	48.6	12.7	60.5	15.2	66.9	4.3	6.4	11.3	133.8	30.8

1 Higher Education Statistics Agency (HESA) higher education institutions include Open University students. Part-time figures include dormant modes, those writing up at home and on sabbaticals.
2 Full-time includes sandwich. Part-time comprises both day and evening, including block release and open/distance learning.
3 Figures for higher education (HE) institutions are based on the HESA 'standard registration' count. Figures for further education (FE) institutions are whole year enrolments.
4 FE institution figures for England include Learning and Skills Council (LSC) funded students only.
5 Includes data for HE students in FE institutions in Wales which cannot be split by level.
6 Including ITT and INSET.

7 Includes Combined and general categories.
8 Includes data for HE students in FE institutions in England, which cannot be split by subject group.

Sources: Department for Education;
Department for Business, Innovation and Skills;
Welsh Assembly Government;
Scottish Government;
Northern Ireland Department of Education;
Northern Ireland Department for Employment and Learning;
01325 391266

6.10 Students[1,2] obtaining higher education qualifications[3,4]: by level, sex and subject group, 2007/08

United Kingdom

Thousands

	Postgraduate			First Degree	Sub-degree[5]	Total higher education
	PhD and equivalent	Masters and Other	Total			
All persons						
Subject group						
Medicine & Dentistry	1.8	4.4	6.1	8.5	0.2	14.8
Subjects Allied to Medicine	1.0	11.7	12.8	32.5	39.4	84.7
Biological Sciences	2.5	6.6	9.1	31.2	4.8	45.1
Vet. Science, Agriculture & related	0.2	1.1	1.3	3.0	1.5	5.8
Physical Sciences	2.2	4.2	6.4	13.0	2.6	22.1
Mathematical & Computer Sciences	1.2	9.3	10.5	20.7	7.1	38.3
Engineering & Technology	2.1	11.5	13.7	20.4	6.0	40.0
Architecture, Building & Planning	0.2	5.9	6.1	8.7	4.3	19.0
Social Studies (inc Law)[6]	1.6	27.5	29.1	48.6	17.2	94.9
Business & Administrative Studies	0.8	43.6	44.4	45.4	15.1	104.9
Mass Communication & Documentation	0.1	4.4	4.5	9.8	1.4	15.6
Languages	0.9	5.4	6.4	21.5	4.9	32.8
Historical and Philosophical Studies	1.0	4.9	5.9	17.1	3.1	26.1
Creative Arts & Design	0.4	7.7	8.1	35.0	7.2	50.3
Education[7]	0.7	43.0	43.7	14.2	17.6	75.5
Combined, general	-	0.1	0.1	5.2	1.2	6.5
All subjects	16.6	191.5	208.1	334.9	133.5	676.5
Males						
Subject group						
Medicine and Dentistry	0.8	1.8	2.7	3.4	-	6.1
Subjects Allied to Medicine	0.4	3.1	3.5	6.1	5.4	15.0
Biological Sciences	1.0	2.2	3.2	11.0	2.1	16.3
Vet. Science, Agriculture & related	0.1	0.5	0.6	0.9	0.6	2.1
Physical Sciences	1.4	2.3	3.7	7.4	1.4	12.5
Mathematical & Computer Sciences	0.9	7.1	8.0	15.4	5.3	28.7
Engineering & Technology	1.7	9.1	10.8	17.0	5.3	33.1
Architecture, Building & Planning	0.1	3.4	3.6	6.0	3.0	12.6
Social Studies (inc Law)[6]	0.8	11.7	12.5	18.5	5.3	36.3
Business & Administrative Studies	0.4	23.0	23.5	22.4	6.9	52.8
Mass Communication & Documentation	-	1.5	1.5	4.1	0.7	6.3
Languages	0.4	1.7	2.1	6.2	1.9	10.1
Historical and Philosophical Studies	0.6	2.4	2.9	8.0	1.1	12.1
Creative Arts & Design	0.2	2.9	3.1	13.2	3.1	19.4
Education[7]	0.2	11.9	12.2	2.0	4.8	18.9
Combined, general	-	-	0.1	2.1	0.4	2.6
All subjects	9.2	84.6	93.8	143.7	47.3	284.8
Females						
Subject group						
Medicine & Dentistry	0.9	2.5	3.5	5.1	0.2	8.7
Subjects Allied to Medicine	0.6	8.7	9.2	26.4	33.9	69.6
Biological Sciences	1.5	4.4	5.9	20.2	2.7	28.8
Vet. Science, Agriculture & related	0.1	0.6	0.7	2.1	0.9	3.7
Physical Sciences	0.8	1.9	2.7	5.6	1.2	9.5
Mathematical & Computer Sciences	0.3	2.2	2.5	5.3	1.7	9.5
Engineering & Technology	0.4	2.5	2.9	3.3	0.7	6.9
Architecture, Building & Planning	0.1	2.4	2.5	2.6	1.2	6.4
Social Studies (inc Law)[6]	0.8	15.8	16.6	30.1	11.9	58.6
Business & Administrative Studies	0.3	20.6	20.9	23.0	8.1	52.0
Mass Communication & Documentation	0.1	2.9	3.0	5.7	0.7	9.3
Languages	0.5	3.7	4.3	15.4	3.0	22.7
Historical and Philosophical Studies	0.4	2.6	3.0	9.1	1.9	14.0
Creative Arts & Design	0.2	4.9	5.0	21.8	4.1	31.0
Education[7]	0.4	31.1	31.5	12.3	12.9	56.6
Combined, general	-	0.1	0.1	3.1	0.7	3.9
All subjects	7.4	106.8	114.3	191.0	86.1	391.4

1 Includes students on Open University courses. The field "gender" has changed to be consistent with the MIAP common data definitions coding frame. Students of indeterminate gender are now included in total figures but not in separate breakdowns. "Indeterminate" means unable to be classified as either male or female and is not related in any way to trans-gender.
2 Includes students qualifying on all modes of study.
3 Excludes qualifications from the private sector, except for the University of Buckingham who returned data to HESA in 2007/08.
4 Includes higher educational qualifications in higher educational institutions in the United Kingdom only. Higher education qualifications in further education institutions are excluded.

5 Excludes students who successfully completed courses for which formal qualifications are not awarded.
6 Including law.
7 Including ITT and INSET
8 Governmant Office Region in England and each UK country by location of study.

Sources: Department for Education;
Department for Business, Innovation and Skills;
Welsh Assembly Government;
Scottish Government;
Northern Ireland Department of Education;
Northern Ireland Department for Employment and Learning;
01325 391266

6.11 Qualified teachers: by type of school and sex[1]

Thousands

	Public sector mainstream schools		Non-maintained mainstream schools	All special schools	Total[6]
	Nursery[2,3,4] and primary	Secondary[5]			
All full-time teachers					
United Kingdom					
1990/91[7]	208.8	233.1	44.9	19.0	505.7
1995/96[7,8]	211.8	222.1	48.6	17.2	499.7
2000/01[9,10]	211.2	225.7	52.3	16.5	505.7
2002/03[11]	210.5	229.7	53.6	19.8	513.6
2003/04	210.6	229.7	55.8	19.8	516.0
2004/05	208.5	232.5	56.3	19.9	517.2
2005/06	208.4	233.8	57.2	20.4	519.8
2006/07	207.0	234.4	58.7	20.5	520.6
2007/08[12]	206.3	231.7	62.0	20.6	520.6
of which:					
England and Wales[1]	176.8	197.8	59.2	17.8	451.6
Scotland	22.0	24.3	2.7	2.2	51.1
Northern Ireland	7.5	9.7	0.1	0.7	18.0
Full-time male teachers					
United Kingdom					
1990/91[7]	37.7	120.7	20.6	5.9	184.9
1995/96[7,8]	35.5	107.9	21.1	5.4	169.8
2000/01[9,10]	32.1	102.9	21.3	5.0	161.3
2002/03[11]	31.7	101.6	21.6	5.9	160.8
2003/04	31.7	101.5	22.7	5.9	161.9
2004/05	31.2	101.6	22.9	5.9	161.6
2005/06	31.0	100.8	23.5	6.0	161.3
2006/07	30.7	99.9	23.9	6.1	160.6
2007/08[12]	30.6	97.5	25.2	6.1	159.3
of which:					
England and Wales[1]	27.7	83.7	24.1	5.4	140.9
Scotland	1.6	10.2	1.0	0.5	13.4
Northern Ireland	1.3	3.6	-	0.1	5.0
Full-time female teachers					
United Kingdom					
1990/91[7]	171.1	112.3	24.3	13.1	320.8
1995/96[7,8]	176.3	114.2	27.4	11.8	329.9
2000/01[9,10]	179.1	122.8	30.9	11.6	344.4
2002/03[11]	178.8	128.2	32.0	13.9	352.8
2003/04	178.9	128.2	33.0	13.9	354.0
2004/05	177.3	130.9	33.4	14.0	355.6
2005/06	175.8	133.1	33.7	14.3	356.8
2006/07	174.6	134.5	34.8	14.4	358.3
2007/08[12]	174.0	134.2	36.8	14.6	359.6
of which:					
England and Wales[1]	149.1	114.1	35.1	12.4	310.7
Scotland	18.6	14.1	1.6	1.6	36.0
Northern Ireland	6.2	6.1	0.1	0.6	12.9
All full time equivalents (FTE) of part-time teachers					
United Kingdom					
1990/91	..	..	..	..	30.0
1995/96[7,8]	19.1	17.7	8.9	1.5	47.2
2000/01[9,10]	21.9	16.7	10.2	1.6	50.4
2002/03[11]	23.8	17.8	11.1	1.7	54.4
2003/04	26.4	19.5	11.4	1.9	59.3
2004/05	27.5	20.6	11.5	1.9	61.4
2005/06	30.1	21.5	11.6	2.0	65.2
2006/07	31.1	22.1	11.8	2.1	67.1
2007/08[12]	33.0	23.0	12.1	2.2	70.2

1 Public sector teachers numbers in England & Wales have been provided from the 618G survey and gender split has been calculated by using the proportions from the Database of Teacher Records (DTR).
2 From 2005/06, data for Scotland include only centres providing pre-school education as a local authority centre or in partnership with the local authority. Figures are not therefore directly comparable with previous years.
3 From 2005/06, for Scotland pre-school education centres, the total full-time equivalent (FTE) of General Teaching Council of Scotland (GTC) registered staff has been provided within the 'full-time' section only because information on full time/part-time split is not available. Teachers are counted once for each centre they work for, so the number of teachers contains some double counting. However, as each centre calculates the teacher's FTE as the time they spend working in that centre, the FTE should not be double-counted. Full-time/part-time figures for 2004/05 are estimates based on the headcount of all GTC registered staff.
4 For Scotland pre-school education centres FTE staff, a gender split is not available. Gender figures for 2004/05 are estimates based on the head-count of all GTC registered staff.

5 From 1993/94 excludes sixth form colleges in England and Wales which were reclassified as further education colleges on 1 April 1993.
6 Excludes Pupil Referral Units (PRUs).
7 Figures for non-maintained mainstream schools refer to Great Britain.
8 Includes 1994/95 data for Northern Ireland.
9 Includes 1999/00 pre-school data for Scotland.
10 Includes 2001/02 data for Northern Ireland.
11 Includes 2001/02 pre-school and 2003/04 school data for Scotland.
12 Provisional.

Sources: Department for Education;
Department for Business, Innovation and Skills;
Welsh Assembly Government;
Scottish Government;
Northern Ireland Department of Education;
Northern Ireland Department for Employment and Learning;
01325 391266

Labour market

Chapter 7

Labour market

Labour Force Survey

(Tables 7.1–7.3, 7.6, 7.9, 7.10–7.11, 7.13 and 7.16–7.18)

Labour Force Survey

Background

The Labour Force Survey (LFS) is the largest regular household survey in the UK, with interviews being conducted continuously throughout the year. In any three-month period, a nationally representative sample of approximately 110,000 people, aged 16 and over, in around 50,000 households are interviewed. Each household is interviewed five times, at three-monthly intervals. The initial interview is done face-to-face by an interviewer visiting the address, except for residents north of the Caledonian Canal in Scotland. The other interviews are done by telephone wherever possible. The survey asks a series of questions about respondents' personal circumstances and their labour market activity. Most questions refer to activity in the week before the interview.

The LFS collects information on a sample of the population. To convert this information to give estimates for the population the data must be grossed. This is achieved by calculating weighting factors (often referred to simply as weights) which can be applied to each sampled individual in such a way that the weighted-up results match estimates or projections of the total population in terms of age distribution, sex and region of residence. There is a considerable amount of ongoing research to improve methodologies. Whenever methodologies are implemented the estimates may be revised.

The concepts and definitions used in the LFS are agreed by the International Labour Organisation (ILO) – an agency of the United Nations. The definitions are used by European Union member countries and members of the Organisation for Economic Co-operation and Development (OECD).

The LFS was carried out every two years from 1973 to 1983. The ILO definition was first used in 1984. This was also the first year in which the survey was conducted on an annual basis with results available for every spring quarter (representing an average of the period from March to May). The survey moved to a continuous basis in spring 1992 in Great Britain and in winter 1994/95 in Northern Ireland, with average quarterly results published four times a year for seasonal quarters: spring (March to May), summer (June to August), autumn (September to November) and winter (December to February). From April 1998, results are published 12 times a year for the average of three consecutive months.

Strengths and limitations of the LFS

The LFS produces coherent labour market information on the basis of internationally standard concepts and definitions. It is a rich source of data on a wide variety of labour market and personal characteristics. It is the most suitable source for making comparisons between countries. The LFS is designed so that households interviewed in each three-month period constitute a representative sample of UK households. The survey covers those living in private households and nurses in National Health Service accommodation. Students living in halls of residence have been included since 1992 as information about them is collected at their parents' address.

However the LFS has its limitations. It is a sample survey and is therefore subject to sampling variability. The survey does not include people living in institutions such as hostels, hotels, boarding houses, mobile home sites or residential homes. 'Proxy' reporting (when members of the household are not present at the interview and another member of the household answers the questions on their behalf) can affect the quality of information on topics such as earnings, hours worked, benefit receipt and qualifications. Around a third of interviews are conducted by proxy, usually by a spouse or partner but sometimes by a parent or other near relation. LFS estimates are also potentially affected by non-response.

Sampling Variability

Survey estimates are prone to *sampling variability*. The easiest way to explain this concept is by example. In the September to November 1997 period, ILO unemployment in Great Britain (seasonally adjusted) stood at 1,847,000. If we drew another sample for the same period we could get a different result, perhaps 1,900,000 or 1,820,000.

In theory, we could draw many samples, and each would give a different result. This is because each sample would be made up of different people who would give different answers to the questions. The spread of these results is the sampling variability. Sampling variability is determined by a number of factors including the sample size, the variability of the population from which the sample is drawn and the sample design. Once we know the sampling variability we can calculate a range of values about the sample estimate that represents the expected variation with a given level of assurance. This is called a confidence interval. For a 95 per cent confidence interval we expect that in 95 per cent of the samples (19 times out of 20) the confidence interval will contain the true value that would be obtained by surveying the entire population. For the example given above, we can be 95 per cent confident that the true value was in the range 1,791,000 to 1,903,000.

Unreliable estimates

Estimates of small numbers have relatively wide confidence intervals making them unreliable. For this reason, ONS does not currently publish LFS estimates below 10,000.

Non-response

All surveys are subject to non-response – that is respondents in the sample who either refuse to take part in the survey or who cannot be contacted. Non-response can introduce bias to a survey, particularly if the people not responding have characteristics that are different from those who do respond.

The LFS has a response rate of around 65 per cent to the first interview, and over 90 per cent of those who are interviewed once go on to complete all five interviews. These are relatively high levels for a household survey.

Any bias from non-response is minimised by weighting the results. Weighting (or grossing) converts sample data to represent the full population. In the LFS, the data are weighted separately by age, sex and area of residence to population estimates based on the census. Weighting also adjusts for people not in the survey and thus minimises non-response bias.

LFS concepts and definitions

Discouraged worker – A sub-group of the economically inactive population who said although they would like a job their main reason for not seeking work was because they believed there were no jobs available.

Economically active – People aged 16 and over who are either in employment or unemployed.

Economic activity rate – The number of people who are in employment or unemployed expressed as a percentage of the relevant population.

Economically inactive – People who are neither in employment nor unemployed. These include those who want a job but have not been seeking work in the last four weeks; those who want a job and are seeking work but are not available to start; and those who do not want a job.

Employment – People aged 16 and over who did at least one hour of paid work in the reference week (as an employee or self-employed); those who had a job that they were temporarily away from; those on government-supported training and employment programmes; and those doing unpaid family work.

Employees – The division between employees and self employed is based on survey respondents' own assessment of their employment status.

Full-time – The classification of employees, self-employed and unpaid family workers in their main job as full-time or part-time is on the basis of self-assessment. However, people on government supported employment and training programmes that are at college in the reference week are classified, by convention, as part-time.

Government-supported training and employment programmes – Comprise all people aged 16 and over participating in one of the government's employment and training programmes (Youth Training, Training for Work and Community Action), together with those on similar programmes administered by Training and Enterprise Councils in England and Wales, or Local Enterprise Companies in Scotland.

Hours worked – Respondents to the LFS are asked a series of questions enabling the identification of both their usual hours and their actual hours. Total hours include overtime (paid and unpaid) and exclude lunch breaks.

- *Actual hours worked* – Actual hours worked statistics measure how many hours were actually worked. These statistics are directly affected by changes in the number of people in employment and in the number of hours that individual works

- *Usual hours worked* – Usual hours worked statistics measure how many hours people usually work per week. Compared with actual hours worked, they are not affected by absences and so can provide a better measure of normal working patterns

Unemployment – The number of unemployed people in the UK is measured through the LFS following the internationally agreed definition recommended by the International Labour Organisation (ILO), an agency of the United Nations.

Unemployed people who are:

1. without a job, have actively sought work in the last four weeks and are available to start work in the next two weeks or

2. out of work, have found a job and are waiting to start in the next two weeks

Unemployment (rate) – The number of unemployed people expressed as a percentage of the relevant economically active population.

Unemployment (duration) – The duration of a respondents' unemployment is defined as the shorter of the following two periods:

- duration of active search for work

- length of time since employment

Part-time – see full-time.

Second jobs – Jobs which LFS respondents hold in addition to a main full-time or part-time job.

Self-employment – See Employees.

Temporary employees – In the LFS these are defined as those employees who say that their main job is non-permanent in one of the following ways: fixed period contract, agency temping, casual work, seasonal work or other temporary work.

Unpaid family workers – Persons doing unpaid work for a business they own or for a business that a relative owns.

International Employment Comparisons

(Table 7.7)

All employment rates for European Union (EU) countries published by Eurostat (including the rate for the UK) are based on the population aged 15–64. The rates for Canada and Japan are also based on the population aged 15–64, but the rate for the US is for those aged 16–64. The employment rate for the UK published by ONS is based on the working age population aged 16–64 (men) and 16–59 (women) and

therefore takes into account both the current school leaving age and state pension ages.

The unemployment rate published by Eurostat for most EU countries (but not for the UK), are calculated by extrapolating from the most recent LFS data using monthly registered unemployment data. A standard population basis (15–74) is used by Eurostat except for Spain and the UK (16–74). The unemployment rate for the US is based on those aged 16 and over, but the rates for Canada and Japan are for those aged 15 and over. All unemployment rates are seasonally adjusted.

The unemployment rate for the UK published by Eurostat is based on the population aged 16–74 while the unemployment rate for the UK published by ONS is based on those aged 16 and over. There are other minor definitional differences.

Jobseekers allowance claimant count

(Tables 7.14 and 7.15)

This is a count of all people claiming Jobseeker's Allowance (JSA) at Jobcentre Plus local offices. People claiming JSA must declare that they are:

- out of work

- capable of work

- available for work

- actively seeking work

during the week in which the claim is made.

All people claiming JSA on the day of the monthly count are included in the claimant count, irrespective of whether they are actually receiving benefits. Also see table 10.6 in Social protection chapter.

Labour disputes

(Table 7.19)

These figures exclude details of stoppages involving fewer than ten workers or lasting less than one day, except any in which the aggregate number of working days lost is 100 or more. There may be some under-recording of small or short stoppages; this would have much more effect on the total of stoppages than of working days lost. Some stoppages which affected more than one industry group have been counted under each of the industries but only once in the totals. Stoppages have been classified using the *Standard Industrial Classification (SIC) 2003*.

The figures for working days lost and workers involved have been rounded and consequently the sum of the constituent items may not agree with the totals. Classifications by size are based on the full duration of stoppages where these continue into the following year. Working days lost per thousand employees are based on the latest available mid-year (June) estimates of employee jobs.

Annual Survey of Hours and Earnings

(Tables 7.20, 7.21, 7.24 and 7.25)

The Annual Survey of Hours and Earnings (ASHE) is based on a one per cent sample of employee jobs taken from HM Revenue & Customs (HMRC) PAYE records. Information on earnings and paid hours worked is obtained from employers and treated confidentially. ASHE does not cover the self-employed nor does it cover employees not paid during the reference period.

The headline statistics for ASHE are based on the median rather than the mean. The median is the value below which 50 per cent of employees fall. It is ONS's preferred measure of average earnings as it is less affected by a relatively small number of very high earners and the skewed distribution of earnings. It therefore gives a better indication of typical pay than the mean.

The earnings information presented relates to gross pay before tax, National Insurance or other deductions, and excludes payments in kind. With the exception of annual earnings, the results are restricted to earnings relating to the survey pay period and so exclude payments of arrears from another period made during the survey period; any payments due as a result of a pay settlement, but not yet paid at the time of the survey, will also be excluded.

More detailed information is available on the ONS website at: www.statistics.gov.uk/StatBase/Product.asp?vlnk=13101

• to increase the estimates of the level of average weekly pay over estimates published from the NES

• for males the increase in estimates of earnings is more than the increase for females. In particular this affects hourly pay excluding overtime, which is used in the calculation of ONS's preferred measure of the gender pay gap. The estimate of hourly pay for males is increased more then the estimate for females, which widens the estimate of the gap between male and female hourly pay

• estimates of the level of earnings for people working in London are increased more than estimates for other regions. This widens the estimate of the difference in pay between London and other regions of the UK

For information about methodological changes to the 2007 ASHE survey see: www.statistics.gov.uk/downloads/theme_labour/ASHE/ChangeInASHE07.pdf

Trade unions

(Table 7.26)

The statistics relate to all organisations of employees known to the Certification Officer with head offices in the UK that fall within the appropriate definition of a trade union in the Trade Union and Labour Relations (Consolidation) Act 1992. Included in the data are home and overseas membership figures of contributory and non-contributory members. Employment status of members is not provided and the

figures may therefore include some people who are self-employed, unemployed or retired.

7.1 Labour force summary:[1] by sex
United Kingdom
At Quarter 2 each year[2]. Seasonally adjusted

Thousands and percentages

All aged 16 & over

	All aged 16 & over	Total economically active	Total in employment	Total unemployed	Economically inactive	Economic activity rate(%)	Employment rate[2] (%)	Unemployment rate[3] (%)	Economic inactivity rate[4] (%)
People									
	MGSL	MGSF	MGRZ	MGSC	MGSI	MGWG	MGSR	MGSX	YBTC
2002	46 787	29 450	27 921	1 529	17 337	63.0	59.7	5.2	37.0
2003	47 087	29 675	28 186	1 489	17 411	63.0	59.9	5.1	37.0
2004	47 448	29 909	28 485	1 424	17 538	63.0	60.0	4.8	37.0
2005	47 871	30 239	28 774	1 465	17 632	63.2	60.1	4.9	36.8
2006	48 268	30 698	29 030	1 669	17 570	63.6	60.2	5.4	36.4
2007	48 668	30 875	29 222	1 653	17 793	63.5	60.0	5.3	36.5
2008	49 059	31 220	29 443	1 776	17 839	63.6	60.0	5.7	36.4
2009	49 468	31 374	28 979	2 395	18 093	63.5	58.6	7.6	36.5
Men									
	MGSM	MGSG	MGSA	MGSD	MGSJ	MGWH	MGSS	MGSY	YBTD
2002	22 600	16 018	15 099	920	6 582	70.8	66.8	5.7	29.1
2003	22 775	16 161	15 262	900	6 614	71.0	67.0	5.6	29.0
2004	22 978	16 240	15 405	836	6 738	70.7	67.1	5.1	29.3
2005	23 214	16 397	15 535	862	6 817	70.6	66.9	5.3	29.4
2006	23 438	16 628	15 662	966	6 811	70.9	66.9	5.8	29.1
2007	23 668	16 757	15 813	944	6 911	70.8	66.8	5.6	29.2
2008	23 891	16 941	15 894	1 047	6 950	70.9	66.5	6.2	29.1
2009	24 104	16 962	15 497	1 465	7 142	70.3	64.3	8.6	29.6
Women									
	MGSN	MGSH	MGSB	MGSE	MGSK	MGWI	MGST	MGSZ	YBTE
2002	24 186	13 432	12 823	609	10 755	55.5	53.0	4.5	44.5
2003	24 311	13 515	12 925	590	10 797	55.6	53.1	4.4	44.4
2004	24 469	13 669	13 080	589	10 800	55.8	53.5	4.3	44.2
2005	24 657	13 842	13 239	603	10 815	56.1	53.7	4.4	43.9
2006	24 830	14 070	13 367	704	10 760	56.7	53.8	5.0	43.3
2007	25 001	14 118	13 409	709	10 883	56.5	53.7	5.1	43.5
2008	25 168	14 278	13 549	729	10 889	56.8	53.8	5.1	43.3
2009	25 364	14 412	13 482	930	10 952	56.8	53.1	6.4	43.2

All aged 16 to 59/64

	All aged 16 to 59/64	Total economically active	Total in employment	Total unemployed	Economically inactive	Economic activity rate(%)	Employment rate(%)	Unemployment rate(%)	Economic inactivity rate(%)
People									
	YBTF	YBSK	YBSE	YBSH	YBSN	MGSO	MGSU	YBTI	YBTL
2002	36 304	28 542	27 034	1 509	7 762	78.6	74.5	5.3	21.4
2003	36 514	28 713	27 240	1 472	7 801	78.6	74.6	5.2	21.3
2004	36 773	28 893	27 486	1 407	7 880	78.6	74.7	4.9	21.4
2005	37 089	29 149	27 705	1 445	7 940	78.6	74.7	5.0	21.4
2006	37 365	29 506	27 863	1 643	7 859	78.9	74.6	5.6	21.0
2007	37 565	29 625	27 996	1 629	7 940	78.9	74.6	5.5	21.1
2008	37 743	29 871	28 120	1 751	7 872	79.1	74.5	5.9	20.9
2009	37 922	29 956	27 597	2 359	7 967	79.0	72.8	7.9	21.0
Men									
	YBTG	YBSL	YBSF	YBSI	YBSO	MGSP	MGSV	YBTJ	YBTM
2002	18 727	15 712	14 801	911	3 015	83.9	79.0	5.8	16.1
2003	18 855	15 823	14 932	891	3 032	83.9	79.2	5.6	16.1
2004	19 010	15 894	15 068	827	3 116	83.6	79.3	5.2	16.4
2005	19 198	16 027	15 175	852	3 171	83.5	79.0	5.3	16.5
2006	19 380	16 228	15 272	955	3 152	83.7	78.8	5.9	16.3
2007	19 549	16 341	15 407	935	3 208	83.6	78.8	5.7	16.4
2008	19 688	16 487	15 452	1 035	3 201	83.8	78.5	6.3	16.3
2009	19 807	16 504	15 055	1 449	3 304	83.3	76.0	8.8	16.7
Women									
	YBTH	YBSM	YBSG	YBSJ	YBSP	MGSQ	MGSW	YBTK	YBTN
2002	17 577	12 830	12 232	598	4 747	73.0	69.6	4.6	27.0
2003	17 660	12 890	12 309	582	4 769	73.0	69.7	4.5	27.0
2004	17 763	12 999	12 419	580	4 765	73.2	69.9	4.4	26.8
2005	17 891	13 123	12 530	592	4 769	73.3	70.0	4.5	26.7
2006	17 985	13 278	12 591	688	4 707	73.8	70.0	5.2	26.1
2007	18 016	13 284	12 589	695	4 732	73.8	69.9	5.3	26.3
2008	18 055	13 384	12 669	716	4 671	74.1	70.2	5.3	25.8
2009	18 116	13 452	12 542	910	4 664	74.3	69.2	6.8	25.7

1 The Labour Force Survey (LFS) is a survey of the population of private households, student halls of residence and NHS accommodation.
2 The headline employment rate is the number of working age people (aged 16 to 59 for women and 16 to 64 for men) in employment divided by the working age population.

3 The headline unemployment rate is the number unemployed people (aged 16+) divided by the economically active population (aged 16+). The economically active population is defined as those in employment plus those who are unemployed.
4 The headline inactivity rate is the number of working age inactive people (aged 16 to 59 for women and 16 to 64 for men) divided by the work population.

Sources: Labour Force Survey: Office for National Statistics;;
Helpline: 01633 456901

7.2 Employment status: full-time, part-time and temporary employees
United Kingdom
Seasonally adjusted

Thousands

| | All in employment | | | | | Total employment[1] | | Employees[1] | | Self-employed[1] | | |
	Total	Employees	Self employed	Unpaid family workers	Government supported training and employment programmes	Full-time	Part-time	Full-time	Part-time	Full-time	Part-time	Workers with second jobs
People												
	MGRZ	MGRN	MGRQ	MGRT	MGRW	YCBE	YCBH	YCBK	YCBN	YCBQ	YCBT	YCBW
2002	27 921	24 386	3 337	95	103	20 809	7 112	18 173	6 213	2 565	772	1 150
2003	28 186	24 427	3 565	95	100	20 915	7 271	18 116	6 311	2 730	834	1 116
2004	28 485	24 645	3 618	97	124	21 131	7 354	18 265	6 381	2 789	830	1 073
2005	28 774	24 929	3 636	96	115	21 484	7 290	18 596	6 333	2 811	825	1 058
2006	29 030	25 098	3 738	97	97	21 642	7 388	18 712	6 386	2 864	874	1 053
2007	29 222	25 204	3 806	102	110	21 801	7 422	18 844	6 360	2 891	915	1 097
2008	29 443	25 407	3 826	101	110	21 938	7 505	18 969	6 438	2 911	915	1 122
2009	28 979	24 937	3 850	87	106	21 362	7 618	18 422	6 515	2 887	963	1 138
Men												
	MGSA	MGRO	MGRR	MGRU	MGRX	YCBF	YCBI	YCBL	YCBO	YCBR	YCBU	YCBX
2002	15 099	12 559	2 444	33	63	13 606	1 493	11 430	1 129	2 131	313	480
2003	15 262	12 566	2 604	34	58	13 691	1 570	11 388	1 178	2 259	345	461
2004	15 405	12 634	2 659	39	73	13 776	1 629	11 413	1 222	2 313	346	456
2005	15 535	12 768	2 666	35	67	13 887	1 649	11 517	1 251	2 322	344	455
2006	15 662	12 857	2 710	38	58	13 975	1 688	11 579	1 279	2 355	356	452
2007	15 813	12 950	2 762	39	61	14 068	1 745	11 650	1 301	2 379	384	454
2008	15 894	13 011	2 780	37	67	14 072	1 822	11 643	1 368	2 393	387	461
2009	15 497	12 657	2 747	34	59	13 635	1 862	11 253	1 404	2 351	396	488
Women												
	MGSB	MGRP	MGRS	MGRV	MGRY	YCBG	YCBJ	YCBM	YCBP	YCBS	YCBV	YCBY
2002	12 823	11 827	893	63	40	7 203	5 620	6 743	5 084	434	459	670
2003	12 925	11 861	961	60	42	7 224	5 701	6 729	5 133	471	490	656
2004	13 080	12 011	960	58	51	7 355	5 726	6 852	5 159	476	484	617
2005	13 239	12 161	970	61	48	7 598	5 642	7 079	5 082	489	481	603
2006	13 367	12 241	1 027	59	39	7 667	5 700	7 133	5 108	510	518	602
2007	13 409	12 254	1 044	63	49	7 732	5 677	7 194	5 060	512	532	643
2008	13 549	12 396	1 047	64	42	7 866	5 683	7 327	5 070	518	529	661
2009	13 482	12 280	1 103	53	46	7 726	5 756	7 168	5 111	536	567	650

| | Temporary employees (reason for temporary working) | | | | | | | Part-time workers (reasons for working part-time)[2] | | | | | |
	Total	Total as % of all employees	Could not find permanent job	% that could not find permanent job	Did not want a permanent job	Had a contract with period of training	Some other reason	Total[3]	Could not find full-time job	% that could not find full-time job	Did not want a full time job	Ill or disabled	Student or at school
People													
	YCBZ	YCCC	YCCF	YCCI	YCCL	YCCO	YCCR	YCCU	YCCX	YCDA	YCDD	YCDG	YCDJ
2002	1 587	6.5	423	26.7	467	82	613	6 985	571	8.2	5 148	138	1 100
2003	1 516	6.2	399	26.3	455	87	577	7 145	567	8.0	5 255	156	1 134
2004	1 509	6.1	384	25.5	430	99	597	7 211	549	7.6	5 291	177	1 163
2005	1 445	5.8	362	25.0	389	100	593	7 157	589	8.2	5 223	167	1 147
2006	1 479	5.9	374	25.3	427	103	576	7 260	637	8.8	5 221	181	1 181
2007	1 500	5.9	396	26.4	426	94	583	7 275	689	9.5	5 226	175	1 152
2008	1 399	5.5	360	25.7	404	85	550	7 353	713	9.7	5 247	197	1 153
2009	1 430	5.7	452	31.6	376	82	520	7 478	971	12.9	5 163	186	1 114
Men													
	YCCA	YCCD	YCCG	YCCJ	YCCM	YCCP	YCCS	YCCV	YCCY	YCDB	YCDE	YCDH	YCDK
2002	721	5.8	233	32.3	186	43	260	1 442	233	16.2	650	60	489
2003	697	5.5	225	32.2	185	38	250	1 523	249	16.4	705	69	489
2004	709	5.6	222	31.3	175	47	265	1 567	246	15.7	745	69	498
2005	681	5.3	204	30.0	169	53	256	1 595	236	14.8	769	74	504
2006	677	5.3	196	29.0	176	53	252	1 634	263	16.1	775	75	511
2007	699	5.4	211	30.1	186	45	258	1 684	283	16.9	820	75	495
2008	641	4.9	184	28.7	165	44	249	1 755	306	17.5	854	76	503
2009	677	5.3	243	36.0	152	43	240	1 800	432	24.0	795	78	478
Women													
	YCCB	YCCE	YCCH	YCCK	YCCN	YCCQ	YCCT	YCCW	YCCZ	YCDC	YCDF	YCDI	YCDL
2002	866	7.3	191	22.0	282	40	354	5 544	337	6.1	4 498	78	611
2003	819	6.9	174	21.2	270	49	327	5 622	318	5.6	4 550	87	645
2004	800	6.7	162	20.3	254	51	333	5 644	303	5.3	4 546	108	666
2005	763	6.3	158	20.7	220	48	338	5 563	353	6.4	4 454	93	643
2006	802	6.6	178	22.1	251	50	324	5 626	375	6.7	4 447	107	671
2007	801	6.5	186	23.2	241	49	325	5 591	405	7.3	4 406	100	657
2008	758	6.1	176	23.2	240	41	301	5 598	407	7.3	4 393	121	650
2009	753	6.1	209	27.8	224	40	280	5 678	540	9.5	4 368	108	637

1 The split between full-time and part-time employment is based on repondents self-classification

2 These series cover employees and self-employed only.
3 The total inclludes those who did not give a reason for working part-time

Sources: Labour Force Survey, Office for National Statistics;
Helpline: 01633 456901

7.3 Employment: by sex and age
United Kingdom
Seasonally adjusted

Thousands and percentages

	All aged 16 and over	16-59/64	16-17	18-24	25-34	35-49	50-64 (m) 50-59 (w)	65+ (m) 60+ (w)
In Employment								
People								
	MGRZ	YBSE	YBTO	YBTR	YBTU	YBTX	MGUW	MGUZ
2003	28 186	27 240	652	3 415	6 362	10 591	6 221	946
2004	28 485	27 486	642	3 528	6 283	10 742	6 293	998
2005	28 774	27 705	607	3 539	6 297	10 885	6 379	1 070
2006	29 030	27 863	559	3 618	6 261	10 975	6 451	1 167
2007	29 222	27 996	534	3 657	6 254	11 039	6 513	1 226
2008	29 443	28 120	525	3 663	6 285	11 065	6 583	1 323
2009	28 979	27 597	430	3 448	6 222	10 916	6 580	1 383
Men								
	MGSA	YBSF	YBTP	YBTS	YBTV	YBTY	MGUX	MGVA
2003	15 262	14 932	316	1 802	3 473	5 659	3 682	330
2004	15 405	15 068	309	1 868	3 417	5 743	3 731	337
2005	15 535	15 175	293	1 879	3 432	5 781	3 790	361
2006	15 662	15 272	260	1 912	3 423	5 845	3 832	390
2007	15 813	15 407	257	1 943	3 443	5 879	3 885	407
2008	15 894	15 452	260	1 935	3 444	5 871	3 943	443
2009	15 497	15 055	196	1 788	3 404	5 744	3 922	443
Women								
	MGSB	YBSG	YBTQ	YBTT	YBTW	YBTZ	MGUY	MGVB
2003	12 925	12 309	336	1 612	2 889	4 932	2 539	616
2004	13 080	12 419	333	1 660	2 866	4 998	2 562	661
2005	13 239	12 530	315	1 660	2 865	5 104	2 589	709
2006	13 367	12 591	299	1 706	2 838	5 130	2 619	776
2007	13 409	12 589	277	1 714	2 812	5 160	2 627	820
2008	13 549	12 669	265	1 729	2 841	5 195	2 640	880
2009	13 482	12 542	234	1 661	2 818	5 171	2 658	940
Employment rates(%)								
People								
	MGSR	MGSU	YBUA	YBUD	YBUG	YBUJ	YBUM	YBUP
2003	59.9	74.6	42.7	66.5	79.5	82.1	69.6	8.9
2004	60.0	74.7	41.2	66.9	79.7	82.2	70.0	9.4
2005	60.1	74.7	38.6	65.6	80.2	82.4	70.4	9.9
2006	60.2	74.6	35.5	65.5	80.1	82.3	70.8	10.7
2007	60.0	74.6	33.7	64.8	80.3	82.3	71.3	11.0
2008	60.0	74.5	33.1	63.8	80.3	82.4	71.9	11.7
2009	58.6	72.8	27.6	59.5	78.3	81.5	71.3	12.0
Men								
	MGSS	MGSV	YBUB	YBUE	YBUH	YBUK	YBUN	YBUQ
2003	67.0	79.2	40.3	69.8	87.6	88.7	71.6	8.4
2004	67.1	79.3	38.7	70.1	87.4	89.0	72.0	8.5
2005	66.9	79.0	36.3	68.8	88.1	88.5	72.4	9.0
2006	66.9	78.8	32.3	68.3	88.1	88.7	72.3	9.6
2007	66.8	78.8	31.5	67.6	88.7	88.8	72.6	9.9
2008	66.5	78.5	31.9	65.9	87.9	88.6	73.0	10.5
2009	64.3	76.0	24.6	60.7	85.2	86.9	71.9	10.3
Women								
	MGST	MGSW	YBUC	YBUF	YBUI	YBUL	YBUO	YBUR
2003	53.1	69.7	45.1	63.1	71.6	75.6	66.8	9.3
2004	53.5	69.9	43.9	63.7	72.1	75.6	67.2	9.9
2005	53.7	70.0	41.0	62.3	72.3	76.4	67.8	10.5
2006	53.8	70.0	39.0	62.8	72.2	76.1	68.5	11.3
2007	53.7	69.9	36.0	62.0	72.0	75.9	69.6	11.8
2008	53.8	70.2	34.3	61.5	72.8	76.3	70.2	12.4
2009	53.1	69.2	30.8	58.2	71.4	76.2	70.4	13.0

1 See chapter text.
  Denominator = all persons in the relevant age group

Sources: Labour Force Survey, Office for National Statistics;
Helpline: 01633 456901

7.4 Distribution of the workforce:[1,2] by sex
At mid-June each year. Seasonally adjusted

Thousands

		1999	2000	2001	2002	2003	2004	2005	2006	2007	2008	2009
United Kingdom												
Claimant count	BCJD	1 248.1	1 088.4	969.9	946.6	933.0	853.3	861.8	945.0	863.6	905.1	1 531.8
Males	DPAE	955.0	831.6	739.6	717.1	700.3	636.2	639.7	697.5	630.9	665.1	1 127.8
Females	DPAF	293.1	256.8	230.3	229.6	232.8	217.1	222.1	247.5	232.8	240.1	404.0
Workforce jobs	DYDC	29 127	29 554	29 890	30 064	30 350	30 671	31 012	31 257	31 471	31 661	30 987
Males	KAMS	15 663	15 772	15 992	16 002	16 245	16 376	16 487	16 662	16 773	16 908	16 405
Females	KAMT	13 464	13 782	13 898	14 061	14 105	14 296	14 525	14 596	14 698	14 753	14 582
HM Forces	KAMU	218	217	214	214	223	218	210	204	198	193	197
Males	KAMV	201	199	196	197	203	199	191	185	180	176	179
Females	KAMW	17	18	18	18	19	19	18	18	18	18	18
Self-employment jobs	DYZN	3 688	3 579	3 604	3 674	3 883	3 964	3 943	4 056	4 169	4 181	4 222
Males	KAMZ	2 642	2 552	2 593	2 637	2 785	2 863	2 840	2 879	2 953	2 961	2 953
Females	KANA	1 046	1 027	1 012	1 037	1 097	1 101	1 103	1 177	1 216	1 220	1 269
Employees jobs	BCAJ	25 091	25 639	25 973	26 085	26 152	26 381	26 763	26 933	27 051	27 232	26 522
Males	KANC	12 740	12 948	13 142	13 114	13 201	13 249	13 398	13 559	13 609	13 739	13 248
Females	KAND	12 351	12 691	12 831	12 971	12 951	13 132	13 365	13 374	13 442	13 493	13 274
of whom												
Total, production and construction industries	KANF	5 382	5 349	5 194	4 952	4 749	4 594	4 475	4 423	4 377	4 378	4 113
Total, all manufacturing industries	KANG	4 059	3 959	3 805	3 599	3 410	3 246	3 102	2 975	2 911	2 867	2 645
Government-supported trainees	KANH	131	119	99	90	92	108	96	65	53	54	46
Males	KANI	81	73	62	55	55	65	58	38	31	32	25
Females	KANJ	50	46	38	36	37	44	38	27	21	22	21
Great Britain												
Claimant count	DPAG	1 197.3	1 046.3	930.5	910.2	898.5	822.5	833.2	917.1	839.3	877.3	1 482.7
Males	ZSDP	915.7	799.6	709.7	689.3	673.9	612.8	618.0	676.6	612.5	643.5	1 089.3
Females	ZSDQ	281.6	246.8	220.8	220.9	224.6	209.8	215.1	240.5	226.8	233.8	393.4
Workforce jobs	KANQ	28 394	28 804	29 127	29 289	29 561	29 870	30 186	30 423	30 632	30 810	30 152
Males	KANR	15 267	15 366	15 580	15 588	15 822	15 946	16 044	16 214	16 327	16 454	15 964
Females	KANS	13 126	13 438	13 547	13 702	13 739	13 924	14 142	14 209	14 305	14 355	14 188
HM Forces	BCAH	218	217	214	214	223	218	210	204	198	193	197
Males	KANU	201	199	196	197	203	199	191	185	180	176	179
Females	KANV	17	18	18	18	19	19	18	18	18	18	18
Self-employment jobs	KANW	3 592	3 480	3 500	3 572	3 774	3 851	3 820	3 933	4 055	4 059	4 100
Males	KANX	2 565	2 470	2 506	2 553	2 695	2 770	2 738	2 780	2 862	2 863	2 855
Females	KANY	1 027	1 011	994	1 019	1 079	1 081	1 082	1 153	1 193	1 196	1 244
Employee jobs	KANZ	24 465	24 997	25 321	25 419	25 478	25 699	26 067	26 227	26 332	26 507	25 813
Males	KAOA	12 429	12 630	12 821	12 788	12 873	12 917	13 062	13 215	13 258	13 386	12 908
Females	KAOB	12 036	12 367	12 500	12 631	12 605	12 782	13 005	13 012	13 074	13 120	12 905
of whom												
Total, production and construction industries	KAOC	5 239	5 205	5 052	4 813	4 616	4 464	4 344	4 290	4 239	4 242	3 991
Total, all manufacturing industries	KAOD	3 954	3 856	3 704	3 501	3 318	3 157	3 015	2 888	2 823	2 778	2 564
Government-supported trainees	KAOE	120	110	92	84	86	102	90	58	46	51	42
Males	KAOF	73	67	57	50	51	60	53	33	27	29	22
Females	KAOG	47	43	35	34	35	42	36	25	19	21	20

Note. Because the figures have been rounded independently totals may differ from the sum of the components. Also the totals may include some employees whose industrial classification could not be ascertained.

1 The data in this table have not been adjusted to reflect the 2001 Census population data. See chapter text.

2 There is a discontinuity in the employee jobs series between December 2005 and September 2006 due to improvements to the annual benchmark. Further information can be found at:
http://www.statistics.gov.uk/statbase/product.asp?vlnk=9765

Sources: Business Statistics Division, Office for National Statistics;
Customer Helpline: 01633 456776

7.5 Employee jobs: by industry[1,2,3]
Standard Industrial Classification 2003
At June each year. Not seasonally adjusted

Thousands

		SIC 2003	United Kingdom						Great Britain				
			2005	2006	2007	2008	2009		2005	2006	2007	2008	2009
All sections	KAOH	A - O	26 735	26 908	27 030	27 211	26 493	LMAB	26 041	26 204	26 312	26 486	25 788
Index of production and construction industries	KAOI	C - F	4 462	4 411	4 365	4 367	4 098	LMAH	4 333	4 278	4 228	4 231	3 978
Index of production industries	KAOJ	C - E	3 258	3 136	3 087	3 049	2 821	LMAF	3 166	3 044	2 994	2 955	2 737
of which, manufacturing industries	KAOK	D	3 102	2 976	2 913	2 869	2 642	KAPQ	3 015	2 889	2 825	2 780	2 564
Service industries	KAOL	G - O	22 023	22 256	22 411	22 574	22 140	LMAJ	21 472	21 697	21 842	21 998	21 567
Agriculture, hunting and forestry and fishing	KAOM	A/B	249	241	254	269	255	KAPS	236	229	242	257	243
Agriculture hunting and forestry	KPHI	A	244	234	247	262	248	KOVW	231	222	235	250	236
Agriculture hunting & related activities	KPHJ	01	234	225	238	251	237	KOVX	221	213	226	239	225
Fishing	KPHK	B	5	7	7	7	7	KOVY	5	7	7	7	7
Mining and quarrying	KPHL	C	57	58	59	58	56	KOVZ	55	56	57	56	55
Mining and quarrying of energy producing materials	KPHM	CA	34	35	35	35	35	KOWA	34	35	35	35	34
Mining	KAPG	10/12	..	..	..	..	..	KOWB	7	6	7	..	..
Extraction of crude petroleum	KPHN	11	..	..	..	..	..	KOWC	27	29	30	..	..
Mining and quarrying except of energy producing materials	KPHO	CB(13/14)	23	22	23	24	22	KOWD	21	20	21	22	20
Energy and water supply industries	KAOO	C/E	156	160	174	180	179	LMAM	151	155	169	175	174
Manufacturing	KPHP	D	3 102	2 976	2 913	2 869	2 642	LMAD	3 015	2 889	2 825	2 780	2 564
Manufacture of food products Beverages and tobacco	KPHQ	DA	428	418	415	413	403	LMAN	409	400	396	395	384
Of food	KPHR	151 to 158	..	..	..	..	..	KOWH	364	356	354	352	345
Of beverages and tobacco	KPHS	159/16	..	..	..	..	..	KOWI	45	44	43	43	40
Manufacture of textiles and textile products	KPHT	DB	123	107	98	94	85	KOWJ	118	103	94	91	82
Of textiles	KPHU	17	84	74	68	65	58	KOWK	81	71	66	63	57
Of made-up textile articles except apparel	KPHV	174	..	..	..	..	..	KOWL	27	25	24	23	21
Of textiles excluding made-up textile	KPHW	Rest of 17	..	..	..	..	..	KOWM	54	46	42	40	36
Of wearing apparel,dressing and dyeing of fur	KPHX	18	39	33	30	29	26	KOWN	38	31	28	28	26
Manufacture of leather and leather products Including footwear	KPHY	DC	11	11	10	9	8	KOWO	11	11	10	8	8
Of leather and leather goods	KPHZ	191/192	..	..	..	..	..	KOWP	5	7	5	4	4
Of footwear	KPIA	193	..	..	..	..	..	KOWQ	5	5	4	4	4
Manufacture of wood and wood products	KPIB	DD(20)	81	77	80	78	70	LMAP	77	73	75	73	67
Manufacture of pulp paper and paper products, publishing and printing	KPIC	DE	400	381	367	353	326	LMAQ	394	375	362	348	321
Of pulp paper and paper products	KPID	21	77	71	67	65	61	KOWT	76	70	66	64	59
Publishing printing and reproduction of recorded media	KPIE	22	322	310	300	288	266	KOWU	318	306	296	284	262
Manufacture of coke refined petroleum products and nuclear fuel	KPIF	DF(23)	23	23	24	24	24	KOWV	23	22	24	24	24
Manufacture of chemicals, chemical products and man-made fibres	KPIG	DG(24)	199	193	186	181	171	LMAR	196	190	182	178	168
Manufacture of rubber and plastics	KPIH	DH(25)	203	196	186	182	162	LMAS	196	189	179	175	156
Manufacture of other non-metallic mineral products	KPII	DI(26)	111	107	105	105	88	KOWZ	105	101	99	98	83
Manufacture of basic metals and fabricated metal products	KPIJ	DJ	398	387	381	374	343	KOXA	391	380	373	366	336
Of basic metals	KPIK	27	74	73	69	68	61	KOXB	73	72	69	67	61
except machinery	KPIL	28	325	314	311	307	282	KOXC	317	307	304	299	275

7.5
Employee jobs: by industry[1,2,3]
Standard Industrial Classification 2003

continued   At June each year. Not seasonally adjusted

Thousands

		SIC 2003	United Kingdom						Great Britain				
			2005	2006	2007	2008	2009		2005	2006	2007	2008	2009
Manufacture of Machinery and Equipment not elsewhere classified	KPIM	DK(29)	280	270	275	276	251	LMAU	273	263	268	269	245
Manufacture of electrical and optical equipment	KPIN	DL	333	315	306	296	272	LMAV	324	306	297	287	264
Of office machinery and computers	KPIO	30	30	26	22	21	20	KOXF	28	24	20	19	18
Of electrical machinery and apparatus	KPIP	31	122	117	115	110	98	KOXG	118	113	111	106	95
Of electric motors etc control apparatus and insulated cable	KPIQ	311 to 313	..	..	..	..	..	KOXH	63	61	60	58	54
Of accumulators, primary cells, batteries, lamps and electrical equipment	KPIR	314 to 316	..	..	..	..	..	KOXI	56	52	51	48	41
Radio television and communication equipment	KPIS	32	66	61	58	55	48	KOXJ	64	59	56	54	47
Of electronic components	KPIT	321	..	..	..	..	..	KOXK	27	24	24	22	19
Of radio TV and telephone apparatus, sound and video recorders	KPIU	322/323	..	..	..	..	..	KOXL	37	35	33	32	28
Of medical precision and optical equipment, watches	KPIV	33	116	111	112	110	106	KOXM	114	109	110	108	104
Manufacture of transport equipment	KPIW	DM	329	316	310	315	285	LMAW	320	306	301	306	276
Of motor vehicles and trailers	KPIX	34	184	172	159	159	132	KOXO	180	168	156	155	129
Of other transport equipment	KPIY	35	146	144	151	157	153	KOXP	139	138	145	150	147
Manufacturing not elsewhere classified	KPIZ	DN(36/37)	182	175	171	169	154	KOXQ	178	170	164	163	148
Electricity gas and water supply	KPJA	E	99	102	115	122	122	KOXR	96	99	112	119	119
Electricity gas steam and hot water supply	KPJB	40	..	..	..	..	..	KOXT	73	73	83	89	89
Collection purification and distribution of water	KPJC	41	..	..	..	..	..	KOXU	24	26	29	30	31
Construction	KPJD	F(45)	1 204	1 275	1 278	1 319	1 277	LMAY	1 166	1 234	1 234	1 275	1 241
Services	KPJE	G - O	22 023	22 256	22 411	22 574	22 140	KOXX	21 472	21 697	21 842	21 998	21 567
Wholesale and retail trade; Repair of motor vehicles, motorcycles and personal household goods	KPJF	G (50 - 52)	4 597	4 554	4 553	4 583	4 435	LMAZ	4 478	4 432	4 429	4 455	4 308
Sale maintenance and repair of motor vehicles, retail of automotive fuel	KPJG	50	565	566	564	561	524	KOXZ	550	549	547	543	508
Sale of motor vehicles, motorcycles and parts, motorcycle repair and sale of automotive fuel	KPJH	501/503 - 505	..	..	..	..	..	KOYA	380	374	373	369	340
Maintenance and repair of motor vehicles	KPJI	502	..	..	..	..	..	KOYB	169	175	174	174	168
Wholesale trade and commission trade except motor vehicles	KPJJ	51	1 131	1 126	1 139	1 151	1 102	KOYC	1 108	1 102	1 115	1 129	1 079
Wholesale on a fee of contract basis	KPJK	511	..	..	..	..	..	KOYD	61	66	70	76	76
Wholesale agricultural raw materials and live animals	KPJL	512	..	..	..	..	..	KPLD	22	19	19	19	18
Wholesale food beverages & tobacco	KPJM	513	..	..	..	..	..	KPLE	190	195	195	196	194
Wholesale household goods	KPJN	514	..	..	..	..	..	KPLF	274	272	274	273	264
Wholesale of non-agricultural intermediate products waste & scrap	KPJO	515	..	..	..	..	..	KPLG	232	230	238	241	219
Wholesale machinery eqpt. & supplies	KPJP	516	..	..	..	..	..	KPLH	238	232	232	236	224
Other wholesale	KPJQ	517	..	..	..	..	..	KPLI	91	89	86	87	84
Retail trade except of motor vehicles and motorcycles;repair of personal and household goods	KPJR	52	2 901	2 862	2 851	2 871	2 808	KPLJ	2 820	2 781	2 767	2 783	2 721
Non-specialised stores selling mainly food beverages & tobacco	KPJS	5211/5221-4,5227	..	..	..	..	..	KPLK	1 140	1 119	1 109	1 125	1 117
Other non-specialised stores second hand shops & sales not in stores	KPJT	5212/525-526	..	..	..	..	..	KPLL	353	337	329	336	331

7.5

continued

Employee jobs: by industry[1,2,3]
Standard Industrial Classification 2003
At June each year. Not seasonally adjusted

Thousands

			United Kingdom						Great Britain				
			2005	2006	2007	2008	2009		2005	2006	2007	2008	2009
		SIC 2003											
Alcoholic & other beverages, tobacco	KPJU	5225 to 5226	..	..	..	..	..	KPLM	49	46	41	39	35
Pharmaceutical & medical goods cosmetics & toilet articles	KPJV	523	..	..	..	..	..	KPLN	103	105	107	111	110
Clothing footwear & leather goods	KPJW	5242/5243	..	..	..	..	..	KPLO	415	416	428	424	409
Textile furniture lighting equipment electrical household appliances radio and TV paints glass hardware and household goods not elsewhere classified	KPJX	5241/5244-46	..	..	..	..	..	KPLP	299	291	293	282	263
Books newspapers and stationery, other retail in specialised stores	KPJY	5247/5248	..	..	..	..	..	KPLQ	435	444	438	446	432
Repair of personal and household goods	KPJZ	527	..	..	..	..	..	KPLR	26	22	22	20	22
Hotels and restaurants	KPKA	H	1 855	1 840	1 826	1 835	1 787	LMBA	1 813	1 797	1 783	1 793	1 746
Hotels camp sites short-stay accom.	KPKB	551/552	..	..	..	..	..	KPLT	387	383	388	392	377
Restaurants	KPKC	553	..	..	..	..	..	KPLU	614	634	628	635	623
Bars	KPKD	554	..	..	..	..	..	KPLV	552	542	536	517	503
Canteens and catering	KPKE	555	..	..	..	..	..	KPLW	261	238	231	249	243
Transport, storage and communication	KPKF	I	1 594	1 588	1 582	1 596	1 530	KPLX	1 565	1 559	1 551	1 565	1 500
Land transport, transport via pipelines	KPKG	60	534	547	549	558	541	KPLY	521	533	535	544	528
Transport via railways	KPKH	601	..	..	..	..	..	KPLZ	53	52	54	54	55
Other land transport and via pipelines	KPKI	602/603	..	..	..	..	..	KPMA	468	481	482	490	473
Water transport	KPKJ	61	19	18	17	17	17	KPMB	18	17	16	16	16
Air transport	KPKK	62	88	90	90	85	79	KPMC	88	89	89	85	78
Supporting and auxiliary transport activities, activities of travel agents	KPKL	63	453	443	452	462	450	KPMD	447	438	446	456	444
Travel agencies and tour operators	KPKM	633	..	..	..	..	..	KPME	120	107	104	106	105
Post and telecommunications	KPKN	64	500	491	474	473	442	LMBC	491	482	465	464	433
National post and courier activities	KPKO	641	..	..	..	..	..	KPMG	275	266	255	260	242
Telecommunications	KPKR	6420	..	..	..	..	..	KPMJ	216	216	209	204	191
Financial intermediation	KPKS	J	1 062	1 059	1 064	1 049	1 002	LMBD	1 044	1 040	1 045	1 030	983
Financial intermediation except insurance and pension funding	KPKT	65	609	603	595	580	544	KPML	596	590	582	567	532
Insurance and pension funding except compulsory social security	KPKU	66	183	181	183	180	178	KPMM	181	179	180	178	176
Activities auxiliary to financial Intermediation	KPKV	67	271	274	287	289	280	KPMN	267	271	283	285	276
Except insurance and pension funding	KPKW	671	..	..	..	..	..	KPMO	136	138	149	150	143
Auxiliary to insurance and pension funding	KPKX	672	..	..	..	..	..	KPMP	131	133	134	135	132
Real estate renting & business activities	KPKY	K	4 336	4 533	4 698	4 766	4 504	KPMQ	4 268	4 462	4 625	4 689	4 429
Real estate activities	KPKZ	70	449	451	450	453	437	LMBE	441	443	442	445	429
Activities with own property, letting of own property	KPLA	701/702	..	..	..	..	..	KPMS	252	249	241	249	252
Activities on a fee or contract basis	KPLB	703	..	..	..	..	..	KPMT	189	194	200	196	177

7.5
Employee jobs: by industry[1,2,3]
Standard Industrial Classification 2003

continued At June each year. Not seasonally adjusted

Thousand

		SIC 2003	United Kingdom						Great Britain				
			2005	2006	2007	2008	2009		2005	2006	2007	2008	2009
Renting of machinery and equipment without operator & of personal & household goods	KPLC	71	157	160	157	156	143	KPMU	155	158	155	154	141
Construction and civil engineering machinery	KOUU	7132	..	..	..	..	..	KPMV	42	45	45	46	39
All other goods and equipment	KOUV	Rest of 71	..	..	..	..	..	KPMW	113	113	110	108	102
Computer and related equipment	KOUW	72	493	525	542	548	542	KPMX	486	518	535	540	534
Research and development	KOUX	73	104	108	109	108	108	KPMY	103	106	108	106	106
Other business activities	KOUY	74	3 133	3 289	3 440	3 501	3 275	KPMZ	3 083	3 238	3 386	3 444	3 220
Legal, accounting, book-keeping & auditing activities	KOUZ	741	..	..	..	..	..	KPNA	889	962	1 005	1 027	972
Legal activities	KOVA	7411	..	..	..	..	..	KPNB	260	280	294	292	264
Accounting, book-keeping auditing, tax consultancy	KOVB	7412	..	..	..	..	..	KPNC	203	218	226	238	230
Market research business and consultancy activities	KOVC	7413/7414	..	..	..	..	..	KPND	316	355	377	389	373
Management activities of holding companies[4]	KOVD	7415	..	..	..	..	..	KPNE	110	109	108	108	106
Architectural engineering activities and related technical consultancy, technical testing	KOVE	742/743	..	..	..	..	..	KPNF	347	374	400	410	386
Advertising	KOVF	744	..	..	..	..	..	KPNG	84	81	87	83	76
Industrial cleaning	KOVG	747	..	..	..	..	..	KPNH	436	449	449	455	440
Public administration and defence, compulsory social security	KOVH	L(75)	1 516	1 514	1 509	1 474	1 465	LMBG	1 456	1 454	1 450	1 415	1 407
Education	KOVI	M(80)	2 348	2 384	2 401	2 420	2 460	LMBH	2 274	2 311	2 328	2 348	2 386
Health and social work	KOVJ	N	3 298	3 345	3 364	3 421	3 527	LOJV	3 188	3 233	3 249	3 305	3 409
Human health, veterinary activities	KOVK	851/852	..	..	..	..	..	KPNL	2 103	2 100	2 095	2 123	2 202
Social work activities	KOVL	853	..	..	..	..	..	KPNM	1 084	1 133	1 153	1 182	1 207
Other community social and personal service activities, private households with employed persons, extra-territorial organisations and bodies	KOVM	O	1 417	1 440	1 414	1 431	1 430	LMBK	1 385	1 408	1 382	1 398	1 398
Sewage and refuse disposal; sanitation	KOVN	90	104	108	110	109	111	KPNO	101	105	106	106	108
Activities of membership organisations	KOVO	91	215	225	215	208	220	KPNP	206	217	207	200	212
Recreational cultural and sporting activities	KOVP	92	779	783	771	789	778	KPNQ	764	767	755	773	762
Motion picture video radio TV news agencies and entertainment activities	KOVQ	921 to 924	..	..	..	..	..	KPNR	222	222	218	232	223
Other service activities, private households with employed persons, extra territorial organisations	KOVT	93/95/99	318	325	319	325	321	KPNU	313	320	314	320	316
Washing, dry cleaning of textile and fur products	KOVU	9301	..	..	..	..	..	KPNV	40	43	40	38	36
Hairdressing, other beauty treatment, physical and well-being activities	KOVV	9302/9304	..	..	..	..	..	KPNW	114	122	122	122	129

Note. Because the figures have been rounded independently totals may differ from the sum of the components. Also the totals may include some employees whose industrial classification could not be ascertained.

1 See chapter text. The data in this table have not been adjusted to reflect the 2001 Census population data.

2 All figures have been revised. For further information see: http://www.statistics.gov.uk/cci/article.asp?id=1340

3 There is a discontinuity in the employee jobs series between December 2005 and September 2006 due to improvements to the annual benchmark. Further information can be found at: http://www.statistics.gov.uk/Statbase/Product.asp?vlnk=9765

Sources: Department of Manpower Services (Northern Ireland);;
Business Statistics Division, ONS: 01633 456776

7.6 Weekly hours worked: by sex[1,2]
United Kingdom
At Quarter 2 each year[3]. Seasonally adjusted

	Total weekly hours (millions)[1,2]	Average(mean) actual weekly hours worked			
		All workers[1]	Full-time workers[3]	Part-time workers[3]	Second jobs
People					
	YBUS	YBUV	YBUY	YBVB	YBVE
1999	892.7	32.9	38.2	15.3	9.1
2000	894.8	32.6	37.9	15.5	9.1
2001	903.5	32.7	37.9	15.6	9.4
2002	901.0	32.3	37.5	15.6	9.4
2003	904.6	32.2	37.4	15.6	9.3
2004	912.1	32.1	37.3	15.6	9.3
2005	923.7	32.2	37.3	15.7	9.5
2006	928.5	32.0	37.1	15.6	9.4
2007	936.1	32.1	37.2	15.6	9.5
2008	940.7	32.0	37.1	15.6	9.7
2009	913.3	31.6	36.8	15.5	9.5
Men					
	YBUT	YBUW	YBUZ	YBVC	YBVF
1999	564.0	38.3	40.2	15.1	9.8
2000	564.2	37.9	39.8	15.3	9.9
2001	567.0	37.8	39.7	15.3	10.3
2002	561.9	37.3	39.3	15.1	10.3
2003	564.3	37.0	39.2	15.3	10.1
2004	569.0	37.0	39.2	15.6	10.3
2005	572.2	36.9	39.1	15.6	10.3
2006	573.6	36.7	38.9	15.5	10.1
2007	580.2	36.8	39.0	15.5	10.6
2008	580.8	36.6	39.0	15.4	10.8
2009	559.0	36.1	38.5	15.5	10.4
Women					
	YBUU	YBUX	YBVA	YBVD	YBVG
1999	328.6	26.5	34.5	15.4	8.6
2000	330.6	26.3	34.2	15.5	8.5
2001	336.5	26.5	34.3	15.7	8.8
2002	339.1	26.5	34.1	15.7	8.8
2003	340.3	26.4	34.0	15.7	8.8
2004	343.1	26.3	33.9	15.6	8.5
2005	351.5	26.6	34.0	15.8	8.9
2006	354.9	26.6	34.0	15.7	8.9
2007	355.9	26.6	33.9	15.6	8.8
2008	359.9	26.6	33.8	15.6	8.9
2009	354.2	26.3	33.7	15.4	8.8

See chapter text.
1 Main and second job
2 Total actual weekly hours worked including paid and unpaid overtime.
3 Main job only. The split between full-time and part-time employment is based on respondents' self-classification.

Sources: Labour Force Survey, Office for National Statistics;
Helpline: 01633 456901

7.7 International comparisons
Employment and unemployment rates[1,2]

		2006 Q4	2007 Q1	2007 Q2	2007 Q3	2007 Q4	2008 Q1	2008 Q2	2008 Q3	2008 Q4	2009 Q1	2009 Q2	2009 Q3
EUROSTAT Employment rates													
Austria	YXSN	70.6	70.3	71.5	72.5	71.3	71.0	72.3	72.8	72.2	70.8	71.7	72.3
Belgium	YXSO	62.1	61.7	61.6	62.1	62.7	62.6	62.0	62.6	62.4	61.7	61.5	61.4
Bulgaria	A495	59.8	59.7	61.6	62.7	62.9	62.6	63.9	65.0	64.3	63.6	63.3	63.1
Cyprus	A4AC	70.4	69.8	71.2	71.3	71.5	70.2	71.1	71.0	71.1	69.5	70.2	70.0
Czech Republic	A4AD	65.6	65.5	66.0	66.3	66.5	66.1	66.6	66.7	66.8	65.6	65.4	65.2
Denmark	YXSP	77.9	76.7	77.3	77.1	77.4	77.0	78.4	78.6	78.3	76.2	76.2	76.3
Estonia	A4AE	68.1	68.6	69.7	70.2	69.1	69.5	69.8	70.4	69.6	65.3	63.8	63.4
Finland	YXSQ	69.0	68.3	71.3	71.7	69.9	69.5	72.3	72.1	70.3	68.5	69.8	69.3
France	YXSR	63.7	63.6	64.4	64.9	64.5	64.6	65.1	65.4	64.7	64.1	64.6	64.6
Germany	YXSS	68.3	68.4	69.1	69.9	70.0	70.0	70.3	71.3	71.3	70.4	70.8	71.0
Greece	YXST	61.0	60.8	61.5	61.8	61.5	61.3	62.2	62.2	61.7	61.7	61.6	61.7
Hungary	A4AF	57.6	56.9	57.6	57.7	57.1	56.1	56.5	57.3	56.7	55.1	55.6	55.5
Ireland	YXSU	68.7	68.5	68.9	69.9	69.0	68.5	68.1	68.0	65.6	62.8	62.2	61.8
Italy	YXSV	58.5	57.9	58.9	59.1	58.7	58.3	59.2	59.0	58.5	57.4	57.9	57.5
Latvia	A4AG	67.4	66.4	67.6	69.0	70.3	69.6	69.5	69.0	66.5	64.3	61.4	59.8
Lithuania	A4AH	63.5	63.9	65.4	66.1	64.4	63.9	64.6	65.0	63.8	61.0	60.3	60.4
Luxembourg	YXSW	63.6	63.9	63.6	64.7	64.4	62.8	64.4	63.9	62.6	64.5	65.7	65.8
Malta	A4AI	53.4	53.9	55.2	54.9	54.5	54.7	55.2	56.1	55.0	54.9	54.9	55.1
Netherlands	YXSX	75.0	75.0	76.0	76.5	76.4	76.4	77.2	77.5	77.6	77.4	77.0	77.0
Poland	A4AJ	55.7	55.4	56.8	57.8	58.1	58.0	58.9	60.0	60.0	58.9	59.3	59.9
Portugal	YXSY	67.6	67.4	67.6	68.1	68.1	68.1	68.6	68.1	67.9	67.0	66.7	66.5
Romania	A494	57.4	57.2	59.6	60.5	57.9	57.7	59.7	60.5	58.3	57.4	59.2	60.4
Slovak Republic	A4AK	60.2	60.1	60.4	60.7	61.6	61.3	61.7	63.1	62.9	61.0	60.4	60.1
Slovenia	A4AL	66.0	66.0	68.3	69.0	67.7	67.1	68.3	70.1	68.8	66.7	67.6	68.3
Spain	YXSZ	65.2	65.1	65.8	66.0	65.5	65.1	65.0	64.5	62.8	60.4	59.9	59.7
Sweden	YXTA	73.2	72.7	74.3	75.7	74.0	73.4	74.8	75.7	73.4	71.9	72.7	72.9
United Kingdom	ANZ6	71.6	71.1	71.2	71.6	71.9	71.6	71.6	71.5	71.3	70.4	69.6	69.8
Total EU[3]	A496	64.8	64.5	65.4	66.0	65.7	65.5	66.0	66.4	65.8	64.6	64.8	64.8
Eurozone[3]	YXTC	65.0	64.8	65.6	66.1	65.9	65.7	66.1	66.4	65.8	64.7	64.9	64.8
National Statistical Offices Employment Rates													
Canada	IUUK	73.0	72.1	74.0	74.6	73.7	72.6	74.3	74.5	73.3	70.7	72.0	72.2
Japan	YXTF	70.1	69.7	71.3	70.8	70.9	70.0	71.3	70.8	70.9	69.8	70.2	70.1
United Kingdom	MGSU	74.5	74.3	74.5	74.6	74.8	74.8	74.8	74.4	74.0	73.5	72.7	72.5
United States	YXTE	72.2	72.1	71.8	71.6	71.5	71.6	71.3	70.7	69.8	68.7	68.1	67.4

		2008 Oct	2008 Nov	2008 Dec	2009 Jan	2009 Feb	2009 Mar	2009 Apr	2009 May	2009 Jun	2009 Jul	2009 Aug	2009 Sep	2009 Oct	2009 Nov
EUROSTAT Unemployment rates															
Austria	ZXDS	3.9	4.0	4.2	4.2	4.4	4.6	4.6	4.8	5.0	5.1	5.2	5.5	5.6	5.5
Belgium	ZXDI	7.0	6.9	7.1	7.5	7.7	7.8	7.7	7.7	7.8	7.9	8.0	8.0	8.0	8.0
Bulgaria	A492	5.1	5.1	5.4	5.6	6.0	6.2	6.3	6.3	6.5	6.7	6.9	7.2	7.4	7.7
Cyprus	A4AN	3.6	3.7	4.0	4.1	4.3	4.6	5.0	5.2	5.3	5.4	5.6	5.9	6.0	6.2
Czech Republic	A4AO	4.3	4.5	4.7	5.2	5.6	5.9	6.2	6.4	6.7	7.0	7.3	7.5	7.7	7.8
Denmark	ZXDJ	3.5	3.7	4.0	4.4	4.7	5.3	5.8	6.0	6.2	6.1	6.1	6.5	6.9	7.1
Estonia	A4AP	7.6	7.6	7.6	11.1	11.1	11.1	13.5	13.5	13.5	15.2	15.2	15.2	15.5	15.5
Finland	ZXDU	6.6	6.7	6.9	7.1	7.4	7.7	8.0	8.2	8.4	8.5	8.6	8.6	8.7	8.8
France	ZXDN	8.1	8.3	8.5	8.7	8.9	9.0	9.2	9.3	9.4	9.5	9.6	9.7	9.9	10.0
Germany	ZXDK	7.1	7.1	7.1	7.2	7.3	7.4	7.6	7.6	7.6	7.6	7.6	7.6	7.5	7.5
Greece	ZXDL	7.9	7.9	7.9	8.8	8.8	8.8	9.2	9.2	9.2	9.7	9.7	9.7	..	..
Hungary	A4AQ	7.8	8.1	8.5	8.8	9.3	9.6	9.6	9.7	9.8	10.2	10.5	10.7	10.8	10.8
Ireland	ZXDO	7.2	7.8	8.3	9.4	10.3	11.1	11.6	12.1	12.0	12.0	12.1	12.5	12.6	13.0
Italy	ZXDP	6.9	7.1	7.0	7.2	7.3	7.6	7.5	7.4	7.6	7.7	7.7	8.0	8.2	8.3
Latvia	A4AR	9.1	10.2	11.3	12.3	13.2	14.3	15.5	16.6	17.2	18.0	18.3	19.9	21.1	22.0
Lithuania	A4AS	8.2	8.2	8.2	10.8	10.8	10.8	13.5	13.5	13.5	14.6	14.6	14.6	..	..
Luxembourg	ZXDQ	5.1	5.2	5.3	5.4	5.4	5.6	5.6	5.7	5.8	5.8	5.8	5.8	5.9	5.9
Malta	A4AT	6.0	6.2	6.0	6.4	6.5	6.7	6.9	7.1	7.2	7.3	7.1	7.1	6.9	7.0
Netherlands	ZXDR	2.7	2.7	2.7	2.8	2.9	3.1	3.2	3.3	3.4	3.5	3.7	3.8	3.9	4.0
Poland	A4AU	6.8	6.9	7.0	7.4	7.7	7.9	8.0	8.0	8.1	8.3	8.4	8.4	8.6	8.7
Portugal	ZXDT	7.8	7.9	8.1	8.5	8.8	9.1	9.3	9.5	9.6	9.8	9.9	10.1	10.2	10.3
Romania	A48Z	5.9	5.9	5.9	6.2	6.2	6.2	6.4	6.4	6.4	7.2	7.2	7.2	..	..
Slovak Republic	A4AV	8.8	9.0	9.3	9.7	10.2	10.6	10.8	11.1	11.6	12.1	12.6	13.0	13.3	13.5
Slovenia	A4AW	4.2	4.2	4.2	4.6	4.9	5.3	5.6	5.9	6.2	6.4	6.4	6.5	6.8	6.8
Spain	ZXDM	13.1	14.0	14.8	15.8	16.7	17.4	17.7	18.0	18.1	18.4	18.7	19.0	19.0	18.9
Sweden	ZXDV	6.4	7.0	6.8	6.9	7.7	7.8	8.0	8.6	8.3	8.4	8.7	8.7	8.8	8.7
United Kingdom	ZXDW	6.2	6.3	6.5	6.8	7.1	7.3	7.5	7.7	7.8	7.8	7.8	7.8	7.8	7.8
Total EU[3]	A493	7.3	7.5	7.6	8.0	8.3	8.5	8.7	8.8	8.9	9.1	9.2	9.3	9.4	9.4
Eurozone[3]	ZXDH	7.8	8.0	8.2	8.5	8.8	9.1	9.2	9.3	9.4	9.5	9.6	9.8	9.8	9.9
National Statistical Offices Unemployment Rates															
Canada	ZXDZ	6.2	6.5	6.8	7.3	8.0	8.1	8.1	8.5	8.6	8.6	8.7	8.3	8.4	8.4
Japan	ZXDY	3.8	4.0	4.3	4.2	4.4	4.8	5.0	5.2	5.4	5.7	5.5	5.3	5.1	5.2
United Kingdom	MGSX	6.2	6.4	6.6	6.8	7.1	7.3	7.6	7.8	7.9	7.9	7.8	7.9	7.8	7.8
United States	ZXDX	6.6	6.9	7.4	7.7	8.2	8.6	8.9	9.4	9.5	9.4	9.7	9.8	10.1	10.0

1 See chapter text.
2 The UK employment rate as published by the Office for National Statistics is seasonally adjusted. All other employment and unemployment rates are not seasonally adjusted.

3 The "Total EU" series consists of all 27 EU countries. The Eurozone series consists of the following EU countries: Austria, Belgium, Cyprus, Finland, France, Germany, Greece, Ireland, Italy, Luxembourg, Malta, Netherlands, Portugal, Slovenia and Spain.

Sources: Office for National Statistics; Eurostat; StatsBLS; StatCan; Stat.go.JP;
Labour Market Statistics Helpline: 01633 456901

7.8 Civil Service employment by department[1]
Great Britain

Full-time equivalents, not seasonally adjusted

		2008 Q3	2008 Q4	2009 Q1	2009 Q2	2009 Q3
Attorney General's Departments	GB3F	9 700	9 610	9 620	9 570	9 510
Cabinet Office	BBGD	1 180	1 210	1 230	1 260	1 270
Other Cabinet Office Agencies	GB3G	1 050	1 180	1 230	1 250	1 270
HM Treasury	GB3H	1 180	1 160	1 240	1 310	1 370
Chancellor's other departments	GB3I	1 630	1 680	1 740	1 730	1 770
Charity Commission	GB3J	460	450	450	460	460
Communities and Local Government	YEGA	5 190	5 170	..	..	..
Ministry of Justice	GB3K	83 610	84 230	84 020	82 480	81 710
Culture, Media and Sport	DMTC	560	560	570	570	570
Defence	BCDW	76 790	75 910	75 630	75 470	75 670
Education and Skills (former)	LNFW	–	–	..	..	..
Children, Schools and Families	I44Z	3 090	3 180	..	..	..
Innovation, Universities and Skills	I452	1 830	1 860	..	..	..
Environment, Food and Rural Affairs	LNFX	10 770	10 840	..	..	..
Export Credits Guarantee Department	GB3L	200	210	210	210	210
Foreign and Commonwealth	BCDK	5 870	5 920	5 990	6 030	6 090
Health	BAKR	3 550	3 610	3 670	3 620	3 710
Food Standards Agency	H6NX	760	760	750	730	720
Meat Hygiene Service	H6NY	1 100	1 050	1 000	980	960
HM Revenue and Customs	GB3M	84 930	85 580	84 970	83 670	82 520
Home Office	BCDL	24 830	24 820	24 520	24 640	24 780
International Development	DMUA	1 590	1 600	1 600	1 630	1 630
Northern Ireland Office	BBGG	120	120	120	110	110
Office for Standards in Education	GB3N	2 510	2 490	2 250	2 220	2 150
Security and Intelligence Services	GB3O	5 270	5 350	5 430	5 550	5 600
Business, Enterprise and Regulatory Reform	BCDQ	8 750	8 840	8 910	10 900	10 980
Transport	BCDR	18 780	18 630	18 610	18 660	18 790
Work and Pensions	LNGA	106 980	107 110	..	..	..
Central Governments Departments Total	GB3P	465 420	466 340	467 340	469 640	475 420
Scottish Government	GB3Q	16 220	16 210	16 400	16 680	16 780
Welsh Assembly	GB3R	5 880	5 890	5 940	5 940	6 030
TOTAL	BCDX	487 520	488 440	489 680	492 260	498 230

1 Numbers are rounded to the nearest ten.

Source: Office for National Statistics

7.9 Unemployment: number by sex and age group[1]
United Kingdom

Seasonally adjusted

Thousands

	All aged 16 and over	16-59/64	16-17	18-24	25-34	35-49	50-64 (m) 50-59 (w)	65+ (m) 60+ (w)
All Persons								
	MGSC	YBSH	YBVH	YBVN	YCGM	YCGS	MGVL	MGVO
2003	1 489	1 472	172	403	318	343	213	18
2004	1 424	1 407	175	409	299	353	195	17
2005	1 465	1 445	179	438	285	338	190	17
2006	1 669	1 643	183	504	341	419	208	27
2007	1 653	1 629	197	507	305	393	223	28
2008	1 776	1 751	184	558	327	405	216	23
2009	2 395	2 359	200	715	512	596	336	36
Men								
	MGSD	YBSI	YBVI	YBVO	YCGN	YCGT	MGVM	MGVP
2003	900	891	100	243	182	211	145	..
2004	836	827	99	240	185	185	137	..
2005	862	852	100	270	160	183	125	..
2006	966	955	107	303	190	229	134	11
2007	944	935	110	306	161	205	149	13
2008	1 047	1 035	101	352	182	218	147	11
2009	1 465	1 449	110	444	313	336	246	16
Women								
	MGSE	YBSJ	YBVJ	YBVP	YCGO	YCGU	MGVN	MGVQ
2003	590	582	73	159	137	132	67	..
2004	589	580	76	169	114	168	57	..
2005	603	592	79	168	125	154	65	..
2006	704	688	76	201	151	191	73	16
2007	709	695	88	201	143	188	74	15
2008	729	716	84	207	145	187	69	12
2009	930	910	90	271	198	260	90	20

See chapter text.

Source: Labour Force Survey, Office for National Statistics; Helpline: 01633 456901

7.10

Unemployment: percentage by sex and age group[1]
United Kingdom
Seasonally adjusted

Percentages

	All aged 16 and over	16-59/64	16-17	18-24	25-34	35-49	50-64 (m) 50-59 (w)	65+ (m) 60+ (w)
People								
	MGSX	YBTI	YBVK	YBVQ	YCGP	YCGV	MGXE	MGXH
2002	5.2	5.3	20.0	10.5	5.0	3.6	3.5	2.4
2003	5.1	5.2	20.9	10.6	4.8	3.1	3.3	1.9
2004	4.8	4.9	21.5	10.4	4.6	3.2	3.0	1.7
2005	4.9	5.0	22.9	11.0	4.3	3.0	2.9	1.6
2006	5.4	5.6	24.6	12.2	5.2	3.7	3.1	2.3
2007	5.3	5.5	27.0	12.2	4.6	3.4	3.3	2.3
2008	5.7	5.9	26.0	13.2	4.9	3.5	2.9	1.7
2009	7.6	7.9	31.9	17.2	7.6	5.2	4.5	2.5
Men								
	MGSY	YBTJ	YBVL	YBVR	YCGQ	YCGW	MGXF	MGXI
2002	5.7	5.8	23.0	12.1	5.1	3.9	4.0	3.2
2003	5.6	5.6	24.0	11.9	4.9	3.6	3.8	..
2004	5.1	5.2	24.3	11.4	5.2	3.1	3.6	..
2005	5.3	5.3	25.6	12.5	4.5	3.1	3.2	..
2006	5.8	5.9	29.0	13.7	5.3	3.8	3.4	2.7
2007	5.6	5.7	30.0	13.6	4.5	3.4	3.7	3.2
2008	6.2	6.3	27.9	15.4	5.0	3.6	3.5	2.3
2009	8.6	8.8	36.2	19.9	8.4	5.5	5.7	3.5
Women								
	MGSZ	YBTK	YBVM	YBVS	YCGR	YCGX	MGXG	MGXJ
2002	4.5	4.6	17.0	8.6	4.8	3.2	2.8	2.1
2003	4.4	4.5	17.8	9.0	4.5	2.6	2.6	..
2004	4.3	4.4	18.6	9.2	3.8	3.3	2.2	..
2005	4.4	4.5	20.1	9.2	4.2	2.9	2.4	..
2006	5.0	5.2	20.4	10.6	5.0	3.6	2.7	2.0
2007	5.1	5.3	24.0	10.5	4.9	3.5	2.7	1.8
2008	5.1	5.3	24.1	10.7	4.9	3.5	2.3	1.4
2009	6.4	6.8	27.9	14.0	6.6	4.8	3.0	2.0

See chapter text.
1 Denominator=economically active for that age group.

Sources: Labour Force Survey, Office for National Statistics;
Helpline: 01633 456901

7.11

Duration of unemployment: by sex
United Kingdom
Seasonally adjusted

Thousands

	All aged 16 and over						All aged 16-59/64					
	All	Up to 6 months	Over 6 and up to 12 months	All over 12 months	%over 12 months	All over 24 months	All	Up to 6 months	Over 6 and up to 12 months	All over 12 months	%over 12 months	All over 24 months
Persons												
	MGSC	YBWF	YBWG	YBWH	YBWI	YBWL	YBSH	YBWO	YBWR	YBWU	YBWX	YBXA
2003	1 489	956	216	318	21.4	157	1 472	947	214	312	21.2	153
2004	1 424	915	222	288	20.2	133	1 407	905	220	282	20.1	129
2005	1 465	926	231	308	21.0	144	1 445	916	228	301	20.8	140
2006	1 669	1 010	288	371	22.2	175	1 643	997	284	363	22.0	169
2007	1 653	997	266	390	23.6	174	1 629	985	262	382	23.5	170
2008	1 776	1 065	286	426	24.0	200	1 751	1 052	281	417	23.9	195
2009	2 395	1 325	483	587	24.5	238	2 359	1 308	476	575	24.3	231
Men												
	MGSD	MGYK	MGYM	MGYO	YBWJ	YBWM	YBSI	YBWP	YBWS	YBWV	YBWY	YBXB
2003	900	534	139	226	25.1	119	891	530	139	222	25.0	116
2004	836	496	141	199	23.8	98	827	492	140	195	23.6	96
2005	862	503	142	216	25.1	106	852	499	141	212	24.9	103
2006	966	537	171	257	26.6	126	955	533	169	253	26.5	123
2007	944	521	157	266	28.2	124	935	517	155	263	28.1	122
2008	1 047	585	167	295	28.2	146	1 035	580	165	290	28.1	144
2009	1 465	767	310	388	26.5	165	1 449	761	306	382	26.3	162
Women												
	MGSE	MGYL	MGYN	MGYP	YBWK	YBWN	YBSJ	YBWQ	YBWT	YBWW	YBWZ	YBXC
2003	590	421	77	92	15.6	38	582	417	75	90	15.4	37
2004	589	419	81	89	15.1	34	580	413	80	87	15.0	33
2005	603	423	89	91	15.2	38	592	417	87	89	15.0	36
2006	704	472	117	114	16.2	49	688	463	115	110	15.9	46
2007	709	476	109	124	17.5	50	695	468	107	120	17.3	48
2008	729	480	118	131	18.0	54	716	472	116	128	17.9	52
2009	930	558	173	199	21.3	73	910	548	170	192	21.1	68

7.11
continued

Duration of unemployment: by sex
United Kingdom
Seasonally adjusted

	Ages 16-17						Ages 18-24					
	All	Up to 6 months	Over 6 and up to 12 months	All over 12 months	%over 12 months	All over 24 months	All	Up to 6 months	Over 6 and up to 12 months	All over 12 months	%over 12 months	All over 24 months
Persons												
	YBVH	YBXD	YBXG	YBXJ	YBXM	YBXP	YBVN	YBXS	YBXV	YBXY	YBYB	YBYE
2003	172	137	23	13	7.2	..	403	299	51	53	13.1	23
2004	175	138	27	..	..	..	409	292	62	55	13.4	19
2005	179	141	26	12	6.7	..	438	306	67	65	14.8	27
2006	183	137	31	15	8.1	..	504	342	84	78	15.4	32
2007	197	149	32	17	8.4	..	507	339	76	93	18.3	33
2008	184	140	32	13	6.8	..	558	370	83	105	18.9	40
2009	200	138	38	24	12.3	..	715	425	142	148	20.6	51
Men												
	YBVI	YBXE	YBXH	YBXK	YBXN	YBXQ	YBVO	YBXT	YBXW	YBXZ	YBYC	YBYF
2003	100	79	14	..	..	..	243	171	35	37	15.2	16
2004	99	76	17	..	..	..	240	161	40	39	16.2	15
2005	100	76	16	..	..	..	270	178	43	50	18.3	23
2006	107	77	20	..	..	..	303	192	53	59	19.3	27
2007	110	80	19	11	10.1	..	306	190	49	67	21.8	26
2008	101	76	17	..	..	..	352	220	54	78	22.2	31
2009	110	73	22	14	13.4	..	444	245	96	104	23.2	38
Women												
	YBVJ	YBXF	YBXI	YBXL	YBXO	YBXR	YBVP	YBXU	YBXX	YBYA	YBYD	YBYG
2003	73	58	..	..	..	..	159	128	16	15	9.7	..
2004	76	62	..	..	..	..	169	131	22	16	9.3	..
2005	79	66	..	..	..	..	168	128	25	16	9.3	..
2006	76	61	..	..	..	..	201	151	31	19	9.6	..
2007	88	69	13	..	..	..	201	148	27	26	12.9	..
2008	84	65	14	..	..	..	207	151	29	28	13.3	..
2009	90	64	16	..	..	..	271	180	46	45	16.4	13

	Ages 25-49						Ages 50 and over					
	All	Up to 6 months	Over 6 and up to 12 months	All over 12 months	%over 12 months	All over 24 months	All	Up to 6 months	Over 6 and up to 12 months	All over 12 months	%over 12 months	All over 24 months
Persons												
	MGVI	YBYH	YBYK	YBYN	YBYQ	YBYT	YBVT	YBYW	YBYZ	YBZC	YBZF	YBZI
2003	685	409	105	171	24.9	85	230	111	36	82	36.0	47
2004	631	378	99	154	24.3	71	210	107	33	70	33.4	42
2005	632	379	104	150	23.6	67	216	101	33	81	37.8	49
2006	748	418	136	194	25.9	90	235	112	38	85	36.1	53
2007	707	393	118	195	27.6	93	242	116	40	86	35.6	47
2008	774	430	129	216	27.9	107	260	125	42	92	35.8	54
2009	1 108	588	224	295	26.6	125	372	174	79	119	32.0	60
Men												
	MGVJ	YBYI	YBYL	YBYO	YBYR	YBYU	YBVU	YBYX	YBZA	YBZD	YBZG	YBZJ
2003	402	216	65	121	30.0	63	154	68	25	62	39.9	38
2004	355	192	61	102	28.6	51	142	67	22	53	37.1	33
2005	350	190	60	100	28.5	47	142	59	24	59	41.3	37
2006	409	209	74	127	30.9	60	147	61	25	62	42.1	40
2007	374	184	63	127	33.8	63	155	67	27	62	40.0	35
2008	424	216	68	140	33.2	73	171	74	28	69	40.9	42
2009	649	333	135	181	27.9	81	262	116	57	89	33.8	46
Women												
	MGVK	YBYJ	YBYM	YBYP	YBYS	YBYV	YBVV	YBYY	YBZB	YBZE	YBZH	YBZK
2003	283	193	40	50	17.6	23	75	43	12	21	27.9	..
2004	276	186	37	52	18.9	20	68	40	11	18	25.6	..
2005	282	189	44	50	17.5	21	74	42	..	23	31.1	..
2006	339	210	62	67	19.8	30	87	52	13	23	26.0	13
2007	333	209	56	69	20.5	31	87	50	13	24	27.6	12
2008	350	214	60	76	21.6	34	89	51	15	23	26.2	12
2009	458	255	90	114	24.8	44	110	58	22	30	27.5	15

See chapter text.

7.12 Claimant count:[1] by age and duration
Computerised claims only
United Kingdom. Seasonally adjusted

Thousands

		2003	2004	2005	2006	2007	2008	2009
Annual averages								
Males								
All ages								
All durations	AGNG	693.0	630.7	635.0	694.2	628.6	662.9	1 124.2
Up to 6 months	AGXK	451.2	408.8	423.4	438.6	405.3	475.9	780.8
Over 6 and up to 12 months	ELNP	127.1	113.7	113.3	136.5	111.1	105.6	225.2
All over 12 months	ELON	114.7	108.2	98.2	119.1	112.2	81.4	118.2
All over 24 months	IKBS	37.6	34.6	33.1	34.5	33.9	21.4	18.9
Aged 18 to 24								
All durations	JLGC	171.9	161.8	174.6	195.6	176.7	191.0	321.6
Up to 6 months	JLGD	143.8	134.3	143.6	155.0	145.7	165.0	263.9
Over 6 and up to 12 months	JLGE	24.5	23.3	25.9	33.1	25.3	22.0	50.9
All over 12 months	JLGF	3.6	4.2	5.0	7.5	5.8	4.0	6.8
All over 24 months	JLGH	0.4	0.5	0.6	0.9	1.1	1.0	1.1
Aged 25 to 49								
All durations	AGMA	404.8	362.3	357.4	387.6	352.6	374.6	633.5
Up to 6 months	JLHG	248.0	221.3	225.9	228.9	211.6	250.0	410.2
Over 6 and up to 12 months	JLHH	82.9	72.9	70.4	83.4	69.6	67.6	138.6
All over 12 months	JLHI	73.8	68.1	61.2	75.2	71.5	57.0	84.7
All over 24 months	JLHK	17.0	14.1	14.2	15.2	14.5	11.5	12.0
Aged 50 and over								
All durations	JLHL	116.2	106.7	103.0	111.0	99.3	97.3	169.1
Up to 6 months	JLHM	59.4	53.2	53.9	54.7	48.0	60.9	106.7
Over 6 and up to 12 months	JLHN	19.7	17.5	17.0	20.0	16.2	16.0	35.7
All over 12 months	JLHO	37.2	35.9	32.0	36.3	35.0	20.4	26.7
All over 24 months	JLHQ	20.2	19.9	18.3	18.4	18.2	8.9	5.7
Females								
All ages								
All durations	JLGI	230.1	214.7	220.0	246.0	231.6	239.2	402.6
Up to 6 months	JLGK	166.3	153.2	159.2	171.5	163.8	182.1	305.0
Over 6 and up to 12 months	JLGJ	37.2	34.9	35.6	43.7	37.6	34.2	67.1
All over 12 months	JLGL	26.5	26.7	25.2	30.8	30.2	22.8	30.5
All over 24 months	JLGN	8.1	8.0	7.9	8.4	8.4	5.8	5.3
Aged 18 to 24								
All durations	JLGO	77.3	74.0	79.1	90.2	85.6	88.7	139.2
Up to 6 months	JLGP	64.9	61.5	65.3	72.3	71.0	76.6	116.3
Over 6 and up to 12 months	JLGQ	10.6	10.4	11.4	14.7	12.0	10.2	20.2
All over 12 months	JLGR	1.8	2.1	2.3	3.3	2.5	1.9	2.7
All over 24 months	JLGT	0.2	0.3	0.4	0.5	0.5	0.5	0.5
Aged 25 to 49								
All durations	JLHR	112.1	102.1	101.9	111.8	105.4	109.9	197.3
Up to 6 months	JLHS	77.3	69.0	70.3	73.6	69.5	78.0	144.0
Over 6 and up to 12 months	JLHT	19.9	18.2	17.7	21.3	18.8	17.6	34.1
All over 12 months	JLHU	14.9	14.9	13.8	16.9	17.1	14.2	19.3
All over 24 months	JLHW	3.1	2.9	3.0	3.3	3.2	2.9	3.1
Aged 50 and over								
All durations	JLHX	40.7	38.7	39.1	43.9	40.6	40.6	66.0
Up to 6 months	JLHY	24.1	22.7	23.5	25.5	23.3	27.5	44.7
Over 6 and up to 12 months	JLHZ	6.8	6.3	6.5	7.8	6.8	6.4	12.8
All over 12 months	JLIA	9.8	9.7	9.1	10.6	10.6	6.7	8.5
All over 24 months	JLIC	4.7	4.8	4.5	4.7	4.7	2.4	1.7

1 Count of claimants of unemployment-related benefits.

Source: Office for National Statistics: 01633 456901

7.13 Unemployment rates: by region[1,2,3]
At Quarter 2 each year[4]. Seasonally adjusted[5]

Percentages

		1999	2000	2001	2002	2003	2004	2005	2006	2007	2008	2009
North East	YCNC	9.3	8.6	7.3	6.8	6.4	5.8	6.4	6.5	6.3	7.6	9.2
North West	YCND	6.3	5.5	5.3	5.4	4.9	4.6	4.6	5.3	5.9	6.7	8.4
Yorkshire and The Humber	YCNE	6.3	6.1	5.3	5.3	5.1	4.7	4.8	5.8	5.6	6.1	8.6
East Midlands	YCNF	5.3	4.8	4.8	4.7	4.3	4.3	4.4	5.4	5.3	5.8	7.2
West Midlands	YCNG	6.8	6.0	5.5	5.7	5.8	5.2	4.8	5.9	6.3	6.7	9.8
East	YCNH	4.2	3.7	3.7	3.8	4.0	3.7	4.1	4.8	4.7	4.8	6.3
London	YCNI	7.4	7.2	6.7	6.9	7.1	7.1	6.9	7.7	6.8	7.1	8.8
South East	YCNJ	3.9	3.3	3.3	3.9	3.9	3.7	3.9	4.5	4.5	4.4	5.9
South West	YCNK	4.5	4.1	3.6	3.8	3.4	3.3	3.6	3.8	3.9	4.1	6.3
Wales	YCNM	7.3	6.3	5.9	5.4	4.8	4.5	4.7	5.3	5.4	6.0	8.2
Scotland	YCNN	7.1	6.8	6.4	6.3	5.7	5.7	5.4	5.3	4.8	4.6	7.0
Northern Ireland	ZSFB	7.1	6.3	6.0	5.8	5.5	5.0	4.6	4.4	4.0	4.5	6.5

1 Total unemployed as a percentage of all economically active persons.
2 All aged 16 and over. See chapter text.
3 In August 2007, ONS published the mid-year population estimates for 2006. These estimates have now been incorporated into the LFS estimates from 2001 onwards. Further details can be found at http://www.statistics.gov.uk/cci/article.asp?id=1919
4 The Labour Force Survey has now moved to calendar quarters from May 2006. More information can be found on page 5 of the Concepts and Definitions.pdf by following this link:- www.statistics.gov.uk/downloads/theme_labour/Concepts_Definitions_HQS.pdf
5 Previously not seasonally adjusted data was shown.

Sources: Labour Force Survey, Office for National Statistics;
Helpline: 01633 456901

7.14 Claimant count rates: by region[1]
Seasonally adjusted annual averages

Percentages

		1999	2000	2001	2002	2003	2004	2005	2006	2007	2008	2009
United Kingdom	BCJE	4.1	3.6	3.1	3.1	3.0	2.7	2.7	3.0	2.7	2.8	4.7
North East	DPDM	7.0	6.3	5.6	5.1	4.5	4.0	3.9	4.1	4.0	4.5	7.0
North West	IBWC	4.6	4.1	3.7	3.5	3.2	2.9	2.9	3.3	3.1	3.4	5.5
Yorkshire and the Humber	DPBI	5.0	4.3	3.9	3.6	3.3	2.8	2.9	3.3	3.0	3.4	5.7
East Midlands	DPBJ	3.6	3.3	3.1	2.9	2.8	2.5	2.5	2.8	2.6	2.8	4.9
West Midlands	DPBN	4.5	4.0	3.7	3.5	3.5	3.3	3.4	3.9	3.7	3.8	6.3
East	DPDP	2.9	2.4	2.0	2.1	2.1	2.0	2.1	2.3	2.1	2.2	4.0
London	DPDQ	4.4	3.7	3.3	3.6	3.6	3.5	3.4	3.5	3.0	2.8	4.3
South East	DPDR	2.3	1.8	1.5	1.6	1.7	1.6	1.6	1.9	1.6	1.7	3.3
South West	DPBM	3.0	2.5	2.0	1.9	1.9	1.6	1.6	1.8	1.6	1.7	3.4
England	VASQ	3.9	3.4	3.0	2.9	2.9	2.6	2.6	2.9	2.7	2.8	4.7
Wales	DPBP	5.0	4.4	3.9	3.5	3.3	3.0	3.0	3.1	2.8	3.2	5.5
Scotland	DPBQ	5.0	4.5	3.9	3.8	3.7	3.4	3.2	3.2	2.8	2.8	4.5
Northern Ireland	DPBR	6.3	5.3	4.9	4.4	4.2	3.6	3.3	3.2	2.8	3.2	5.7
Great Britain	DPAJ	4.0	3.5	3.1	3.0	3.0	2.7	2.7	2.9	2.7	2.8	4.7

1 The number of unemployment-related benefit claimants as a percentage of the estimated total workforce (the sum of claimants, employee jobs, self-employed, participants on work-related government training programmes and HM Forces) at mid-year. Excluded are claimants under 18, consistent with current coverage. See chapter text.

Source: Office for National Statistics: 01633 456901

Labour Market

7.15 Claimant count:[1] by region
Seasonally adjusted

Thousands

	North East	North West	Yorkshire and the Humber	East Midlands	West Midlands	East	London	South East	South West	England	Wales	Scotland	Great Britain	Northern Ireland	United Kingdom
	DPDG	IBWA	DPAX	DPAY	DPBC	DPDJ	DPDK	DPDL	DPBB	IBWK	DPBE	DPBF	DPAG	DPBG	BCJD
1994 Jan	145.6	325.1	233.7	174.7	262.3	210.0	451.4	296.7	203.6	2 302.3	126.7	236.0	2 665.8	100.2	2 766.0
Apr	141.6	314.5	227.4	170.7	252.0	200.4	440.4	280.9	194.5	2 221.7	123.3	231.7	2 577.4	98.9	2 676.3
Jul	139.1	304.2	222.7	166.3	242.3	191.0	428.1	268.1	188.1	2 148.8	119.0	227.4	2 496.3	97.2	2 593.5
Oct	136.0	291.7	215.9	160.1	230.5	180.5	415.4	251.1	178.9	2 059.0	112.9	218.1	2 391.1	93.8	2 484.9
1995 Jan	133.0	280.1	210.6	153.2	218.5	172.3	401.4	237.9	171.4	1 977.5	108.3	209.3	2 296.0	91.3	2 387.3
Apr	130.0	270.8	206.8	148.1	211.0	167.1	395.0	229.7	166.0	1 923.8	106.2	200.3	2 231.0	88.6	2 319.6
Jul	128.2	266.1	204.6	145.3	206.9	165.0	390.2	225.1	162.5	1 892.8	106.7	195.3	2 195.9	87.6	2 283.5
Oct	126.4	260.9	200.7	142.3	201.3	160.7	383.2	219.1	159.4	1 852.7	105.4	193.5	2 152.9	85.8	2 238.7
1996 Jan	123.1	255.8	197.0	140.0	196.5	157.2	376.8	213.3	155.6	1 814.6	104.0	193.2	2 112.5	85.9	2 198.4
Apr	121.7	254.9	195.7	137.7	194.2	153.5	367.9	207.6	152.3	1 785.1	104.6	194.9	2 085.0	86.1	2 171.1
Jul	116.9	248.2	188.8	131.8	187.6	146.8	357.5	198.9	146.8	1 722.5	101.8	191.9	2 017.0	86.4	2 103.4
Oct	110.5	238.4	181.1	124.9	177.8	138.5	341.6	185.5	137.9	1 635.0	98.2	186.3	1 920.7	81.7	2 002.4
1997 Jan	101.0	218.5	166.4	111.8	160.1	123.5	312.6	163.3	126.0	1 483.2	90.3	173.8	1 747.3	71.1	1 818.4
Apr	95.2	201.3	154.7	102.4	147.3	110.6	284.9	144.4	112.1	1 352.9	82.5	162.2	1 597.6	65.0	1 662.6
Jul	92.4	188.9	148.2	95.0	138.0	102.5	264.3	131.0	100.7	1 261.0	78.1	153.6	1 492.7	61.4	1 554.1
Oct	90.4	177.6	142.0	87.6	131.7	94.3	246.4	120.4	93.0	1 183.4	73.6	146.5	1 403.5	60.6	1 464.1
1998 Jan	87.6	170.6	137.2	82.8	126.1	88.5	234.3	112.3	88.7	1 128.1	70.9	141.6	1 340.6	59.9	1 400.5
Apr	84.1	165.4	134.1	79.9	122.3	85.2	229.4	108.0	85.1	1 093.5	69.3	138.7	1 301.5	57.9	1 359.4
Jul	81.8	163.7	133.3	80.0	121.4	83.7	225.2	105.5	84.1	1 078.7	68.6	139.4	1 286.7	57.3	1 344.0
Oct	82.1	160.9	130.9	79.9	121.4	82.0	219.3	102.5	81.8	1 060.8	68.1	136.9	1 265.8	56.1	1 321.9
1999 Jan	82.6	159.5	129.5	79.0	122.6	80.3	214.5	101.2	81.2	1 050.4	67.8	135.6	1 253.8	55.9	1 309.7
Apr	82.5	157.2	127.0	78.2	123.1	79.1	207.8	98.8	78.4	1 032.1	67.1	133.9	1 233.1	55.0	1 288.1
Jul	80.3	153.8	122.4	75.9	120.2	76.6	202.2	94.4	74.9	1 000.7	63.8	130.2	1 194.7	50.0	1 244.7
Oct	76.7	150.0	118.3	73.6	115.9	73.6	196.5	91.1	71.4	967.1	61.0	126.1	1 154.2	46.5	1 200.7
2000 Jan	75.7	145.7	114.6	73.2	112.1	70.3	189.4	87.2	68.0	936.2	59.3	123.2	1 118.7	44.2	1 162.9
Apr	73.6	139.9	108.9	70.0	108.1	66.9	181.6	81.3	63.8	894.1	57.8	119.0	1 070.9	42.4	1 113.3
Jul	72.0	135.4	104.9	68.7	107.2	62.5	172.0	77.5	61.1	861.3	57.1	115.1	1 033.5	41.2	1 074.7
Oct	69.5	131.0	102.5	67.7	106.5	60.7	165.0	74.3	58.1	835.3	56.4	111.7	1 003.4	41.3	1 044.7
2001 Jan	66.2	127.4	99.9	66.6	104.0	57.2	158.2	69.7	54.9	804.1	54.9	108.8	967.8	40.8	1 008.6
Apr	63.2	124.9	97.6	65.1	100.8	54.8	151.8	66.1	53.6	777.9	52.4	105.3	935.6	39.9	975.5
Jul	61.4	121.5	95.1	63.0	97.4	53.7	151.0	65.1	52.1	760.3	49.8	102.4	912.5	39.3	951.8
Oct	61.5	121.4	93.2	61.6	95.7	54.3	156.3	65.9	51.1	761.0	49.2	104.2	914.4	38.6	953.0
2002 Jan	60.9	121.3	91.4	60.6	95.4	55.4	163.1	68.6	51.1	767.8	48.1	104.3	920.2	38.0	958.2
Apr	59.2	119.4	89.4	59.4	93.6	56.4	166.2	71.0	50.9	765.5	47.5	104.4	917.4	37.5	954.9
Jul	58.5	118.1	89.1	58.6	93.4	57.5	167.3	72.3	50.1	764.9	46.8	101.9	913.6	36.4	950.0
Oct	55.9	116.1	87.6	57.9	93.7	57.2	167.6	72.3	49.3	757.6	46.7	100.1	904.4	35.1	939.5
2003 Jan	54.8	115.9	87.0	58.0	94.3	57.4	168.6	72.9	48.9	757.8	46.3	100.2	904.3	35.0	939.3
Apr	53.5	112.7	84.1	58.8	94.7	58.5	171.3	75.6	48.6	757.8	45.2	99.1	902.1	34.0	936.1
Jul	52.6	112.5	84.2	59.9	94.9	58.7	171.7	76.4	49.1	760.0	45.0	100.6	905.6	34.6	940.2
Oct	51.1	108.7	81.6	58.8	94.2	57.3	170.2	76.0	47.4	745.3	43.1	98.9	887.3	34.7	922.0
2004 Jan	49.8	104.6	78.3	56.2	93.0	56.7	167.8	75.0	45.3	726.7	42.0	97.0	865.7	33.5	899.2
Apr	47.5	101.3	75.6	53.7	89.7	56.0	165.5	72.3	42.7	704.3	41.4	94.4	840.1	31.8	871.9
Jul	45.4	96.7	71.6	51.1	86.7	54.6	162.0	68.5	40.4	677.0	39.5	90.0	806.5	29.9	836.4
Oct	45.1	96.5	71.1	50.9	86.0	55.0	158.8	69.2	40.6	673.2	39.2	89.5	801.9	29.6	831.5
2005 Jan	44.0	94.4	70.1	50.8	85.7	55.1	158.8	68.4	40.9	668.2	38.9	87.4	794.6	29.1	823.7
Apr	44.9	98.0	73.2	52.1	88.0	56.4	162.1	69.7	41.5	685.9	39.6	86.1	811.7	28.6	840.3
Jul	46.1	102.2	76.1	54.5	97.1	58.9	162.4	71.6	42.5	711.4	41.7	84.9	838.1	28.6	866.7
Oct	47.4	105.9	79.9	56.5	99.2	60.2	166.0	73.7	43.0	731.8	42.8	85.8	860.0	28.2	888.2
2006 Jan	47.2	109.4	84.2	59.1	102.6	62.2	168.2	78.5	44.3	755.7	43.9	85.7	885.4	28.2	913.7
Apr	49.4	115.0	86.9	62.1	109.2	64.9	167.8	81.2	44.7	784.3	45.1	88.1	917.5	28.0	945.5
Jul	50.8	117.0	88.3	62.5	109.8	65.9	168.4	83.5	49.2	795.4	44.3	89.0	928.8	28.0	956.7
Oct	51.6	118.2	89.0	63.3	110.2	68.0	166.4	82.5	49.7	799.0	44.3	87.3	930.6	28.0	958.6
2007 Jan	51.0	115.8	86.1	62.4	109.8	66.0	159.5	78.7	47.5	776.8	42.4	82.7	901.8	26.1	927.9
Apr	49.8	111.0	83.1	59.8	104.1	62.1	151.1	74.5	43.7	739.1	41.0	78.7	858.7	24.7	883.5
Jul	49.7	108.6	80.9	58.0	100.6	60.9	143.3	70.7	42.2	714.7	40.3	75.0	830.0	23.8	853.8
Oct	48.2	108.1	78.1	56.3	100.3	58.9	137.1	67.6	40.8	695.5	40.2	72.8	808.5	23.8	832.3
2008 Jan	46.9	106.0	75.4	53.3	95.1	55.5	131.8	65.8	38.0	667.4	38.6	69.6	775.7	23.7	799.3
Apr	48.1	107.4	76.9	53.7	95.5	54.7	128.3	66.0	37.8	668.5	39.7	69.9	778.1	24.2	802.3
Jul	52.2	116.0	85.0	58.8	102.2	61.3	132.9	72.9	44.9	726.4	44.0	76.3	846.6	27.1	873.7
Oct	59.8	132.4	99.1	68.7	116.2	71.9	145.9	86.8	55.4	836.4	51.2	87.9	975.4	31.5	1 006.8
2009 Jan	72.1	161.0	123.1	89.1	144.6	92.7	170.5	117.8	73.7	1 044.7	65.7	104.3	1 214.7	39.1	1 253.8
Apr	82.9	188.7	147.1	107.6	172.2	116.0	205.4	147.5	93.3	1 260.7	76.9	121.8	1 459.4	46.1	1 505.5
Jul	86.6	198.7	154.7	111.6	179.2	120.8	219.0	155.1	96.1	1 321.8	79.4	130.7	1 531.9	51.1	1 583.0
Oct	88.0	203.7	160.2	115.3	185.0	123.4	229.6	160.9	96.6	1 362.7	81.3	134.7	1 578.7	53.8	1 632.5

1 The figures are based on the number of claimants receiving unemployment related benefits and are adjusted for seasonality and discontinuities to be consistent with current coverage. See chapter text.

The latest national and regional seasonally adjusted claimant count figures are provisional and subject to revision in the following month.

Source: Office for National Statistics: 01633 456901

7.16 Economic activity: by sex and age[1]
United Kingdom
Seasonally adjusted

Thousands and percentages

	All aged 16 and over	16-59/64	16-17	18-24	25-34	35-49	50-64 (m) 50-59 (w)	65+ (m) 60+ (w)
Economically active								
People								
	MGSF	YBSK	YBZL	YBZO	YBZR	YBZU	YBZX	YCAD
2003	29 675	28 713	825	3 817	6 684	10 953	6 434	963
2004	29 909	28 893	817	3 936	6 581	11 074	6 485	1 016
2005	30 239	29 149	786	3 977	6 584	11 229	6 574	1 090
2006	30 698	29 506	741	4 122	6 593	11 391	6 660	1 193
2007	30 875	29 625	731	4 164	6 562	11 437	6 731	1 250
2008	31 220	29 871	709	4 221	6 629	11 495	6 816	1 349
2009	31 374	29 956	630	4 164	6 734	11 512	6 916	1 419
Men								
	MGSG	YBSL	YBZM	YBZP	YBZS	YBZV	YBZY	YCAE
2003	16 161	15 823	417	2 046	3 664	5 870	3 828	338
2004	16 240	15 894	408	2 108	3 593	5 922	3 863	346
2005	16 397	16 027	393	2 149	3 592	5 971	3 922	370
2006	16 628	16 228	367	2 215	3 605	6 072	3 969	401
2007	16 757	16 341	366	2 249	3 611	6 083	4 032	416
2008	16 941	16 487	361	2 286	3 635	6 104	4 101	455
2009	16 962	16 504	306	2 232	3 718	6 080	4 167	459
Women								
	MGSH	YBSM	YBZN	YBZQ	YBZT	YBZW	YBZZ	YCAF
2003	13 515	12 890	408	1 772	3 021	5 084	2 606	625
2004	13 669	12 999	409	1 828	2 989	5 151	2 621	670
2005	13 842	13 123	393	1 828	2 992	5 258	2 652	720
2006	14 070	13 278	375	1 907	2 988	5 319	2 691	792
2007	14 118	13 284	365	1 915	2 951	5 354	2 700	834
2008	14 278	13 384	348	1 935	2 994	5 391	2 715	894
2009	14 412	13 452	324	1 931	3 016	5 432	2 749	960
Economic activity rates (%)[1]								
People								
	MGWG	MGSO	YCAG	YCAJ	YCAM	YCAP	MGWP	MGWS
2003	63.0	78.6	53.9	74.3	83.5	84.9	72.0	9.1
2004	63.0	78.6	52.4	74.7	83.4	84.8	72.1	9.5
2005	63.2	78.6	50.0	73.7	83.8	85.0	72.6	10.1
2006	63.6	78.9	47.2	74.7	84.3	85.4	73.1	10.9
2007	63.5	78.9	46.1	73.8	84.3	85.3	73.7	11.3
2008	63.6	79.1	44.8	73.5	84.8	85.6	74.4	11.9
2009	63.5	79.0	40.5	71.8	84.8	85.9	74.9	12.3
Men								
	MGWH	MGSP	YCAH	YCAK	YCAN	YCAQ	MGWQ	MGWT
2003	71.0	83.9	53.0	79.2	92.4	92.0	74.5	8.6
2004	70.7	83.6	51.1	79.1	91.9	91.8	74.5	8.7
2005	70.6	83.5	48.8	78.6	92.3	91.4	74.9	9.2
2006	70.9	83.7	45.4	79.1	92.9	92.2	74.9	9.9
2007	70.8	83.6	44.9	78.2	93.0	91.9	75.3	10.1
2008	70.9	83.8	44.3	77.9	92.8	92.2	76.0	10.9
2009	70.3	83.3	38.5	75.8	92.9	92.0	76.4	10.6
Women								
	MGWI	MGSQ	YCAI	YCAL	YCAO	YCAR	MGWR	MGWU
2003	55.6	73.0	54.8	69.4	74.8	77.9	68.6	9.4
2004	55.8	73.2	53.9	70.1	75.1	77.9	68.8	10.0
2005	56.1	73.3	51.3	68.6	75.6	78.7	69.4	10.6
2006	56.7	73.8	49.0	70.1	75.9	78.8	70.4	11.6
2007	56.5	73.8	47.3	69.3	75.6	78.8	71.4	11.9
2008	56.8	74.1	45.2	68.9	76.7	79.2	72.2	12.6
2009	56.8	74.3	42.7	67.7	76.5	80.0	72.8	13.2

See chapter text.
1 Denominator = economically active for that age group.

Sources: Labour Force Survey, Office for National Statistics;
Helpline: 01633 456901

7.17 Economically inactive: by sex and age[1]
United Kingdom
Seasonally adjusted   Thousands and percentages

	All aged 16 and over	16-59/64	16-17	18-24	25-34	35-49	50-64 (m) 50-59 (w)	65+ (m) 60+ (w)
Economically inactive								
All Persons								
	MGSI	YBSN	YCAS	YCAV	YCAY	YCBB	MGWA	MGWD
2003	17 411	7 801	705	1 320	1 320	1 954	2 503	9 610
2004	17 538	7 880	741	1 336	1 306	1 990	2 509	9 659
2005	17 632	7 940	786	1 421	1 270	1 984	2 480	9 692
2006	17 570	7 859	831	1 399	1 224	1 947	2 459	9 711
2007	17 793	7 940	856	1 478	1 226	1 980	2 400	9 854
2008	17 839	7 872	876	1 523	1 195	1 936	2 343	9 967
2009	18 093	7 967	923	1 637	1 210	1 884	2 314	10 126
Men								
	MGSJ	YBSO	YCAT	YCAW	YCAZ	YCBC	MGWB	MGWE
2003	6 614	3 032	369	538	303	512	1 311	3 582
2004	6 738	3 116	391	557	316	533	1 320	3 623
2005	6 817	3 171	412	583	302	561	1 313	3 646
2006	6 811	3 152	441	586	278	518	1 329	3 659
2007	6 911	3 208	449	627	272	539	1 322	3 703
2008	6 950	3 201	453	649	283	521	1 296	3 748
2009	7 142	3 304	490	715	282	528	1 289	3 838
Women								
	MGSK	YBSP	YCAU	YCAX	YCBA	YCBD	MGWC	MGWF
2003	10 797	4 769	336	782	1 018	1 442	1 192	6 027
2004	10 800	4 765	351	779	989	1 457	1 189	6 036
2005	10 815	4 769	374	837	968	1 424	1 166	6 047
2006	10 760	4 707	390	812	946	1 429	1 130	6 052
2007	10 883	4 732	406	851	954	1 442	1 079	6 151
2008	10 889	4 671	423	875	911	1 415	1 047	6 219
2009	10 952	4 664	434	921	928	1 356	1 025	6 288
Economic inactivity rates (%)[1]								
All Persons								
	YBTC	YBTL	LWEX	LWFA	LWFD	LWFG	LWFJ	LWFM
2003	37.0	21.3	46.1	25.7	16.5	15.1	28.0	90.9
2004	37.0	21.4	47.6	25.3	16.5	15.2	27.9	90.5
2005	36.8	21.4	50.0	26.3	16.2	15.0	27.4	89.9
2006	36.4	21.0	52.8	25.4	15.6	14.6	27.0	89.1
2007	36.5	21.1	53.9	26.2	15.7	14.8	26.3	88.8
2008	36.4	20.9	55.3	26.5	15.3	14.4	25.6	88.1
2009	36.5	21.0	59.5	28.2	15.2	14.1	25.1	87.7
Men								
	YBTD	YBTM	LWEY	LWFB	LWFE	LWFH	LWFK	LWFN
2003	29.0	16.1	47.0	20.8	7.6	8.0	25.5	91.4
2004	29.3	16.4	48.9	20.9	8.1	8.2	25.5	91.3
2005	29.4	16.5	51.2	21.4	7.8	8.6	25.1	90.8
2006	29.1	16.3	54.6	20.9	7.1	7.8	25.0	90.2
2007	29.2	16.4	55.1	21.8	7.0	8.1	24.7	89.9
2008	29.1	16.3	55.7	22.1	7.2	7.9	24.0	89.1
2009	29.6	16.7	61.5	24.2	7.1	8.0	23.6	89.3
Women								
	YBTE	YBTN	LWEZ	LWFC	LWFF	LWFI	LWFL	LWFO
2003	44.4	27.0	45.2	30.6	25.2	22.1	31.4	90.6
2004	44.2	26.8	46.1	29.9	24.9	22.0	31.2	90.0
2005	43.9	26.7	48.7	31.4	24.5	21.3	30.6	89.4
2006	43.3	26.1	51.0	29.9	24.0	21.2	29.6	88.4
2007	43.5	26.3	52.7	30.8	24.5	21.2	28.5	88.1
2008	43.3	25.8	54.8	31.1	23.4	20.8	27.8	87.4
2009	43.2	25.7	57.3	32.3	23.5	20.0	27.1	86.8

See chapter text.
1 Denominator = all persons in the relevant age group.

Sources: Labour Force Survey, Office for National Statistics;
Helpline: 01633 456901

7.18 Economically inactive: by reason and sex
United Kingdom
Seasonally adjusted

Thousands and percentages

| | Economic inactivity by reason: | | | | | | | by: | | All economically inactive |
	Student	Looking after family/home	Temporary sick	Long-term sick	Discouraged workers[4]	Retired	Other	Does not want a job	Wants a job[1]	
Thousands										
All Persons										
	BEDZ	BEEC	BEBK	BEBN	YCFO	BEEI	BEEL	YBVZ	YBWC	YBSN
2002	1 543	2 398	188	2 203	37	585	810	5 505	2 258	7 762
2003	1 655	2 393	187	2 136	35	582	814	5 669	2 133	7 801
2004	1 717	2 347	190	2 158	32	595	842	5 841	2 040	7 880
2005	1 836	2 335	189	2 126	37	594	825	5 892	2 048	7 940
2006	1 837	2 325	191	2 068	37	593	808	5 781	2 079	7 859
2007	1 926	2 315	199	2 043	37	604	815	5 843	2 097	7 940
2008	1 995	2 267	177	2 019	42	597	776	5 732	2 140	7 872
2009	2 166	2 243	173	2 009	66	578	732	5 767	2 201	7 967
Men										
	BEEX	BEAQ	BEDI	BEDL	YCFP	BEDR	BEDU	YBWA	YBWD	YBSO
2002	763	180	90	1 226	23	396	337	2 072	943	3 015
2003	828	185	90	1 170	20	396	344	2 129	903	3 032
2004	873	189	96	1 180	21	407	351	2 249	866	3 116
2005	913	193	97	1 171	23	414	362	2 324	848	3 171
2006	919	194	94	1 134	26	433	351	2 263	889	3 152
2007	966	197	98	1 131	21	443	352	2 312	896	3 208
2008	1 002	194	85	1 118	24	435	343	2 286	916	3 201
2009	1 104	210	84	1 114	40	431	321	2 343	961	3 304
Women										
	BEBL	BEBO	BEEG	BEEJ	YCFQ	BEEP	BEES	YBWB	YBWE	YBSP
2002	779	2 218	98	977	14	189	474	3 433	1 314	4 747
2003	827	2 208	98	966	15	186	469	3 540	1 230	4 769
2004	844	2 158	94	978	..	189	490	3 592	1 173	4 765
2005	923	2 142	93	955	14	180	463	3 569	1 200	4 769
2006	918	2 131	97	933	..	160	458	3 518	1 190	4 707
2007	959	2 119	101	912	16	161	464	3 531	1 201	4 732
2008	993	2 073	91	901	18	162	433	3 447	1 224	4 671
2009	1 061	2 034	89	896	26	148	412	3 424	1 240	4 664
Percentages[5]										
All Persons										
	BEDJ	BEDM	BEDP	BEDS	BEDV	BEDY	BEEB	BEEE	BEBM	BEAR
2002	19.9	30.9	2.4	28.4	0.5	7.5	10.5	70.9	29.1	100
2003	21.2	30.7	2.4	27.4	0.4	7.5	10.4	72.7	27.4	100
2004	21.8	29.8	2.4	27.4	0.4	7.6	10.7	74.1	25.9	100
2005	23.1	29.4	2.4	26.8	0.4	7.5	10.4	74.2	25.8	100
2006	23.4	29.6	2.4	26.3	0.5	7.6	10.3	73.6	26.4	100
2007	24.3	29.2	2.5	25.8	0.4	7.6	10.3	73.6	26.4	100
2008	25.3	28.8	2.3	25.6	0.5	7.6	9.9	72.8	27.2	100
2009	27.2	28.1	2.2	25.2	0.9	7.2	9.2	72.4	27.6	100
Men										
	BEEH	BEEK	BEEN	BEEQ	BEET	BEEW	BEEZ	BEAS	BEGT	BEBP
2002	25.3	5.9	3.0	40.7	0.8	13.1	11.1	68.7	31.3	100
2003	27.3	6.1	3.0	38.6	0.7	13.0	11.4	70.2	29.8	100
2004	28.0	6.1	3.1	37.9	0.6	13.1	11.3	72.2	27.8	100
2005	28.8	6.1	3.0	36.9	0.8	13.1	11.4	73.3	26.7	100
2006	29.1	6.2	3.0	36.0	0.8	13.7	11.1	71.8	28.2	100
2007	30.1	6.2	3.0	35.3	0.6	13.8	11.0	72.1	27.9	100
2008	31.3	6.1	2.7	34.9	0.8	13.6	10.7	71.4	28.6	100
2009	33.4	6.3	2.5	33.7	1.2	13.0	9.7	70.9	29.0	100
Women										
	BEGZ	BEHC	BEHF	BEHI	BEHL	BEHO	BEBQ	BEHR	BEHU	BEGW
2002	16.4	46.7	2.0	20.5	0.3	4.0	10.0	72.3	27.7	100
2003	17.4	46.3	2.0	20.3	0.3	3.9	9.8	74.2	25.8	100
2004	17.7	45.3	2.0	20.5	..	4.0	10.3	75.4	24.6	100
2005	19.3	44.9	1.9	20.0	0.3	3.8	9.7	74.8	25.1	100
2006	19.5	45.3	2.0	19.9	..	3.4	9.7	74.8	25.3	100
2007	20.3	44.8	2.2	19.3	0.4	3.4	9.8	74.6	25.4	100
2008	21.3	44.4	2.0	19.3	0.4	3.5	9.3	73.8	26.2	100
2009	22.8	43.6	1.9	19.2	0.6	3.2	8.8	73.4	26.6	100

1 This series comprises those who have not been looking for work in the last four weeks, but who say they would like a regular paid job, plus those who have been looking for work but who were unable to start within two weeks.

Sources: Labour Force Survey, Office for National Statistics;
Helpline: 01633 456901

7.19 Labour disputes: by industry[1]
United Kingdom
Standard Industrial Classification 2003

Thousands and numbers

		2001	2002	2003	2004	2005	2006	2007	2008
Working days lost through all stoppages in progress (thousands)	KBBZ	525	1 323	499	905	157	755	1 041	759
Analysis by industry									
Mining, quarrying, electricity, gas and water	DMME	25	..	..	5	6	12	..	1
Manufacturing	BBFX	43	21	63	31	16	18	16	7
Construction	DMMG	10	17	14	..	2	15	2	3
Transport, storage and communication	BBFY	107	96	126	44	33	41	658	25
Public administration and defence	BBFZ	216	488	138	437	23	627	325	614
Education	BBGA	43	376	131	379	43	31	31	103
Health and social work	BBGB	73	148	15	4	..	5	5	2
Other community, social and personal services	DMML	4	107	10	4	6	2	4	3
All other industries and services	DMMM	4	70	2	2	29	5	2	2
Analysis by number of working days lost in each stoppage									
Under 250 days	KBFC	9	7	6	7	5	7	6	8
250 and under 500 days	KBFJ	11	8	6	5	4	8	6	5
500 and under 1,000 days	KBFL	15	15	13	12	7	8	11	8
1,000 and under 5,000 days	KBFY	59	47	69	51	80	66	50	27
5,000 and under 25,000 days	KBFZ	140	104	46	59	61	69	76	54
25,000 and under 50,000 days	KBGS	72	122	112	–	–	–	..	..
50,000 days and over	KBGT	220	1 021	248	770	..	597	892	656
Working days lost per 1 000 employees all industries and services	KBHA	20	51	19	34	6	28	39	28
Workers directly and indirectly involved (thousands)	KBHB	180	943	151	293	93	713	745	511
Analysis by industry									
Mining, quarrying, electricity, gas and water	DMMN	3	..	..	1	6	1	..	1
Manufacturing	DMMO	17	10	18	14	3	11	13	5
Construction	DMMP	3	17	2	..	1	2	1	3
Transport, storage and communications	DMMQ	69	33	52	12	13	14	399	19
Public administration and defence	DMMR	46	171	56	207	15	654	317	370
Education	DMMS	34	388	15	55	43	28	9	110
Health and social work	DMMT	6	144	3	1	..	2	2	..
Other community, social and personal services	DMMU	1	103	3	3	6	1	2	2
All other industries and services	DMMV	1	76	1	1	5	2	2	1
Analysis by duration of stoppage									
Not more than 5 days	KBHM	98	828	78	222	89	705	357	511
Over 5 but not more than 10 days	KBHN	43	57	23	47	3	5	288	..
Over 10 but not more than 20 days	KBJQ	4	3	31	1	1	2	6	..
Over 20 but not more than 30 days	KBJR	–	1	..	3	..	1	94	..
Over 30 but not more than 50 days	KBJS	6	1	..	..	1	–	..	..
Over 50 days	KBJT	30	55	20	20	–	–	..	..
Numbers of stoppages in progress: total	KBLG	194	146	133	130	116	158	142	144
Analysis by industry									
Mining, quarrying, electricity, gas and water	DMMW	3	2	1	3	2	2	..	1
Manufacturing	DMMX	32	33	43	30	19	25	22	21
Construction	DMMY	9	3	4	1	3	5	4	4
Transport, storage and communications	DMMZ	94	51	45	46	42	30	55	28
Public administration and defence	DMNA	22	20	12	19	13	18	20	16
Education	DMNB	16	16	15	16	22	53	21	40
Health and social work	DMNC	12	14	7	4	1	4	12	4
Other community, social and personal services	DMND	10	11	9	12	5	8	11	18
All other industries and services	DMNE	9	12	4	4	10	13	7	12
Analysis of number of stoppages by duration									
Not more than 5 days	KBNH	162	118	113	111	102	126	119	136
Over 5 but not more than 10 days	KBNI	15	16	10	10	8	19	12	5
Over 10 but not more than 20 days	KBNJ	7	3	5	4	3	10	6	1
Over 20 but not more than 30 days	KBNK	1	3	1	2	..	1	1	..
Over 30 but not more than 50 days	KBNL	4	1	1	1	3	2	2	1
Over 50 days	KBNM	5	5	3	2	..	..	2	1

1 See chapter text.

Source: Labour Market Statistics, Office for National Statistics: 01633 456721

7.20 Median[1] weekly and hourly earnings of full-time employees [2] by industry division[3] United Kingdom

April 2008 to 2009. Standard Industrial Classification 2007[3]

	Agriculture, forestry and fishing	Mining and Quarrying	Manufacturing	Electricity, gas, steam and air conditioning supply	Water supply, sewerage, waste management and remediation activities	Construction	Wholesale and retail trade; repair of motor vehicles and motorcycles	Transport and storage	Accommodation and food service activities
Median gross weekly earnings									
All employees									
	JR89	JR8A	JR8B	JR8C	JR8D	JR8E	JR8F	JR8G	JR8H
2008	356.8	649.0	486.3	661.5	500.0	516.7	380.0	470.6	296.8
2009	439.0	409.7	802.9	562.7	696.6	592.9	482.2	375.9	567.6
Men									
	JR8S	JR8T	JR8U	JR8V	JR8W	JR8X	JR8Y	JR8Z	JR92
2008	375.4	674.8	513.6	715.8	512.6	533.3	421.6	480.1	316.2
2009	402.5	726.5	510.4	636.2	531.2	550.0	428.0	488.3	317.3
Women									
	JR9D	JR9E	JR9F	JR9G	JR9H	JR9I	JR9J	JR9K	JR9L
2008	301.1	499.6	365.4	399.9	447.2	398.4	317.7	421.6	272.9
2009	345.0	568.0	370.5	405.4	474.1	403.9	325.8	436.5	278.3
Median hourly earnings (excluding overtime)									
All employees									
	JR9W	JR9X	JR9Y	JR9Z	JRA2	JRA3	JRA4	JRA5	JRA6
2008	7.69	15.27	11.44	16.12	10.94	11.79	9.18	10.48	7.00
2009	8.24	16.67	11.76	14.97	11.80	12.22	9.46	11.00	7.10
Men									
	JRB9	JRC2	JRC3	JRC4	JRC5	JRC6	JRC7	JRC8	JRC9
2008	7.69	15.27	11.44	16.12	10.94	11.79	9.18	10.48	7.00
2009	8.24	16.67	11.76	14.97	11.80	12.22	9.46	11.00	7.10
Women									
	JRE4	JRE5	JRE6	JRE7	JRE8	JRE9	JRF2	JRF3	JRF4
2008	7.21	15.07	9.20	10.53	11.03	10.49	8.10	10.59	6.63
2009	8.25	16.17	9.50	10.68	12.23	10.50	8.38	11.02	6.90
Median total paid hours worked									
All employees									
	JS5P	JS5Q	JS5R	JS5S	JS5T	JS5U	JS5V	JS5W	JS5X
2008	40.0	39.9	39.1	37.0	40.0	40.0	39.1	40.0	40.0
2009	40.0	37.5	38.9	37.0	40.0	40.0	39.1	40.0	40.0
Men									
	JS6A	JS6B	JS6C	JS6D	JS6E	JS6F	JS6G	JS6H	JS6I
2008	40.0	40.0	39.8	37.2	40.5	40.0	40.0	40.5	40.0
2009	40.0	39.9	39.0	37.0	40.7	40.0	40.0	40.0	40.0
Women									
	JS6T	JS6U	JS6V	JS6W	JS6X	JS6Y	JS6Z	JS72	JS73
2008	40.0	37.5	37.8	37.0	37.2	37.5	37.6	38.9	39.8
2009	39.1	37.0	37.5	36.9	37.0	37.5	37.6	37.5	39.5

7.20
continued

Median[1] weekly and hourly earnings of full-time employees [2] by industry division[3]
United Kingdom
April 2008 to 2009. Standard Industrial Classification 2007[3]

	Information and communication	Financial and insurance activities	Real estate activities	Professional and scientific and technical activities	Administrative and support service activities	Public administration and defence	Education	Human Health and social work activities	Arts,entertainment and recreation	Other service activities
Median gross weekly earnings										
All employees										
	JR8I	JR8J	JR8K	JR8L	JR8M	JR8N	JR8O	JR8P	JR8Q	JR8R
2008	634.8	597.2	451.9	579.7	383.6	533.5	525.6	458.4	380.6	414.7
2009	806.9	651.8	583.4	568.8	542.6	524.9	541.6	473.0	387.8	424.3
Men										
	JR93	JR94	JR95	JR96	JR97	JR98	JR99	JR9A	JR9B	JR9C
2008	687.8	766.6	528.8	680.4	402.7	595.0	575.5	542.6	406.9	464.1
2009	682.8	799.4	526.0	689.9	415.2	605.8	587.4	563.2	404.8	470.5
Women										
	JR9M	JR9N	JR9O	JR9P	JR9Q	JR9R	JR9S	JR9T	JR9U	JR9V
2008	536.6	450.4	391.7	479.1	350.0	443.9	484.5	433.8	351.9	361.5
2009	542.5	484.3	408.3	496.0	353.6	463.7	500.5	441.0	366.4	364.1
Median hourly earnings (excluding overtime)										
All employees										
	JRA7	JRA8	JRA9	JRB2	JRB3	JRB4	JRB5	JRB6	JRB7	JRB8
2008	16.39	16.43	11.92	15.26	8.82	13.34	14.56	11.99	9.25	10.75
2009	16.73	17.38	12.18	15.84	9.20	13.83	15.06	12.34	9.76	11.10
Men										
	JRD2	JRD3	JRD4	JRD5	JRD6	JRD7	JRD8	JRD9	JRE2	JRE3
2008	16.39	16.43	11.92	15.26	8.82	13.34	14.56	11.99	9.25	10.75
2009	16.73	17.38	12.18	15.84	9.20	13.83	15.06	12.34	9.76	11.10
Women										
	JRF5	JRF6	JRF7	JRF8	JRF9	JRG2	JRG3	JRG4	JRG5	JRG6
2008	14.23	12.45	10.56	12.86	8.83	11.57	13.79	11.34	8.73	9.45
2009	14.64	13.54	10.95	13.29	9.07	12.25	14.30	11.51	9.24	9.56
Median total paid hours worked										
All employees										
	JS5Y	JS5Z	JS62	JS63	JS64	JS65	JS66	JS67	JS68	JS69
2008	37.5	35.0	37.4	37.5	40.0	37.6	36.1	37.5	39.9	37.5
2009	37.5	35.0	37.0	37.5	39.9	37.1	36.1	37.5	39.6	37.5
Men										
	JS6J	JS6K	JS6L	JS6M	JS6N	JS6O	JS6P	JS6Q	JS6R	JS6S
2008	37.5	35.0	37.5	37.5	40.0	39.9	36.9	37.5	40.0	38.6
2009	37.5	35.0	37.4	37.5	40.0	39.1	36.9	37.5	40.0	37.5
Women										
	JS74	JS75	JS76	JS77	JS78	JS79	JS7A	JS7B	JS7C	JS7D
2008	37.5	35.0	37.0	37.0	37.5	37.0	35.0	37.5	38.3	37.5
2009	37.5	35.0	37.0	37.0	37.5	37.0	35.0	37.5	37.7	37.3

1 See chapter text. Median values are less affected by extremes of earnings at either ends of the scale with half the employees earning above the stated amount and half below. Previous editions of Annual Abstract published means.

2 Data relate to full-time employeeson adult rates whose pay for the survey-period was not affected by absence.

3 Classification is based on Standard Industrial Classification 2007.

Sources: Annual Survey of Hours and Earnings;
Office for National Statistics: 01633 456120

7.21 Median[1] weekly and hourly earnings and total paid hours of full-time employees:[2]
United Kingdom
April 2008 to 2009

	Manufacturing industries				All industries and services			
			Hourly earnings(£)				Hourly earnings(£)	
	Gross weekly earnings	Total paid hours	including overtime pay	excluding overtime pay	Gross weekly earnings(£)	Total paid hours	including overtime	excluding overtime
SIC 2007[3]								
All								
	JR7J	JR7K	JR7L	JR7M	JR7V	JR7W	JR7X	JR7Y
2008	486.3	39.1	11.72	11.44	479.1	37.5	11.98	11.88
2009	484.9	38.9	11.94	11.76	488.7	37.5	12.43	12.34
Men								
	JR7N	JR7O	JR7P	JR7Q	JR7Z	JR82	JR83	JR84
2008	513.6	39.8	12.21	11.95	522.0	39.0	12.63	12.50
2009	510.4	39.0	12.47	12.27	531.1	38.7	13.09	12.97
Women								
	JR7R	JR7S	JR7T	JR7U	JR85	JR86	JR87	JR88
2008	365.4	37.8	9.25	9.20	412.4	37.1	10.94	10.92
2009	370.5	37.5	9.54	9.50	426.4	37.0	11.42	11.40

1 Median values are less affected by extremes of earnings at either ends of the scale with half the employees earning above the stated amount and half below. Previous editions of Annual Abstract published means.
2 Data relate to full-time employees on adult rates whose pay for the survey pay-period was not affected by absence.
3 Classification is based on Standard Industrial Clasification 2007.

Source: Annual Survey of Hours and Earnings: 01633 456120

7.22 Average weekly earnings: main industrial sectors
Great Britain
Standard Industrial Classification 2007

	Whole economy		Manufacturing		Construction		Services		Distribution Hotels and Restuarants	
	Actual	Seasonally adjusted	Actual	Seasonally adjusted	Actual	Seasonally adjusted	Actual	Seasonally adjusted	Actual	Seasonally adjusted
	KA46	KAB9	KA49	KAE3	KA4C	KAE6	KA4F	KAD2	KA4I	KAE9
2000	321	320	371	371	386	386	306	306	224	224
2001	338	337	385	385	418	417	323	322	233	233
2002	348	348	399	399	427	427	334	333	242	241
2003	359	359	414	413	445	445	345	344	247	247
2004	375	374	434	433	458	458	360	360	255	255
2005	392	391	450	449	472	471	378	377	264	264
2006	410	410	466	465	501	501	396	396	274	273
2007	431	430	484	483	535	535	416	416	290	290
2008	446	445	500	499	546	545	433	431	297	297
2009	445	445	506	505	553	553	431	430	301	301

	Finance and Business Industries		Private Sector		Public Sector		Private Sector Excl Financial Services	
	Actual	Seasonally adjusted	Actual	Seasonally adjusted	Actual	Seasonally adjusted	Actual	Seasonally adjusted
	KA4L	KAD5	KA4O	KAC4	KA4R	KAC7	KA4U	KAD8
2000	410	412	322	322	314	313	314	313
2001	443	443	339	339	331	329	331	329
2002	451	452	349	349	344	342	344	342
2003	463	464	359	359	360	358	360	358
2004	486	487	374	374	376	374	375	374
2005	511	511	391	390	396	394	395	394
2006	546	546	410	410	410	408	410	408
2007	574	572	432	432	424	421	424	421
2008	603	600	448	447	439	437	438	436
2009	583	584	443	443	453	451	450	448

1 See chapter text.

Source: Office for National Statistics: 01633 819024

Labour Market

7.23 Average weekly earnings : by industry
Great Britain
Not seasonally adjusted

£ per employee per week

	Agriculture, forestry and fishing	Mining and quarrying	Food products, beverages and tobacco	Textiles, leather and clothing	Chemicals and man-made fibres	Basic metals and metal products	Engineering and allied industries	Other manufacturing	Electricity, gas and water supply	Construction
Excluding bonuses										
SIC 1992										
	JT7X	JT7Y	JT7Z	JT82	JT83	JT84	JT85	JT86	JT87	JT88
2008	303	883	436	346	562	476	526	448	584	522
2009	314	915	446	360	602	475	527	458	608	534
2007 Aug	283	856	421	357	561	452	510	425	554	518
Sep	278	835	418	355	564	453	510	430	557	526
Oct	280	854	426	353	566	459	514	435	571	517
Nov	281	859	422	340	575	458	515	435	567	521
Dec	277	871	431	340	570	451	514	438	576	518
2008 Jan	289	875	418	344	566	479	518	443	569	509
Feb	299	878	431	355	565	469	518	447	569	518
Mar	302	859	436	343	550	465	530	450	584	513
Apr	303	862	435	344	565	475	531	445	569	523
May	304	888	434	345	557	476	527	448	571	521
Jun	303	900	438	342	566	478	526	449	569	528
Jul	298	881	435	345	563	481	529	448	583	525
Aug	302	882	434	343	550	477	525	444	618	511
Sep	310	895	435	347	566	478	520	449	585	527
Oct	313	887	437	349	564	479	527	450	583	530
Nov	306	883	443	354	562	486	529	454	598	530
Dec	310	910	452	346	570	474	529	449	604	527
2009 Jan	311	885	447	354	578	479	523	448	592	534
Feb	301	904	442	359	574	471	521	447	595	531
Mar	314	904	449	357	585	471	525	451	607	536
Apr	308	924	449	361	587	478	527	453	596	534
May	322	916	447	359	612	475	522	460	605	531
Jun	319	912	445	354	622	474	522	460	607	527
Jul	303	922	444	356	616	463	520	456	612	532
Aug	314	906	435	359	609	467	527	459	607	531
Sep	319	925	443	355	593	474	527	461	607	534
Oct	313	927	438	366	610	475	536	464	616	540
Nov	323	928	437	371	613	484	537	465	629	540
Dec	325	930	476	373	623	486	541	466	626	541
2010 Jan	321	905	475	379	620	478	536	476	622	544
Feb	309	937	457	370	620	505	536	471	620	539
Mar	318	927	469	392	617	509	543	479	640	544
Percentage change on the year										
	JT8R	JT8S	JT8T	JT8U	JT8V	JT8W	JT8X	JT8Y	JT8Z	JT92
2008 Aug	6.7	3.0	3.1	–3.9	–2.0	5.5	2.9	4.5	11.6	–1.4
Sep	11.5	7.2	4.1	–2.3	0.4	5.5	2.0	4.4	5.0	0.2
Oct	11.8	3.9	2.6	–1.1	–0.4	4.4	2.5	3.4	2.1	2.5
Nov	8.9	2.8	5.0	4.1	–2.3	6.1	2.7	4.4	5.5	1.7
Dec	11.9	4.5	4.9	1.8	–	5.1	2.9	2.5	4.9	1.7
2009 Jan	7.6	1.1	6.9	2.9	2.1	–	1.0	1.1	4.0	4.9
Feb	0.7	3.0	2.6	1.1	1.6	0.4	0.6	–	4.6	2.5
Mar	4.0	5.2	3.0	4.1	6.4	1.3	–0.9	0.2	3.9	4.5
Apr	1.7	7.2	3.2	4.9	3.9	0.6	–0.8	1.8	4.7	2.1
May	5.9	3.2	3.0	4.1	9.9	–0.2	–0.9	2.7	6.0	1.9
Jun	5.3	1.3	1.6	3.5	9.9	–0.8	–0.8	2.4	6.7	–0.2
Jul	1.7	4.7	2.1	3.2	9.4	–3.7	–1.7	1.8	5.0	1.3
Aug	4.0	2.7	0.2	4.7	10.7	–2.1	0.4	3.4	–1.8	3.9
Sep	2.9	3.4	1.8	2.3	4.8	–0.8	1.3	2.7	3.8	1.3
Oct	–	4.5	0.2	4.9	8.2	–0.8	1.7	3.1	5.7	1.9
Nov	5.6	5.1	–1.4	4.8	9.1	–0.4	1.5	2.4	5.2	1.9
Dec	4.8	2.2	5.3	7.8	9.3	2.5	2.3	3.8	3.6	2.7
2010 Jan	3.2	2.3	6.3	7.1	7.3	–0.2	2.5	6.3	5.1	1.9
Feb	2.7	3.7	3.4	3.1	8.0	7.2	2.9	5.4	4.2	1.5
Mar	1.3	2.5	4.5	9.8	5.5	8.1	3.4	6.2	5.4	1.5

7.23
continued

Average weekly earnings : by industry
Great Britain

Not seasonally adjusted

£ per employee per week

	Wholesale trade	Retail trade and repairs	Hotels and restaurants	Transport, storage and communication	Financial interm-ediation	Real estate renting and business activities	Public admini-stration	Education	Health and social work	Other services
Excluding bonuses										
SIC 1992										
	JT89	JT8A	JT8B	JT8C	JT8D	JT8E	JT8F	JT8G	JT8H	JT8I
2008	472	249	209	497	656	474	496	377	383	370
2009	480	256	209	502	686	482	509	390	392	366
2007 Aug	455	248	208	494	633	453	490	368	364	368
Sep	452	246	207	483	638	453	487	371	365	368
Oct	461	242	209	481	635	456	485	368	368	358
Nov	455	239	213	487	638	459	490	372	383	358
Dec	458	238	214	496	640	461	496	376	377	354
2008 Jan	470	247	206	492	636	461	496	366	377	368
Feb	466	243	206	493	646	465	497	367	376	367
Mar	472	247	214	500	654	464	490	368	377	376
Apr	473	256	207	502	654	471	496	372	381	369
May	471	252	210	501	653	469	494	373	379	374
Jun	471	250	209	501	662	475	494	372	380	369
Jul	470	248	208	490	671	479	495	375	385	378
Aug	468	251	212	492	657	484	496	378	392	378
Sep	475	252	210	494	653	480	495	382	385	366
Oct	473	249	209	499	663	480	495	381	387	367
Nov	474	245	204	497	659	481	507	395	389	366
Dec	478	248	211	499	667	479	503	393	391	367
2009 Jan	480	254	205	500	664	480	502	386	389	366
Feb	479	254	209	497	675	482	524	386	384	363
Mar	479	256	209	498	675	482	506	383	388	365
Apr	476	256	210	501	689	488	510	388	393	371
May	478	258	211	504	683	487	510	387	395	364
Jun	479	257	209	505	682	487	504	390	399	366
Jul	479	257	211	499	685	485	506	393	394	368
Aug	478	257	210	503	689	483	509	394	389	367
Sep	478	259	208	505	690	480	503	397	393	367
Oct	484	257	209	505	693	478	508	396	394	365
Nov	484	252	208	502	714	478	512	392	393	366
Dec	488	253	214	505	696	479	511	393	396	369
2010 Jan	484	261	210	503	699	483	519	389	391	386
Feb	479	259	215	502	718	484	520	388	395	370
Mar	486	264	215	511	723	487	518	389	392	370
Percentage change on the year										
	JT93	JT94	JT95	JT96	JT97	JT98	JT99	JT9A	JT9B	JT9C
2008 Aug	2.9	1.2	1.9	−0.4	3.8	6.8	1.2	2.7	7.7	2.7
Sep	5.1	2.4	1.4	2.3	2.4	6.0	1.6	3.0	5.5	−0.5
Oct	2.6	2.9	–	3.7	4.4	5.3	2.1	3.5	5.2	2.5
Nov	4.2	2.5	−4.2	2.1	3.3	4.8	3.5	6.2	1.6	2.2
Dec	4.4	4.2	−1.4	0.6	4.2	3.9	1.4	4.5	3.7	3.7
2009 Jan	2.1	2.8	−0.5	1.6	4.4	4.1	1.2	5.5	3.2	−0.5
Feb	2.8	4.5	1.5	0.8	4.5	3.7	5.4	5.2	2.1	−1.1
Mar	1.5	3.6	−2.3	−0.4	3.2	3.9	3.3	4.1	2.9	−2.9
Apr	0.6	–	1.4	−0.2	5.4	3.6	2.8	4.3	3.1	0.5
May	1.5	2.4	0.5	0.6	4.6	3.8	3.2	3.8	4.2	−2.7
Jun	1.7	2.8	–	0.8	3.0	2.5	2.0	4.8	5.0	−0.8
Jul	1.9	3.6	1.4	1.8	2.1	1.3	2.2	4.8	2.3	−2.6
Aug	2.1	2.4	−0.9	2.2	4.9	−0.2	2.6	4.2	−0.8	−2.9
Sep	0.6	2.8	−1.0	2.2	5.7	–	1.6	3.9	2.1	0.3
Oct	2.3	3.2	–	1.2	4.5	−0.4	2.6	3.9	1.8	−0.5
Nov	2.1	2.9	2.0	1.0	8.3	−0.6	1.0	−0.8	1.0	–
Dec	2.1	2.0	1.4	1.2	4.3	–	1.6	–	1.3	0.5
2010 Jan	0.8	2.8	2.4	0.6	5.3	0.6	3.4	0.8	0.5	5.5
Feb	–	2.0	2.9	1.0	6.4	0.4	−0.8	0.5	2.9	1.9
Mar	1.5	3.1	2.9	2.6	7.1	1.0	2.4	1.6	1.0	1.4

Labour Market

7.23 Average weekly earnings : by industry
Great Britain

Not seasonally adjusted

£ per employee per week

	Agriculture, forestry and fishing	Mining and quarrying	Food products, beverages and tobacco	Textiles, leather and clothing	Chemicals and man-made fibres	Basic metals and metal products	Engineering and allied industries	Other manufacturing	Electricity, gas and water supply	Construction

Including bonuses

SIC 1992

	KA5Z	KA64	KA67	KA6A	KA6D	KA6G	KA6J	KA6M	KA6P	KA6S
2008	310	996	460	368	600	499	547	469	622	546
2009	321	1 013	466	384	641	492	548	475	652	553
2007 Aug	289	910	427	382	576	462	520	438	576	532
Sep	282	923	437	391	591	468	519	440	582	555
Oct	282	906	437	368	582	480	525	450	595	538
Nov	286	946	429	357	588	479	531	452	593	555
Dec	287	991	461	362	613	504	549	473	591	584
2008 Jan	297	957	428	369	586	499	534	458	587	531
Feb	300	987	469	370	603	491	556	466	594	539
Mar	311	1 384	488	374	696	492	591	492	697	561
Apr	308	965	457	355	667	506	546	466	628	541
May	308	951	482	356	569	497	544	470	598	539
Jun	305	999	456	402	593	495	543	469	627	548
Jul	300	957	462	357	580	520	543	471	629	541
Aug	309	920	442	350	558	492	535	457	635	527
Sep	318	972	458	364	576	489	532	461	621	553
Oct	316	932	446	369	575	507	538	465	604	547
Nov	308	943	450	369	588	497	540	468	623	553
Dec	346	984	479	378	607	501	564	483	619	567
2009 Jan	318	1 004	457	369	596	497	539	460	617	547
Feb	311	995	458	375	607	493	556	460	625	546
Mar	321	1 298	520	387	753	505	587	487	731	576
Apr	311	1 031	465	378	711	499	554	468	651	553
May	323	972	456	374	622	489	537	473	633	543
Jun	321	972	460	452	644	489	535	476	673	543
Jul	313	969	459	367	631	484	533	474	667	548
Aug	316	970	442	365	615	475	536	472	631	543
Sep	326	967	464	365	601	480	537	474	634	550
Oct	318	981	447	375	622	486	545	479	643	555
Nov	326	977	448	389	625	507	547	479	663	560
Dec	352	1 024	511	411	669	506	568	494	651	574
2010 Jan	325	993	484	402	644	499	548	492	649	560
Feb	330	1 092	472	390	682	533	566	495	648	554
Mar	330	1 586	580	435	825	593	610	529	772	614

Percentage change on the year

	JT9D	JT9E	JT9F	JT9G	JT9H	JT9I	JT9J	JT9K	JT9L	JT9M
2008 Aug	6.9	1.1	3.5	−8.4	−3.1	6.5	2.9	4.3	10.2	−0.9
Sep	12.8	5.3	4.8	−6.9	−2.5	4.5	2.5	4.8	6.7	−0.4
Oct	12.1	2.9	2.1	0.3	−1.2	5.6	2.5	3.3	1.5	1.7
Nov	7.7	−0.3	4.9	3.4	–	3.8	1.7	3.5	5.1	−0.4
Dec	20.6	−0.7	3.9	4.4	−1.0	−0.6	2.7	2.1	4.7	−2.9
2009 Jan	7.1	4.9	6.8	–	1.7	−0.4	0.9	0.4	5.1	3.0
Feb	3.7	0.8	−2.3	1.4	0.7	0.4	–	−1.3	5.2	1.3
Mar	3.2	−6.2	6.6	3.5	8.2	2.6	−0.7	−1.0	4.9	2.7
Apr	1.0	6.8	1.8	6.5	6.6	−1.4	1.5	0.4	3.7	2.2
May	4.9	2.2	−5.4	5.1	9.3	−1.6	−1.3	0.6	5.9	0.7
Jun	5.2	−2.7	0.9	12.4	8.6	−1.2	−1.5	1.5	7.3	−0.9
Jul	4.3	1.3	−0.6	2.8	8.8	−6.9	−1.8	0.6	6.0	1.3
Aug	2.3	5.4	–	4.3	10.2	−3.5	0.2	3.3	−0.6	3.0
Sep	2.5	−0.5	1.3	0.3	4.3	−1.8	0.9	2.8	2.1	−0.5
Oct	0.6	5.3	0.2	1.6	8.2	−4.1	1.3	3.0	6.5	1.5
Nov	5.8	3.6	−0.4	5.4	6.3	2.0	1.3	2.4	6.4	1.3
Dec	1.7	4.1	6.7	8.7	10.2	1.0	0.7	2.3	5.2	1.2
2010 Jan	2.2	−1.1	5.9	8.9	8.1	0.4	1.7	7.0	5.2	2.4
Feb	6.1	9.7	3.1	4.0	12.4	8.1	1.8	7.6	3.7	1.5
Mar	2.8	22.2	11.5	12.4	9.6	17.4	3.9	8.6	5.6	6.6

7.23
continued

Average weekly earnings : by industry
Great Britain
Not seasonally adjusted

£ per employee per week

	Wholesale trade	Retail trade and repairs	Hotels and restaurants	Transport, storage and communication	Financial interm-ediation	Real estate renting and business activities	Public admini-stration	Education	Health and social work	Other services
Including bonuses										
SIC 1992										
	KA6V	KA6Y	KA73	KA76	KA79	KA7C	KA7F	KA7I	KA7L	KA7O
2008	517	264	214	525	970	507	500	378	384	387
2009	520	271	214	526	886	512	511	391	393	383
2007 Aug	486	259	212	511	714	482	502	369	365	386
Sep	487	259	210	494	739	479	488	372	366	382
Oct	495	259	214	492	681	480	486	369	369	372
Nov	502	252	219	502	707	484	495	373	383	375
Dec	512	252	224	531	780	508	506	378	377	378
2008 Jan	516	258	209	505	1 402	490	497	367	377	387
Feb	530	259	216	519	1 984	498	498	368	377	383
Mar	558	277	225	534	1 390	525	492	369	378	406
Apr	513	276	210	521	740	506	499	373	381	385
May	504	270	218	564	785	498	495	374	379	384
Jun	518	267	212	571	801	507	496	373	381	385
Jul	510	264	212	510	744	521	505	377	386	396
Aug	501	262	215	513	724	514	507	379	393	394
Sep	505	261	212	505	752	502	498	383	385	377
Oct	502	261	211	512	736	507	496	382	388	378
Nov	521	257	209	511	706	503	511	396	390	378
Dec	526	261	216	531	870	516	510	394	391	389
2009 Jan	520	266	207	512	1 028	508	503	387	390	386
Feb	541	273	216	513	1 235	517	527	386	385	379
Mar	551	282	214	537	1 182	539	507	384	389	394
Apr	511	274	213	525	807	517	511	389	394	387
May	508	273	218	564	761	513	511	388	396	376
Jun	514	276	212	549	851	513	505	390	399	380
Jul	512	273	214	514	757	513	509	394	395	388
Aug	507	271	212	521	751	505	512	396	389	378
Sep	505	269	210	516	788	502	504	398	394	376
Oct	512	271	212	516	756	499	509	397	395	376
Nov	522	265	214	517	783	499	515	393	394	383
Dec	536	264	220	525	927	515	521	394	397	388
2010 Jan	527	275	214	515	895	509	520	390	392	405
Feb	539	283	223	522	1 709	519	521	389	396	389
Mar	621	311	222	564	1 337	557	521	390	393	422
Percentage change on the year										
	JT9N	JT9O	JT9P	JT9Q	JT9R	JT9S	JT9T	JT9U	JT9V	JT9W
2008 Aug	3.1	1.2	1.4	0.4	1.4	6.6	1.0	2.7	7.7	2.1
Sep	3.7	0.8	1.0	2.2	1.8	4.8	2.0	3.0	5.2	−1.3
Oct	1.4	0.8	−1.4	4.1	8.1	5.6	2.1	3.5	5.1	1.6
Nov	3.8	2.0	−4.6	1.8	−0.1	3.9	3.2	6.2	1.8	0.8
Dec	2.7	3.6	−3.6	–	11.5	1.6	0.8	4.2	3.7	2.9
2009 Jan	0.8	3.1	−1.0	1.4	−26.7	3.7	1.2	5.4	3.4	−0.3
Feb	2.1	5.4	–	−1.2	−37.8	3.8	5.8	4.9	2.1	−1.0
Mar	−1.3	1.8	−4.9	0.6	−15.0	2.7	3.0	4.1	2.9	−3.0
Apr	−0.4	−0.7	1.4	0.8	9.1	2.2	2.4	4.3	3.4	0.5
May	0.8	1.1	–	–	−3.1	3.0	3.2	3.7	4.5	−2.1
Jun	−0.8	3.4	–	−3.9	6.2	1.2	1.8	4.6	4.7	−1.3
Jul	0.4	3.4	0.9	0.8	1.7	−1.5	0.8	4.5	2.3	−2.0
Aug	1.2	3.4	−1.4	1.6	3.7	−1.8	1.0	4.5	−1.0	−4.1
Sep	–	3.1	−0.9	2.2	4.8	–	1.2	3.9	2.3	−0.3
Oct	2.0	3.8	0.5	0.8	2.7	−1.6	2.6	3.9	1.8	−0.5
Nov	0.2	3.1	2.4	1.2	10.9	−0.8	0.8	−0.8	1.0	1.3
Dec	1.9	1.1	1.9	−1.1	6.6	−0.2	2.2	–	1.5	−0.3
2010 Jan	1.3	3.4	3.4	0.6	−12.9	0.2	3.4	0.8	0.5	4.9
Feb	−0.4	3.7	3.2	1.8	38.4	0.4	−1.1	0.8	2.9	2.6
Mar	12.7	10.3	3.7	5.0	13.1	3.3	2.8	1.6	1.0	7.1

1 See chapter text.

Source: Office for National Statistics: 01633 819024

7.24 Median[1] Gross weekly and hourly earnings of full-time employees[2] by sex:
United Kingdom
At April

£

	Gross weekly earnings					Gross hourly earnings				
	Lowest decile	Lower quartile	Median	Upper quartile	Highest decile	Lowest decile	Lower quartile	Median	Upper quartile	Highest decile
All employees										
	C5U9	C5UC	C5UF	C5UI	C5UL	C5UO	C5UR	C5UU	C5V2	C5UX
2006	243.8	315.2	443.6	630.5	881.6	6.24	7.93	11.12	16.39	23.49
2007	252.9	325.8	457.6	650.5	907.1	6.47	8.22	11.47	16.87	24.17
2008	262.2	338.8	479.1	677.9	950.7	6.67	8.51	11.98	17.59	25.12
2009	270.6	347.5	488.7	692.8	971.0	6.95	8.83	12.43	18.19	25.90
Male employees										
	C5UA	C5UD	C5UG	C5UJ	C5UM	C5UP	C5US	C5UV	C5V3	C5UY
2006	264.5	346.0	484.3	687.5	980.5	6.50	8.37	11.76	17.38	25.64
2007	274.0	358.0	498.3	706.0	1 008.1	6.73	8.65	12.09	17.89	26.40
2008	283.0	371.5	522.0	737.7	1 055.5	6.96	8.95	12.63	18.69	27.54
2009	290.8	379.5	531.1	752.7	1 080.4	7.21	9.25	13.09	19.28	28.40
Female employees										
	C5UB	C5UE	C5UH	C5UK	C5UN	C5UQ	C5UT	C5UW	C5V4	C5UZ
2006	226.3	282.1	383.3	550.0	724.9	5.98	7.42	10.16	14.92	20.39
2007	233.5	289.8	394.8	565.4	749.0	6.18	7.67	10.48	15.33	20.95
2008	241.0	302.9	412.4	590.8	777.9	6.37	7.95	10.94	16.01	21.65
2009	250.4	313.0	426.4	612.9	812.2	6.63	8.28	11.42	16.62	22.64

1 Median values are less affected by extremes of earnings at either ends of the scale with half the employees earning above the stated amount and half below.

2 Data relate to full-time employees on adult rates whose pay for the survey pay-period was not affected by absence.

Sources: Annual Survey of Hours and Earnings;
Office for National Statistics: 01633 456120

7.25 Median[1] weekly and hourly earnings of full-time emloyees:[2] by age group: United Kingdom
April 2006 to 2009

£

	Full time employees on adult rates whose pay was unaffected by absence						
	18-21	22-29	30-39	40-49	50-59	60+	All ages
Median gross weekly earnings							
All							
	JRG9	JRH2	JRH3	JRH4	JEH5	JRH6	JRH7
2006	250.6	376.5	496.1	502.5	465.4	400.0	443.6
2007	265.5	387.8	509.0	517.3	479.1	418.7	457.6
2008	271.6	400.0	532.7	539.9	504.1	437.5	479.1
2009	277.7	407.5	541.7	550.6	514.1	447.4	488.7
Men							
	JRH8	JRH9	JRI2	JRI3	JRI4	JRI5	JRI6
2006	261.5	390.6	525.0	558.7	516.0	421.6	484.3
2007	275.9	402.5	539.0	574.9	534.4	440.9	498.3
2008	280.0	416.7	566.3	599.1	563.6	462.6	522.0
2009	285.5	421.6	571.1	605.9	569.7	470.5	531.1
Women							
	JRI7	JRI8	JRI9	JRJ2	JRJ3	JRJ4	JRJ5
2006	240.4	362.7	444.0	410.2	385.0	343.7	383.3
2007	254.3	374.1	460.6	420.3	395.6	356.1	394.8
2008	258.8	384.7	480.9	437.3	419.7	376.4	412.4
2009	268.3	392.9	497.5	457.7	434.1	383.2	426.4
Median hourly earnings(excluding overtime)							
All							
	JRJ6	JRJ7	JRJ8	JRJ9	JRK2	JRK3	JRK4
2006	6.31	9.50	12.43	12.49	11.50	9.72	11.03
2007	6.60	9.80	12.77	12.77	11.87	10.09	11.36
2008	6.75	10.12	13.34	13.31	12.53	10.57	11.88
2009	7.00	10.44	13.80	13.84	12.95	11.00	12.34
Men							
	JRK5	JRK6	JRK7	JRK8	JRK9	JRL2	JRL3
2006	6.37	9.51	12.78	13.46	12.28	9.96	11.64
2007	6.65	9.80	13.10	13.77	12.79	10.31	11.97
2008	6.85	10.13	13.70	14.37	13.52	10.89	12.50
2009	7.06	10.47	14.15	14.96	13.90	11.28	12.97
Women							
	JRL4	JRL5	JRL6	JRL7	JRL8	JRL9	JRM2
2006	6.24	9.48	11.87	10.95	10.24	9.17	10.14
2007	6.55	9.79	12.28	11.14	10.54	9.48	10.48
2008	6.64	10.12	12.78	11.57	11.10	9.82	10.92
2009	6.94	10.40	13.27	12.20	11.55	10.25	11.39

1 Median values are less affected by extremes of earnings at either ends of the scale with half the employees earning above the stated amount and half below.
2 Data relate to full-time employees on adult rates whose pay for the survey pay-period was not affected by absence.

Source: Annual Survey of Hours and Earnings: 01633 456120

7.26 Trade unions[1]
United Kingdom
Year ending 31st March[2]

Percentages

		2000 /01	2001 /02	2002 /03	2003 /04	2004 /05	2005 /06	2006 /07	2007 /08	2008 /09
Number of trade unions	KCLB	237	226	216	213	206	193	192	193	185
Analysis by number of members:										
Under 100 members	KCLC	18.60	22.10	19.00	20.70	19.90	17.60	17.70	17.10	17.80
100 and under 500	KCLD	20.70	18.10	18.50	18.80	17.50	20.70	18.20	19.20	17.30
500 and under 1,000	KCLE	9.30	9.30	11.60	10.30	10.70	9.30	9.90	10.90	13.00
1,000 and under 2,500	KCLF	14.30	12.40	10.20	10.80	11.70	13.00	12.50	11.40	10.80
2,500 and under 5,000	KCLG	9.70	9.30	11.60	10.80	10.70	10.90	11.50	12.40	12.40
5,000 and under 10,000	KCLH	5.10	5.30	4.20	4.70	5.30	5.70	6.30	6.20	5.90
10,000 and under 15,000	KCLI	1.70	1.80	2.80	3.30	2.40	2.10	1.60	1.60	1.10
15,000 and under 25,000	KCLJ	4.20	5.30	6.00	4.20	4.90	4.10	4.70	4.10	4.90
25,000 and under 50,000	KCLK	7.60	6.60	6.50	7.00	7.30	7.80	8.90	8.30	8.10
50,000 and under 100,000	KCLL	2.10	2.70	2.30	1.90	2.40	1.60	1.60	1.00	1.10
100,000 and under 250,000	KCLM	2.10	2.20	2.30	2.80	2.40	2.60	2.60	3.10	3.20
250,000 and over	KCLN	4.60	4.90	5.10	4.70	4.90	4.70	4.70	4.70	4.30
All sizes	KCLP	100	100	100	100	100	100	100	100	100
Membership										
Analysis by size of union:										
Under 100 members	KCLQ	–	–	–	–	–	–	–	–	–
100 and under 500	KCLR	0.20	0.20	0.20	0.20	0.10	0.10	0.10	0.10	0.10
500 and under 1,000	KCLS	0.20	0.20	0.20	0.20	0.20	0.20	0.20	0.20	0.20
1,000 and under 2,500	KCLT	0.70	0.60	0.50	0.50	0.50	0.60	0.50	0.50	0.40
2,500 and under 5,000	KCLU	1.10	1.00	1.20	1.10	1.00	1.00	1.00	1.10	1.00
5,000 and under 10,000	KCLV	1.20	1.10	0.90	0.90	1.10	1.20	1.20	1.20	1.10
10,000 and under 15,000	KCLW	0.70	0.60	0.90	1.10	0.80	0.60	0.50	0.50	0.30
15,000 and under 25,000	KCLX	2.30	2.90	3.30	2.20	2.50	1.90	2.20	2.00	2.30
25,000 and under 50,000	KCLY	7.80	6.60	6.30	6.70	6.90	7.10	8.10	7.40	7.00
50,000 and under 100,000	KCLZ	3.80	4.60	4.00	3.10	4.40	2.60	2.70	1.80	1.80
100,000 and under 250,000	KCMA	10.00	9.80	9.60	10.20	9.00	10.60	10.60	12.20	12.20
250,000 and over	KCMB	72.10	72.40	73.00	73.90	73.30	74.10	72.90	73.00	73.50
All sizes	KCMC	100	100	100	100	100	100	100	100	100
Total membership (thousands)	KCMD	7 897 519	7 779 393	7 750 990	7 735 983	7 559 062	7 473 000	7 602 842	7 627 693	7 656 156

1 See chapter text.
2 Data derived from trade union annual returns with periods which ended between October and September each year. The majority, however, ended in December. In the case of year 2004/05, for example, the data derived from annual returns with periods which ended between October 2004 and September 2005 - approximately 73% ended in December.

Source: Certification Office

Personal income, expenditure and wealth

Chapter 8

Personal income, expenditure and wealth

Distribution of total incomes

(Table 8.1)

The information shown in Table 8.1 comes from the Survey of Personal Incomes for the financial years from 2000/01 to 2007/08. This is an annual survey that covers approximately 600,000 individuals across the whole of the UK. It is based on administrative data held by HMRC offices on individuals who could be liable to tax.

The table relates only to those individuals who are taxpayers. The distributions cover only incomes as computed for tax purposes and above a level which for each year corresponds approximately to the single person's allowance. Incomes below these levels are not shown because the information about them is incomplete.

Some components of Investment income (for example, interest and dividends) from which tax has been deducted at source is not always held on HMRC business systems. Estimates of missing bank and building society interest and dividends from UK companies are included in these tables. The missing investment income is distributed to cases so that the population as a whole has amounts consistent with evidence from other sources. For example, amounts of tax accounted for by deposit takers and the propensity to hold interest bearing accounts as indicated by household surveys.

Superannuation contributions are estimated and included in total income. They have been distributed among earners in the Survey of Personal Incomes sample by a method consistent with information about the number of employees who are contracted in or out of the State Earnings Related Pension Scheme and the proportion of their earnings contributed.

When comparing results of these surveys across years, it should be noted that the Survey of Personal Incomes is not a longitudinal survey. However, sample sizes have increased in recent years to increase precision.

Average incomes of households

(Table 8.2)

Original income is the total income in cash of all the members of the household before receipt of state benefits or the deduction of taxes. It includes income from employment, self-employment, investment income and occupational pensions. Gross income is original income plus cash benefits received from government (retirement pensions, child benefit, etc). Disposal income is the income available for consumption. It is equal to gross income less direct taxes which include income tax, national insurance contributions, and council tax. By further allowing for taxes paid on goods and services purchased, such as VAT, an estimate of post-tax income is derived. These income figures are derived from estimates made by the Office for National Statistics, based largely on information from the Living Costs and Food Survey (LCF), and published each year in *Economic & Labour Market Review*, and available on the Office for National Statistics website.

For the purposes of table 8.2, a retired household is defined as one where the combined income of retired members amounts to at least half the total gross income of the household, where a retired person is defined as anyone who describes themselves as 'retired' or anyone over the minimum National Insurance (NI) pension age describing themselves as 'unoccupied' or 'sick or injured but not intending to seek work'.

Children are defined as persons under 16 or aged between 16 and 18, unmarried and receiving full-time non-advanced further education.

Living Costs and Food Survey

(Tables 8.3 to 8.5)

The Living Costs and Food Survey (LCF) is a sample survey of 11,484 private households in the UK, with an achieved response of around 5,845 private households. The survey, formerly the Expenditure and Food Survey (EFS), was renamed in 2008. The LCF sample is representative of all regions of the UK and of different types of households. The survey is continuous with interviews spread evenly over the year to ensure that estimates are not biased by seasonal variation. The survey results show how households spend their money – how much goes on food, clothing and so on – how spending patterns vary depending upon income, household composition, and regional location of households. From January 2006 the survey has been conducted on a calendar year basis; therefore the latest results refer to the January to December 2008 period.

One of the main purposes of the LCF is to define the 'basket of goods' for the Retail Prices Index (RPI) and the Consumer Prices Index (CPI). The RPI has a vital role in the up-rating of state pensions and welfare benefits, while the CPI is a key instrument pf the Government's monetary policy. Information from the survey is also a major source for estimates of household expenditure in the UK National Accounts. In addition, many other government departments use LCF data as a basis for policy making, for example in the areas of housing and transport. The Department for Environment, Food and Rural Affairs (Defra) uses LCF data to report on trends in food consumption and nutrient intake within the UK. Users of the LCF outside government include independent research institutes, academic researchers and business and market researchers. Like all surveys based on a sample of the population, its results are subject to sampling variability and potentially to some bias due to non-response. The results of the survey are published in an annual report, the latest being *Family Spending 2009 edition*. The report includes a list of definitions used in the survey, items on which information is collected and a brief account of the fieldwork procedure.

Personal income, expenditure and wealth

8.1 Distribution of total income before and after tax
United Kingdom
Years ending 5 April

| | 2004/2005 Annual Survey | | | | | 2005/06 Annual Survey | | | |
| | Number of individuals (Thousands) | £ million | | | | Number of individuals (Thousands) | £ million | | |
		Total income before tax	Total tax	Total income after tax			Total income before tax	Total tax	Total income after tax
Lower limit of range of income					**Lower limit of range of income**				
All incomes[1]	30 300	691 000	123 000	568 000	All incomes[1]	31 100	756 000	138 000	618 000
Income before tax (£)					Income before tax (£)				
4 745	329	1 600	4	1 600	4 895	112	555	-	555
5 000	1 110	6 090	80	6 010	5 000	1 040	5 750	62	5 690
6 000	2 760	19 500	600	18 900	6 000	2 540	18 000	522	17 500
8 000	2 950	26 500	1 600	24 900	8 000	2 920	26 200	1 450	24 800
10 000	2 760	30 300	2 580	27 700	10 000	2 810	30 900	2 500	24 800
12 000	2 470	32 100	3 350	28 700	12 000	2 550	33 100	3 380	29 700
14 000	2 280	34 200	4 080	30 100	14 000	2 340	35 000	4 140	30 900
16 000	2 050	34 800	4 520	30 300	16 000	2 100	35 700	4 610	31 100
18 000	1 790	34 100	4 720	29 300	18 000	1 880	35 700	4 930	30 800
20 000	6 000	146 000	22 700	124 000	20 000	6 200	152 000	23 400	128 000
30 000	4 090	152 000	27 300	125 000	30 000	4 540	170 000	29 900	140 000
50 000	1 270	83 700	21 600	62 100	50 000	1 500	98 800	25 000	73 700
100 000	300	40 000	12 600	27 400	100 000	366	49 300	15 300	34 000
200 000 and over	111	49 500	17 300	32 200	200 000 and over	144	66 000	22 900	43 000
Income after tax (£)					Income after tax (£)				
4 745	364	1 770	5	1 1770	4 895	129	636	1	636
5 000	1 220	6 830	98	6 730	5 000	1 160	6 500	77	6 420
6 000	3 270	24 100	902	23 200	6 000	3 000	22 000	767	21 300
8 000	3 600	34 800	2 510	32 300	8 000	3 590	34 600	2 300	32 300
10 000	3 280	40 000	3 920	36 000	10 000	3 390	41 100	3 890	37 200
12 000	2 920	43 000	5 050	37 900	12 000	3 020	44 300	5 120	39 200
14 000	2 540	43 700	5 730	38 000	14 000	2 650	45 600	5 940	39 600
16 000	2 180	43 200	6 090	37 100	16 000	2 260	44 600	6 270	38 300
18 000	1 850	41 400	6 210	35 200	18 000	1 850	41 300	6 140	35 100
20 000	5 320	154 000	25 100	129 000	20 000	5 630	163 000	26 400	137 000
30 000	2 840	131 000	27 100	104 000	30 000	3 310	152 000	30 700	121 000
50 000	681	63 200	18 300	44 800	50 000	817	75 500	21 600	53 900
100 000	143	28 400	9 420	19 000	100 000	188	37 100	12 100	24 900
200 000 and over	53	35 500	12 500	23 000	200 000 and over	69	47 900	16 800	31 000

8.1
continued

Distribution of total income before and after tax
United Kingdom
Years ending 5 April

| | 2006/07 Annual Survey | | | | | 2007/08 Annual Survey | | | |
| | Number of individuals (Thousands) | £ million | | | | Number of individuals (Thousands) | £ million | | |
		Total income before tax	Total tax	Total income after tax			Total income before tax	Total tax	Total income after tax
Lower limit of range of income					**Lower limit of range of income**				
All incomes[1]	31 800	810 000	150 000	661 000	All incomes[1]	32 500	870 000	163 000	708 000
Income before tax (£)					**Income before tax (£)**				
5 035	919	5 090	43	5 050	5 225	719	4 050	27	4 020
6 000	2 440	17 200	451	16 800	6 000	2 210	15 600	371	15 200
8 000	2 920	26 200	1 330	24 900	8 000	2 760	24 800	1 140	23 700
10 000	2 790	30 600	2 390	28 200	10 000	2 720	30 000	2 190	27 800
12 000	2 570	33 400	3 310	30 100	12 000	2 650	34 400	3 230	31 100
14 000	2 400	36 000	4 180	31 800	14 000	2 420	36 300	4 050	32 200
16 000	2 140	36 300	4 630	31 700	16 000	2 220	37 800	4 690	33 100
18 000	1 970	37 300	5 110	32 200	18 000	2 020	38 400	5 140	33 200
20 000	6 530	160 000	24 460	135 000	20 000	6 850	168 000	25 500	142 000
30 000	4 900	184 000	32 000	152 000	30 000	5 340	201 000	34 500	167 000
50 000	1 670	110 000	27 400	82 600	50 000	1 900	125 000	30 700	94 100
100 000	406	54 700	16 700	38 000	100 000	456	61 600	18 800	42 800
200 000 and over	170	79 700	27 400	52 300	200 000 and over	192	93 900	32 400	61 500
Income after tax (£)					**Income after tax (£)**				
5 035	1 040	5 800	55	5 750	5 225	802	4 550	34	4 520
6 000	2 860	20 900	656	20 200	6 000	2 540	18 500	512	18 000
8 000	3 550	34 000	2 090	31 900	8 000	3 390	32 300	1 800	30 500
10 000	3 410	41 200	3 770	37 500	10 000	3 430	41 300	3 560	37 700
12 000	3 120	45 600	5 160	40 500	12 000	3 160	45 900	4 950	41 000
14 000	2 710	46 700	5 990	40 700	14 000	2 820	48 300	6 010	42 300
16 000	2 370	46 800	6 530	40 200	16 000	2 470	48 500	6 610	41 800
18 000	1 920	42 700	6 320	36 400	18 000	2 030	45 100	6 550	38 500
20 000	5 980	173 000	28 000	145 000	20 000	6 370	184 000	29 600	155 000
30 000	3 650	168 000	33 200	134 000	30 000	4 080	188 000	36 400	151 000
50 000	914	83 800	23 600	60 200	50 000	1 040	95 200	26 600	68 600
100 000	220	43 300	13 900	29 400	100 000	247	48 400	15 600	32 800
200 000 and over	82	58 600	20 200	38 300	200 000 and over	95	70 600	24 600	46 100

1 See chapter text. All figures have been independently rounded.

Sources: Survey of Personal Incomes;
Board of HM Revenue & Customs: 020 7438 7055

Personal income, expenditure and wealth

8.2 Average incomes of households before and after taxes and benefits,[1] 2007/08
United Kingdom

	Retired households		Non-retired households									
	1 adult	2 or more adults	1 adult	2 adults	3 or more adults	1 adult with children	2 adults with 1 child	2 adults with 2 children	2 adults with 3 or more children	3 or more adults with children	All house-holds
Number of households in the population (thousands)	3 580	3 063	3 521	5 834	1 953	1 445	1 830	2 172	784	1107	25 289
Average per household (£ per year)											
Original income	5 092	13 095	21 345	43 156	48 908	11 038	40 861	51 449	40 483	48 391	30 390
Gross income	12 847	23 431	23 763	45 190	51 848	18 921	43 669	54 714	47 176	54 094	35 164
Disposable income	11 445	19 909	18 240	34 387	40 965	16 784	33 835	41 908	38 224	43 634	27 769
Post-tax income	9 588	15 714	15 065	28 648	32 989	13 269	28 056	35 038	31 962	35 699	22 865

1 See chapter text. Figures taken from the article "Effects of taxes and bene-fits on household income, 2007/08", published on the National Statistics website *www.statistics.gov.uk/taxesbenefits*

Sources: Office for National Statistics: 01633 455951; household.income.and.expenditure@ons.gsi.gov.uk

8.3 Sources of gross household income
United Kingdom

		1997 /98	1998 /99	1999 /00	2000 /01	2001[1] /02	2002 /03	2003 /04	2004 /05	2005[2] /06	2006[3]	2007	2008
Weighted number of households (thousands)	GH92	24 560	24 660	25 330	25 030	24 450	24 350	24 670	24 430	24 800	25 440	25 350	25 690
Number of households supplying data	KPDA	6 409	6 630	7 097	6 637	7 473	6 927	7 048	6 798	6 785	6 650	6 140	5 850
Average weekly household income by source (£)													
Wages and salaries	KPCB	280.20	309.20	315.40	336.70	369.30	373.90	383.90	409.70	414.80	428.20	444.90	476.30
Self-employment	KPCC	32.90	37.20	46.00	44.50	43.10	44.50	49.80	49.00	50.80	55.20	53.50	66.10
Investments	KPCD	18.70	18.80	21.80	20.00	20.00	18.80	16.70	16.50	19.50	20.90	23.20	27.80
Annuities and pensions (other than social security benefits)	KPCE	28.90	30.30	32.80	35.00	37.00	39.90	40.90	41.70	45.50	44.40	47.60	48.70
Social security benefits[4]	KPCF	55.00	55.80	58.00	60.10	64.50	68.50	72.50	76.90	78.00	79.40	83.30	88.70
Other sources	KPCH	5.20	5.70	5.90	6.20	6.70	6.70	6.40	6.90	7.40	6.50	7.00	5.50
Total[5]	KPCI	420.80	457.00	479.90	502.50	540.60	552.30	570.30	600.70	615.90	634.70	659.40	713.10
Sources of household income as a percentage of total household income													
Wages and salaries	KPCJ	67	68	66	67	68	68	67	68	67	67	67	67
Self-employment	KPCK	8	8	10	9	8	8	9	8	8	9	8	9
Investments	KPCL	4	4	5	4	4	3	3	3	3	3	4	4
Annuities and pensions (other than social security benefits)	KPCM	7	7	7	7	7	7	7	7	7	7	7	7
Social security benefits[4]	KPCN	13	12	12	12	12	12	13	13	13	13	13	12
Other sources	KPCP	1	1	1	1	1	1	1	1	1	1	1	1
Total[5]	KPCQ	100	100	100	100	100	100	100	100	100	100	100	100

1 From 2001/02 onwards, weighting is based on the population estimates from the 2001 census.
2 From 1995/96 to 2005, figures shown are based on weighted data, including children's expenditure, using non-response weights based on the 1991 Census and population figures from the 1991 and 2001 Census.
3 From 2006, figures shown are based on weighted data, including children's expenditure, using updated weights, with non-response weights and population figures based on the 2001 Census.
4 Excluding housing benefit and council tax benefit (rates rebate in Northern Ireland) and their predecessors in earlier years.
5 Does not include imputed income from owner-occupied and rent-free occu-pancy.

Sources: Living Costs and Food Survey; (previously Expenditure and Food Survey); Office for National Statistics; 01633 455282

8.4 Household expenditure based on FES classification[1]
United Kingdom

		1997 /98	1998 /99	1999 /00	2000 /01	2001[2] /02	2002 /03	2003 /04	2004 /05	2005[3] /06	2006[4]	2007	2008
Weighted number of households (thousands)	GH92	24 560	24 660	25 330	25 030	24 450	24 350	24 670	24 430	24 800	25 440	25 350	25 690
Number of households supplying data	KPDA	6 409	6 630	7 097	6 637	7 473	6 927	7 048	6 798	6 785	6 650	6 140	5 850

Average weekly household expenditure on commodities and services (£)

		1997 /98	1998 /99	1999 /00	2000 /01	2001[2] /02	2002 /03	2003 /04	2004 /05	2005[3] /06	2006[4]	2007	2008
Housing (NET)[5]	KPEV	51.50	57.20	57.00	63.90	65.90	66.70	69.90	76.70	80.90	83.20	92.00	94.00
Fuel and power	KPEW	12.70	11.70	11.30	11.90	11.70	11.70	12.00	12.50	13.90	15.80	17.20	18.90
Food and non-alcoholic drinks	KPEX	55.90	58.90	59.60	61.90	61.90	64.30	64.90	67.30	67.90	69.60	71.40	74.50
Alcoholic drink	KPEY	13.30	14.00	15.30	15.00	14.30	14.80	14.70	14.80	14.80	14.70	14.70	13.40
Tobacco	KPEZ	6.10	5.80	6.00	6.10	5.50	5.40	5.50	5.00	4.50	4.70	4.60	4.60
Clothing and footwear	KCWC	20.00	21.70	21.00	22.00	22.30	22.00	22.40	23.50	22.40	22.60	21.60	21.20
Household goods	KCWH	26.90	29.60	30.70	32.60	33.00	33.80	35.10	35.60	33.50	34.00	34.60	34.00
Household services	KCWI	17.90	18.90	18.90	22.00	23.60	23.30	24.90	26.30	27.10	26.40	26.50	27.30
Personal goods and services	KCWJ	12.50	13.30	13.90	14.70	14.90	15.20	16.20	16.00	16.90	17.50	17.80	17.20
Motoring	KCWK	46.60	51.70	52.60	55.10	57.90	61.70	62.40	62.60	63.80	61.10	62.00	63.60
Fares and other travel costs	KCWL	8.10	8.30	9.20	9.50	9.50	9.70	9.60	9.50	11.10	11.00	10.90	14.20
Leisure goods	KCWM	16.40	17.80	18.50	19.70	19.60	20.50	21.40	21.40	19.40	19.40	20.10	19.00
Leisure services	KCWN	38.80	41.90	43.90	50.60	51.90	53.60	55.00	59.60	63.00	65.30	61.70	65.90
Miscellaneous	KCWO	2.00	1.20	1.40	0.70	1.90	2.00	1.90	2.00	2.20	2.10	1.90	2.00
Total	KCWP	328.80	352.20	359.40	385.70	393.90	404.70	415.70	432.90	441.40	447.40	456.80	469.70

Expenditure on commodity or service as a percentage of total expenditure

		1997 /98	1998 /99	1999 /00	2000 /01	2001[2] /02	2002 /03	2003 /04	2004 /05	2005[3] /06	2006[4]	2007	2008
Housing (NET)[5]	KPFH	16	16	16	17	17	16	17	18	18	19	20	20
Fuel and power	KPFI	4	3	3	3	3	3	3	3	3	4	4	4
Food and non-alcoholic drinks	KPFJ	17	17	17	16	16	16	16	16	15	16	16	16
Alcoholic drink	KPFK	4	4	4	4	4	4	4	3	3	3	3	3
Tobacco	KPFL	2	2	2	2	1	1	1	1	1	1	1	1
Clothing and footwear	KPFM	6	6	6	6	6	5	5	5	5	5	5	5
Household goods	KCWQ	8	8	9	8	8	8	8	8	8	8	8	7
Household services	KCWR	5	5	5	6	6	6	6	6	6	6	6	6
Personal goods and services	KCWS	4	4	4	4	4	4	4	4	4	4	4	4
Motoring	KCWT	14	15	15	14	15	15	15	14	14	14	14	14
Fares and other travel costs	KCWU	2	2	3	2	2	2	2	2	3	2	2	3
Leisure goods	KCWV	5	5	5	5	5	5	5	5	4	4	4	4
Leisure services	KCWW	12	12	12	13	13	13	13	14	14	15	13	14
Miscellaneous	KPFR	1	–	–	–	–	–	–	–	–	–	–	–
Total	KPFS	100	100	100	100	100	100	100	100	100	100	100	100

1 Data are based on the Family Expenditure Survey (FES) classification and not the Expenditure and Food Survey (EFS) standard classification: Classification of Individual Consumption by Purpose (COICOP). This has been done to preserve an historical time-series, as COICOP data are only available from 2001/02.

2 From 2001/02 onwards, commodities and services are based on COICOP codes broadly mapped to FES.

3 From 1995/96 to 2005, figures shown are based on weighted data, including children's expenditure, using non-response weights based on the 1991 Census and population figures from the 1991 and 2001 Census.

4 From 2006, figures shown are based on weighted data, including children's expenditure, using updated weights, with non-response weights and population figures based on the 2001 Census.

5 An improvement to the imputation of mortgage interest payments has been implemented for 2007 and 2007 data which should lead to more accurate figures. This will lead to a slight discontinuity. An error was discovered in the derivation of mortgage capital repayments which was leading to double counting.

Sources: Living Costs and Food Survey;
(previously Expenditure and Food Survey);
Office for National Statistics;
01633 455282

8.5 Percentage of households with certain durable goods
United Kingdom

Percentages

		1997 /98	1998 /99	1999 /00	2000 /01	2001[1] /02	2002 /03	2003 /04	2004 /05	2005[2] /06	2006[3]	2007	2008
Weighted number of households (thousands)	GH92	24 560	24 660	25 330	25 030	24 450	24 350	24 670	24 430	24 800	25 440	25 350	25 690
Number of households supplying data	KPDA	6 409	6 630	7 097	6 637	7 473	6 927	7 048	6 798	6 785	6 650	6 140	5 850
Car/van	KPDB	70	72	71	72	74	74	75	75	74	74	75	74
One	KPDC	44	44	43	44	44	44	44	42	46	43	44	43
Two	KPDD	21	23	21	22	23	25	25	27	23	25	25	25
Three or more	KPDE	5	5	6	6	6	6	6	6	5	6	6	6
Central heating, full or partial	KPDF	89	89	90	91	92	93	94	95	94	95	95	95
Washing machine	KPDG	91	92	91	92	93	94	94	95	95	96	96	96
Tumble dryer	J803	51	51	52	53	54	56	57	58	58	59	57	59
Fridge/freezer or deep freezer	KPDI	90	92	91	94	95	96	96	96	97	97	97	97
Dishwasher	GPTL	22	23	23	25	27	29	31	33	35	37	37	38
Microwave	J804	77	79	80	84	86	87	89	90	91	91	91	92
Telephone	KPDL	94	95	95	93	94	94	92	93	92	91	89	90
Mobile phone	GH96	20	27	44	47	64	70	76	78	79	79	78	79
Home computer	KPDM	29	33	38	44	49	55	58	62	65	67	70	72
Video recorder	KPDN	84	85	86	87	90	90	90	88	86	82	75	70
DVD player	J805	..	..	..	..	..	31	50	67	79	83	86	88
CD player	J806	63	68	72	77	80	83	86	87	88	87	86	86
Digital television service[4]	GH97	26	28	32	40	43	45	49	58	65	70	77	82
Internet connection	ZBUZ	..	10	19	32	39	45	49	53	55	58	61	66

1 From 2001/02 onwards, weighting is based on the population estimates from the 2001 census.

2 From 1995-96 to 2005, figures shown are based on weighted data, including children's expenditure, using non-response weights based on the 1991 Census and poulation figures from the 1991 and 2001 Census.

3 From 2006, figures shown are based on weighted data, including children's expenditure, using updated weights, with non- response weights and population figures based on the 2001 Census.

4 Includes digital, satellite and cable receivers.

Sources: Living Costs and Food Survey;
(previously Expenditure and Food Survey);
Office for National Statistics;
01633 455282

Health

Chapter 9

Health

Deaths: analysed by cause

(Table 9.6)

All figures in this table for England and Wales represent the number of deaths **occurring** in each calendar year. All data for Scotland and Northern Ireland relate to the number of deaths **registered** during each calendar year. From 2001, all three constituent countries of the United Kingdom are coding their causes of death using the latest, tenth, revision of the International Statistical Classification of Diseases and Related Health Problems (ICD-10). All cause of death information from 2001 (also for 2000 for Scotland) presented in this table is based on the revised classification.

To assist users in assessing any discontinuities arising from the introduction of the revised classification, bridge-coding exercises were carried out on all deaths registered in 1999 in England and Wales and also in Scotland. For further information about ICD-10 and the bridge-coding carried out by The Office for National Statistics (ONS), see the ONS Report: Results of the ICD-10 bridge-coding study, England and Wales, 1999. *Health Statistics Quarterly* 14 (2002), pages 75–83 or log on to the National Statistics website at: www.statistics.gov.uk.

For information on the Scottish bridge-coding exercise, consult the Annual Report of the General Register Office for Scotland or log on to their website at: www.gro-scotland.gov.uk. No bridge-coding exercise was conducted for Northern Ireland.

Neonatal deaths and homicide and assault

For England and Wales, neonatal deaths (those at age under 28 days) are included in the number of total deaths but excluded from the cause figures. This has particular impact on the totals shown for the chapters covered by the ranges P and Q, 'Conditions originating in the perinatal period' and 'Congenital malformations, deformations and chromosomal abnormalities'. These are considerably lower than the actual number of deaths because it is not possible to assign an underlying cause of death from the neonatal death certificate used in England and Wales.

Also, for England and Wales only, the total number shown for Homicide and assault, X85–Y09, will not be a true representation because the registration of these deaths is often delayed by adjourned inquests.

Occupational ill-health

(Tables 9.8 and 9.9)

There are a number of sources of data on the extent of occupational or work-related ill health in Great Britain. For some potentially severe lung diseases caused by exposures which are highly unlikely to be found in a non-occupational setting, it is useful to count the number of death certificates issued each year. This is also true for mesothelioma, a cancer affecting the lining of the lungs and stomach, for which the number of cases with non-occupational causes is likely to be larger (although still a minority). **Table 9.9** shows the number of deaths for mesothelioma and asbestosis (linked to exposure to asbestos), pneumoconiosis (linked to coal dust or silica), byssinosis (linked to cotton dust) and some forms of allergic alveolitis (including farmer's lung). For asbestos-related diseases the figures are derived from a special register maintained by HSE.

Most conditions which can be caused or made worse by work can also arise from other factors. The remaining sources of data on work-related ill health rely on attribution of individual cases of illness to work causes. In The Health and Occupation Reporting Network (THOR), this is done by specialist doctors, either occupational physicians or those working in particular disease specialisms (covering musculoskeletal, psychological, respiratory, skin, audiological and infectious disease). **Table 9.8** presents data from THOR for the last three years. It should be noted that not all cases of occupational disease will be seen by participating specialists; for example, the number of deaths due to mesothelioma (shown in Table 9.9) is known to be greater than the number of cases reported to THOR.

Injuries at work

(Table 9.10)

The appropriate 'responsible person' is required to report injuries arising from workplace activities to HSE or the local authority under the Reporting of Injuries, Diseases and Dangerous Occurrences Regulations 1995 (RIDDOR 95). This includes fatal injuries, nonfatal major injuries, as defined by the Regulations, and other injuries causing incapacity for work for more than 3 days. As of 1 April 2001, reports are to be made to an Incident Centre (ICC), based at Caerphilly.

HSE gets to know about virtually all workplace fatalities. However, it is known that employers and others do not report all non-fatal reportable injuries. To estimate the level of under-reporting by employers, HSE place questions each year with the Labour Force Survey (LFS), asking respondents if they have suffered a workplace injury in the past year.

The results from the latest LFS show that in Great Britain employers report around 49 per cent of reportable injuries (2004/05). When compared to the previous year, these results also indicate a drop of in the non-fatal injury rate of 10.0 per cent. The self-employed report between 5 and 10 per cent of reportable non-fatal injuries.

Health

9.1 Ambulance Staff by Type : by country

Headcount

		2004	2005	2006[1]	2007	2008	2009
England							
Qualified ambulance staff:							
Total Amubulance Staff	JF83	26 902	28 180	28 648	28 471	30 518	32 284
Manager	JF85	789	773	614	598	685	692
Emergency care practitioner	JF87	..	..	438	646	705	750
Paramedic	JF89	7 536	8 311	8 222	8 241	9 203	10 089
Ambulance Technician	JF8B	..	..	6 902	7 543	6 858	6 391
Ambulance Personnel	JF8D	8 947	9 033	..	..	..	..
Support to Ambulance Staff							
Trainee Ambulance Technician	JF8F	..	..	1 829	1 147	1 258	1 415
Trainee Ambulance Personnel	JF8H	2 047	2 201	..	..	..	..
Wales							
Qualified ambulance staff:							
Total Amubulance Staff	JF84	1 354	1 401	1 458	1 397	1 413	..
Manager	JF86	144	136	125	99	89	..
Emergency care practitioner	JF88	..	..	..	2	4	..
Paramedic	JF8A	668	749	804	818	847	..
Ambulance Technician	JF8C	..	..	..	477	462	..
Ambulance Personnel	JF8E	385	385	489	..	..	..
Support to Ambulance Staff							
Trainee Ambulance Technician	JF8G	..	..	..	1	11	..
Trainee Ambulance Personnel	JF8I	157	131	40	..	..	..
Scotland							
Total Ambulance staff	JHQ3	2 779	2 883	..	3 655	3 681	3 836
Paramedic	JHQ4	1 023	1 153	..	1 247	1 269	1 323
Technician	JHQ5	982	899	..	1 010	989	1 051
Driver/chauffeur	JHQ6	53	55	..	103	91	97
Care assistant	JHQ7	722	776	..	931	948	961
Other[2]	JHQ8	–	–	..	364	384	404
Northern Ireland							
Total Ambulance staff	JHQ9	867	889	934	988	1 038	1 033
Emergency Medical Technicians and Paramedics	JHR2	687	722	753	557	621	635
Other/Patient care services	JHR3	122	126	121	339	328	327
Ambulance officers	JHR4	45	28	48	79	89	71
Manager	JHR5	11	12	12	11	..	..

Note: In 2006 ambulance staff were collected under new, more detailed, occupational codes. As a result, qualified totals and support to ambulance staff totals are not directly comparable with previous years.

1 Scottish ambulance service 2006 data is unavailable.

2 Includes EMDC/control from 2007, newly identified from Agenda for Change.

Sources: The NHS Information Centre for health and social care;
Welsh Assembly Government;
ISD Scotland;
Department of Health, Social services and Public Safety Northern Ireland

9.2 Hospital and primary care services
Scotland

			1999 /00	2000 /01	2001 /02	2002 /03	2003 /04	2004 /05	2005 /06	2006 /07	2007 /08	2008 /09
Hospital and community services												
In-patients:[1,2]												
Average available staffed beds	KDEA	Thousands	33.5	32.1	30.9	29.8	28.9	28.1	27.4	26.8	26.3	–
Average occupied beds:												
All departments	KDEB	"	26.9	25.8	25.1	24.2	23.2	22.5	22.1	21.7	20.9	–
Psychiatric and learning disability	KDEC	"	8.3	7.6	7.0	6.4	5.9	5.5	5.2	4.9	4.6	–
Discharges or deaths[3]	KDED	"	980.0	972.0	969.0	959.0	989.0	1 003.0	1 014.0	1 036.0	1 067.0	–
Outpatients:[2,4]												
New cases	KDEE	"	2 766.0	2 749.0	2 728.0	2 731.0	2 750.0	2 718.0	2 763.0	2 818.0	2 911.8	–
Total attendances	KDEF	"	6 451.0	6 382.0	6 254.0	6 193.0	6 147.0	5 983.0	6 066.0	6 030.0	6 131.6	–
Medical and dental staff:[5,6]	JYXO	Numbers	9 273	9 325	9 644	10 256	10 407	10 658	10 871	11 201	11 823	12 534
Whole-time	KDEG	"	7 185	7 216	7 530	8 115	8 349	8 612	8 796	9 201	9 826	9 971
Part-time	KDEH	"	1 632	1 648	1 681	1 697	1 636	1 630	1 670	1 607	1 597	2 257
Honorary	JYXN	"	495	495	468	468	437	431	418	411	418	377
Professional and technical staff:[6,7]												
Whole-time	KDEI	"	11 261	11 261	11 705	12 265	12 942	13 258	13 750	14 323	13 647	14 550
Part-time	KDEJ	"	5 218	5 483	5 852	6 273	6 708	6 968	7 440	7 990	8 313	8 788
Nursing and midwifery staff:[6,8]												
Whole-time	KDEK	"	32 356	32 401	33 334	34 294	34 939	35 338	36 093	37 104	37 075	37 664
Part-time	KDEL	"	29 242	29 131	29 004	29 015	29 354	29 484	29 688	29 995	30 270	30 301
Administrative and clerical staff:[6,9]												
Whole-time	KDEM	"	14 541	14 710	15 361	16 200	17 260	17 806	18 434	18 907	18 192	18 163
Part-time	KDEN	"	7 456	7 677	8 075	8 630	9 307	9 943	10 707	11 375	11 174	11 592
Domestic, transport, etc, staff:[6,10]												
Whole-time	KDEO	"	7 972	7 848	7 625	7 768	8 234	8 305	8 516	8 697	10 206	10 625
Part-time	KDEP	"	12 424	12 272	11 522	11 915	12 588	12 324	12 545	12 675	13 094	13 142
Primary care services												
Primary Medical services												
General medical practitioners (GPs):[11]	JX4B	Numbers	4 072	4 253	4 346	4 360	4 447	4 456	4 553	4 626	4 721	4 916
Performer[12]	KDET	"	3 702	3 710	3 761	3 769	3 805	3 782	3 801	3 807	3 826	3 818
Performer salaried[13]	KDEU	"	88	99	108	114	155	188	267	330	408	451
Performer registrar	JX4C	"	283	261	283	284	281	282	302	310	316	486
Performer retainee[14]	JX4D	"	–	184	196	194	209	208	190	184	178	168
Expenditure on Primary Medical Services[15]	KDEW	£ million	377.5	404.7	429.6	467.5	519.0	628.4	701.0	699.8	704.6	701.0
Pharmaceutical services[16]												
Prescriptions dispensed	KDEX	Millions	62.34	65.56	69.13	71.83	74.66	76.74	79.03	81.89	85.17	–
Payments to pharmacists (gross)	KDEY	£ million	731.0	788.6	868.9	946.3	988.0	993.7	1 043.0	1 063.9	1 095.1	–
Average gross cost per prescription	KDEZ	£	11.7	12.0	12.6	13.2	13.2	12.9	13.2	13.0	12.9	–
Dental services												
Dentists on list[17]	KDFA	Numbers	1 808	1 808	1 844	1 869	1 882	1 900	1 936	2 009	2 099	2 204
Number of courses of treatment completed	KDFB	Thousands	3 338	3 389	3 359	3 420	3 359	3 375	3 348	3 387	3 401	3 548
Payments to dentists (gross)	KDFC	£ million	160.6	162.9	165.1	172.3	170.4	173.5	179.0	188.3	198.7	219.8
Payments by patients	KDFD	"	48.8	50.6	52.3	54.7	53.3	53.9	54.1	46.0	46.5	49.8
Payments out of public funds	KDFE	"	111.8	112.3	112.9	117.6	117.1	119.6	124.9	142.6	152.2	169.9
Average gross cost per course	KDFF	£	37.6	38.0	38.4	39.7	39.7	40.4	41.3	41.9	43.1	44.5
General ophthalmic services Number of Eye Exams given[18,19]	KDFG	Thousands	850	861	877	907	920	935	960	1 573	1 626	1 728
Number of pairs of glasses supplied[20]	KDFH	"	494	439	463	458	450	457	457	443	451	468
Payments out of public funds for sight testing and dispensing[21]	KDFK	£ million	..	..	..	34.9	35.5	37.8	39.4	65.5	79.4	86.3

1 Excludes joint user and contractual hospitals.
2 In year to 31 March.
3 Includes transfers out and emergency inpatients treated in day bed units.
4 Including attendances at accident and emergency consultant clinics.
5 As at 30 September. Figures exclude officers holding honorary locum appointments. Part-time includes maximum part-time appointments. There is an element of double counting of "heads" in this table as doctors can hold more than one contract. For example, they may hold contracts of different type, eg part time and honorary. Doctors holding two or more contracts of the same type, eg part time, are not double counted. Doctors, whose sum of contracts amounts to whole time, are classed as such. Figures have been revised due to coding changes.
6 The change in both collection and presentation of workforce data due to changes in staff groupings under Agenda for Change has inevitably meant that the amount of historical trend analysis of data is limited, though still available for some high level groupings.
7 As at 30 September. Comprises Therapeutics, Healthcare Science, Technical and pharmacy, Allied health professionals and Medical and dental staff.
8 As at 30 September. Includes Health Care Assistants. Figures post 2003 have been amended due to a coding error resulting in some staff previously in this group being moved to the admin and clerical group.
9 As at 30 September. Comprises Senior Management and Administrative and Clerical staff. Figures for 2003 onwards have been amended due to the inclusion of some staff previously in the nursing and midwifery staff group.
10 As at 30 September. Comprises Ambulance, Works, Ancillary and Trades.

11 Contracted GP's in post in Scottish general practices, at 1 October up to 2003/04 and Sept for 2004/05 onwards. Excludes GP locums and GPs working only in Out of Hours services. The total may not equal the sum of the figures for individual GP designations as some GPs hold more than one contract. Source: www.isdscotland.org/workforce
12 For 2004/05 onwards this group comprised mainly of Provider (partner) GPs. Known prior to 2004/05 as Principal GPs.
13 Up to 2003/04 this group comprises salaried GPs plus associates, assistants and 'other' GPs. Terminology changed with the introduction of the new GMS contract in April 2004.
14 Data on the number of GP retainees not available prior to 2000.
15 Total expenditure on General Medical Services/Primary Medical Services Source: NHS Scotland Costs Book "R390" tables, www.isdscotland.org/costs Note, the contractual arrangements for payments to many general practices changed with the introduction of the new GMS contract in April 2004.
16 For prescriptions dispensed in calendar year by all community pharmacists (including stock orders), dispensing doctors and appliance suppliers. Gross total excludes patient charges.
17 Comprises of non-salaried GDS principal dentists only as at 31 March.
18 Figures represent eye examinations paid for by health boards, hospital eye service referrals and GOS(s) ST (v) claimants.
19 Free NHS eye examinations were extended to all on 1st April 2006.
20 Does not include hospital eye service.
21 OPTIX, the electronic system for recording ophtalmic payment information, was introduced in 2002. Information for previous years is now not centrally available from ISD

Sources: ISD Scotland, NHS National Services Scotland; 0131 275 7777

9.3 Hospital and general health services
Northern Ireland

			1999	2000	2001	2002	2003	2004	2005	2006	2007	2008
Hospital services[1]												
In-patients:												
Beds available[2]	KDGA	Numbers	8 639	8 571	8 419	8 301	8 347	8 323	8 238	8 049	7 873	7 706
Average daily occupation of beds	KDGB	Percentages	*81.5*	*82.0*	*83.3*	*84.3*	*84.1*	*84.2*	*83.6*	*83.2*	*82.5*	*82.3*
Discharges or deaths[3]	KDGC	Thousands	332	333	328	327	332	337	343	359	370	372
Out-patients:[4]												
New cases	KDGD	"	984	994	997	992	1 014	1 027	1 040	1 081	1 115	1 154
Total attendances	KDGE	"	2 111	2 114	2 131	2 122	2 161	2 175	2 219	2 233	2 283	2 296
General health services												
Medical services[1]												
Doctors (principals) on the list[5,6]	KDGF	Numbers	1 054	1 066	1 073	1 076	1 076	1 078	1 084	1 100	1 127	1 156
Number of patients per doctor	KDGG	"	1 678	1 661	1 651	1 652	1 658	1 663	1 655	1 631	1 626	1 618
GrossPayments to doctors[7]	KDGH	£ thousand	78 604	82 471	84 664	88 194	96 894	..	..	..	..	..
Pharmaceutical services[8]												
Prescription forms dispensed	KDGI	Thousands	13 454	13 666	14 277	14 622	15 158	15 283	15 860	16 393	17 280	18 055
Number of prescriptions	KDGJ	"	23 249	23 985	24 705	25 501	26 656	27 401	28 417	29 599	30 864	32 150
Gross Cost[9]	KDGK	£ thousand	266 535	278 405	303 489	327 045	362 401	382 789	390 763	408 771	425 440	445 921
Charges[10]	KDGL	"	8 183	8 499	9 074	9 597	9 798	10 262	10 676	11 298	11 943	10 254
Net Cost[9]	KDGM	"	258 353	269 906	294 415	317 448	352 602	372 527	380 087	397 473	413 497	435 667
Average gross cost per prescription[9]	KDGN	£	11.46	11.61	12.28	12.82	13.60	13.97	13.75	13.81	13.78	13.87
Dental services[8,11]												
Dentists on the list[5]	KDGO	Numbers	632	661	673	689	696	720	722	751	763	795
Number of courses of paid treatment	KDGP	Thousands	1 086	1 113	1 126	1 123	1 107	1 086	1 084	1 064	1 002	1 034
Gross cost	KDGQ	£ thousand	58 712	61 237	64 454	66 201	66 910	67 294	69 480	65 172	68 775	71 401
Patients	KDGR	Thousands	14 358	15 302	16 041	930	919	907	910	900	859	868
Contributions (Net cost)	KDGS	£ thousand	44 354	46 152	48 413	49 376	50 282	50 498	52 308	50 068	53 301	55 801
Average gross cost per paid treatment	KDGT	£	54	55	57	59	60	62	64	61	69	69
Ophthalmic services[8]												
Number of sight tests given[12]	KDGU	Thousands	305	307	326	334	346	347	360	368	385	404
Number of optical appliances supplied[13]	KDGV	"	178	181	187	190	192	189	194	196	200	210
Cost of service (gross)[14]	KDGW	£ thousand	11 509	12 035	12 738	13 473	13 981	14 395	15 868	16 280	16 970	18 468
Health and social services[15]												
Medical and dental staff:												
Whole-time	KDGZ	Numbers	2 231	2 224	2 281	2 411	2 607	2 749	2 948	3 152	3 254	3 280
Part-time	KDHA	"	1 014	580	597	626	620	627	562	556	589	605
Nursing and midwifery staff:												
Whole-time	KDHB	"	10 135	9 926	9 828	10 248	10 729	11 137	11 416	11 477	11 641	11 542
Part-time	KDHC	"	8 813	7 591	7 814	8 395	8 706	8 887	9 047	9 107	9 362	9 318
Administrative and clerical staff:												
Whole-time	KDHD	"	7 230	7 373	7 536	7 966	8 370	8 846	9 047	9 113	8 782	8 351
Part-time	KDHE	"	2 910	2 972	3 136	3 372	3 609	3 858	4 190	4 249	4 261	4 242
Professional and technical staff:												
Whole-time	KDHF	"	3 177	3 642	3 762	3 975	4 163	4 528	4 695	4 772	4 954	4 632
Part-time	KDHG	"	1 226	1 283	1 369	1 499	1 616	1 731	1 827	2 032	2 093	2 365
Social services staff(excluding casual home helps):												
Whole-time	KDHH	"	3 319	3 017	3 127	3 284	3 461	3 716	3 777	3 893	4 024	4 454
Part-time	KDHI	"	2 358	868	911	986	1 105	1 207	1 297	1 429	2 061	2 835
Ancillary and other staff:												
Whole-time	KDHJ	"	3 426	3 506	3 472	3 426	3 418	3 470	3 725	3 836	3 861	3 870
Part-time	KDHK	"	3 913	4 508	4 925	5 125	5 420	5 588	5 498	5 904	5 685	4 766
Cost of services (gross)[14]	KDHL	£ thousand	1 422 920	1 576 657	1 639 283	1 868 538	2 113 453	..	..	..	..	..
Payments by recipients	KDHM	Thousands	65 533	71 411	78 478	88 860	87 999	..	..	..	..	..
Payments out of public funds	KDHN	£ thousand	1 357 387	1 505 246	1 560 805	1 779 678	2 025 454	..	..	..	..	..

1 Financial Year.

2 Average available beds in wards open overnight during the year.

3 Includes transfers to other hospitals.

4 Includes consultant outpatient clinics and Accident and Emergency departments.

5 At beginning of period for Dentists. Doctors numbers at 2002 (Oct), 2003 (Nov), 2004, 2005 & 2006 (Oct).

6 From 2003 onwards (UPE's).

7 These costs refer to the majority of non-cash limited services: further expenditure under GMS is allocated through HSS Boards on a cash limited basis. Change between 2002 and 2003 is due to advance payments being made in relation to the new GMS contract introduced in April 2004.

8 From 1995 onwards figures are taken from financial year.

9 Gross cost is defined as net ingredient costs plus on-cost, fees and other payments.

10 Excludes amount paid by patients for pre-payment certificates.

11 Due to changes in the Dental Contract which came into force in October 1990 dentists are paid under a combination of headings relating to Capitation and Continuing Care patients. Prior to this, payment was simply on an item of service basis.

12 Excluding sight tests given in hospitals and under the school health service and in the home.

13 Relates to the number of vouchers supplied and excludes repair/replace spectacles.

14 Figures relate to the costs of the hospital, community health and personal social services, and have been estimated from financial year data.

15 Workforce figures until 1999 refer to 31st December and are taken from the Trust and Board payroll system. Figures from 2000 onwards are at 30th September and are taken from the Trust and Board Human Resource Management Systems. Some figures for 2000 have been revised. Figures for 2000 onwards exclude all home helps and all agency /bank staff Figures include Ambulance and Works staff in the Ancillary & Other Staff category and from 2008 this category also includes staff grouped as 'Generic ' who are multidisciplinary staff. Due to Agenda for Change new grade codes have been gradually introduced which have resulted in some staff moving between categories. This will be seen from 2007 onwards. Backward comparison of the workforce is therefore not advisable as definitions differ.

Sources: Central Services Agency Northern Ireland: 028 9053 2975; Dept of Health, Social Services & Public Safety Northern Ireland: 028 9052 2509; (Figures on Hospital Services: 028 9052 2800)

9.4 Health services: workforce summary
England
As at 30 September each year

headcount

		2000	2001	2002	2003	2004	2005	2006	2007	2008	2009
Total	JHR6	1 118 958	1 167 166	1 224 934	1 283 901	1 331 857	1 366 030	1 338 779	1 331 109	1 368 693	1 431 996
Total HCHS medical and dental staff (excl HPCA's)[3]	JX5A	66 067	68 484	72 168	76 400	82 951	87 043	90 243	91 790	95 942	100 628
Total HCHS non-medical staff	JX5B	919 252	962 528	1 013 199	1 063 846	1 101 797	1 130 949	1 092 886	1 085 524	1 120 548	1 176 831
Total GPs	JX5C	31 369	31 835	32 292	33 564	34 855	35 944	36 008	36 420	37 720	40 269
Total GP practice staff	JX5D	102 270	104 319	107 275	110 091	112 254	112 094	119 642	117 375	114 483	114 268
Professionally qualified clinical staff (excl retainers)	JHR8	554 053	575 796	604 187	634 346	661 476	679 799	675 260	681 811	701 831	725 579
All doctors	JHR9	97 436	100 319	104 460	109 964	117 806	122 987	126 251	128 210	133 662	140 897
Consultants (including directors of public health)	JHS3	24 401	25 782	27 070	28 750	30 650	31 993	32 874	33 674	34 910	36 950
Registrars	JHS4	12 730	13 220	13 770	14 619	16 823	18 006	18 808	30 759	35 042	37 108
Other doctors in training	JHS5	19 192	19 572	21 145	22 701	24 874	26 305	27 461	16 024	14 136	14 394
Hospital practitioners and clinical assistants (non-dental specialities)[3]	JHS6	5 621	5 362	4 863	4 451	4 045	3 587	3 077	2 848	2 761	2 333
Other medical and dental staff	JHS7	9 744	9 910	10 183	10 330	10 604	10 739	11 100	11 333	11 854	12 176
GPs total	JX5E	31 369	31 835	32 292	33 654	34 855	35 944	36 008	36 420	37 720	40 269
GP Providers	JHT2	27 791	27 938	28 117	28 646	28 781	29 340	27 691	27 342	27 347	28 607
Other GPs	JHT3	802	864	1 085	1 712	2 742	3 398	5 400	6 022	6 663	7 310
GP registrars[5]	JHT4	1 659	1 883	1 980	2 235	2 562	2 564	2 278	2 491	3 203	3 881
GP retainers	JHT5	1 117	1 150	1 110	971	770	642	639	565	507	471
Total qualified nursing staff[1]	JHT6	335 952	350 381	367 520	386 359	397 515	404 161	398 335	399 597	408 160	417 164
Qualified nursing, midwifery & health visiting staff	JHT7	289 381	300 499	314 879	326 579	336 615	344 677	343 184	340 859	346 377	353 570
Bank nursing, midwifery & health visiting staff	JX5F	27 371	30 036	31 658	38 113	38 756	36 580	31 354	35 878	39 735	41 659
GP pratice nurses	JHT8	19 200	19 846	20 983	21 667	22 144	22 904	23 797	22 860	22 048	21 935
Total qualified scientific, therapeutic & technical staff[2]	JHT9	105 910	110 241	116 598	122 066	128 883	134 534	134 498	136 976	142 558	149 596
Qualified Allied Health Professions	JHU2	54 788	57 001	59 415	62 189	65 515	67 841	67 483	68 687	71 301	73 953
Other qualified scientific, therapeutic & technical staff	JHU3	51 122	53 240	57 183	59 877	63 368	66 693	67 015	68 289	71 257	75 643
Qualified ambulance staff[4]	JHU4	14 755	14 855	15 609	15 957	17 272	18 117	16 176	17 028	17 451	17 922
Support to clinical staff	JHU5	307 225	325 890	344 524	360 666	368 285	376 219	357 877	346 596	355 010	377 617
Support to doctors & nursing staff	JHU6	232 007	243 979	255 305	265 549	271 389	279 193	267 934	259 547	266 070	278 390
Bank support to doctors & nursing staff	JX5G	25 129	27 999	31 793	33 203	32 241	31 248	23 164	22 347	20 184	25 034
Support to scientific, therapeutic & technical staff	JHU7	41 800	44 602	48 030	52 230	55 025	55 715	54 307	53 259	55 689	59 831
Support to ambulance staff	JHU8	8 289	9 310	9 396	9 684	9 630	10 063	12 472	11 443	13 067	14 362
NHS infrastructure support	JHU9	173 733	179 783	189 274	199 808	211 489	220 387	209 387	207 778	219 064	236 103
Central functions	JHV2	77 628	81 439	85 706	92 257	99 831	105 565	101 860	100 177	105 354	115 818
Hotel, property & estates	JHV3	70 849	70 920	71 274	72 230	73 932	75 431	70 776	71 102	73 797	75 624
Manager & senior manager	JHV4	25 256	27 424	32 294	35 321	37 726	39 391	36 751	36 499	39 913	44 661
Other non-medical staff or unknown classification	JHV5	877	1 224	657	657	497	435	410	409	353	364
Other GP pratice staff	JHV6	83 070	84 473	86 292	88 424	90 110	89 190	95 845	94 515	92 436	92 333

1 Nursing and midwifery figures exclude students on training courses leading to a first qualification as a nurse or midwife.

2 To make the census data comparable with the Review Body for Nursing Staff and Other Health Professionals definitions, qualified Allied Health Professional (AHPs) now include Speech & Language Therapists (previously these were included on Other Qualified ST&T staff). For comparability historical data has been reassigned to match the revised definition. The numbers of AHPs will not match those published in previous years.

3 In order to avoid double counting Hospital Practitioners & Clinical Assistants (HPCAs) are excluded from the all doctors totals, as they are predominantly GPs that work part time in hospitals (applies to headcount data only).

4 In 2006 ambulance staff were collected under new, more detailed, occupation codes. As a result, qualified totals and support to ambulance staff totals are not directly comparable with previous years.

5 GP Registrar count for 2008 & 2009 represents an improvement in data collection processes and comparisons with previous years should be treated with caution.

Source: NHS Information centre for health and social care

131

9.5 Health service: workforce summary
Wales

Whole-time equivalent

		2004	2005	2006	2007	2008
Directly employed NHS staff[1]:						
Medical and dental staff[2]						
Hospital medical staff	JHV7	4 381	4 546	..	5 182	5 272
Of which consultants	JHV8	1 503	1 584	..	1 820	1 893
Community/Public health medical staff	JHV9	78	79	..	98	102
Hospital dental staff	JHW2	142	138	..	149	149
Of which consultants	JHW3	46	43	..	49	40
Community/Public health dental staff	JHW4	115	97	..	89	48
Total	JHW5	4 715	4 859	..	5 520	5 571
Nursing, midwifery and health visiting staff[3]	JHW6	27 407	28 152	27 901	28 060	27 806
of which qualified	JHW7	20 126	20 698	20 980	21 443	24 126
Scientific, therapeutic and technical staff	JHW8	9 394	9 699	10 242	10 654	10 843
Health care assistants and other support staff	JHW9	8 305	8 584	9 904	9 015	9 488
Administration and estates staff	JHX2	14 677	15 421	16 417	16 031	16 056
Ambulance staff	JHX3	1 347	1 394	1 444	1 377	1 398
Other[4]	JHX4	159	163	161	170	210
Unknown	JHX5	–	–	–	80	94
Total	JHX6	66 004	68 272	..	70 907	71 467
Family Practitioners:						
General medical practitioners[5]	JHX7	1 816	1 849	1 882	1 936	1 940
GP Registrars	JHX8	115	103	152	165	198
GP retainers	JHX9	70	70	61	73	70
General dental practitioners[6]	JHY2	1 026	1 027	1 087	1 141	1 247
Ophthalmic medical practitioners[7]	JHY3	34	33	25	27	23
Ophthalmic opticians	JHY4	638	640	648	681	711

1 Whole-time equivalent at 30 September. The majority of the information on NHS staff has been obtained as a by-product of personnel systems. Some staff may be undergoing temporary regrading at the time and these staff are excluded from the figures.
2 Excludes locum staff.
3 Excludes pre-registration learners.
4 Health Authority professional advisors and staff on general payments, eg Macmillan and Marie Curie nurses.
5 Numbers at 1 October. All practitioners excluding GP registrars, GP Retainers and locums.
6 Numbers at 31 March. Number of performers (dentists) on an open contract recorded by Local Health Boards on the Dental Practice Division's Payments Online system Data for 2006 are not comparable with previous years.
7 Numbers at 31 December.

Source: Welsh Assembly Government

9.6 Deaths: by cause
International Statistical Classification of Diseases, Injuries and Causes of Death[1]
Tenth Revision 2001

Numbers

		England and Wales					
	ICD-10 code	2003	2004	2005	2006	2007	2008
Total deaths		538 254	512 541	512 692	502 599	504 052	509 090
Deaths from natural causes	A00-R99	519 297	493 835	494 054	482 745	484 350	488 743
Certain infectious and parasitic diseases	A00-B99	4 763	5 009	6 141	7 632	8 169	6 499
Intestinal infectious diseases	A00-A09	1 063	1 382	2 221	3 630	4 225	2 690
Respiratory and other tuberculosis including late effects	A15-A19,B90	451	388	406	432	335	384
Meningococcal infection	A39	118	72	86	52	75	77
Viral hepatitis	B15-B19	209	197	205	205	223	218
AIDS (HIV - disease)	B20-B24	224	209	230	235	256	249
Neoplasms	C00-D48	139 360	138 062	138 454	138 777	140 080	141 143
Malignant neoplasms	C00-97	135 955	134 856	135 252	135 635	136 804	137 831
Malignant neoplasm of oesophagus	C15	6 427	6 298	6 490	6 495	6 424	6 609
Malignant neoplasm of stomach	C16	5 285	5 098	4 927	4 562	4 587	4 546
Malignant neoplasm of colon	C18	9 152	9 130	9 076	8 954	8 854	8 958
Malignant neoplasm of rectum and anus	C20-C21	3 982	3 917	3 995	3 870	3 795	3 872
Malignant neoplasm of pancreas	C25	6 242	6 294	6 509	6 584	6 845	6 929
Malignant neoplasm of trachea, bronchus and lung	C33-C34	28 765	28 328	28 792	29 332	29 660	30 326
Malignant neoplasm of skin	C43	1 585	1 597	1 622	1 649	1 825	1 847
Malignant neoplasm of breast	C50	11 276	11 031	11 121	11 011	10 727	10 779
Malignant neoplasm of cervix uteri	C53	951	957	911	831	820	830
Malignant neoplasm of prostate	C61	9 166	9 169	9 042	9 057	9 230	9 157
Leukaemia	C91-C95	3 916	3 828	3 910	3 859	3 935	3 924
Diseases of the blood and blood-forming organs and certain disorders involving the immune mechanism	D50-D89	1 065	1 014	1 096	1 013	1 029	952
Endocrine, nutritional and metabolic diseases	E00-E90	8 016	7 519	7 433	7 153	7 214	7 426
Diabetes mellitus	E10-E14	6 316	5 837	5 677	5 490	5 433	5 541
Mental and behavioural disorders	F00-F99	14 846	14 299	14 563	14 863	16 582	18 438
Vascular and unspecified dementia	F01,F03	13 401	12 756	12 995	13 289	14 948	16 610
Alcohol abuse (inc. alcoholic psychosis)	F10	469	538	523	545	533	685
Drug dependence and non-dependent abuse of drugs	F11-F16,F18-F19	655	718	762	739	781	844
Diseases of the nervous system and sense organs	G00-H95	15 793	14 645	15 253	15 218	16 375	17 554
Meningitis (including meningococcal)	G00-G03	229	182	187	164	164	159
Alzheimer's disease	G30	5 055	4 821	4 914	4 901	5 697	6 231
Diseases of the circulatory system	I00-I99	205 508	190 603	183 997	174 637	170 338	168 238
Ischaemic heart diseases	I20-I25	99 790	92 528	88 271	82 619	79 910	76 985
Cerebrovascular diseases	I60-I69	57 808	52 899	50 772	48 389	46 597	46 446
Diseases of the respiratory system	J00-J99	75 138	69 213	72 517	68 599	68 974	71 751
Influenza	J10-J11	77	25	44	17	31	39
Pneumonia	J12-J18	34 400	30 649	31 443	28 674	28 152	28 929
Bronchitis, emphysema and other chronic obstructive pulmonary diseases	J40-J44	25 765	23 204	24 230	23 319	23 727	24 816
Asthma	J45-J46	1 284	1 243	1 186	1 082	1 033	1 071
Diseases of the digestive system	K00-K93	24 948	24 912	25 213	25 786	25 670	25 997
Gastric and duodenal ulcer	K25-K27	3 678	3 495	3 266	3 145	2 833	2 912
Chronic liver disease	K70,K73-K74	5 844	5 824	5 873	6 250	6 326	6 470
Diseases of the skin and subcutaneous tissue	L00-L99	1 661	1 670	1 788	1 812	1 822	1 895
Diseases of the musculo-skeletal system and connective tissue	M00-M99	4 634	4 393	4 378	4 238	4 304	4 398
Rheumatoid arthritis and juvenile arthritis	M05-M06,M08	907	794	835	743	734	753
Osteoporosis	M80-M81	1 583	1 478	1 416	1 390	1 509	1 420
Diseases of the genito-urinary system	N00-N99	9 120	9 397	10 231	10 722	11 301	11 886
Diseases of the kidney and ureter	N00-N29	4 135	4 024	3 967	3 988	4 386	4 381
Complications of pregnancy, childbirth and the puerperium	O00-O99	45	46	36	41	47	44
Certain conditions originating in the perinatal period (excluding neonatals)[1]	P00-P96	207	213	205	160	180	234
Congenital malformations, deformations and chromosomal abnormalities (excluding neonatals)[1]	Q00-Q99	1 299	1 274	1 292	1 214	1 235	1 139
Congenital malformations of the nervous system	Q00-Q07	142	116	123	117	124	118
Congenital malformations of the circulatory system	Q20-Q28	540	527	535	484	527	444
Symptoms, signs and abnormal clinical and laboratory findings not elsewhere classified	R00-R99	12 894	11 566	11 457	10 880	11 030	11 149
Senility without mention of psychosis (old age)	R54	11 394	9 905	9 785	9 169	9 195	9 320
Sudden infant death syndrome	R95	136	148	164	143	170	176
Deaths from external causes	V01-Y89	16 693	16 497	16 411	17 509	17 000	17 628
All accidents	V01-X59,Y85,Y86	10 979	10 735	11 053	11 824	11 883	12 306
Land transport accidents	V01-V89	2 943	2 693	2 697	2 990	2 919	2 626
Accidental falls	W00-W19	2 732	2 915	3 006	3 226	3 318	3 459
Accidental poisonings	X40-X49	835	927	910	1 072	1 207	1 429
Suicide and intentional self-harm	X60-X84,Y87.0	3 270	3 306	3 172	3 331	3 165	3 438
Homicide and assault[1]	X85-Y09,Y87.1	318	363	326	342	370	340
Event of undetermined intent	Y10-Y34, Y87.2	1 776	1 685	1 486	1 616	1 161	1 172

9.6
continued

Deaths: by cause
International Statistical Classification of Diseases, Injuries and Causes of Death[1]
Tenth Revision 2001

Numbers

	ICD-10 code	Scotland					
		2003	2004	2005	2006	2007	2008
Total deaths		58 472	56 187	55 747	55 093	55 986	55 700
Deaths from natural causes	A00-R99	56 161	53 759	53 535	52 856	53 683	53 439
Certain infectious and parasitic diseases	A00-B99	660	688	719	791	949	936
Intestinal infectious diseases	A00-A09	85	104	99	128	164	183
Respiratory and other tuberculosis including late effects	A15-A19,B90	59	52	49	43	41	46
Meningococcal infection	A39	5	8	4	6	8	4
Viral hepatitis	B15-B19	23	20	16	20	22	24
AIDS (HIV - disease)	B20-B24	33	16	31	19	21	18
Neoplasms	C00-D48	15 412	15 336	15 408	15 360	15 570	15 525
Malignant neoplasms	C00-C97	15 116	15 047	15 135	15 084	15 274	15 269
Malignant neoplasm of oesophagus	C15	776	801	798	765	786	831
Malignant neoplasm of stomach	C16	579	615	590	552	506	511
Malignant neoplasm of colon	C18	966	917	966	922	899	940
Malignant neoplasm of rectum and anus	C20-21	368	383	367	390	394	379
Malignant neoplasm of pancreas	C25	641	615	603	567	713	642
Malignant neoplasm of trachea, bronchus and lung	C33-34	3 893	3 923	4 009	4 062	4 115	4 080
Malignant neoplasm of skin	C43	146	151	158	158	164	171
Malignant neoplasm of breast	C50	1 149	1 093	1 151	1 112	1 067	1 050
Malignant neoplasm of cervix uteri	C53	120	102	127	92	105	102
Malignant neoplasm of prostate	C61	786	802	765	779	793	792
Leukaemia	C91-C95	367	352	351	362	348	366
Diseases of the blood and blood-forming organs and certain disorders involving the immune mechanism	D50-D89	148	111	118	113	111	85
Endocrine, nutritional and metabolic diseases	E00-E90	958	972	988	1 018	980	991
Diabetes mellitus	E10-E14	709	760	745	751	726	733
Mental and behavioural disorders	F00-F99	2 637	2 670	2 454	2 817	3 117	3 362
Vascular and unspecified dementia	F01,F03	1 997	1 955	1 835	2 101	2 446	2 590
Alcohol abuse (inc. alcoholic psychosis)	F10	356	421	343	378	321	342
Drug dependence and non-dependent abuse of drugs	F11-F16,F18-F19	228	238	217	293	310	395
Diseases of the nervous system and sense organs	G00-H95	1 303	1 254	1 306	1 333	1 555	1 619
Meningitis (including meningococcal)	G00-G03	19	25	18	15	16	20
Alzheimer's disease	G30	354	399	415	452	549	624
Diseases of the circulatory system	I00-I99	22 102	20 837	20 060	18 771	18 579	17 849
Ischaemic heart diseases	I20-I25	11 441	10 778	10 331	9 532	9 343	8 841
Cerebrovascular diseases	I60-I69	6 497	6 155	5 789	5 466	5 333	5 367
Diseases of the respiratory system	J00-J99	7 454	6 743	7 093	7 183	7 362	7 443
Influenza	J10-J11	15	3	11	2	5	10
Pneumonia	J12-J18	2 859	2 399	2 483	2 513	2 444	2 453
Bronchitis, emphysema and other chronic obstructive pulmonary diseases	J40-J44	3 014	2 752	2 857	2 848	2 901	2 848
Asthma	J45-J46	98	94	100	82	112	103
Diseases of the digestive system	K00-K93	3 215	3 065	3 221	3 208	3 076	3 119
Gastric and duodenal ulcer	K25-K27	316	305	230	262	206	220
Chronic liver disease	K70,K73-K74	1 170	1 044	1 152	1 162	1 080	1 059
Diseases of the skin and subcutaneous tissue	L00-L99	131	131	127	130	131	159
Diseases of the musculo-skeletal system and connective tissue	M00-M99	369	350	326	354	395	351
Rheumatoid arthritis and juvenile arthritis	M05-M06,M08	103	107	109	108	139	107
Osteoporosis	M80-M81	70	52	47	40	64	58
Diseases of the genito-urinary system	N00-N99	1 056	965	1 063	1 112	1 149	1 279
Diseases of the kidney and ureter	N00-N29	670	574	617	578	598	653
Complications of pregnancy, childbirth and the puerperium	O00-O99	7	6	4	7	8	5
Certain conditions originating in the perinatal period	P00-P96	149	151	164	139	157	134
Congenital malformations, deformations and chromasomal abnormalities	Q00-Q99	172	134	159	151	150	144
Congenital malformations of the nervous system	Q00-Q07	23	21	15	25	22	18
Congenital malformations of the circulatory system	Q20-Q28	63	53	58	46	47	46
Symptoms, signs and abnormal clinical and laboratory findings not elsewhere classified	R00-R99	388	346	325	369	394	438
Senility without mention of psychosis (old age)	R54	236	193	210	206	221	235
Sudden infant death syndrome	R95	43	28	20	27	31	22
Deaths from external causes	V01-Y89	2 311	2 428	2 212	2 237	2 303	2 261
All accidents	V01-X59,Y85,Y86	1 326	1 390	1 284	1 264	1 289	1 261
Land transport accidents	V01-V89	357	325	293	326	294	280
Accidental falls	W00-W19	668	690	676	642	658	634
Accidental poisonings	X40-X49	30	57	48	70	63	82
Suicide and intentional self-harm	X60-X84,Y87.0	560	606	547	542	517	569
Homicide and assault	X85-Y09,Y87.1	101	121	80	115	88	88
Event of undetermined intent	Y10-Y34, Y87.2	234	229	216	223	321	274

9.6
continued

Deaths: by cause
International Statistical Classification of Diseases, Injuries and Causes of Death[1]
Tenth Revision 2001

Numbers

	ICD-10 code	Northern Ireland					
		2003	2004	2005	2006	2007	2008
Total deaths		14 462	14 354	14 224	14 532	14 649	14 907
Deaths from natural causes	A00-R99	13 912	13 711	13 463	13 679	13 876	14 053
Certain infectious and parasitic diseases	A00-B99	157	149	162	188	184	183
Intestinal infectious diseases	A00-A09	13	16	16	39	35	69
Respiratory and other tuberculosis including late effects	A15-A19,B90	11	13	4	7	10	6
Meningococcal infection	A39	4	5	1	1	3	2
Viral hepatitis	B15-B19	-	1	2	4	4	2
AIDS (HIV - disease)	B20-B24	2	-	5	-	-	-
Neoplasms	C00-D48	3 882	3 835	3 826	3 959	3 992	4 086
Malignant neoplasms	C00-C97	3 757	3 757	3 735	3 848	3 870	3 971
Malignant neoplasm of oesophagus	C15	154	138	162	161	161	176
Malignant neoplasm of stomach	C16	165	180	161	159	161	132
Malignant neoplasm of colon	C18	313	286	293	280	319	290
Malignant neoplasm of rectum and anus	C20-C21	103	94	99	99	96	106
Malignant neoplasm of pancreas	C25	173	152	173	194	205	228
Malignant neoplasm of trachea, bronchus and lung	C33-C34	810	837	824	850	863	927
Malignant neoplasm of skin	C43	40	36	43	48	56	57
Malignant neoplasm of breast	C50	291	320	307	300	311	312
Malignant neoplasm of cervix uteri	C53	31	37	20	29	16	28
Malignant neoplasm of prostate	C61	217	241	222	212	235	226
Leukaemia	C91-C95	85	95	92	91	94	102
Diseases of the blood and blood-forming organs and certain disorders involving the immune mechanism	D50-D89	37	34	36	31	39	36
Endocrine, nutritional and metabolic diseases	E00-E90	246	248	302	281	299	254
Diabetes mellitus	E10-E14	190	189	224	197	210	181
Mental and behavioural disorders	F00-F99	341	370	408	418	514	575
Vascular and unspecified dementia	F01,F03	284	298	316	335	405	520
Alcohol abuse (inc. alcoholic psychosis)	F10	52	68	86	79	94	46
Drug dependence and non-dependent abuse of drugs	F11-F16,F18-F19	3	2	2	1	5	2
Diseases of the nervous system and sense organs	G00-H95	481	487	484	557	588	600
Meningitis (including meningococcal)	G00-G03	3	1	2	1	5	3
Alzheimer's disease	G30	224	251	207	265	291	293
Diseases of the circulatory system	I00-I99	5 448	5 272	5 002	4 879	4 838	4 752
Ischaemic heart diseases	I20-I25	2 843	2 775	2 708	2 556	2 494	2 410
Cerebrovascular diseases	I60-I69	1 531	1 435	1 307	1 326	1 325	1 329
Diseases of the respiratory system	J00-J99	2 082	1 950	1 921	1 982	1 992	2 096
Influenza	J10-J11	4	1	-	1	1	2
Pneumonia	J12-J18	1 025	909	895	895	859	900
Bronchitis, emphysema and other chronic obstructive pulmonary diseases	J40-J44	660	609	596	616	639	680
Asthma	J45-J46	32	44	32	35	28	31
Diseases of the digestive system	K00-K93	587	691	584	646	711	682
Gastric and duodenal ulcer	K25-K27	77	70	60	57	53	52
Chronic liver disease	K70,K73-K74	156	189	150	171	193	204
Diseases of the skin and subcutaneous tissue	L00-L99	15	19	20	21	26	24
Diseases of the musculo-skeletal system and connective tissue	M00-M99	93	66	95	79	76	85
Rheumatoid arthritis and juvenile arthritis	M05-M06,M08	26	15	28	36	25	18
Osteoporosis	M80-M81	16	10	12	11	12	15
Diseases of the genito-urinary system	N00-N99	327	364	351	359	381	400
Diseases of the kidney and ureter	N00-N29	225	252	210	219	232	246
Complications of pregnancy, childbirth and the puerperium	O00-O99	3	1	1	3	-	-
Certain conditions originating in the perinatal period	P00-P96	62	64	81	54	50	67
Congenital malformations, deformations and chromasomal abnormalities	Q00-Q99	69	61	82	84	61	74
Congenital malformations of the nervous system	Q00-Q07	12	10	10	9	8	16
Congenital malformations of the circulatory system	Q20-Q28	16	17	20	19	19	16
Symptoms, signs and abnormal clinical and laboratory findings not elsewhere classified	R00-R99	82	100	108	138	125	139
Senility without mention of psychosis (old age)	R54	63	70	71	98	95	107
Sudden infant death syndrome	R95	-	-	2	1	4	3
Deaths from external causes	V01-Y89	550	643	761	853	773	854
All accidents	V01-X59,Y85,Y86	364	448	492	525	499	525
Land transport accidents	V01-V89	120	161	175	184	172	147
Accidental falls	W00-W19	44	63	99	117	112	127
Accidental poisonings	X40-X49	30	17	40	22	37	63
Suicide and intentional self-harm	X60-X84,Y87.0	132	128	186	249	215	252
Homicide and assault	X85-Y09,Y87.1	30	32	32	30	30	40
Event of undetermined intent	Y10-Y34, Y87.2	12	18	27	42	27	30

1 See chapter text.

*Sources: Office for National Statistics;
General Register Office, Scotland;
Northern Ireland Statistics and Research Agency*

9.7 Notifications of infectious diseases: by country

Numbers

		1998	1999	2000	2001	2002	2003	2004	2005	2006	2007	2008
United Kingdom												
Measles	KHQD	4 540	2 951	2 865	2 661	3 675	2 726	2 703	2 326	4 016	3 869	5 331
Mumps	KWNN	1 917	2 000	3 367	3 433	2 333	4 565	20 742	66 541	15 963	10 101	8 682
Rubella	KWNO	4 064	2 575	2 064	1 782	2 002	1 525	1 548	1 327	1 407	1 254	1 230
Whooping cough	KHQE	1 902	1 461	866	1 059	1 051	509	619	679	645	1 203	1 676
Scarlet fever	KHQC	4 708	2 956	2 544	2 320	2 749	3 252	2 642	2 075	2 653	2 477	3 983
Dysentery	KHQG	1 934	1 630	1 613	1 495	1 167	1 144	1 301	1 346	1 241	1 383	1 289
Food poisoning	KHQH	105 060	96 866	98 076	95 752	81 562	79 073	78 812	78 959	79 407	80 889	77 854
Typhoid and Paratyphoid fevers	KHQB	252	278	205	254	183	277	282	300	390	341	418
Hepatitis	KWNP	3 781	4 365	4 530	4 419	5 035	5 203	5 054	5 246	5 290	5 306	6 515
Tuberculosis	KHQI	6 605	6 701	7 100	7 204	7 239	6 978	7 259	8 017	8 083	7 461	7 878
Malaria	KWNQ	1 163	1 038	1 166	1 118	866	820	634	700	637	445	403
England and Wales[1]												
Measles	KHRD	3 728	2 438	2 378	2 250	3 187	2 488	2 356	2 089	3 705	3 670	5 088
Mumps	KWNR	1 587	1 691	2 162	2 741	1 997	4 204	16 367	56 256	12 841	7 196	7 827
Rubella	KWNS	3 208	1 954	1 653	1 483	1 660	1 361	1 287	1 155	1 221	1 082	1 096
Whooping cough	KHRE	1 577	1 139	712	888	883	409	504	594	550	1 089	1 512
Scarlet fever	KHRC	3 339	2 086	1 933	1 756	2 159	2 553	2 201	1 678	2 166	1 948	2 920
Dysentery	KHRG	1 813	1 538	1 494	1 388	1 087	1 047	1 203	1 237	1 122	1 217	1 166
Food poisoning	KHRH	93 932	86 316	86 528	85 468	72 649	70 895	70 311	70 407	70 603	72 382	68 962
Typhoid and Paratyphoid fevers	KHRB	243	276	204	250	175	275	280	298	386	334	410
Viral hepatitis	KWNT	3 183	3 424	3 541	3 388	3 859	4 004	3 932	4 109	4 007	3 857	4 756
Tuberculosis[2]	KHRJ	6 087	6 144	6 572	6 714	6 753	6 518	6 723	7 628	7 621	6 989	7 319
Malaria	KWNU	1 110	1 005	1 128	1 081	847	791	609	679	613	426	386
Total meningitis	KHRO	2 072	2 094	2 432	2 623	1 545	1 472	1 267	1 381	1 494	1 251	1 181
Meningococcal meningitis	KHRP	1 152	1 145	1 164	1 020	706	646	554	579	618	557	499
Meningococcal septicaemia	KWNV	1 509	1 822	1 614	1 238	842	732	691	721	657	673	528
Ophthalmia neonatorum	KHRI	198	163	176	115	91	102	85	87	100	83	77
Scotland												
Measles	KHSE	700	434	395	315	399	181	257	186	259	168	219
Mumps	KWNW	251	216	199	155	259	181	3 595	5 698	2 917	2 741	720
Rubella	KWNX	745	548	349	234	292	130	222	141	153	146	106
Whooping cough	KHSF	225	214	93	106	99	60	87	51	67	98	134
Scarlet fever	KHSD	883	438	301	281	376	395	213	208	274	315	890
Dysentery	KHSH	103	82	95	85	73	83	90	103	112	156	107
Food poisoning	KHSI	9 186	8 517	9 263	8 640	7 693	6 910	6 835	6 918	7 335	7 186	7 625
Typhoid and Paratyphoid fevers	KHSB	6	2	1	3	4	2	2	1	3	4	7
Viral hepatitis	KWNY	490	863	943	1 008	1 165	1 159	1 063	1 002	1 235	1 397	1 684
Tuberculosis[3]	KHSL	457	496	469	442	418	422	463	389	414	409	502
Malaria	KWUC	30	20	27	24	17	28	20	20	18	15	15
Meningococcal infection	KWUD	313	329	301	256	175	117	147	139	140	150	120
Erysipelas	KHSC	66	64	41	39	41	28	28	17	25	20	23
Northern Ireland												
Measles	KHTD	112	79	92	96	89	57	90	56	52	31	24
Mumps	KHTR	79	93	1 006	537	77	180	780	4 556	205	164	135
Rubella	KHTQ	111	73	62	65	50	34	39	31	33	26	28
Whooping cough	KHTE	100	108	61	65	69	40	28	28	28	16	30
Scarlet fever	KHTC	486	432	310	283	214	304	228	186	213	214	173
Dysentery	KHTG	18	10	24	22	7	14	8	7	7	10	16
Food poisoning	KHTH	1 942	2 033	2 285	1 644	1 220	1 268	1 666	1 409	1 469	1 321	1 267
Typhoid and Paratyphoid fevers	KHTB	3	–	–	1	4	–	–	1	1	3	1
Infective hepatitis	KHTO	108	78	46	23	11	40	59	74	48	52	75
Tuberculosis	KHTI	61	61	59	48	68	38	73	68	48	63	57
Malaria	KWUE	23	13	11	13	2	1	5	2	6	4	2
Acute encephalitis/meningitis	KHTM	64	99	130	97	98	78	64	66	58	36	41
Meningococcal septicaemia	KWUF	87	145	123	90	98	76	82	66	75	42	33
Gastro-enteritis (children under 2 years)	KHTP	1 371	1 121	1 205	1 106	882	867	697	736	718	762	758

1 The figures show the corrected number of notifications, incorporating revisions of diagnosis, either by the notifying registered medical practitioner or by the medical superintendent of the infectious diseases hospital. Cases notified in Port Health Authorities are included.

2 Formal notifications of new cases only. The figures exclude chemoprophylaxis.

3 Figures include cases of tuberculosis not notified before death.

Sources: Health Protection Scotland;
Communicable Disease Surveillance Centre (Northern Ireland);
Health Protection Agency, Centre for Infections, IM&T Dept: 020 8200 6868

9.8 Estimated number of cases of work-related disease reported by specialist physicians to THOR[1]

Great Britain

Numbers

	All physicians				Disease specialist				Occupational physicians			
	2005	2006	2007	2008	2005	2006	2007	2008	2005	2006	2007	2008
Musculoskeletal disorders					MOSS				OPRA			
Upper limb	3 654	3 328	2 391	2 203	1 521	1 503	1 049	1 121	2 133	1 825	1 342	922
Spine/ back	1 761	1 348	1 243	1 120	447	392	297	227	1 314	956	946	893
Lower limb	441	406	487	224	122	158	150	125	319	248	337	99
Other	221	204	149	190	33	55	28	41	188	149	121	149
Total number of diagnoses	6 205	5 347	4 394	3 769	2 204	2 131	1 608	1 533	4 001	3 216	2 786	2 236
Total number of individuals[2]	5 932	5 160	4 226	3 619	2 064	2 036	1 521	1 469	3 868	3 124	2 705	2 150
Mental ill health					SOSMI				OPRA			
Stress/ anxiety/ depression	6 063	5 648	5 467	4 812	1 751	1 423	1 014	1 028	4 312	4 225	4 453	3 724
Other	912	908	803	289	702	660	507	151	210	248	296	138
Total number of diagnoses	6 975	6 556	6 270	5 393	2 453	2 083	1 521	1 473	4 522	4 473	4 749	3 920
Total number of individuals[2]	6 396	5 916	5 753	5 126	2 223	1 975	1 421	1 396	4 173	3 941	4 332	3 730
Respiratory disease					SWORD				OPRA			
Asthma	492	596	306	350	374	451	250	295	118	145	56	55
Malignant mesothelioma	762	653	873	623	754	637	872	609	8	16	1	14
Benign pleural disease	1 496	1 293	968	1 063	1 481	1 281	968	1 063	15	12	-	-
Other	906	564	592	147	620	506	424	67	286	58	54	80
Total number of diagnoses	3 656	3 106	2 739	2 586	3 229	2 875	2 514	2 436	427	231	225	150
Total number of individuals[2]	3 609	3 059	2 711	2 548	3 207	2 829	2 486	2 399	402	230	225	149
Skin disease					EPIDERM				OPRA			
Contact dermatitis	2 285	2 406	1 780	1 573	1 698	1 810	1 365	1 251	587	596	415	322
Skin neoplasia	434	760	614	406	434	760	614	406	-	-	-	-
Other	361	390	223	66	176	295	154	30	185	95	69	36
Total number of diagnoses	3 080	3 556	2 617	2 180	2 308	2 865	2 133	1 771	772	691	484	409
Total number of individuals[2]	3 045	3 507	2 589	2 162	2 275	2 828	2 106	1 753	770	679	483	409
Audiological disease					OSSA				OPRA			
Sensorineural hearing loss	315	264	..	..	53	28	..	..	262	236	..	..
Other	48	31	..	..	22	15	..	..	26	16	..	..
Total number of diagnoses	363	295	..	..	75	43	..	..	288	252	..	..
Total number of individuals[2]	340	280	..	..	54	28	..	..	286	252	..	..
Infections					SIDAW				OPRA			
Diarrhoeal diseases	1 429	1 408	..	..	1 396	1 408	..	..	33	-	..	..
Other	149	168	..	..	121	165	..	..	28	3	..	..
Total number of diagnoses	1 578	1 576	..	..	1 517	1 573	..	..	61	3	..	..
Total number of individuals[2]	1 578	1 576	..	..	1 517	1 573	..	..	61	3	..	..

1 THOR: The Health and Occupation Reporting Network (formerly know as ODIN) comprises of the following schemes: MOSS: Musculoskeletal Occupation Surveillance Scheme; SOSMI: Surveillance of Occupational Stress and Mental Illness; SWORD: Surveillance or Work-related and Occupational Respiratory Disease; EPIDERM: Occupational Skin Disease Surveillance by Dermatologists; OSSA: Occupational Surveillance Scheme for Audiologists; SIDAW: Surveillance of Infectious Disease at Work.

2 Individuals may have more than one diagnosis.

Sources: Health and Safety Executive: 0151 951 4842; statisticsrequestteam@hse.gsi.gov.uk

Health

9.9 Deaths due to occupationally related lung disease
Great Britain

Numbers

		1997	1998	1999	2000	2001	2002	2003	2004	2005	2006	2007
Asbestosis (without mesothelioma)[1,3]	KADY	191	165	171	186	233	234	235	266	301	324	314
Mesothelioma[2]	KADZ	1 367	1 541	1 615	1 633	1 862	1 868	1 887	1 979	2 047	2 056	2 156
Pneumoconiosis (other than asbestosis)	KAEA	230	268	321	279	240	271	231	214	194	167	142
Byssinosis	KAEB	5	5	6	4	2	–	3	4	3	5	2
Farmer's lung and other occupational allergic alveolitis	KAEC	5	8	9	7	7	6	7	5	13	10	3
Total	KAED	1 798	1 987	2 122	2 109	2 344	2 373	2 362	2 467	2 548	2 562	2 617

1 By definition every case of asbestosis is due to asbestos; the association with mesothelioma is also very strong, though there is thought to be a low natural background incidence.
2 For the inclusion into the Mesothelioma register the cause of death on the death certificate must mention the word Mesothelioma.
3 For inclusion into the Asbestosis register the cause of death on the death certificate must mention the word Asbestosis.

Sources: Office for National Statistics; Health and Safety Executive: 0151 951 4842; statisticsrequestteam@hse.gsi.gov.uk

9.10 Injuries to workers:[1] by industry and severity of injury
Great Britain
As reported to all enforcing authorities

Numbers

				Fatal				Major				Over 3 Days[2]		
		Section	SIC (92)	2006/07	2007/08	2008/09		2006/07	2007/08	2008/09		2006/07	2007/08	2008/09
Agriculture, hunting, forestry and fishing[3]	KSYS	A,B	01,02,05	36	46	26	KSZN	488	569	589	KTAZ	863	1 103	1 178
Energy and water supply industries	KSYT	C,E	10-14,40/41	10	9	6	KSZO	397	402	361	KTBH	1 366	1 306	1 206
Mining and quarrying	KSYU	C	10-14	9	5	4	KSZP	196	201	154	KTBI	615	626	576
Mining and quarrying of energy producing materials	KSON	CA	10-12	7	3	2	KSZQ	117	129	99	KTBJ	385	447	433
Mining and quarrying except energy producing materials	KSOO	CB	13/14	2	2	2	KSZR	79	72	55	KTBK	230	173	143
Electricity, gas and water supply	KSOP	E	40/41	1	4	2	KSZS	201	201	207	KTBL	751	680	630
Manufacturing	KSOQ	D	15-37	36	33	32	KSZT	5 200	5 205	4 549	KTBM	21 968	20 852	17 858
of food products; beverages and tobacco	KSOR	DA	15/16	3	2	2	KSZU	927	918	827	KTBN	5 281	4 866	4 395
of textile and textile products	KSOS	DB	17/18	–	1	..	KSZV	131	101	91	KTBO	441	450	370
of leather and leather products	KSOT	DC	19	–	–	..	KSZW	5	4	4	KTBP	24	27	21
of wood and wood products	KSOU	DD	20	3	1	..	KSZX	228	271	204	KTBQ	702	720	558
of pulp, paper and paper products; publishing and printing	KSOV	DE	21/22	2	2	3	KSZY	340	321	270	KTBR	1 330	1 228	1 056
of coke, refined petroleum products and nuclear fuel	KSOW	DF	23	1	–	1	KSZZ	23	9	13	KTBS	50	61	44
of chemicals, chemical products and man-made fibres	KSOX	DG	24	2	2	..	KTAE	222	252	208	KTBT	985	953	843
of rubber and plastic products	KSOY	DH	25	–	4	2	KTAF	368	383	280	KTBU	1 530	1 349	1 183
of other non-metallic mineral products	KSOZ	DI	26	2	2	2	KTAG	268	291	218	KTBV	994	925	743
of basic metals and fabricated metal products	KSYV	DJ	27/28	10	10	7	KTAH	1 206	1 226	1 120	KTBW	3 873	3 792	3 203
of machinery and equipment not elsewhere classified	KSYW	DK	29	7	1	8	KTAI	322	368	314	KTBX	1 387	1 475	1 198
of electrical and optical equipment	KSYX	DL	30-33	1	2	..	KTAJ	197	191	206	KTBY	944	857	753
of transport equipment	KSYY	DM	34/35	3	2	1	KTAK	473	477	416	KTBZ	2 391	2 127	1 835
Manufacturing not elsewhere classified	KSYZ	DN	36/37	2	4	6	KTAL	490	393	378	KTCA	2 036	1 970	1 656
Construction	KSZA	F	45	79	72	53	KTAM	4 457	4 415	3 913	KTCB	7 915	8 188	7 351
Total service industries	KSZB	G-Q	50-99	86	73	63	KTAN	19 196	18 798	19 280	KTCC	83 687	79 726	77 629
Wholesale and retail trade, and repairs	KSZC	G	50-52	7	15	14	KTAO	3 671	3 505	3 427	KTCD	14 206	9 954	13 467
Hotel and restaurants	KSZD	H	55	4	2	4	KTAP	1 099	1 198	1 213	KTCE	4 102	4 134	4 308
Transport, storage and communication[4]	KSZE	I	60-64	34	21	21	KTAQ	3 362	3 468	3 349	KTCF	20 746	19 498	18 328
Financial intermediation	KSZF	J	65-67	–	–	..	KTAR	277	289	300	KTCG	736	769	774
Real estate, renting and business activities	KSZG	K	70-74	9	12	5	KTAS	2 489	2 356	2 314	KTCH	7 227	6 597	6 608
Public administration and defence	KSZH	L	75	6	10	7	KTAT	3 438	2 246	2 151	KTCI	16 565	11 480	10 127
Education	KSZI	M	80	4	2	2	KTAU	1 186	3 672	3 994	KTCJ	2 989	9 590	10 106
Health and social work	KSZJ	N	85	4	4	..	KTAV	2 428	5 038	5 952	KTCK	14 133	19 693	29 856
Other community, social and personal services activities	KSZK	O-Q	90-99	18	10	11	KTAW	1 246	1 381	1 513	KTCL	2 983	4 052	4 036
All industries	KSZM			247	233	180	KTAY	29 738	29 389	28 692	KTCN	115 799	111 175	105 222

1 See chapter text.
2 Injuries causing incapacity for normal work for more than 3 days.
3 Excludes sea fishing.

4 Injuries arising from shore based services only. Excludes incidents reported under merchant shipping legislation.

Sources: Health and Safety Executive (HSE): 0151 951 4842; statisticsrequestteam@hse.gsi.gov.uk

Social protection

Chapter 10

Social protection

(Tables 10.2 to 10.11, 10.13 and 10.15 to 10.19)

Tables 10.2 to 10.6, 10.9 to 10.11 and 10.13 to 10.19 give details of contributors and beneficiaries under the National Insurance and Industrial Injury Acts, supplementary benefits and war pensions.

There are four classes of National Insurance Contributions (NICs):

Class 1   Earnings-related contributions paid on earnings from employment. Employees pay primary Class 1 contributions and employers pay secondary Class 1 contributions. Payment of Class 1 contributions builds up entitlement to contributory benefits which include Basic State Pension; Additional State Pension (State Earnings Related Pension Scheme SERPS and from April 2002, State Second Pension, S2P); Contribution Based Jobseeker's Allowance; Bereavement Benefits; Incapacity Benefit and the new Employment and Support Allowance.

Primary class 1 contributions stop at State Pension age, but not Class 1 secondary contributions paid by employers. There are reduced contribution rates where the employee contracts out of S2P (previously SERPS). They still receive a Basic State Pension but an Occupational or Personal Pension instead of the Additional State Second Pension.

Class 2   Flat rate contributions paid by the self-employed whose profits are above the small earnings exception. Payment of Class 2 contributions builds up entitlement to the contributory benefits, which include Basic State Pension, Bereavement Benefits, Maternity Allowance and Incapacity Benefit and the Employment and Support Allowance, but not Additional State Second Pension or Contribution Based Jobseeker's Allowance (JSA).

Class 2 contributions stop at State Pension age.

Class 3   Flat rate voluntary contributions, which can be paid by someone whose contribution record is insufficient. Payment of Class 3 contributions builds up entitlement to contributory benefits which include Basic State Pension and Bereavement Benefits. (Tables 10.2 to 10.11, 10.13 and 10.15 to 10.19) Tables 10.2 to 10.6, 10.9 to 10.11 and 10.13 to 10.19 give details of contributors and beneficiaries under the National Insurance and Industrial Injury Acts, supplementary benefits and war pensions.

Class 4   Profit-related contributions paid by the self employed in addition to Class 2 contributions. Class 4 contributions stop at State Pension age. Under some circumstances people who are not in employment do not have to make voluntary contributions to accrue a qualifying year for Basic State Pension.

Home Responsibilities Protection

Home Responsibilities Protection (HRP) helps to protect the basic State Pension of those precluded from regular employment because they are caring for children or a sick or disabled person at home. To be entitled to HRP, a person must have been precluded from regular employment for a full tax year. HRP reduces the amount of qualifying years a person would otherwise need for a Basic State Pension.

National Insurance Credits

In addition to paying, or being treated as having paid contributions, a person can be credited with National Insurance. Contribution credits help to protect people's rights to State Retirement Pension and other Social Security Benefits.

A person is likely to be entitled to contributions credits if they are: a student in full time education or training, in receipt of Jobseeker's Allowance, unable to work due to sickness or disability, entitled to Statutory Maternity Pay or Statutory Adoption Pay, or they have received Carer's Allowance.

Credits are automatically awarded for men aged 60 to 65 provided they are not liable to pay Class 1 or 2 NICs, and to young people for the tax years containing their 16th, 17th and 18th birthdays.

Jobseeker's Allowance

(Table 10.6)

Jobseeker's Allowance (JSA) replaced Unemployment Benefit and Income Support for unemployed claimants on 7 October 1996. It is a unified benefit with two routes of entry: contribution-based, which depends mainly upon National Insurance contributions, and income-based, which depends mainly upon a means test. Some claimants can qualify by either route. In practice they receive income-based JSA but have an underlying entitlement to the contribution based element.

Employment and support allowance, Invalidity Benefit and Incapacity Benefit

(Tables 10.7)

Incapacity Benefit replaced Sickness Benefit and Invalidity Benefit from 13 April 1995. The first condition for entitlement to these contributory benefits is that the claimants are incapable of work because of illness or disablement. The second is that they satisfy the contribution conditions, which depend on contributions paid as an employed (Class 1) or self-employed person (Class 2). Under Sickness and Invalidity Benefits the contribution conditions were automatically treated as satisfied if a person was incapable of work because of an industrial accident or prescribed disease. Under Incapacity Benefit those who do not satisfy the contribution conditions do not have them treated as satisfied. Class 1A contributions paid by employers are in respect of the benefit of cars provided for the private use of employees, and the free fuel provided for private use. These contributions do not provide any type of benefit cover.

Since 6 April 1983, most people working for an employer and paying National Insurance contributions as employed persons receive Statutory Sick Pay (SSP) from their employer when they are off work sick. Until 5 April 1986 SSP was payable for a maximum of eight weeks, since this date SSP has been payable for 28 weeks. People who do not work for an employer, and employees who are excluded from the SSP scheme, or those who have run out of SSP before reaching the maximum of 28 weeks and are still sick, can claim benefit. Any period of SSP is excluded from the tables.

Spells of incapacity of three days or less do not count as periods of interruption of employment and are excluded from the tables. Exceptions are where people are receiving regular weekly treatment by dialysis or treatment by radiotherapy, chemotherapy or plasmapheresis where two days in any six consecutive days make up a period of interruption of employment, and those whose incapacity for work ends within three days of the end of SSP entitlement.

At the beginning of a period of incapacity, benefit is subject to three waiting days, except where there was an earlier spell of incapacity of more than three days in the previous eight weeks. Employees entitled to SSP for less than 28 weeks and who are still sick can get Sickness Benefit or Incapacity Benefit Short Term (Low) until they reach a total of 28 weeks provided they satisfy the conditions.

After 28 weeks of SSP and/or Sickness Benefit (SB), Invalidity Benefit (IVB) was payable up to pension age for as long as the incapacity lasted. From pension age, IVB was paid at the person's State Pension rate, until entitlement ceased when SP was paid, or until deemed pension age (70 for a man, 65 for a woman). People who were on Sickness or Invalidity Benefit on 12 April 1995 were automatically transferred to Incapacity Benefit, payable on the same basis as before.

For people on Incapacity Benefit under State Pension age there are two short-term rates: the lower rate is paid for the first 28 weeks of sickness and the higher rate for weeks 29 to 52. From week 53 the Long Term rate Incapacity Benefit is payable. The Short Term rate Incapacity Benefit is based on State Pension entitlement for people over State Pension age and is paid for up to a year if incapacity began before pension age.

The long-term rate of Incapacity Benefit applies to people under State Pension age who have been sick for more than a year. People with a terminal illness, or who are receiving the higher rate care component of Disability Living Allowance, will get the Long Term rate. The Long Term rate is not paid for people over pension age.

Under Incapacity Benefit, for the first 28 weeks of incapacity, people previously in work will be assessed on the 'own occupation' test – the claimant's ability to do their own job. Otherwise, incapacity will be based on a personal capability assessment, which will assess ability to carry out a range of work-related activities. The test will apply after 28 weeks of incapacity or from the start of the claim for people who did not previously have a job. Certain people will be exempted from this test.

The tables exclude all men aged over 65 and women aged over 60 who are in receipt of State Pension, and all people over deemed pension age (70 for a man and 65 for a woman), members of the armed forces, mariners while at sea, and married women and certain widows who have chosen not to be insured for sickness benefit. The tables include a number of individuals who were unemployed prior to incapacity.

The Short Term (Higher) and Long Term rates of Incapacity Benefit are treated as taxable income. There were transitional provisions for people who were on Sickness or Invalidity Benefit on 12 April 1995. They were automatically transferred to Incapacity Benefit, payable on the same basis as before. Former IVB recipients continue to get Additional Pension entitlement, but frozen at 1994 levels. Also their IVB is not subject to tax. If they were over State Pension age on 12 April 1995 they may get Incapacity Benefit for up to five years beyond pension age.

141

Social protection

Employment and Support Allowance

Employment and Support Allowance (ESA) replaced Incapacity Benefit and Income Support paid on the grounds of incapacity for new claims from 27 October 2008. ESA consists of two phases. The first, the assessment phase rate, is paid for the first 13 weeks of the claim whilst a decision is made on the claimants capability through the 'Work Capability Asessment'. The second, or main phase begins after 14 weeks, but only if the 'Work Capability Assesment' has deemed the claimants illness or disability as a limitation on their ability to work.

Within the main phase there are two groups, 'The Work Related Activity Group' and 'The Support Group'. If a claimant is placed in the first, they are expected to take part in work focused interviews with a personal advisor. They will be given support to help them prepare for work and on gaining work will receive a work related activity component in addition to their basic rate. If the claimant is placed in the second group due to their illness or disability having a sever effect upon their ability to work, the claimant will not be expected to work at all, but can do so on a voluntary basis. These claimants will recive a support component in addition to their basic rate.

Child Benefits

(Table 10.9)

Child Benefit (CB) is paid to those responsible for children (aged under 16) or qualifying young people. The latter includes:

a) a person under the age of 19 in full-time non-advanced education or (from April 2006) on certain approved vocational training programmes

b) a person who is aged 19 who began their course of full-time, non-advanced education or approved training before reaching age 19 (note: those reaching 19 up to 9 April 2006 ceased to qualify on their 19th birthday)

c) a person who has reached the age of 16 until the 31 August following their 16th birthday

d) a person aged 16 or 17 who has left education and training who is registered with the Careers service or with Connexions and is awaiting a placement in employment or training for the limited period of up to 20 weeks from the date they left education or training. Entitlement for a qualifying young person continues until the terminal date following the date they leave full-time education or approved training. The terminal dates are at the end of August, November, February and May (there is a slight variation for Scotland). Entitlement is also maintained for a person who is entered for external examinations connected with their course throughout the period

between a person leaving education or training and completing those examinations. Entitlement in all cases ceases when a person reaches the age of 20.

Guardian's Allowance is an additional allowance for people bringing up a child because one or both of their parents has died. They must be getting Child Benefit (CB) for the child. The table shows the number of families in the UK in receipt of CB. The numbers shown in the table are estimates based on a random 5 per cent sample of awards current at 31 August, and are therefore subject to sampling error. The figures take no account of new claims, or revisions to claims that were received or processed after 31 August, even if they are backdated to start before 31 August.

Family Credit/ Working Families' Tax Credit

(Table 10.10)

Working Families' Tax Credit (WFTC) replaced Family Credit from 5 October 1999.

Family Credit was, and Working Families' Tax Credit is, available to families with at least one adult in remunerative work for at least 16 hours per week and who is responsible for at least one child under 16 (under 19 if in full-time education up to A-level or equivalent standard). The rate of payment of WFTC depends on the number of such children and expenditure incurred on eligible childcare. It is also higher if the worker works for at least 30 hours per week, or if there are disabled children or severely disabled adults in the family. It is tapered away above an income threshold. Further details can be obtained from HM Revenue & Customs (HMRC).

Child and Working Tax Credits (New Tax Credits)

(Table 10.11)

Child and Working Tax Credits (CTC and WTC) replaced Working Families' Tax Credit (WFTC) from 6th April 2003. CTC and WTC are claimed by individuals, or jointly by couples, whether or not they have children.

CTC provides support to families for the children (up to the 31 August after their 16th birthday) and the 'qualifying' young people (in full-time non-advanced education until their 19th birthday) for which they are responsible. It is paid in addition to CB.

WTC tops up the earnings of families on low or moderate incomes. People working for at least 16 hours a week can claim it if they: (a) are responsible for at least one child or qualifying young person, (b) have a disability which puts them at a disadvantage in getting a job or, (c) in the first year of work, having returned to work aged at least 50 after a period of at least six months receiving out-of-work benefits. Other adults also qualify if they are aged at least 25 and work for at least 30 hours a week.

Widow's Benefit and Bereavement Benefit

(Table 10.12 and 10.13)

Widow's Benefit is payable to women widowed on or after 11 April 1988 and up to and including 8 April 2001. There are three types of Widow's Benefits: Widow's Payment, Widowed Mother's Allowance and Widow's Pension. Women widowed before 11 April 1988 continue to receive Widow's Benefit based on the rules that existed before that date. Bereavement Benefit was introduced on 9 April 2001 as a replacement for Widow's Benefit, payable to both men and women widowed on or after 9 April 2001. There are three types of Bereavement Benefits available: Bereavement Payment, Widowed Parent's Allowance and Bereavement Allowance.

Government expenditure on social services and housing

(Table 10.20 to 10.25)

The tables of general government expenditure on social services and housing in the UK comprise a summary table followed by separate tables for each of the social services and housing categories. The definition of government expenditure used in the tables is consistent with Table 5.2.4S of the *Blue Book* 2009 edition, and covers both current and capital expenditure of central government (including the National Insurance Fund) and local authorities. The figures in the tables have been compiled based on the United Nations Classification of the Functions of Government (COFOG) and are consistent with the European System of Accounts 1995 (ESA95). The format of the tables was revised in the 2007 edition. As such they may not be comparable with earlier editions of the *Annual Abstract of Statistics*, which were based on information supplied directly by government departments. This information from government departments is generally no longer available and, as such, the tables are compiled under the categories of National Accounts.

Useful links

National Accounts Blue Book: www.statistics.gov.uk/cci/article. asp?id=2055

UN CoFoG classification: http://unstats.un.org/unsd/cr/registry/regcst.asp?Cl=4

The main categories of expenditure now used are:

Final Consumption Expenditure – The expenditure on goods and services that are used for the direct satisfaction of individual needs or the collective needs of members of the community as distinct from their purchase for use in the productive process. It may be contrasted with actual final consumption, which is the value of goods consumed but not necessarily purchased by that sector.

Compensation of Employees – Total remuneration payable to employees in cash or in kind. Includes the value of social contributions payable by the employer Net Procurement – current expenditure less receipts for sales and charges.

Gross Capital Formation – acquisition less disposals of fixed assets and the improvement of land.

Subsidies – current unrequited payments made by general government or the European Union to enterprises. Those made on the basis of a quantity or value of goods or services are classified as 'subsidies on products'. Other subsidies based on levels of productive activity (for example, numbers employed) are designated, 'Other subsidies on production'.

Capital Transfers – transfers which are related to the acquisition or disposal of assets by the recipient or payer. They may be in cash or kind, and may be imputed to reflect the assumption or forgiveness of debt.

Non-produced financial or non financial assets – assets produced either through production or otherwise of a non-financial nature.

Non-market capital consumption – output of own account production of goods and services provided free or at price that are not economically significant. Non-market output is produced mainly by the general government and Non-profit Institutions Serving Household sectors.

Education

(Table 10.21)

Table 10.21 includes expenditure by the education departments, local education authorities and the University Grants Committee on education in schools, training colleges, technical institutions and universities. Compensation of employees' figures are based on revenue outturn returns produced by Department for Communities and Local Government, Welsh Assembly Government and the Scottish Government.

Social protection

National Health Service

(Table 10.22)

Table 10.22 includes expenditure by central government on hospital and community health, family practitioner and other health services. The figures are based on departmental expenditure reported to HM Treasury.

Welfare services

(Table 10.23)

Personal social services: this table covers local authority and central government expenditure on such things as the aged, handicapped, homeless, child care, care of mothers and young children, mental health, domestic help, etc.

Social security

(Table 10.24)

Table 10.24 comprises both benefits under the Social Security schemes and non-contributory benefits and allowances, administered by the Department for Work and Pensions (DWP). Benefits paid overseas are also included, as are unfunded social benefits such as voluntary employer social contributions. The analysis by type of Income Support is not exact; the estimates are derived from average numbers in receipt of benefit and average amounts paid. War pensions which are now administered by the Ministry of Defence are included in this table. Child and Working Tax Credits (NTCs) replaced Working Families' Tax Credit (WFTC) from 6 April 2003 and are administered by the HMRC.

Housing

(Table 10.25)

The table shows government expenditure on housing. It includes expenditure made by central and local government sectors, but excludes expenditure by public corporations. The Housing Revenue Account is classified as a quasi-public corporation, so that most of its current and capital expenditure and income is included in the corporate rather than government sector. All overhead and administration expenses are included in final current expenditure. Non-capitalised support for public corporations and other market bodies relating to housing is recorded as subsidies. Capital transfers are paid mainly by local government to individuals for repair and improvement of privately owned housing. Current transfers paid include insurance premiums. Gross capital formation includes that of the council houses administered by the Housing Revenue Account. This is net of any sales of housing either through Right to Buy or Large Scale Voluntary Transfers. Housing benefit in the form of rent rebates and rent allowances is not included in the table, as they are regarded as forms of social security.

10.1 National Insurance Fund
(Great Britain and Northern Ireland)
Years ended 31 March

£ million

		2000/01	2001/02	2002/03	2003/04	2004/05	2005/06	2006/07	2007/08	2008/09
Receipts										
Opening balance	KJFB	14 909	19 868	24 177	27 267	27 816	29 804	34 940	39 243	49 306
Contributions	JXVM	55 627	58 050	59 658	59 827	62 863	67 786	69 599	77 224	76 107
State Scheme Premiums[1]	C59W	..	..	194	147	115	117	76	79	68
Compensation for SSP/SMP	KJQM	688	710	775	1 346	1 470	1 392	1 197	1 919	1 724
Transfers from Great Britian	KOTG	200	110	350	260	270	185	630	452	505
Income from investments	KJFE	884	1 146	1 457	1 292	1 288	1 399	1 867	2 453	2 026
Other receipts	KJFF	112	67	80	82	72	66	54	57	53
Redundancy receipts	KIBQ	23	22	24	28	32	38	43	37	39
Total	JYJO	72 442	79 972	86 716	90 249	93 926	100 787	108 406	121 464	129 830
Expenditure										
Total benefits	JYJP	50 960	54 550	54 201	56 255	58 572	61 304	63 695	67 443	72 366
Jobseeker's Allowance (Contributory)	LUQW	449	478	519	512	455	497	493	435	723
Incapacity	JYXL	6 982	7 074	7 104	7 116	6 910	7 028	7 009	6 945	6 937
Maternity	KETY	46	57	70	128	153	128	180	250	329
Bereavement Benefits	KEWU	1 008	1 132	1 142	1 033	946	903	826	759	708
Guardian's allowances and Child's special allowance[2]	KJFK	2	2	2	2	1	2	2	2	2
Retirement pensions[3]	JYJV	42 350	45 677	45 240	47 339	49 979	52 578	55 053	58 921	62 764
Other payments	KAAZ	21	29	27	34	30	33	40	61	97
Administration	KABE	1 197	873	1 280	1 794	1 521	1 464	1 473	1 430	1 371
Transfers to Northern Ireland	KABF	200	110	350	260	270	185	630	452	505
Redundancy payments	KIBR	195	232	255	243	222	295	248	215	431
Personal Pensions	C59X	..	..	3 336	3 847	3 508	2 566	3 076	2 557	2 680
Total	JYJU	52 574	55 795	59 449	62 433	64 123	65 847	69 161	72 027	76 549
Accumulated funds	KABH	19 868	24 177	27 267	27 816	29 804	34 940	39 245	49 437	53 281

1 State Scheme Premiums are payable in respect of employed persons who cease to be covered, in certain circumstances, by a contracted out pension scheme.
2 Includes Child's special allowance for Northern Ireland.
3 Includes personal pensions up to 2001/02.

Sources: HM Revenue and Customs: 01702 367480;
Department for Work and Pensions: 01253 856123 Ext 62436

10.2 Persons[1] who paid National Insurance contributions[2,3] in a tax year:[4] by sex
United Kingdom

Millions

		Total				Men				Women		
		2005/06	2006/07	2007/08		2005/06	2006/07	2007/08		2005/06	2006/07	2007/08
Total	KABI	29.02	28.91	28.98	KEYF	15.89	15.83	15.82	KEYP	13.13	13.08	13.17
Class 1	KABJ	24.50	24.50	24.77	KEYG	13.03	13.03	13.16	KEYQ	11.47	11.47	11.61
Not contracted out[5]	KABK	17.47	17.88	18.54	KEYH	9.69	9.95	10.35	KEYR	7.79	7.93	8.19
Contracted out	KABL	7.03	6.62	6.23	KEYI	3.35	3.08	2.81	KEYS	3.68	3.54	3.42
Mixed contracted in/out[6]	KABM	1.18	1.10	1.06	KEYJ	0.50	0.48	0.43	KEYT	0.68	0.63	0.63
Class 1 Reduced rate (including standard rate)	KABO	0.04	0.03	0.02	KEYL	–	–	–	KEYV	0.04	0.03	0.02
Class 2 exclusively[7]	KABP	2.38	2.40	2.36	KEYM	1.80	1.79	1.75	KEYW	0.59	0.60	0.62
Mixed Class 1 and Class 2	KABQ	0.71	0.70	0.70	KEYN	0.47	0.46	0.45	KEYX	0.24	0.25	0.25
Class 3 exclusively[8]	KABR	0.16	0.13	0.07	KEYO	0.07	0.06	0.03	KEYY	0.09	0.07	0.04
Mixed Class 1, 2 and 3[9]	I6CH	0.06	0.05	0.01	I6CK	0.02	0.02	–	I6CN	0.03	0.03	0.01

1 Based on all persons making contributions and not only if they have a qualifying year.
2 Estimates obtained from DWP Information Directorate: Lifetime Labour Market Data Tabulation Tool which uses a 1% sample of the National Insurance Recording System (NIRS2) summer 2008 extract.
3 Components may not sum to totals as a result of rounding.
4 The tax year commences on 6 April and ends on 5 April the following year.
5 Includes those persons with an Appropriate Personal Pension (such persons pay contributions at the not contracted out rate but then receive a rebate paid directly to their scheme).
6 Not included in the above rows.
7 Persons who paid a mixture of Class 2 contributions and others are not included in this category.
8 Persons who paid a mixture of Class 3 contributions and others are not included in this category.
9 Persons with a mixture of class1, 2 or 3 contributions.

Source: HM:Revenue and Customs:020 7147 3045

10.3 National Insurance contributions
United Kingdom

	Employee's standard contibutions[1]		Employer's standard contributions[1]	
	not contracted-out rate	contracted-out rate[2]	not contracted-out rate	contracted-out rate[3]

Class 1

Weekly earnings

2003/04
Below 77.00 (LEL)	-	-	-	-
77.00-89.00 (PT/ST)	-	See note 4	-	See note 5
89.01-595.00 (UEL)	11.0%	9.4%	12.8%	9.3%
	£55.66	£47.37		
Above 595.00 (UEL)	1%	1%	12.8%	12.8%

2004/05
Below 79.00 (LEL)	-	-	-	-
79.00-91.00 (PT/ST)	-	See note 4	-	See note 5
91.01-610.00 (UEL)	11.0%	9.4%	12.8%	9.3%
	£57.09	£48.59		
Above 610.00(UEL)	1.0%	1.0%	12.8%	12.8%

2005/06
Below 82.00 (LEL)	-	-	-	-
82.00-94.00 (PT/ST)	-	See note 4	-	See note 5
94.01-630.00 (UEL)	11.0%	9.4%	12.8%	9.3%
	£58.96	£50.38		
Above 630.00(UEL)	1.0%	1.0%	12.8%	12.8%

2006/07
Below 84.00 (LEL)	-	-	-	-
84.00-97.00 (PT/ST)	-	See note 4	-	See note 5
97.01-645.00 (UEL)	11.0%	9.4%	12.8%	9.3%
	£60.28	£51.51		
Above 645.00(UEL)	1.0%	1.0%	12.8%	12.8%

2007/08
Below 87.00 (LEL)	-	-	-	-
87.00-100.00 (PT/ST)	-	See note 4	-	See note 6
100.01-670.00 (UEL)	11.0%	9.4%	12.8%	9.1%
	£62.70	£53.58		
Above 670.00(UEL)	1.0%	1.0%	12.8%	12.8%

2008/09
Below 90.00 (LEL)	-	-	-	-
90.00-105.00 (PT/ST)	-	See note 4	-	See note 6
105.01-770.00 (UEL)	11.0%	9.4%	12.8%	9.1%
	£73.15	£62.51		
Above 770.00(UEL)	1.0%	1.0%	12.8%	12.8%

2009/10
Below 95.00 (LEL)	-	-	-	-
95.00-110.00 (PT/ST)	-	See note 4	-	See note 6
110.01-844.00 (UEL)	11.0%	9.4%	12.8%	9.1%
	£xx.xx	£xx.xx		
Above 844.00(UEL)	1.0%	1.0%	12.8%	12.8%

	2003/04	2004/05	2005/06	2006/07	2007/08	2008/09	2009/10
Class 2							
Flat rate weekly	£2.00	£2.05	£2.10	£2.10	£2.20	£2.30	£2.40
Small earnings exception[7] (per annum)	£4,095	£4,215	£4,345	£4,465	£4,635	£4,825	£5,075
Class 3							
Flat-rate voluntary weekly contributions	£6.95	£7.15	£7.35	£7.55	£7.80	£8.10	£12.05
Class 4 (Self-employed; profit-related)							
Rate on profits between LPL and UPL	8.0%	8.0%	8.0%	8.0%	8.0%	8.0%	8.0%
Rate on profits above UPL	1.0%	1.0%	1.0%	1.0%	1.0%	1.0%	1.0%
Lower profits limit (LPL)	£4,615	£4,745	£4,895	£5,035	£5,225	£5435	£5715
Upper profits limit (UPL)	£30,940	£31,720	£32,760	£33,540	34,840	£40,040	£43875

Note: LEL: Lower Earnings Limit; UEL: Upper Earnings Limit. PT: Primary Threshold; ST: Secondary Threshold.

1 Married women opting to pay contributions at the reduced rate at 3.85% before 2003-04 and 4.85% from 2003-04 earn no entitlement to contributory National Insurance benefits as a result of these contributions. No women have been allowed to exercise this option since 1977, but around 70,000 women who have been continually married or widowed and in the labour market since that time have retained their right to pay the reduced rate.

2 The contracted-out rebate for employees' contributions is applied only between LEL and UEL. Earnings below LEL are charged at the appropriate not contracted-out rate (which depends on total earnings). Earnings above the UEL are not subject to employee NICs before 2003-04.

3 The rates shown only apply to Contracted-Out Salary Related schemes (COSR).

Earnings below the LEL and above the UEL are charged at the appropriate not-contracted out rate. The employers' contracted-out rate applies only between the LEL and the UEL.

4 The contracted-out rebate for primary contributions is 1.6% of earnings between the LEL and the UEL for all forms of contracting-out.

5 The contracted-out rebate for secondary contributions is 3.5% of earnings between the LEL and the UEL up to 2006-07.

6 Since 2007-08 the contracted-out rebate for secondary contributions is 3.7% of earnings between the LEL and UEL.

7 If earnings from self-employment are below this annual limit and the contributor applies for and is granted a small earnings exception Class 2 contributions need not be paid. Class 2 or 3 contributions may be paid voluntarily.

Source: HM Revenue and Customs: 020 7147 3045

10.4 Weekly rates of principal social security benefits[1]
Great Britain and Overseas (excluding Northern Ireland)

At April

£

		2000	2001	2002	2003	2004	2005	2006	2007	2008	2009
Jobseeker's Allowance:											
Personal allowances											
Single											
Aged under 18[2]	KXDH	31.45	31.95	32.50	32.90	33.50	33.85	34.60	35.65	47.95	50.95
Aged 18 - 24	KXDJ	41.35	42.00	42.70	43.25	44.05	44.50	45.50	46.85	47.95	50.95
Aged 25 or over	KXDK	52.20	53.05	53.95	54.65	55.65	56.20	57.45	59.15	60.50	64.30
Lone parent											
Aged under 18 - usual rate	F92E	31.45	31.95	32.50	32.90	33.50	33.85	34.60	35.65	47.95	50.95
Aged under 18 - higher rate payable in specific circumstances	F92F	41.35	42.00	42.70	43.25	44.05	44.50	45.50	46.85	47.95	50.95
Aged 18 or over	F92G	52.20	53.05	53.95	54.65	55.65	56.20	57.45	59.15	60.50	64.30
Couple											
Both aged under 18	KXDL	31.45	31.95	32.50	32.90	33.50	33.85	34.60	35.65	47.95	50.95
Both under 18, one disabled	KXDI	41.35	42.00	42.70	43.25	44.05	44.50	45.50	46.85	47.95	50.95
Both under 18, with a child	F92H	62.35	63.35	64.45	65.30	66.50	67.15	68.65	70.70	72.35	76.90
One under 18, one 18 - 24	KXDI	41.35	42.00	42.70	43.25	44.05	44.50	45.50	46.85	47.95	50.95
One under 18, one 25+	F92I	52.20	53.05	53.95	54.65	55.65	56.20	57.45	59.15	60.50	64.30
Both aged 18 or over	KXDM	81.95	83.25	84.65	85.75	87.30	88.15	90.10	92.80	94.95	100.95
Dependant children and young people											
Aged under 11 - 16	KXDN	26.60	31.45	33.50	38.50	42.27	43.88	45.58	47.45	52.59	56.11
Aged 16 - 18	KXDP	31.75	32.25	34.30	38.50	42.27	43.88	45.58	47.45	52.59	56.11
Invalidity allowance											
High rate	KJND	14.20	14.65	14.90	15.15	15.55	16.05	16.50	17.10	17.75	15.65
Middle rate	KJNE	9.00	9.30	9.50	9.70	10.00	10.30	10.60	11.00	11.40	9.10
Low rate	KJNF	4.50	4.65	4.75	4.85	5.00	5.15	5.30	5.50	5.70	5.35
Increase for dependants											
Adult	KJNG	40.40	41.75	42.45	43.15	44.35	45.70	46.95	48.65	50.55	53.10
Each child[3]	KJNH	11.35	11.35	11.35	11.35	11.35	11.35	11.35	11.35	11.35	11.35
Incapacity Benefit:											
Short term (Lower) Under pension age	KOSB	50.90	52.60	53.50	54.40	55.90	57.65	59.20	61.35	63.75	67.75
Increase for adult dependant	KOSC	31.50	32.55	33.10	33.65	34.60	35.65	36.60	37.90	39.40	41.35
Short term (Lower) Over pension age	KOSD	64.75	66.90	68.05	69.20	71.15	73.35	75.35	78.05	81.10	86.20
Increase for adult dependant	KOSE	38.80	40.10	42.45	41.50	42.65	43.95	45.15	46.80	48.65	51.10
Short term (Higher)	KOSF	60.20	62.20	63.25	64.35	66.15	68.20	70.05	72.55	75.40	80.15
Increase for dependants:											
Adult	KOSG	31.50	32.55	33.10	33.65	34.60	35.65	36.60	37.90	39.40	41.35
Child[3]	KOSH	11.35	11.35	11.35	11.35	11.35	11.35	11.35	11.35	11.35	11.35
Long term	KOSI	67.50	69.75	70.95	72.15	74.15	76.45	78.50	81.35	84.50	89.80
Increase for dependants:											
Adult	KOSJ	40.40	41.75	42.45	43.15	44.35	45.70	46.95	48.65	50.55	53.10
Child[3]	KOSK	11.35	11.35	11.35	11.35	11.35	11.35	11.35	11.35	11.35	11.35
Incapacity age addition:[4]											
Higher rate	KOSL	14.20	14.65	14.90	15.15	15.55	16.05	16.50	17.10	17.75	15.65
Lower rate	KOSM	7.10	7.35	7.45	7.60	7.80	8.05	8.25	8.55	8.90	6.55
Employment and Support Allowance:[5]											
Single											
Aged under 18[2]	JTM6	..	..	..	..	..	..	..	..	..	50.95
Aged 18 - 24	JTM7	..	..	..	..	..	..	..	..	..	50.95
Aged 25 and over	JTM8	..	..	..	..	..	..	..	..	..	64.3
Lone parent											
Aged under 18 - usual rate	JTM9	..	..	..	..	..	..	..	..	..	50.95
Aged 18 or over	JTN2	..	..	..	..	..	..	..	..	..	64.3
Couple											
Both aged under 18	JTN3	..	..	..	..	..	..	..	..	..	50.95
Both under 18, with a child	JTN4	..	..	..	..	..	..	..	..	..	76.9
Both aged under 18(main phase)	JTN5	..	..	..	..	..	..	..	..	..	64.3
Both under 18, with a child (main phase)	JTN6	..	..	..	..	..	..	..	..	..	100.95
One under 18, one 18-24	JTN7	..	..	..	..	..	..	..	..	..	50.95
One under 18, one 25+	JTN8	..	..	..	..	..	..	..	..	..	64.3
Both aged 18 or over	JTN9	..	..	..	..	..	..	..	..	..	100.95
Attendance Allowance:											
Higher rate	KJNI	53.55	55.30	56.25	57.20	58.80	60.60	62.25	64.50	67.00	70.35
Lower rate	KJNJ	35.80	37.00	37.65	38.30	39.35	40.55	41.65	43.15	44.85	47.10
Carer's Allowance											
Standard Rate	J8T6	..	..	..	43.15	44.35	45.70	46.95	48.65	50.55	53.10
Disability Living Allowance:											
Care component											
Higher rate	KXDC	53.55	55.30	56.25	57.20	58.80	60.60	62.25	64.50	67.00	70.35
Middle rate	KXDD	35.80	37.00	37.65	38.30	39.35	40.55	41.65	43.15	44.85	47.10
Lower rate	KXDE	14.20	14.65	14.90	15.15	15.55	16.05	16.50	17.10	17.75	18.65
Mobility component											
Higher rate	KXDF	37.40	38.65	39.30	39.95	41.05	42.30	43.45	45.00	46.75	49.10
Lower rate	KXDG	14.20	14.65	14.90	15.15	15.55	16.05	16.50	17.10	17.75	18.65

10.4

Weekly rates of principal social security benefits[1]
Great Britain and Overseas (excluding Northern Ireland)
At April

£

		2000	2001	2002	2003	2004	2005	2006	2007	2008	2009
Maternity Benefit:											
Maternity allowances for insured women[6]											
Higher rate	KOSN	60.20	..	..	..	..	..	..	..	..	..
Lower rate[7]	KJNL	52.25	..	..	..	..	..	..	..	..	..
Standard rate	GPTJ	..	62.20	75.00	100.00	102.80	106.00	108.85	112.75	117.18	123.06
Threshold	GPTK	..	30.00	30.00	30.00	30.00	30.00	30.00	30.00	30.00	30.00
Guardian's Allowance	KJNN	11.35	11.35	11.35	11.55	11.85	12.20	12.50	12.95	13.45	14.10
Widow's Benefit:											
Widow's pension	KJNO	67.50	72.50	75.50	77.45	79.60	82.05	84.25	87.30	90.70	95.25
Widowed mother's allowance	KJNP	67.50	72.50	75.50	77.45	79.60	82.05	84.25	87.30	90.70	95.25
Addition for each child[3]	KJNQ	11.35	11.35	11.35	11.35	11.35	11.35	11.35	11.35	11.35	11.35
Bereavement Benefit:											
Bereavement allowance	WMPF	..	72.50	75.50	77.45	79.60	82.05	84.25	87.30	90.70	95.25
Widowed parent's allowance	WMOZ	..	72.50	72.50	77.45	79.60	82.05	84.25	87.30	90.70	95.25
Addition for each child[3]	WMPA	..	11.35	11.35	11.35	11.35	11.35	11.35	11.35	11.35	11.35
State Pension contributory:[8]											
Single person	KJNR	67.50	72.50	75.50	77.45	79.60	82.05	84.25	87.30	90.70	95.25
Married couple	KJNS	107.90	115.90	120.70	122.80	127.25	131.20	134.75	139.60	145.05	152.30
State Pension non contributory:											
Man or woman	KJNT	40.40	43.40	45.20	45.45	47.65	49.15	50.50	52.30	54.35	57.05
Married woman	KJNU	24.15	24.95	27.00	27.70	28.50	29.40	30.20	31.30	32.50	34.15
Industrial Injuries Benefit:											
Disablement pension at 100 per cent rate	KJNW	109.30	112.90	114.80	116.80	120.10	123.80	127.10	131.70	136.80	143.60
Child Benefit:											
First child	KJOA	15.00	15.50	15.75	16.05	16.50	17.00	17.45	18.10	18.80	20.00
Subsequent children	KETZ	10.00	10.35	10.55	10.75	11.05	11.40	11.70	12.10	12.55	13.20
War pension:											
Ex-private (100 per cent assessment)	KJOJ	116.00	116.00	119.80	121.79	123.90	127.38	130.20	133.60	138.34	152.40
War widow	KJOK	87.55	86.74	89.55	91.00	92.69	95.27	98.09	101.43	105.09	115.55

10.4
continued

Weekly rates of principal social security benefits[1]
Great Britain and Overseas (excluding Northern Ireland)

At April

£

		2000	2001	2002	2003	2004	2005	2006	2007	2008	2009
Income Support:											
Personal allowances[9]											
Single											
aged 16-17 usual rate	KJOW	31.45	31.95	32.50	32.90	33.50	33.85	34.60	35.65	47.95	50.95
aged 16-17 higher rate in specific circumstances	KABS	41.35	42.00	42.70	43.25	44.05	44.50	45.50	46.85	47.95	50.95
aged 18-24	KJOX	41.35	42.00	42.70	43.25	44.05	44.50	45.50	46.85	47.95	50.95
aged 25 or over	KJOY	52.20	53.05	53.95	54.65	55.65	56.20	57.45	59.15	60.50	64.30
Couple											
both aged under 18	KJOZ	31.45	31.95	32.50	32.90	33.50	33.85	34.60	35.65	47.95	50.95
both aged under 18, one disabled	F92J	41.35	42.00	42.70	43.25	44.05	44.50	45.50	46.85	47.95	50.95
both aged under 18, with a child	F92K	62.35	63.35	64.45	65.30	66.50	67.15	68.65	70.70	72.35	76.90
One aged under 18, one 18-24	F92L	41.35	42.00	42.70	43.25	44.05	44.50	45.50	46.85	47.95	50.95
One aged under 18, one 25+	F92M	52.20	53.05	53.95	54.65	55.65	56.20	57.45	59.15	60.50	64.30
Both aged 18 or over	KJPA	81.95	83.25	84.65	85.75	87.30	88.15	90.10	92.80	94.95	100.95
Lone parent											
aged 16-17 usual rate	KJPB	31.45	31.95	32.50	32.90	33.50	33.85	34.60	35.65	47.95	50.95
aged 16-17 higher rate in specific circumstances	KABT	41.35	42.00	42.70	43.25	44.05	44.50	45.50	46.85	47.95	50.95
aged 18 or over	KJPC	52.20	53.05	53.95	54.65	55.65	56.20	57.45	59.15	60.50	64.30
Pension Credit[10]											
Standard minimum guarantee:											
single	C59Y	..	..	..	102.10	105.45	109.45	114.05	119.05	124.05	130.00
couple	C59Z	..	..	..	155.80	160.95	167.05	174.05	181.70	189.35	198.45
Additional amount for severe disability											
single	C5A2	..	..	..	42.95	44.15	45.50	46.75	48.45	50.35	52.85
couple (one qualifies)	C5A3	..	..	..	42.95	44.15	45.50	46.75	48.45	50.35	52.85
couple (both qualifies)	C5A4	..	..	..	85.90	88.30	91.00	93.50	96.90	100.70	105.70
Additional amount for carers	C5A8	..	..	..	25.10	25.55	25.80	26.35	27.15	27.75	29.50
savings credit											
threshold single	C5A9	..	..	..	77.45	79.60	82.05	84.25	87.30	91.20	96.00
threshold couple	C5AA	..	..	..	123.80	127.25	131.20	134.75	139.60	145.80	153.40
maximum single	C5AB	..	..	..	14.79	15.51	16.44	17.88	19.05	19.71	20.40
maximum couple	C5AC	..	..	..	19.20	20.22	21.51	23.58	25.26	26.13	27.03

1 See chapter text.
2 Persons under 18 are entitled to the appropriate adult rate.
3 The rate of child dependency increase is adjusted where it is payable for the eldest child for whom child benefit (ChB) is also paid. The weekly rate in such cases is reduced by the difference (less £3.65) between the ChB rates for the eldest and subsequent children.
4 The rate of age addition depends on age at date of onset of incapacity: higher rate for under age 35 and lower rate for age 35-44.
5 Employment and Support Allowance (ESA) replaced Incapacity Benefit and Income Support paid on the grounds of incapacity for new claims from 27 October 2008.
6 Following an EU Directive, employee's maternity benefit is aligned with the state benefit they would receive if off work sick.
7 Women who are either not employed or self-employed receive the lower rate.
8 Retirement pensioners over 80 receive 25p addition.
9 In addition to personal allowances, a claimant may also be entitled to premiums. The types of premiums are family, lone parent, pensioner, higher pensioner, disability, severe disability and disabled child.
10 Pension Credit replaced Minimum Income Guarantee (MIG) for Income Support for those aged 60 and over on 6th Ocotober 2003.

Sources: Department for Work and Pensions;
Information Directorate;
HM Revenue and Customs: 020 7438 7370;
Ministry of Defence/DASA (Pay & Pensions): 020 7218 4271

10.5 Social Security Acts: number of persons receiving benefit[1]
Great Britain and Overseas (excluding Northern Ireland)

At any one time

Thousands

		2000	2001	2002	2003	2004	2005	2006	2007	2008	2009
Persons receiving:											
Jobseeker's Allowance[3]	JYXM	1 037.01	909.15	877.38	885.78	777.40	800.66	895.88	807.27	787.87	1 443.00
Employment and Support Allowance[4]	JTM5	..	..	..	..	..	..	..	..	..	288.27
Incapacity benefit[2,4,5]	KXDT	2 352.53	2 420.87	2 471.15	2 494.90	2 508.78	2 490.85	2 449.99	2 417.71	2 382.01	2 130.12
Severe Disablement Allowance	J8T2	375.56	374.45	336.48	320.76	305.94	292.87	280.01	267.61	255.56	244.09
Attendance Allowance	KXDU	1 556.10	1 570.90	1 290.77	1 315.64	1 377.35	1 419.42	1 465.59	1 507.50	1 546.68	1 585.79
Disability Living Allowance	KXDW	2 193.10	2 306.40	2 424.35	2 547.09	2 644.28	2 729.72	2 799.16	2 881.83	2 973.54	3 070.61
Carers' Allowance	J8T3	..	..	..	..	421.18	441.03	453.54	464.67	480.73	507.97
Child Benefit[6]	J8T4	7 305.00	7 297.10	7 296.10	7 297.50	7 301.30	7 311.40	7 365.40	7 449.60	..	..
Widows' Benefits	KJHF	265.11	254.97	223.41	191.50	163.43	138.96	117.65	96.89	77.90	62.14
Bereavement Benefits	VQAA	..	..	41.49	47.68	51.18	55.24	57.66	58.54	59.85	61.91
National Insurance											
State pension contributory:											
Males[2]	KJHH	4 039.40	4 083.90	4 149.15	4 211.36	4 275.68	4 336.81	4 374.17	4 432.29	4 520.56	4 626.96
Females[2]	KJHL	6 928.00	6 959.70	6 972.19	7 037.15	7 117.78	7 197.93	7 245.69	7 391.11	7 529.40	7 650.40
Total[2]	KJHG	10 967.40	11 043.60	11 121.34	11 248.52	11 393.45	11 534.73	11 619.88	11 823.40	12 049.97	12 277.36
State pension non contributory:											
Males	KJHI	5.20	5.10	5.26	5.37	5.39	5.34	5.36	5.68	6.23	6.67
Females	KJHJ	18.00	18.20	18.06	17.73	17.31	16.74	16.58	17.34	18.80	20.04
Total	KJHK	23.20	23.30	23.32	23.10	22.70	22.08	21.94	23.03	25.03	26.71
Industrial Injuries Disablement[2,7]											
Pensions assessments[5]	KJHN	274.60	275.40	273.70	267.13	266.48	267.12	266.45	264.88	262.73	260.69
Reduced Earnings Allowance/											
Retirement Allowance assessments[8]	KEYC	82.90	82.60	81.00	76.22	74.81	73.15	71.38	69.36	67.19	65.16
Income Support (Excluding MIG)	KABV	2 237.13	2 260.63	2 238.76	2 236.38	2 192.64	2 139.78	2 114.77	2 117.70	2 091.52	1 979.80
Minimum Income Guaranteed	J8T5	1 607.48	1 714.37	1 737.53	1 777.79	12.09	10.98	10.27	10.65	10.74	10.19
Pension Credit	C5AP	..	..	..	..	2 490.76	2 682.73	2 717.39	2 733.50	2 719.14	2 730.56
Housing Benefit and Council Tax Benefit											
Housing Benefit Total[9,10]	EW3X	4 033.30	3 874.40	3 812.63	3 796.42	3 879.42	3 956.82	3 990.03	4 031.81	..	4 412.99
Social Landlord[11]	KABY	3 218.35	3 131.14	3 093.80	3 081.67	3 135.49	3 165.89	3 152.25	3 108.73	..	3 186.40
Private Landlord	KABZ	814.95	743.26	718.83	714.75	743.93	790.93	837.79	923.07	..	1 221.42
Council tax benefit[12]	KJPO	4 830.06	4 673.37	4 601.73	4 627.78	4 800.22	4 959.69	5 049.97	5 076.94	..	5 440.06
War pensions[13]	KADG	295.67	284.33	272.78	260.79	247.59	235.30	223.85	212.54	201.27	190.75

1 See chapter text. Figures as at May each year unless otherwise stated.
2 Due to rounding errors several figures have been revised for May 2008.
3 Totals include 'credits only' cases.
4 Employment and Support Allowance (ESA) replaced Incapacity Benefit and Income Support paid on the grounds of incapacity for new claims from 27th October 2008.
5 Totals also include 'Credits only' cases.
6 Figures for Child Benefit in 2008 and 2009 are delayed due to extraction system updates.
7 Figures for IIDB include those receiving both IIDB and REA, at March.
8 Figures show REA cases only and are at March each year.
9 The DWP have implemented an improvement to the way in which HB and CTB caseload statistics are compiled. Historic statistics for the period up to August 2008 are based on clerical returns made by Local Authorities (LAs) of the aggregate number of people claiming HB and CTB as a specific point in time. This has gradually transitioned into a monthly electronic scan of claimant level data direct from the LA computer systems. This data source (the Single Housing Benefit Extract (SHBE)) has been designed to provide sufficient information for all current and future statistical purposes and is now the single source of HB and CTB data.
10 Housing Benefit figures excludes any Extended Payment cases.
11 Social landlord figures include registered social landlord tenants.
12 Figure excludes Second Adult Rebate Claims.
13 Figures for War pensions are at March each year.

Sources: DWP Information Directorate: Work and Pensions Longitudinal Study
100% data;
HM Revenue and Customs: 020 7438 7370;
Ministry of Defence/DASA (Pay & Pensions): 020 7218 4271

10.6 Jobseeker's Allowance[1,2,3] claimants: by benefit entitlement
Great Britain and Overseas (excluding Northern Ireland)
As at May

Thousands

		2003	2004	2005	2006	2007	2008	2009
All Persons								
All with benefit - total	KXDX	797.9	699.6	728.3	812.0	730.8	718.0	1 316.4
Contribution-based JSA only	KXDY	160.4	131.0	139.5	134.6	113.6	127.8	341.8
Contribution based JSA & income-based JSA	KXDZ	18.1	13.5	13.5	13.0	11.9	12.8	34.6
Income-based JSA only payment	KXEA	619.4	555.1	575.3	664.5	605.3	577.4	940.0
No benefit in payment	KXEB	87.9	77.8	72.4	83.9	76.4	69.9	126.6
Total	KXEC	885.8	777.4	800.7	895.9	807.4	788.0	1 443.0
Males								
All with benefit - total	KXED	605.6	527.2	545.3	606.8	537.8	529.9	978.9
Contribution-based JSA only	KXEE	114.1	93.8	99.5	95.8	79.6	90.6	248.7
Contribution based JSA & income-based JSA	KXEF	15.9	12.3	12.6	12.0	10.7	11.7	31.2
Income-based JSA only payment	KXEG	475.6	421.1	433.2	498.9	447.5	427.6	698.9
No benefit in payment	KXEH	60.3	52.7	49.8	56.6	51.7	46.7	88.8
Total	KXEI	665.9	580.0	595.1	663.4	589.6	576.7	1 067.7
Females								
All with benefit - total	KXEJ	192.3	172.4	182.9	205.3	193.0	188.1	337.6
Contribution-based JSA only	KXEK	46.3	37.2	40.0	38.7	34.0	37.2	93.1
Contribution based JSA & income-based JSA	KXEL	2.2	1.2	0.8	1.0	1.2	1.2	3.4
Income-based JSA only payment	KXEM	143.8	134.0	142.1	165.5	157.8	149.8	241.1
No benefit in payment	KXEN	27.6	25.0	22.6	27.2	24.8	23.2	37.7
Total	KXEO	219.8	197.4	205.5	232.5	217.8	211.3	375.3

1 See chapter text. Jobseeker's Allowance (JSA) has two routes of entry: contribution-based which depends mainly upon national insurance contributions and income-based which depends mainly on a means test. Some claimants can qualify by either route. In practice they receive income-based JSA but have an underlying entitlement to the contribution-based element.

2 Figures are given at May each year and have been derived by applying 5% proportions to 100% totals taken from the DWP 100% Work and Pensions Longitudinal Study (WPLS).

3 Figures are rounded to the nearest hundred and quoted in thousands. They not sum due to rounding.

Sources: Department for Work and Pensions;
Information Directorate

10.7 Employment and Support Allowance and Incapacity Benefit claimants by age and duration of spell[1,2,3]

Great Britain and Overseas (excluding Northern Ireland). At end of May

Thousands

		2004	2005	2006	2007	2008[4]	2009
Males							
All durations: All ages	KJJA	1 517.62	1 492.38	1 455.52	1 428.65	1 399.58	1 419.43
Under 20	KJJB	22.04	21.45	19.95	18.66	17.25	18.09
20-29	KJJC	142.68	143.24	141.80	146.07	149.47	159.10
30-39	KJJD	253.32	245.61	233.70	224.29	215.51	215.95
40-49	KJJE	318.04	320.77	319.77	320.24	319.22	330.96
50-59	KJJF	463.37	451.93	439.54	418.26	404.76	405.59
60-64	KJJG	318.12	309.36	300.73	301.10	293.33	289.57
65 and over	KJJH	0.05	0.04	0.02	0.03	0.04	0.17
Over six months: All ages	KJJI	1 359.08	1 347.43	1 323.20	1 291.32	1 266.80	1 253.91
Under 20	KJJJ	13.78	13.51	12.85	11.70	10.90	10.42
20-29	KJJK	110.85	114.57	115.21	117.83	121.90	124.50
30-39	KJJL	217.81	213.91	205.36	195.22	188.25	182.41
40-49	KJJM	285.90	290.72	291.36	289.94	289.72	293.13
50-59	KJJN	427.06	418.60	409.46	387.76	374.75	368.48
60-64	KJJO	303.64	296.10	288.93	288.85	281.25	274.93
65 and over	KJJP	0.04	0.02	0.02	0.03	0.03	0.05
Females							
All durations: All ages	KJJQ	990.84	998.20	994.33	988.93	982.33	998.74
Under 20	KJJR	21.48	20.51	18.92	17.86	16.79	15.68
20-29	KJJS	105.02	108.61	109.73	114.42	117.91	121.50
30-39	KJJT	177.91	173.45	167.36	162.39	156.95	156.85
40-49	KJJU	270.90	276.62	279.32	283.45	285.84	296.87
50-59	KJJV	415.52	418.99	418.99	410.80	404.82	407.82
60 and over	KJJW	0.02	0.02	0.02	0.02	0.02	0.02
Over six months: All ages	KJJX	880.52	894.57	896.33	885.69	881.41	882.94
Under 20	KJJY	12.40	12.10	11.13	10.20	9.55	8.75
20-29	KJJZ	84.02	88.98	90.99	93.60	97.24	99.15
30-39	KJKA	154.95	152.48	148.00	142.28	137.59	134.90
40-49	KJKB	243.52	250.11	253.50	255.99	258.74	263.70
50-59	KJKC	385.61	390.88	392.69	383.60	378.27	376.43
60 and over	KJKD	0.02	0.02	0.02	0.02	0.02	0.02
Unknown Gender							
All durations	EW44	0.31	0.26	0.15	0.13	0.11	0.23
Over 6 months	EW45	0.16	0.13	0.10	0.09	0.09	0.10

Definitions and conventions. Caseload figures are rounded to the nearest ten and displayed in thousands. Totals may not sum due to rounding.

1 See chapter text. Figures are given at May each year.

2 Table includes Employment and Support Allowance and Incapacity Benefit ONLY claimants and not those claiming Severe Disablement Allowance (SDA).

3 From 27th October 2008, new claims to Incapacity Benefit can also be allocated, on incapacity grounds, to the newly introduced Employment and Support Allowance (ESA).

4 Due to rounding errors several figures have been revised for May 2008.

Sources: Department for Work and Pensions; Information Directorate

10.8 Attendance allowance - cases in payment[1]: Age and gender of claimant

Great Britain

At May each year

Thousands

		2003	2004	2005	2006	2007	2008	2009
Males: All ages	JT9Z	393.9	418.5	436.9	459.5	478.4	497.2	516.5
Unknown age	JTA2	–	–	–	–	–	–	–
65 - 69	JTA3	19.5	21.4	22.0	22.3	22.8	23.5	24.4
70 - 74	JTA4	56.6	59.8	61.6	64.2	66.8	70.2	73.7
75 - 79	JTA5	100.9	103.8	104.2	104.8	106.3	109.1	112.4
80 - 84	JTA6	110.1	121.7	125.3	130.4	133.1	135.4	137.8
85 - 89	JTA7	68.5	70.1	78.7	89.4	98.5	107.7	116.0
90 and over	JTA8	38.3	41.7	45.1	48.4	50.8	51.2	52.2
Females: All ages	JTA9	921.8	958.9	982.6	1 006.2	1 029.1	1 049.5	1 069.3
Unknown age	JTB2	0.1	–	–	–	–	–	–
65 - 69	JTB3	25.1	27.3	27.7	28.3	28.4	29.1	30.0
70 - 74	JTB4	88.2	91.5	92.0	93.6	96.4	99.6	103.5
75 - 79	JTB5	189.1	190.9	189.1	186.8	185.8	186.7	188.4
80 - 84	JTB6	260.7	282.5	282.0	279.4	278.3	277.7	277.7
85 - 89	JTB7	206.1	204.7	221.4	241.6	259.3	276.7	290.9
90 and over	JTB8	152.6	162.0	170.4	176.4	180.9	179.6	178.8

1 Totals show the number of people in receipt of allowance, and exclude people with entitlement where the payment has been suspended, for example if they are in hospital.

Sources: Department for Work and Pensions; Information Directorate

10.9 Child benefits[1]

Thousands

		United Kingdom As at 31 August									
		2000	2001	2002	2003	2004	2005	2006	2007	2008	2009
Families receiving allowances:[2]											
Total	VOWX	7 340	7 335	7 336	7 246	7 296	7 315	7 413	7 475	7 583	7 770
With 1 child	VOWY	3 128	3 143	3 162	3 067	3 165	3 187	3 266	3 345	3 468	3 606
2 children	VOWZ	2 898	2 891	2 894	2 907	2 891	2 891	2 910	2 904	2 903	2 936
3 children	VOXA	977	970	954	947	926	921	919	910	899	906
4 or more children	VOXB	251	247	242	325	315	316	318	317	313	320
Families receiving Guardian's Allowance[3]	VOXH	2.5	2.3	2.5	2.6	2.9	2.8	3.2	3.3	..	..

1 See chapter text.
2 Data revised from 2003, updates to previous years not available.
3 Latest data not available.

Source: HM Revenue and Customs: 020 7147 3021

10.10 Family Credit/ Working Families' Tax Credit[1,2]

Thousands

		Great Britain As at 31 December						United Kingdom As at 30 November			
		1994	1995	1996	1997	1998		1999	2000	2001	2002
Families in receipt:											
Total	KJTO	578.0	646.5	716.7	751.4	779.7	ZCMK	965.3	1 167.8	1 293.7	1 377.3
Two-parent families: total	KJTP	324.6	356.9	390.2	388.0	383.4	ZCML	467.6	565.9	617.2	639.8
With 1 child	KJTQ	80.1	89.7	98.6	96.6	95.4	ZCMM	116.8	144.8	151.6	159.0
2 children	KJTR	122.4	135.1	146.1	144.4	141.7	ZCMN	178.4	220.1	243.5	252.7
3 children	KJTS	76.4	83.4	91.1	91.4	89.1	ZCMO	107.8	129.2	142.9	147.3
4 children or more children	ZIYM	45.8	48.6	54.4	55.6	57.3	ZCMP	64.6	71.8	79.2	80.8
One-parent families: total	KJTW	253.4	289.6	326.5	363.4	396.3	ZIYI	497.8	601.8	676.5	737.6
With 1 child	KJTX	133.8	152.2	170.4	189.3	203.4	ZIYJ	259.6	313.7	349.5	381.2
2 children	KJTY	86.0	99.1	111.2	121.8	136.1	ZIYK	169.6	207.6	238.7	261.6
3 or more children	KJTZ	33.5	38.3	45.0	52.3	56.9	ZIYL	68.6	80.5	88.3	94.8

1 See chapter text. Family Credit was replaced by Working Families Tax Credit (WFTC) in October 1999. The WFTC figures for December 1999 include Family Credit awards made before October 1999 and still current (both FC and WFTC awards last for 26 weeks).
2 WFTC was replaced by Child Credit and Working Tax Credit on 6th April 2003. See table 10.11.

Sources: HM Revenue and Customs: 020 7438 7370;
Department for Work and Pensions;
Information Directorate

10.11 In-work families with Child Tax Credit or Working Tax Credit awards
United Kingdom
As at December

Thousands

		2003[1]	2004	2005	2006	2007	2008	2009
In-work families with positive award:	C5PF	4 423	4 519	4 538	4 526	4 541	4 630	4 712
With children	C5PG	4 208.0	4 261.0	4 218.0	4 204.0	4 189.0	4 205.0	4 200.0
Receiving Working Tax Credit and Child Tax Credit	C5PH	1 548.0	1 492.0	1 497.0	1 596.0	1 650.0	1 763.0	1 870.0
Receiving Child Tax Credit only	C5PI	2 660.0	2 769.0	2 721.0	2 608.0	2 539.0	2 442.0	2 330.0
Without children								
Working Tax Credit only	C5PL	215.0	258.0	320.0	323.0	352.0	426.0	511.0

1 Child and Working Tax Credits replaced Working Families' Tax Credit on 6th April 2003. Figures for 2003 are based on awards current at 5th January 2004. All other figures at December each year. See chapter text.

Source: HM Revenue and Customs: 020 7147 3083

10.12 Widows' Benefit (excluding bereavement payment[1,2,3]): by type of benefit Great Britain

Number in receipt of widows benefit as at May each year

Thousands

		2004	2005	2006	2007	2008	2009
All Widows' Benefit (excluding bereavement allowance)							
All ages	KJGA	163.40	139.00	117.70	96.89	77.90	62.14
Unknown Age	EW4O	–	–	–	0.02	–	–
18 - 24	EW4P	–	–	–	–	–	–
25 - 29	EW4Q	0.20	0.10	0.10	0.04	0.02	0.01
30 - 34	EW4R	1.20	0.80	0.50	0.32	0.20	0.13
35 - 39	EW4S	3.90	2.90	2.10	1.53	1.08	0.74
40 - 44	EW4T	7.50	6.10	4.90	3.93	3.04	2.31
45 - 49	EW4U	13.20	11.00	9.10	7.58	6.26	5.14
50 - 54	EW4V	33.30	26.90	21.80	17.69	14.42	11.72
55 - 59	EW4W	77.70	66.90	57.30	45.78	36.86	30.37
60 - 64	EW4X	26.40	24.30	21.80	20.01	16.01	11.71
Widowed parents' allowance - with dependant children							
All ages	KJGG	28.20	23.20	19.00	15.60	12.60	9.98
Unknown Age	EW4Y	–	–	–	–	–	–
18 - 24	EW4Z	–	–	–	–	–	–
25 - 29	EW52	0.20	0.10	0.10	0.03	0.02	0.01
30 - 34	EW53	1.10	0.80	0.50	0.31	0.19	0.12
35 - 39	EW54	3.80	2.80	2.10	1.49	1.05	0.72
40 - 44	EW55	7.00	5.70	4.60	3.75	2.92	2.23
45 - 49	EW56	7.80	6.70	5.60	4.71	3.87	3.13
50 - 54	EW57	5.70	4.80	4.10	3.58	3.10	2.53
55 - 59	EW58	2.30	2.00	1.80	1.57	1.33	1.13
60 - 64	EW59	0.30	0.30	0.20	0.17	0.13	0.10
Widowed parents' allowance - without dependant children							
All ages	KJGM	1.40	1.10	0.80	0.69	0.54	0.46
Unknown Age	EW5A	–	–	–	–	–	–
18 - 24	EW5B	–	–	–	–	–	–
25 - 29	EW5C	–	–	–	–	–	–
30 - 34	EW5D	–	–	–	0.01	0.01	0.01
35 - 39	EW5E	0.10	0.10	0.10	0.04	0.03	0.02
40 - 44	EW5F	0.30	0.20	0.20	0.13	0.09	0.07
45 - 49	EW5G	0.40	0.30	0.20	0.21	0.17	0.15
50 - 54	EW5H	0.30	0.30	0.20	0.17	0.13	0.13
55 - 59	EW5I	0.20	0.20	0.10	0.11	0.10	0.07
60 - 64	EW5J	–	–	–	0.02	0.01	0.01
Age -related bereavement allowance							
All ages	KJGS	110.10	96.60	84.00	70.13	57.37	46.58
Unknown Age	EW5K	–	–	–	0.01	–	–
18 - 24	EW5L	–	–	–	–	–	–
25 - 29	EW5M	–	–	–	–	–	–
30 - 34	EW5N	–	–	–	–	–	–
35 - 39	EW5O	–	–	–	–	–	–
40 - 44	EW5P	0.20	0.20	0.10	0.06	0.03	0.01
45 - 49	EW5Q	5.10	4.00	3.30	2.66	2.23	1.86
50 - 54	EW5R	26.70	21.40	17.20	13.75	11.08	9.01
55 - 59	EW5S	66.30	59.00	50.90	40.57	32.61	26.83
60 - 64	EW5T	11.90	12.00	12.50	13.08	11.42	8.87
Bereavement allowance (Not age related)							
All ages	KJGW	23.70	18.10	13.90	10.47	7.39	5.12
Unknown Age	EW5U	–	–	–	–	–	–
18 - 24	EW5V	–	–	–	–	–	–
25 - 29	EW5W	–	–	–	–	–	–
30 - 34	EW5X	–	–	–	–	–	–
35 - 39	EW5Y	–	–	–	–	–	–
40 - 44	EW5Z	–	–	–	–	–	–
45 - 49	EW62	–	–	–	–	–	–
50 - 54	EW63	0.60	0.50	0.30	0.20	0.11	0.05
55 - 59	EW64	8.80	5.60	4.40	3.53	2.82	2.33
60 - 64	EW65	14.20	12.00	9.10	6.74	4.45	2.74

1 Definitions and Conventions: "-" Nil or Negligible; "." Not applicable; Caseload figures are rounded to the nearest hundred and displayed in thousands.

2 Caseload (Thousands) All Claimants of Widows Benefit are female. No new claims for WB have been accepted since April 2001 when it was replaced by Bereavement Benefit.

3 Figures include overseas cases.

Sources: DWP Information Directorate: Work and Pensions Longitudinal Study 100% data; Information Directorate

10.13 Bereavement Benefit[1,2] (excluding bereavement payment): by sex, type of benefit and age of widow/er

Great Britain.

Thousands

		Males				Females		
		2007	2008	2009		2007	2008	2009
All Bereavement Benefit (excluding bereavement allowance)								
All ages	WLSX	17.77	17.82	18.60	WLTC	40.77	42.04	43.32
18 - 24	EVW9	..	..	..	EVY2	0.07	0.08	0.06
25 - 29	EVX2	0.05	0.06	0.06	EVY3	0.53	0.53	0.53
30 - 34	EVX3	0.28	0.25	0.25	EVY4	1.63	1.66	1.68
35 - 39	EVX4	1.15	1.11	1.06	EVY5	4.05	4.31	4.30
40 - 44	EVX5	2.50	2.50	2.47	EVY6	7.01	7.33	7.61
45 - 49	EVX6	3.61	3.69	3.92	EVY7	8.92	9.54	10.22
50 - 54	EVX7	3.47	3.51	3.68	EVY8	8.65	9.10	9.64
55 - 59	EVX8	3.43	3.33	3.38	EVY9	9.90	9.49	9.28
60 - 64	EVX9	3.29	3.36	3.77	EVZ2	..	..	..
Widowed parents' allowance - with dependant children								
All ages	WLUD	11.27	11.51	11.81	WLUH	26.86	29.18	31.08
18 - 24	EVZ3	..	..	..	EW24	0.07	0.08	0.06
25 - 29	EVZ4	0.05	0.06	0.06	EW25	0.52	0.52	0.53
30 - 34	EVZ5	0.28	0.25	0.25	EW26	1.61	1.64	1.66
35 - 39	EVZ6	1.14	1.11	1.06	EW27	4.01	4.27	4.26
40 - 44	EVZ7	2.48	2.49	2.46	EW28	6.93	7.25	7.54
45 - 49	EVZ8	3.13	3.26	3.39	EW29	7.23	7.99	8.70
50 - 54	EVZ9	2.36	2.48	2.62	EW2A	4.61	5.29	5.97
55 - 59	EW22	1.29	1.32	1.38	EW2B	1.89	2.14	2.36
60 - 64	EW23	0.53	0.54	0.59	EW2C	..	..	..
Widowed parents' allowance - without dependant children								
All ages	WLVK	0.05	0.04	0.04	WMMR	0.34	0.32	0.28
18 - 24	EW2D	..	..	..	EW2M	..	..	..
25 - 29	EW2E	..	..	..	EW2N	0.01	0.01	0.01
30 - 34	EW2F	..	..	..	EW2O	0.02	0.02	0.02
35 - 39	EW2G	0.01	..	..	EW2P	0.05	0.04	0.04
40 - 44	EW2H	0.02	0.01	0.01	EW2Q	0.08	0.08	0.06
45 - 49	EW2I	0.01	0.01	0.01	EW2R	0.08	0.09	0.08
50 - 54	EW2J	0.01	0.01	0.01	EW2S	0.06	0.05	0.05
55 - 59	EW2K	0.01	–	0.01	EW2T	0.04	0.04	0.03
60 - 64	EW2L	..	..	..	EW2U	..	..	..
Age-related bereavement allowance								
All ages	WMOB	1.71	1.59	1.74	WMOC	6.17	5.76	5.59
18 - 24	EW2V	..	..	..	EW36	..	..	..
25 - 29	EW2W	..	..	..	EW37	..	..	..
30 - 34	EW2X	..	..	..	EW38	..	..	..
35 - 39	EW2Y	..	..	..	EW39	..	..	..
40 - 44	EW2Z	..	..	..	EW3A	..	..	..
45 - 49	EW32	0.46	0.42	0.52	EW3B	1.61	1.46	1.45
50 - 54	EW33	1.10	1.03	1.06	EW3C	3.97	3.76	3.62
55 - 59	EW34	0.15	0.14	0.16	EW3D	0.58	0.54	0.52
60 - 64	EW35	..	..	..	EW3E	..	..	..
Bereavement allowance (not age related)								
All ages	WMOX	4.74	4.68	5.01	WMOY	7.39	6.77	6.36
18 - 24	EW3F	..	..	..	EW3O	..	..	..
25 - 29	EW3G	..	..	..	EW3P	..	..	..
30 - 34	EW3H	..	..	..	EW3Q	..	..	..
35 - 39	EW3I	..	..	..	EW3R	..	..	..
40 - 44	EW3J	..	..	..	EW3S	..	..	..
45 - 49	EW3K	..	..	..	EW3T	..	..	..
50 - 54	EW3L	..	..	..	EW3U	..	..	..
55 - 59	EW3M	1.98	1.86	1.83	EW3V	7.39	6.77	6.36
60 - 64	EW3N	2.76	2.81	3.18	EW3W	..	..	..

1 Figures include overseas cases.
2 Figures are given at May each year and are taken from the DWP 100% Work and Pensions Longitudinal Study (WPLS).

Sources: Department for Work and Pensions;
Work and Pensions Longitudinal Study (WPLS);
Information Directorate

10.14 Contributory and non-contributory retirement pensions:[1,2] by sex and age of claimant

Great Britain and Overseas. At May each year.

Thousands and percentages

		2005	2006	2007	2008	2009
Men:						
Age-groups:						
65-69	KJSB	1 364.10	1 341.50	1 332.77	1 350.61	1 389.85
Percentage	KJSC	*31.40*	*30.60*	*30.03*	*29.84*	*29.99*
70-74	KJSD	1 150.00	1 160.10	1 177.96	1 205.70	1 232.97
Percentage	KJSE	*26.50*	*26.50*	*26.54*	*26.63*	*26.61*
75-79	KJSF	887.10	903.00	918.47	932.17	942.03
Percentage	KJSG	*20.40*	*20.60*	*20.70*	*20.59*	*20.33*
80-84	KJSH	593.30	596.90	604.74	614.77	627.28
Percentage	KJSI	*13.70*	*13.60*	*13.63*	*13.58*	*13.54*
85-89	KJSJ	246.40	273.10	296.36	317.90	335.49
Percentage	KJSK	*5.70*	*6.20*	*6.68*	*7.02*	*7.24*
90 and over	KJSL	100.20	103.60	106.13	105.33	105.62
Percentage	KJSM	*2.30*	*2.40*	*2.39*	*2.33*	*2.28*
Unknown age	EW3Y	1.10	1.20	1.45	0.19	0.24
Percentage	EW3Z	*–*	*–*	*–*	*..*	*..*
Total all ages	KJSA	4 342.20	4 379.50	4 437.99	4 526.79	4 633.62
Women:						
Age-groups:						
60-64	KJSO	1 498.70	1 524.00	1 628.19	1 695.88	1 734.92
Percentage	KJSP	*20.80*	*21.00*	*21.98*	*22.47*	*22.62*
65-69	KJSQ	1 464.20	1 453.10	1 456.08	1 484.80	1 527.47
Percentage	KJSR	*20.30*	*20.00*	*19.65*	*19.67*	*19.91*
70-74	KJSS	1 314.50	1 312.70	1 322.14	1 343.22	1 366.91
Percentage	KJST	*18.20*	*18.10*	*17.85*	*17.80*	*17.82*
75-79	KJSU	1 158.60	1 165.50	1 168.86	1 170.01	1 166.20
Percentage	KJSV	*16.10*	*16.00*	*15.78*	*15.50*	*15.20*
80-84	KJSW	951.60	933.30	923.70	919.11	921.01
Percentage	KJSX	*13.20*	*12.90*	*12.47*	*12.18*	*12.01*
85-89	KJSY	511.00	552.70	587.91	621.15	643.50
Percentage	KJSZ	*7.10*	*7.60*	*7.94*	*8.23*	*8.39*
90 and over	KJTA	314.90	319.40	319.90	313.66	310.07
Percentage	KJTB	*4.40*	*4.40*	*4.32*	*4.16*	*4.04*
Unknown age	EW42	1.30	1.50	1.67	0.37	0.38
Percentage	EW43	*–*	*–*	*–*	*..*	*..*
Total all ages	KJSN	7 214.70	7 262.30	7 408.44	7 548.20	7 670.44

1 See chapter text.
2 Caseloads include both contributory and non-contributory state pensioners.

Sources: Department for Work and Pensions;
Work and Pensions Longitudinal Study (WPLS);
Information Directorate

10.15 War pensions: estimated number of pensioners[1]
Great Britain

At 31 March each year

Thousands

		1999	2000	2001	2002	2003	2004	2005	2006[2]	2007	2008	2009
Disablement	KADH	248.93	240.76	231.62	221.80	212.18	201.55	191.75	182.80	173.85	165.17	157.13
Widows and dependants	KADI	55.85	54.92	52.71	50.98	48.61	46.04	43.55	41.05	38.69	36.10	33.62
Total	KADG	306.06	295.67	284.33	272.78	260.79	247.59	235.30	223.85	212.54	201.27	190.75

1 See chapter text. From 1914 war, 1939 war and later service.
2 The discontinuity between 2005 and 2006 is due to improvements in data processing.

Source: Ministry of Defence/DASA (Health Information): 01225 467801

10.16 Income support[1,2] by statistical group[3]: number of claimants receiving weekly payment
Great Britain

Thousands[4]

		2004	2005	2006	2007	2008	2009
All income support claimants[5]	F8YY	2 192.6	2 139.8	2 114.8	2 117.7	2 091.5	1 979.8
Incapacity Benefits	F8YZ	1 205.2	1 193.8	1 183.2	1 184.7	1 182.5	1 088.5
Lone Parent	F8Z2	823.3	789.3	774.9	765.6	738.6	720.5
Carer	F8Z3	78.40	79.00	80.20	82.80	85.70	92.10
Others on Income Related Benefits	F8Z4	85.90	77.70	76.50	84.60	84.70	78.70

1 Figures are given at May each year and are taken from the DWP 100% Work and Pensions Longitudinal Study (WPLS).
2 From 27th October 2008, new claims to Income Support can also be allocated, on incapacity grounds, to the newly introduced Employment and Support Allowance (ESA).
3 Statistical groups are defined as follows:
  Incapacity Benefits- claimants aged under 60 on Incapacity Benefit or Severe Disablement Allowance;
  Lone Parent - single claimants aged under 60 with dependants not in receipt of IB/SDA;
  Carer- claimants aged under 60 entitled to Carer's Allowance;
  Other Income Related Benefit- claimants not in one of the above categories.
4 Figures are rounded to the nearest hundred and quoted in thousands.
5 Totals may not sum due to rounding.

Sources: Department for Work and Pensions; Information Directorate

10.17 Pension Credit[1]: number of claimants
Great Britain

End of May

Thousands[2]

		2004	2005	2006	2007	2008	2009
All Pension Credit	F8Z5	2 490.8	2 682.7	2 717.4	2 733.5	2 719.1	2 730.6
Guarantee Credit Only	F8Z6	735.0	767.3	775.6	805.7	882.1	925.7
Guarantee Credit Only and Savings Credit	F8Z7	1 269.5	1 321.7	1 343.2	1 330.1	1 246.2	1 205.2
Savings Credit	F8Z8	486.0	593.7	598.6	597.7	590.8	599.6

1 Source: DWP 100% Work and Pensions Longitudinal study (WPLS).
2 All figures are rounded to the nearest hundred and expressed in thousands.

Sources: Department for Work and Pensions; Information Directorate

Social protection

10.18 Income support: average weekly amounts of benefit[1,2,3]
Great Britain

As at May

£ per week

		2004	2005	2006	2007	2008	2009
All income support claimants	F8ZF	91.14	85.81	83.41	82.29	82.35	84.94
Incapacity benefits[4]	F8ZG	77.70	76.93	78.12	79.78	81.55	88.90
Lone Parent[4]	F8ZH	114.96	102.85	94.88	89.70	87.37	82.79
Carer[4]	F8ZI	76.78	72.42	70.40	69.97	69.28	70.92
Others on income related benefits[4]	F8ZJ	64.25	62.69	62.62	62.33	62.87	66.22

1 Figures are given at May each year and are taken from the DWP 100% Work and Pensions Longitudinal Study (WPLS).
2 From 27th October 2008, new claims to Income Support can also be allocated, on incapacity grounds, to the newly introduced Employment and Support Allowance (ESA).
3 Average amounts are rounded to the nearest penny.
4 Statistical groups are defined as follows:
Incapacity Benefits- claimants under 60 on incapacity benefit or Severe Disablement Allowance;
Lone Parent- single claimants aged under 60 with dependants not in receipt of IB/SDA;
Carer- claimants aged under 60 entitled to Carer's Allowance;
Other Income Related Benefit- claimants not in one of the above categories.

Sources: Department for Work and Pensions; Information Directorate

10.19 Pension Credit: average weekly amounts of benefit[1]
Great Britain

As at May

£ per week[2]

		2004	2005	2006	2007	2008	2009
All Pension Credit	F8ZA	42.30	43.62	46.75	50.04	52.69	55.56
Guarantee Credit Only	F8ZB	71.91	75.43	79.56	83.74	85.07	88.86
Guarantee Credit and Savings Credit	F8ZC	37.51	39.87	43.11	46.11	48.29	50.81
Savings Credit only	F8ZD	10.03	10.83	12.39	13.36	13.62	13.71

1 Figures are given in each May and are taken from the DWP 100% Work and Pensions Longitudinal Study (WPLS).
2 Average amounts are shown as pounds per week and rounded to the nearest penny.

Sources: Department for Work and Pensions; Information Directorate

10.20 Summary of government expenditure on social services and housing[1]
Years ended 31 March

£ million

		2001 /02	2002 /03	2003 /04	2004 /05	2005 /06	2006 /07	2007 /08	2008 /09
Final Consumption Expenditure									
Education	QYWZ	53 779	58 505	63 866	69 216	75 368	78 830	82 564	89 018
Health	QYXA	62 263	68 794	75 844	83 637	89 998	95 980	103 512	110 435
Personal social services	GB7F	15 033	17 232	19 927	21 906	23 413	24 315	25 354	26 908
Social benefits	GG5O	121 098	126 345	135 591	142 004	145 268	149 793	159 832	173 476
Housing	QYXD	8 043	9 276	11 768	14 527	14 391	16 055	18 396	17 734
Total government expenditure	GH2K	260 216	280 152	306 996	331 290	348 438	364 973	389 658	417 571
Total government expenditure on social services and housing as a percentage of GDP	GGN7	25.2	25.7	26.6	27.2	27.4	27.2	27.5	29.2

1 See chapter text.

Source: Office for National Statistics: 0207 014 2125

10.21 Summary of Government expenditure on education[1]
Years ended 31 March

£ million

		2001 /02	2002 /03	2003 /04	2004 /05	2005 /06	2006 /07	2007 /08	2008 /09
Education									
Final consumption expenditure									
Current expenditure									
Compensation of employees									
Local Authorities[2]									
Nursery and primary schools	G8ZX	10 034	10 812	11 576	12 294	12 840	13 531	14 168	14 511
Secondary schools	G8ZY	10 007	10 783	11 545	12 262	12 806	13 495	14 130	14 473
Special schools	G8ZZ	1 258	1 356	1 452	1 452	1 610	1 697	1 777	1 820
Central Government									
Northern Ireland wages and salaries	HMPM	769	841	928	959	997	1 251	1 162	1 190
Other wages and salaries[3]	GB7H	391	445	494	513	670	872	1 291	1 322
Total Central Government expenditure	MMTF	1 160	1 286	1 422	1 472	1 667	2 123	2 453	2 513
Tertiary Education & Other Education[4]	G922	2 167	2 300	2 344	2 715	3 144	2 596	2 257	2 311
Total Compensation of employees	QYSA	25 786	27 853	29 761	31 727	33 674	35 564	37 238	38 141
Net procurement									
Local Government Net procurement[5]	QTKJ	6 407	7 620	7 688	8 916	10 261	10 810	11 452	12 347
Central Government Net procurement[6]	QTLN	1 835	2 034	2 112	2 034	2 154	2 446	2 476	3 593
Nursery/Primary schools									
secondary schools									
Tertiary education									
Total	QYSB	8 242	9 654	9 800	10 950	12 415	13 256	13 928	15 940
Non-market capital consumption	QYSD	1 200	1 248	1 305	1 409	1 568	1 778	1 858	2 045
Total final consumption expenditure	QYSE	35 108	38 205	41 223	44 069	47 715	50 565	53 467	57 041
Other current transfers	QZNU	13 791	14 743	16 467	17 818	18 975	19 215	20 169	20 830
Gross capital formation	QYVD	2 920	3 134	3 775	4 812	5 479	5 745	5 315	7 102
Non-produced non-financial assets	QYWM	−187	−191	−205	−216	−231	−237	−230	−235
Capital transfers	QZKJ	802	1 108	1 384	1 500	2 101	1 605	1 737	2 013
Subsidies	YBBL	153	168	184	192	212	206	205	205
Property Income	YBBN	–	–	–	–	–	–	–	–
Social Benefits	UGNA	1 192	1 338	1 038	1 041	1 117	1 731	1 901	2 062
Total Central Government Expediture	G924	21 770	23 819	26 333	28 851	31 551	32 878	33 876	37 725
Total Local Government Expediture	G925	32 009	34 686	37 533	40 365	43 817	45 952	48 688	51 293
Total government expenditure	QYWZ	53 779	58 505	63 866	69 216	75 368	78 830	82 564	89 018
Total government education expenditure as a percentage of GDP	GGN8	5.2	5.4	5.5	5.7	5.9	5.9	5.8	6.2

1 See chapter text.
2 Based on pay figures published by Dept for Communities and Local Government , Scottish Executive and National Assembly for Wales.
3 Includes wages/salaries for Scotland, Wales and Non-Departmental Public Bodies (NDPBs).
4 Includes Higher, Further, Adult and Continuing education.
5 Net of VAT.
6 Includes Central Government Net Procurement on NDPBs, Scotland, Wales, Northern Ireland and Education in Healthcare.

Sources: Office for National Statistics: 0207 014 2125;
Department for Communities and Local Government;
Scottish Government;
Welsh Assembly Government

Social protection

10.22 Summary of Government expenditure on Health[1]
Years ended 31 March

£ million

		2001/02	2002/03	2003/04	2004/05	2005/06	2006/07	2007/08	2008/09
Final Consumption expenditure[2]									
Current expenditure[3]									
Compensation of employees	QWWQ	31 043	34 159	38 402	43 116	45 824	48 651	49 303	53 690
non-market capital consumption	QYOB	1 574	1 680	1 787	1 884	2 113	2 342	2 359	1 754
other	QTLP	25 755	28 682	30 890	33 433	36 869	39 673	45 371	47 865
Total Final consumption expenditure	QYOT	58 372	64 521	71 079	78 433	84 806	90 666	97 033	103 309
Subsidies	CBRA	34	33	21	83	62	38	52	36
other current transfers	QZMR	1 291	1 176	1 262	1 289	1 658	1 222	1 451	1 599
Grosss capital formation	QYVE	2 566	2 930	3 332	3 593	3 215	3 813	4 731	5 299
Non produced non financial assets	QYWN	−140	−182	−143	−17	2	4	47	11
Capital transfers	HMSF	140	316	293	256	255	237	198	181
total outlays	QYXA	62 263	68 794	75 844	83 637	89 998	95 980	103 512	110 435
Total NHS expenditure as a percentage of GDP	GGN9	6.0	6.3	6.6	6.9	7.1	7.1	7.3	7.7

1 See chapter text.
2 Figures are based on Departmental Expenditure reported to HM Treasury Statistics database.
3 Includes expenditure by Dept. of Health, NHS Trusts, Scottish Government, Welsh Assembly Government and Northern Ireland Executive.

Source: Office for National Statistics: 0207 014 2125

10.23 Summary of Government expenditure on personal social services[1]
Years ended 31 March

£ million

		2001/02	2002/03	2003/04	2004/05	2005/06	2006/07	2007/08	2008/09
Personal social services									
Central government Current Expenditure									
Compensation of employees	ADQ7	331	376	462	482	519	537	560	594
Net Procurement	ADR2	343	532	489	667	634	548	571	606
Total	GB7D	674	908	951	1 149	1 153	1 085	1 131	1 200
Local Authorities Current Expenditure									
Compensation of employees	CFCR	5 936	6 385	6 940	7 449	7 889	8 230	8 436	8 938
Net Procurement	QWSB	8 349	9 859	11 951	13 207	14 250	14 864	15 637	16 610
Total	GB7E	14 285	16 244	18 891	20 656	22 139	23 094	24 073	25 548
Capital Expenditure	GDZU	74	80	85	101	121	136	150	160
Total Final Consumption Expenditure	GB7F	15 033	17 232	19 927	21 906	23 413	24 315	25 354	26 908
Total government expenditure as a percentage of GDP	GGO2	1.5	1.6	1.8	1.8	1.9	1.8	1.8	1.9

1 See chapter text.

Source: Office for National Statistics: 0207 014 2125

10.24 Summary of Government expenditure on social security benefits[1] and administration

Years ended 31 March

£ million

		2001 /02	2002 /03	2003 /04	2004 /05	2005 /06	2006 /07	2007 /08	2008 /09
Social benefits									
Social security benefits in cash									
National Insurance fund									
Retirement pensions	CSDG	42 128	44 580	46 692	48 958	51 567	53 769	57 734	62 421
Widows and Guardians allowances	CSDH	1 099	1 090	1 006	922	873	792	728	674
Unemployment Benefit	CSDI	−2	−2	−1	−1	−3	–	–	–
Jobseeker's Allowance	CJTJ	472	517	507	444	486	474	419	727
Incapacity Benefit	CUNL	6 669	6 754	6 713	6 647	6 635	6 563	6 568	6 556
Maternity Benefit	CSDL	56	69	128	150	164	175	247	322
Statutory sick pay	CSDQ	22	18	72	75	80	85	75	96
Statutory maternity pay	GTKZ	665	737	1 261	1 339	1 295	1 303	1 306	1 706
Payment in lieu of benefits foregone	GTKV	–	–	–	–	–	–	–	–
Total national insurance fund benefits	ACHH	51 109	53 763	56 378	58 534	61 097	63 161	67 077	72 502
Redundancy fund benefit	GTKN	205	280	240	186	253	205	175	393
Maternity fund benefit	GTKO	–	–	–	–	–	–	–	–
Social fund benefit	GTLQ	1 883	1 925	2 159	2 200	2 249	2 279	2 337	3 185
Benefits paid to overseas residents	FJVZ	1 262	1 357	1 449	1 533	1 619	1 721	1 802	1 950
Total social security benefits in cash	QYRJ	54 459	57 325	60 226	62 453	65 218	67 366	71 391	78 030
Total unfunded social benefits[2]:	QYJT	15 229	15 232	16 484	16 761	18 086	19 368	21 722	23 010
Social assistance benefits in cash									
War pensions and allowances[3]	CSDD	1 200	1 186	1 089	1 052	1 009	983	1 016	1 002
Income Support	CSDE	14 066	14 159	15 151	15 975	15 506	15 616	16 121	16 301
Income tax credits and reliefs	RYCQ	5 745	6 711	9 485	11 566	12 938	14 315	15 642	18 530
Child benefit	EKY3	8 795	8 955	9 374	9 566	9 756	10 132	10 641	11 198
Non-contributory job seekers allowance	EKY4	2 212	2 276	2 187	1 859	1 890	2 082	2 012	2 268
Care allowances	EKY5	5 237	5 363	5 619	5 888	6 218	6 487	6 886	7 292
Disability benefits	EKY6	7 306	7 784	8 307	8 822	9 376	9 997	10 699	11 360
Other benefits	EKY7	4 387	3 924	4 310	4 231	5 214	3 392	3 649	4 434
Benefits paid to overseas residents	RNNF	55	48	51	57	57	55	53	51
Total social assistance benefits in cash	NZGO	48 310	50 706	55 226	59 016	61 964	63 059	66 719	72 436
Total social benefits	NMDR	117 037	122 511	131 819	138 230	145 268	149 793	159 832	173 476
Administration[4]	KJEE	4 061	3 834	3 772	3 774	–	–	–	–
Total benefits and administration	GG5O	121 098	126 345	135 591	142 004	145 268	149 793	159 832	173 476
Total government benefit expenditure as a percentage of GDP	GGO3	12.2	12.2	11.7	11.7	11.4	11.1	11.3	12.1

1 See chapter text. Figures are based on table 5.2.4s of the Blue Book 2007. They are not fully comparable with earlier editions of the Annual Abstract.
2 Includes Civil & Defence, voluntary employer social contributions, teachers & NHS inflationary pensions increase payments.
3 From 2002/03 War Pensions are administered by the Ministry of Defence.
4 Figures published by HM Treasury in Public Expenditure Statistical Analyses. A separate figure for administration is no longer published.

Sources: Office for National Statistics: 0207 014 2125; Department for Work and Pensions; HM Treasury

Social protection

10.25 Summary of Government expenditure on housing[1]
Years ended 31 March

£ million

		2001/02	2002/03	2003/04	2004/05	2005/06	2006/07	2007/08	2008/09
Housing									
Final consumption expenditure									
Compensation of employees	QYSV	954	1 145	1 534	1 514	1 722	1 851	1 921	2 138
Other current expenditure on goods and services	QYSW	1 811	2 191	3 786	3 964	3 692	3 888	3 833	4 566
Capital consumption	QYSY	1 301	1 407	1 454	1 632	1 563	1 596	1 690	1 832
Total	QYSZ	4 066	4 743	6 774	7 110	6 977	7 335	7 444	8 536
Subsidies	QYVP	604	558	481	944	1 892	1 827	1 785	1 448
Other current transfers	QZNY	295	349	675	262	363	284	262	160
Gross Fixed Capital Formation	QYVH	643	482	424	750	842	874	902	1 384
Non-produced financial assets	QYWQ	−5	−7	−110	−128	−193	−170	−144	−34
Capital transfers	GVFX	2 440	3 151	3 524	5 589	4 510	5 905	8 147	6 240
Total government expenditure	QYXD	8 043	9 276	11 768	14 527	14 391	16 055	18 396	17 734
Total public sector housing expenditure as a percentage of GDP	GGO4	0.8	0.9	1.0	1.2	1.1	1.2	1.3	1.2

1 See chapter text.

Source: Office for National Statistics: 0207 014 2125

Crime and Justice

Chapter 11

Crime and Justice

There are differences in the legal and judicial systems of England and Wales, Scotland and Northern Ireland which make it impossible to provide tables covering the UK as a whole in this section. These differences concern the classification of offences, the meaning of certain terms used in the statistics, the effects of the several Criminal Justice Acts and recording practices.

Recorded crime statistics

(Table 11.3)

Crimes recorded by the police provide a measure of the amount of crime committed. The statistics are based on counting rules, revised with effect from 1 April 1998, which are standard for all the police forces in England, Wales and Northern Ireland. They now include all indictable and triable-either-way offences together with a few summary offences which are closely linked to these offences. The new rules have changed the emphasis of measurement more towards one crime per victim and have also increased the coverage of offences. These changes have particularly impacted on the offences of violence against the person, fraud and forgery, drugs offences and other offences.

For a variety of reasons many offences are either not reported to the police or not recorded by them. The changes in the number of offences recorded do not necessarily accurately reflect the changes in the amount of crime committed.

In order to further improve the consistency of recorded crime statistics and to take a more victim oriented approach to crime recording, the National Crime Recording Standard (NCRS) was introduced across all forces in England, Wales and Northern Ireland with effect from 1 April 2002. Some police forces implemented the principles of NCRS in advance of its introduction across all forces. The NCRS had the effect of increasing the number of offences recorded by the police.

Similarly, the Scottish Crime Recording Standard (SCRS) was introduced by the eight Scottish police forces with effect from 1 April 2004. This means that no corroborative evidence is required initially to record a crime-related incident as a crime if so perceived by the victim. Again, the introduction of this new recording standard was expected to increase the numbers of minor crimes recorded by the police, such as minor crimes of vandalism, minor thefts, offences of petty assault and breach of the peace. However, it was expected that the SCRS would not have much impact on the figures for the more serious crimes of serious assault, sexual assault, robbery or housebreaking.

The Sexual Offences Act 2003, introduced in May 2004, altered the definition and coverage of sexual offences. In particular, it redefined indecent exposure as a sexual offence, which is likely to account for much of the increase in sexual offences.

Further information is available from *Crime in England and Wales 2007/2008* (Home Office, Sian Nicholas, Chris Kershaw and Alison Walker, editors).

Court proceedings and police cautions

(Tables 11.4–11.8, 11.13–11.17, 11.20–11.22)

The statistical basis of the tables of court proceedings is broadly similar in England and Wales, Scotland and Northern Ireland. The tables show the number of persons found guilty, recording a person under the heading of the principal offence of which he/she was found guilty, but excluding additional findings of guilt at the same proceedings. A person found guilty at a number of separate court proceedings is included more than once.

The statistics on offenders cautioned in England and Wales cover only those who, on admission of guilt, were given a formal caution by, or on the instructions of, a senior police officer as an alternative to prosecution. Written warnings given by the police for motor offences and persons paying fixed penalties for certain motoring offences are excluded. Formal cautions are not issued in Scotland. There are no statistics on cautioning available for Northern Ireland.

The Crime and Disorder Act 1998 provides for reprimands and final warnings, which are new offences and orders implemented nationally from 1 June 2000. They replace the system of cautioning for offenders under the age of 18. Reprimands can be given to first-time offenders for minor offences. Any further offending results in either a final warning or a charge.

For persons proceeded against in Scotland, the statistics relate to the High Court of Justiciary, the sheriff courts and the district courts. The High Court deals with serious solemn offences (requiring trial by jury) and has unlimited sentencing power. Sheriff courts deal with solemn offences where imprisonment is limited to 3 years or summary offences (not requiring a jury) where imprisonment is limited to 3 months (6 months when specified in legislation for second or subsequent offences and 12 months for certain statutory offences). District courts deal only with summary cases and are limited to 60 days imprisonment and level 4 fines. Stipendiary magistrates sit in Glasgow District Court and have the summary sentencing powers of a sheriff.

In England and Wales, indictable offences are offences which are:

- *triable only on indictment.* that is by the Crown Court. ('indictable-only' offences include murder, manslaughter, rape and robbery)

- *triable either way.* that is by the Crown Court or a magistrates' court

The Criminal Justice Act 1991 resulted in the following changes being made to the sentencing system in England and Wales:

- the introduction of combination orders

- the introduction of the 'unit fine scheme' at magistrates' courts

- the abolition of the sentence of detention in a young offender institution for 14-year-old boys and to a change in the minimum and maximum lengths of sentence to 10 and 12 months respectively to which 15 to 17-year-olds might be subjected, and

- the abolition of partly suspended sentences of imprisonment and to a restriction in the use of fully suspended sentences

The Criminal Justice Act 1993 abolished the unit fine scheme in magistrates' courts, which had been introduced under the Criminal Justice Act 1991.

A charging standard for assault was introduced in England and Wales on 31 August 1994, the aim being to promote consistency between the police and prosecution on the appropriate level of charge to be brought.

The Criminal Justice and Public Order Act 1994 created several new offences in England and Wales, mainly in the area of public order, but also including male rape (there is no statutory offence of male rape in Scotland, although such a crime may be charged as serious assault). The Act also:

- extended the provisions of section 53 of the Children and Young Persons Act 1993 to 10 to 13-year-olds

- increased the maximum sentence length for 15 to 17-year-olds to 2 years

- increased the upper limit from £2,000 to £5,000 for offences of criminal damage proceeded against as if triable only summarily

- introduced provisions for the reduction of sentences for early guilty pleas and

- increased the maximum sentence length for certain firearm offences

Provisions within the Crime (Sentences) Act 1997 (as amended by the Powers of Criminal Courts Sentencing Act 2000) in England and Wales, and the Crime and Punishment (Scotland) Act 1997 allow for:

- an automatic life sentence for a second serious violent or sexual offence unless exceptional circumstances exist (this provision has not been enacted in Scotland)

- a minimum sentence of 7 years for an offender convicted for a third time of a 'class A' drug trafficking offence unless the court considers this to be unjust in all the circumstances, and

- in England and Wales, section 38A of the Magistrates' Courts' Act 1980 (which extends the circumstances in which a magistrates' court may commit a person convicted of an offence triable-either-way to the Crown Court for sentence) was implemented in conjunction with section 49 of the Criminal Procedure and Investigations Act 1996 (when the magistrates' court requires a defendant to indicate a plea before a decision can be taken on the mode of trial and which compels the court to sentence or commit for sentence any defendant who indicates a guilty plea)

Under the Criminal Justice and Court Service Act 2000 new terms were introduced for certain orders. 'Community rehabilitation order' is the new name given to a probation order. A community service order is now known as a 'community punishment order'. Finally, the new term for a combination order is 'community punishment and rehabilitation order'. In April 2000 the secure training order was replaced by the 'detention and training order'. Section 53 of the Children and Young Persons Act 1993 was repealed on 25 August 2000 and its provisions re-enacted in sections 90 to 92 of the Powers of Criminal Courts (Sentencing) Act 2000. 'Reparation and action plan orders' were implemented nationally from 1 June 2000. 'Drug treatment and testing orders' were introduced in England, Scotland and Wales with effect from October 2000. 'Referral orders' were introduced in England, Scotland and Wales with effect from April 2000. These changes are now reflected in Table 11.8.

Following the introduction of the Libra case management system during 2008, offenders at magistrates' courts can now be recorded as sex 'Not Stated'. In 2008 one per cent of offenders sentenced were recorded as sex 'Not Stated'. Amendments to the data tables have been made to accommodate this new category.

Crime and Justice

The system of magistrates' courts and Crown Courts in Northern Ireland operates in a similar way to that in England and Wales. A particularly significant statutory development, however, has been the Criminal Justice (NI) Order 1996, which introduces a new sentencing regime to Northern Ireland and largely replicates that introduced to England and Wales by the Criminal Justice Acts of 1991 and 1993. The order makes many changes to both community and custodial sentences and introduces new orders such as the combination order, the custody probation order, and orders for release on licence of sexual offenders.

Expenditure on penal establishments in Scotland

(Table 11.19)

The results shown in this table are reported on a cash basis for financial years 1996/97 to 2000/01 in line with funding arrangements. Financial year 2001/02 is reported on a resource accounting basis in line with the introduction of resource budgeting. Capital charges were introduced with resource accounting and budgeting.

11.1 Police Officer Strength[1]: by country and sex
As at 31 March

Numbers

		1999	2000	2001	2002	2003	2004	2005	2006	2007	2008	2009
England and Wales												
Regular Police(FTE)												
Strength:												
Men	KERB	103 956	101 801	102 139	104 483	106 996	110 150	110 597	109 327	108 118	106 866	106 996
Women	KERC	19 885	20 155	21 174	22 784	24 430	26 956	28 898	30 307	31 914	32 861	34 651
Seconded:[2,3]												
Men	KERD	2 017	1 965	1 914	2 031	1 689	1 811	1 514	1 545	422	432	438
Women	KERE	238	249	292	305	251	284	222	203	60	70	66
Additional Officers:[4]												
Men	KERF	324	361	493	567	375	394	522	676	657	661	653
Women	KERG	582	519	509	564	709	969	1 042	1 213	1 203	1 471	1 470
Special constables												
Strength:[5]												
Men	KERH	10 860	9 623	8 630	8 014	7 718	7 645	8 074	8 829	9 327	9 719	9 544
Women	KERI	5 624	4 724	4 108	3 584	3 319	3 343	3 844	4 350	4 694	4 828	4 707
Scotland												
Regular police												
Strength:[6]												
Men	KERK	12 545	12 374	12 547	12 513	12 590	12 685	12 798	12 820	12 687	12 532	12 328
Women	KERL	2 265	2 325	2 602	2 738	2 897	2 898	3 203	3 401	3 547	3 689	3 991
Central service:[7]												
Men	KERM	88	95	87	116	131	166	195	171	153	219	180
Women	KERN	9	13	10	12	17	29	29	21	28	44	37
Seconded:[8]												
Men	KERO	85	130	140	133	166	192	216	200	195	196	291
Women	KERP	12	18	14	18	24	30	31	27	28	30	69
Additional regular police:												
Men	HFVM	85	80	83	80	79	88	79	85	107	106	129
Women	HFVN	6	4	5	12	10	13	21	15	12	14	24
Special constables												
Strength:												
Men	KERS	1 229	981	924	812	711	773	718	888	886	884	..
Women	KERT	422	355	336	307	280	328	437	432	471	510	..
Northern Ireland												
Regular police[9,10]												
Strength:												
Men	KERU	7 406	6 844	6 227	6 057	6 171	6 108	6 016	5 992	5 949	5 761	5 669
Women	KERV	987	966	1 009	1 080	1 266	1 418	1 547	1 534	1 600	1 653	1 735
Reserve[11]												
Strength:												
Men	KERW	3 199	2 962	2 629	2 223	1 983	1 824	1 431	1 424	1 212	1 119	930
Women	KERX	641	607	556	510	453	485	410	402	400	382	345

1 Figures for England and Wales are as 31 March and are based on full-time equivalent strength excluding those on career breaks or maternity/paterntiy leave. Figures for Scotland are as 31 March. From 1999, figures for Northern Ireland reflect the position at the end of the financial year, ie 1999 and 2000 figures are as 31 March 2000 and 31 March 2001 respectively. Prior to this figures were as at 31 December.

2 Figures exclude secondments outside the police service in England and Wales (eg to the private sector or to law enforcement agencies overseas).

3 From 31 March 2007 onwards details of officers seconded to NCIS and NCS will no longer appear following the launch of Serious Organised Crime Agency (SOCA) in April 2006.

4 Figures include those officers on career breaks or maternity/paternity leave. Prior to 2003, these figures were not collected centrally.

5 Special constable figures are given as a headcount measure.

6 'Strength' is WTE police strength, only excluding special constables.

7 Instructors at Training Establishments, etc, formerly shown as secondments.

8 Includes Scottish Crime and Drug Enforcement Agency .

9 Does not include officers on secondment.

10 Also includes student officers.

11 Includes part-time reserve and full-time reserve, FTR -515 as at 31 March 2009 (481 males and 34 females). Con PT - 760 as at 31 March 2009 (449 males and 311 females). FTR -382 as at 31 March 2010 (362 males and 20 females) Con PT -703 as at 31 March 2010 (412 males and 291 female)

Sources: Home Office: 020 7035 0289;
Scottish Government Justice Department: 0131 244 2148;
The Police Service of Northern Ireland: 0845 6008000 ext 24070

Crime and justice

11.2 Prison Population[1] international comparisons

Country	2001	2002	2003	2004	2005	2006	2007	% change 2006-2007	Rate[16] per 100,000 population in 2007
England & Wales[5]	67 056	71 324	72 992	75 057	76 896	79 085	80 692	2	149
Northern Ireland[3]	910	1 026	1 160	1 274	1 301	1 433	1 468	2	83
Scotland[7]	6 137	6 404	6 524	6 805	6 792	7 111	7 291	3	142
Austria	6 915	7 511	7 816	9 000	8 767	8 780	8 887	1	107
Belgium[12]	8 544	8 605	9 308	9 245	9 375	9 635	10 008	4	94
Bulgaria[3]	8 971	8 994	9 422	10 066	10 871	11 436	11 058	-3	144
Croatia[3]	2 623	2 584	2 732	2 803	3 022	3 485	3 833	10	86
Cyprus	369	345	355	546	536	599	673	12	85
Czech Republic[6]	19 320	16 213	17 277	18 343	18 937	18 578	18 901	2	182
Denmark	3 150	3 439	3 577	3 762	4 132	3 759	3 406	-9	62
Estonia[3]	4 803	4 775	4 352	4 576	4 565	4 411	4 327	-2	322
Finland[6]	3 110	3 469	3 463	3 535	3 883	3 477	3 370	-3	64
France[10]	47 005	53 463	57 440	56 271	56 595	55 754	60 677	9	95
Germany[4]	80 333	74 904	81 176	81 166	80 410	78 581	75 719	-4	92
Greece[9]	8 343	8 284	8 555	8 760	9 589	10 113	10 700	6	96
Hungary[6]	17 275	17 838	16 507	16 543	15 720	14 821	14 353	-3	143
Iceland	110	107	112	115	119	119	115	-3	37
Ireland (Eire)[13]	3 025	3 028	2 986	3 083	3 022	3 080	3 325	8	76
Italy[6]	57 203	56 723	56 845	56 068	59 523	39 005	48 693	25	82
Latvia[3]	8 831	8 531	8 366	8 179	7 646	6 965	6 548	-6	287
Lithuania[3]	9 516	11 566	11 070	8 063	8 125	8 137	8 079	-1	239
Luxembourg	357	380	498	548	693	756	745	-1	155
Malta[11]	257	283	278	277	298	346	387	12	95
Netherlands	15 246	16 239	18 242	20 075	21 826	20 463	18 103	-12	110
Norway	2 666	2 662	2 914	2 975	3 097	3 164	3 280	4	69
Poland[5]	80 004	80 610	80 692	79 344	82 656	87 669	90 199	3	237
Portugal[6]	13 260	13 918	13 835	13 152	12 889	12 636	11 587	-8	109
Romania[6]	49 840	48 081	42 815	39 031	36 700	34 038	29 390	-14	137
Russian Federation[3]	925 072	980 151	877 393	847 004	763 115	823 451	871 693	6	613
Slovakia[6]	7 433	7 758	8 873	9 422	8 897	8 249	7 986	-3	148
Slovenia	1 155	1 120	1 099	1 126	1 132	1 301	1 336	3	66
Spain	46 962	50 994	55 244	59 224	61 269	64 120	66 400	4	148
Sweden[15]	6 089	6 506	6 755	7 332	7 054	7 175	6 770	-6	74
Switzerland[14]	5 137	4 937	5 214	5 977	6 137	5 888	5 715	-3	76
Turkey	61 336	60 091	64 051	71 148	54 296	67 795	85 865	27	122
Ukraine	198 885	198 946	198 386	193 489	179 519	165 716	154 055	-7	332
Australia[2]	22 458	22 492	23 555	24 171	25 353	25 790	27 224	6	130
Canada[8]	35 533	35 736	35 868	34 155	34 365	35 110	-	-	108
Japan[3]	61 242	65 508	69 502	73 734	76 413	79 052	81 255	3	63
Korea(Rep. of)[7]	62 235	61 084	58 945	57 184	52 403	46 721	46 313	-1	96
Mexico[6]	165 687	172 888	182 530	193 889	205 821	210 140	212 841	1	193
New Zealand[7]	5 887	5 738	6 059	6 556	7 100	7 595	7 959	5	188
South Africa[4]	170 959	178 998	189 748	187 640	187 394	150 302	161 639	8	339
U.S.A.[2]	1 961 247	2 033 331	2 081 580	2 129 802	2 186 230	2 245 189	2 299 116	2	762
European Union 27	581 419	592 331	607 522	609 873	620 099	601 513	611 078	2	123

1 At 1 September: number of prisoners, including pre-trial detainees/remand prisoners.
2 At 30 June.
3 At 1 January.
4 At 31 March.
5 At 31 August.
6 At 31 December.
7 Annual averages. Countries calculate these on the basis of daily, weekly or monthly figures.
8 Annual averages by financial year (e.g. 2006=1 April 2005-31 March 2006). Rate per 100,000 population reflects the position in 2006.
9 At 1 September (2001-03, 2005-06). At 16 December (2004). At 30 June (2007).
10 Metropolitan and overseas departments and territories.
11 At 1 September (2001-06). Annual average (2007).
12 At 1 March.
13 At 1 September (2001-06). At 26 October (2007).
14 At third Wednesday in March (2001). At first Wednesday in September (2002-07).
15 At 1 October.
16 Based on estimates of national population.

Sources: Ministries responsible for prisons, national prison administrations; national statistical offices, Council of Europe Annual Penal Statistics (SPACE); World Prison Population List and World Prison Brief; (International Centre for Prison Studies King's College, London)

11.3 Recorded crime statistics: by offence group[1]
England and Wales

Thousands

			1997	1998[2,3]		1999/00	2000/01	2001[4]/02	2002[4,6]/03	2003/04	2004/05	2005/06	2006[8]/07	2007/08	2008/09
Violence against the person	BEAB		250.8	230.8	LQMP	581.0	600.9	650.3	845.1	967.2	1 048.1	1 059.6	1 046.4	961.1	903.4
Sexual offences[7]	BEAC		33.2	34.9	LQMQ	37.8	37.3	41.4	58.9	62.5	62.9	62.1	57.5	53.5	51.4
Burglary	BEAD		1 015.1	951.9	LQMR	906.5	836.0	878.5	890.1	820.0	680.4	645.1	622.0	583.7	581.5
Robbery	BEAE		63.1	66.2	LQMS	84.3	95.2	121.4	110.3	103.7	91.0	98.2	101.4	84.7	80.1
Theft and handling stolen goods (of which):	BEAF		2 165.0	2 126.7	LQMT	2 223.6	2 145.4	2 267.0	–	–	–	–	–	–	–
Offences against vehicles					I8RM	..	..	..	1 074.7	985.0	820.1	792.8	765.0	656.4	591.9
Other theft offences					I8RN	..	..	..	1 336.9	1 327.9	1 247.6	1 226.2	1 180.8	1 121.0	1 080.0
Fraud and forgery	BEAG		134.4	173.7	LQMU	334.8	319.3	314.9	331.1	319.6	280.1	232.8	199.7	155.3	163.1
Criminal damage	BEAH		877.0	834.4	LQMV	945.7	960.1	1 064.5	1 120.6	1 218.5	1 197.5	1 184.3	1 185.0	1 036.2	936.4
Drug offences[5]	LQMO		..	21.3	LQYT	121.9	113.5	121.3	143.3	143.5	145.8	178.5	194.2	229.0	243.4
Other offences[5]	BEAI		36.6	42.0	LQYU	65.7	63.2	65.3	64.0	65.7	64.0	75.6	75.7	69.3	69.4
Total	BEAA		4 598.3	4 481.8	LQYV	5 301.2	5 170.8	5 527.1	5 975.0	6 013.8	5 637.5	5 555.2	5 427.6	4 951.2	4 702.5

1 See chapter text.
2 Estimates.
3 Figures from this period are not directly comparable with data prior to 1998/99 and from 2002/03 onwards.
4 The National Crime Recording Standard (NCRS) was introduced in England and Wales from 1 April 2002. These figures are not directly comparable with those for earlier years.

5 Prior to 1 April 1998 the offence of drug trafficking was included in the 'Other offences' group. From 1 April 1999, under the new counting rules, drug trafficking became part of a new 'Drug offences' group which, now also includes possession and other drug offences.
6 Includes the British Transport Police (BTP) from 2002/03 onwards.
7 The Sexual Offences Act 2003, introduced in May 2004, altered the definitions and coverage of sexual offences.
8 The offence groupings were revised in 2006/07 and backdated to 2002/03.

Source: Home Office: 020 7035 0307

11.4 Offenders found guilty: by offence group[1,2,3], England and Wales

Magistrates' courts and the Crown Court

Thousands

		1998	1999	2000	2001	2002	2003	2004	2005	2006	2007	2008[6]
All ages[4]												
Indictable offences												
Violence against the person:	KJEJ	37.1	35.7	35.3	35.3	37.7	38.0	39.1	40.9	41.9	42.0	41.5
Murder	KESB	0.3	0.3	0.3	0.3	0.3	0.3	0.4	0.4	0.4	0.4	0.4
Manslaughter	KESC	0.3	0.2	0.2	0.3	0.3	0.2	0.3	0.3	0.2	0.2	0.2
Wounding	KESD	35.2	33.9	33.5	33.5	35.7	35.9	36.9	38.6	39.8	39.8	39.3
Other offences of violence against the person	KESE	1.3	1.4	1.3	1.2	1.4	1.6	1.6	1.6	1.5	1.5	1.5
Sexual offences	KESF	4.6	4.3	3.9	4.0	4.4	4.4	4.8	4.8	4.9	5.1	5.1
Burglary	KESG	30.8	29.3	26.2	24.8	26.7	25.7	24.3	23.0	23.0	23.8	23.9
Robbery	KESH	5.5	5.6	5.9	6.8	7.7	7.3	7.5	7.1	8.1	8.8	8.5
Theft and handling stolen goods	KESI	125.7	131.2	128.0	127.0	127.3	119.1	110.6	103.8	99.0	106.0	110.9
Fraud and forgery	KESJ	19.8	20.3	19.2	18.3	18.1	18.0	18.1	18.5	18.2	19.9	19.8
Criminal damage	KESK	10.9	10.9	10.3	10.7	11.0	11.2	11.7	11.7	12.7	12.5	9.6
Drug offences	KBWX	48.8	48.7	44.6	45.6	49.0	51.2	39.2	39.1	39.6	44.6	52.9
Other offences (excluding motoring)	KESL	49.6	47.9	44.5	44.0	48.0	51.4	54.5	53.1	50.0	45.3	40.1
Motoring offences	KESM	9.0	8.1	7.6	7.7	8.2	8.7	8.0	6.6	5.9	5.4	4.5
Total	KESA	341.7	342.0	325.5	324.2	338.3	335.1	317.8	308.5	303.2	313.3	316.9
Summary offences												
Summary assaults	KESO	35.3	37.5	37.4	37.7	40.7	45.6	53.4	60.4	64.5	68.9	67.7
Offences against Public Order	JW94	31.3	30.8	29.8	28.6	29.0	31.0	33.5	32.6	34.9	38.7	37.0
Firearms Acts	JW95	0.5	0.4	0.4	0.3	0.3	0.3	0.5	0.8	0.6	0.7	0.5
Interference with a motor vehicle	JW96	2.7	2.8	2.6	2.6	2.6	2.6	2.5	2.4	2.3	2.3	1.9
Stealing or unauthorised taking of a conveyance	JW97	6.9	7.5	7.0	6.9	7.2	6.6	5.9	5.2	4.8	4.6	3.9
Social Security Offences	JW98	5.9	5.0	6.5	7.5	6.8	7.0	6.9	6.3	4.0	3.3	3.4
Intoxicating Liquor Laws: Drunkenness	KESR	30.8	28.7	27.2	26.2	26.9	27.7	21.1	16.1	15.7	17.4	18.9
Education Acts	KEST	5.0	5.1	5.1	5.6	5.8	5.8	6.5	6.4	7.4	8.4	8.5
Summary offences of criminal Criminal Damage - £5,000 or less	KESW	26.5	27.9	28.0	26.9	28.3	29.8	31.5	31.1	30.2	32.1	33.3
Offences by prostitutes	KESX	5.2	3.4	3.4	2.8	2.7	2.6	1.7	1.1	0.7	0.5	0.5
TV licence evasion	KETC	76.6	55.8	105.7	83.8	96.6	79.9	89.3	105.0	115.5	121.0	122.0
Motoring offences (summary)	KETA	665.2	632.9	607.5	583.3	595.8	662.6	707.9	667.1	622.5	611.1	552.2
Other summary non-motoring offences	JX2K	236.0	228.8	237.5	213.2	240.3	254.6	270.1	241.6	215.0	193.6	196.5
Total	KESN	1 128.00	1 066.50	1 098.20	1 025.50	1 083.00	1 156.10	1 230.70	1 175.90	1 118.20	1 102.60	1 046.30
Persons aged 10 to under 18[5]												
Indictable offences												
Violence against the person:	KETF	6.0	6.0	6.4	6.9	6.9	6.6	6.9	7.4	7.5	7.7	7.4
Wounding	KBXC	5.9	5.9	6.3	6.8	6.8	6.5	6.8	7.3	7.4	7.6	7.3
Other offences of violence against the person	KCAA	0.1	0.1	0.1	0.1	0.1	0.1	0.1	0.1	0.1	0.1	0.1
Sexual offences	KETG	0.5	0.5	0.5	0.5	0.6	0.4	0.6	0.6	0.5	0.5	0.5
Burglary	KETH	8.5	7.8	6.8	6.3	6.4	5.8	5.9	6.0	6.2	6.1	5.4
Robbery	KETI	2.2	2.0	2.2	2.8	2.8	2.6	3.0	3.1	3.7	4.1	3.6
Theft and handling stolen goods	KETJ	21.9	22.7	21.0	20.6	18.4	16.5	16.8	17.1	16.3	18.2	16.0
Fraud and forgery	KETK	1.0	1.1	1.0	1.0	0.9	0.8	0.8	0.7	0.6	0.7	0.5
Criminal damage	KETL	2.3	2.7	2.6	2.9	2.9	2.9	3.2	3.3	3.7	3.6	2.6
Drug offences	KCAB	2.7	3.1	3.7	4.3	5.0	5.1	4.5	4.6	4.5	5.3	6.4
Other offences (excluding motoring)	KETM	4.2	4.3	4.4	4.3	4.4	4.3	4.6	4.5	4.1	4.2	3.5
Motoring	KETN	0.4	0.4	0.6	0.7	0.8	0.8	0.7	0.6	0.5	0.4	0.3
Total	KETE	49.7	50.6	49.2	50.3	49.1	46.0	47.0	47.8	47.6	50.9	46.3
Summary offences												
Summary assaults	JW99	5.0	5.8	6.3	6.8	7.3	7.9	9.5	11.0	12.0	13.0	11.8
Offences against Public Order	JW9A	3.9	4.1	4.4	4.5	4.3	4.6	5.3	5.4	6.0	6.8	6.2
Firearms Acts	JW9B	0.1	0.1	0.2	0.1	0.1	0.1	0.2	0.3	0.2	0.2	0.2
Interference with a motor vehicle	JW9N	0.9	1.0	1.1	1.0	1.0	1.0	0.9	0.9	0.8	0.7	0.6
Stealing or unauthorised taking of a conveyance	JW9P	3.0	3.5	3.4	3.5	3.5	3.0	2.6	2.4	2.0	1.8	1.4
Criminal Damage - £5,000 or less	KETS	5.2	6.1	6.7	6.9	7.0	7.2	8.3	8.8	8.6	9.2	8.7
Intoxicating liquor laws Drunkenness	JW9E	1.6	1.8	1.9	1.9	1.8	2.0	1.9	1.5	1.5	1.7	1.8
Motoring offences (summary)	KCAC	11.3	12.6	14.5	16.7	17.1	17.8	17.0	14.8	12.1	9.9	7.7
Other summary non-motoring offences	JX3D	5.8	4.6	3.8	3.8	3.3	2.8	3.3	3.2	3.0	3.2	3.8
Total	KETO	36.8	39.6	42.2	45.2	45.4	46.6	49.2	48.3	46.1	46.6	42.1

1 See chapter text.
2 Data provided on the principal offence basis.
3 Every effort is made to ensure that the figures presented are accurate and complete. However, it is important to note that these data have been extracted from large administrative data systems generated by the courts and police forces. As a consequence, care should be taken to ensure data collection processes and their inevitable limitations are taken into account when those data are used.
4 Includes 'Companies', etc.
5 Figures for persons aged 10 to under 18 are included in the totals above.
6 2008 figures exclude data for Cardiff magistrates' court for April, July and August 2008.

Source: Justice Statistics Analytical Services in the Ministry of Justice 020 3334 4969

11.5 Offenders cautioned: by offence group[1,2,3]
England and Wales

Thousands

		1998	1999	2000	2001	2002	2003	2004	2005	2006	2007	2008
All ages[4]												
Indictable offences												
Violence against the person:	KELB	23.5	21.2	19.9	19.6	23.6	28.8	36.6	51.0	57.3	52.3	37.6
Wounding	KCAF	22.9	20.6	19.3	18.9	22.9	27.9	35.4	49.6	55.7	50.8	36.1
Other violence against the person	KCAG	0.6	0.6	0.6	0.6	0.7	0.9	1.2	1.4	1.5	1.6	1.6
Sexual offences	KELC	1.7	1.5	1.3	1.2	1.2	1.4	1.6	1.8	1.9	2.0	1.7
Burglary	KELD	8.4	7.7	6.6	6.4	5.8	5.6	5.6	6.5	7.7	7.0	5.4
Robbery	KELE	0.6	0.6	0.6	0.5	0.4	0.4	0.5	0.6	0.7	0.6	0.4
Theft and handling stolen goods	KELF	83.6	75.4	67.6	63.5	54.2	54.5	61.9	67.6	72.4	72.8	63.8
Fraud and forgery	KELG	7.4	7.2	6.2	5.8	5.3	5.5	6.0	6.9	8.0	8.6	8.2
Criminal damage	KELH	2.7	3.0	3.2	3.4	3.1	3.7	5.5	7.2	9.0	8.8	7.7
Drug offences	KCAI	58.7	49.4	41.1	39.4	44.9	45.7	32.6	34.4	37.4	43.1	46.9
Other offences	KELI	5.0	4.6	4.4	4.1	4.4	5.3	6.0	6.9	9.4	10.0	8.6
Total	KELA	191.7	170.6	150.9	143.9	142.9	150.7	156.3	182.9	203.8	205.1	180.3
Summary offences												
Summary assaults	KELK	13.2	17.0	17.2	18.2	17.3	19.8	26.1	40.8	64.6	72.6	69.5
Offences against Public Order	JW9W	14.5	14.6	13.4	13.0	12.7	15.1	15.4	15.3	18.5	20.6	19.0
Firearms Acts	JW9X	0.9	0.7	0.6	0.4	0.3	0.2	0.8	1.1	1.0	1.1	0.6
Interference with a motor vehicle	JW9Y	0.5	0.6	0.5	0.5	0.5	0.5	0.4	0.5	0.6	0.6	0.4
Stealing or unauthorised taking of a conveyance	JW9Z	4.5	4.5	4.3	4.4	3.9	3.7	3.3	3.2	3.3	3.2	2.6
Social Security Offences	JWA2	0.1	0.1	0.2	0.2	0.5	0.4	0.4	0.5	0.5	0.6	0.7
Intoxicating Liquor Laws:												
Drunkenness	KELN	47.0	45.9	42.4	41.7	39.7	44.4	45.8	45.8	48.3	49.8	44.4
Education Acts	KELP	–	–	–	–	–	0.1	0.1	0.1	0.1	0.1	0.1
Offences by prostitutes	KELT	0.1	0.1	–	–	–	–	–	–	–	–	–
TV licence evasion	KELY	6.4	5.7	5.0	4.5	4.2	4.0	4.5	6.3	7.1	7.3	7.3
Other summary non-motoring offences	JX6L	9.1	6.4	4.5	3.0	3.1	3.0	2.8	2.4	2.2	2.1	2.2
Total	KELJ	96.2	95.6	88.1	85.9	82.4	91.1	99.5	116.0	146.2	157.8	146.6
Persons aged 10 to under 18[5]												
Indictable offences												
Violence against the person:	KEMB	9.5	8.5	8.3	8.7	9.3	11.0	13.6	16.5	16.6	13.9	9.3
Wounding	KCAP	9.4	8.4	8.2	8.6	9.3	10.9	13.5	16.4	16.5	13.8	9.3
Other violence against the person	KCCE	–	0.1	0.1	0.1	0.1	0.1	0.1	0.1	0.1	0.1	0.1
Sexual offences	KEMC	0.6	0.6	0.5	0.5	0.4	0.5	0.5	0.6	0.6	0.7	0.5
Burglary	KEMD	6.7	6.1	5.4	5.3	4.6	4.4	4.2	4.6	5.0	4.5	3.2
Robbery	KEME	0.5	0.5	0.5	0.5	0.4	0.4	0.4	0.5	0.6	0.5	0.3
Theft and handling stolen goods	KEMF	44.0	39.6	36.9	35.2	28.1	28.3	33.1	36.8	39.4	39.7	30.0
Fraud and forgery	KEMG	1.6	1.7	1.5	1.3	1.1	1.0	1.0	1.1	1.3	1.4	1.1
Criminal damage	KEMH	1.7	1.9	2.1	2.3	1.9	2.3	3.1	3.9	4.7	4.5	3.5
Drug offences	KCCF	11.0	9.6	7.9	8.5	9.5	9.6	8.3	7.8	7.1	8.1	8.5
Other offences	KEMI	1.5	1.4	1.3	1.3	1.3	1.4	1.6	1.6	1.9	2.0	1.6
Total	KEMA	77.2	69.8	64.3	63.5	56.6	58.7	65.9	73.4	77.1	75.2	58.1
Summary offences												
Summary assaults	JWA3	4.3	5.8	6.4	6.9	6.2	6.8	8.8	12.2	16.2	16.8	14.2
Offences against Public Order	JWA5	4.2	4.3	4.0	4.1	3.8	4.6	5.8	6.2	7.4	7.3	5.8
Firearms Acts	JWA4	0.6	0.5	0.4	0.3	0.2	0.1	0.4	0.6	0.5	0.6	0.3
Interference with a motor vehicle	JWA6	0.3	0.4	0.4	0.4	0.4	0.4	0.3	0.3	0.3	0.3	0.2
Stealing or unauthorised taking of a conveyance	JWA7	3.5	3.6	3.5	3.7	3.3	3.1	2.6	2.3	2.0	1.7	1.3
Criminal Damage - £5,000 or less	KEMN	14.2	14.7	14.4	15.2	12.6	14.3	17.1	19.8	21.9	21.7	15.1
Intoxicating liquor laws:												
Drunkenness	JWA8	2.9	2.6	2.3	2.3	2.1	2.4	2.5	1.9	1.5	1.6	1.5
Other summary non-motoring offences	JX6M	2.5	2.3	1.9	1.7	1.4	1.5	1.6	2.1	2.1	2.2	1.6
Total	KEMJ	32.5	34.2	33.2	34.5	29.9	33.3	39.1	45.5	52.0	52.1	39.9

1 See chapter text.
2 Data provided on the principal offence basis.
3 Every effort is made to ensure that the figures presented are accurate and complete. However, it is important to note that these data have been extracted from large administrative data systems generated by police forces. As a consequence, care should be taken to ensure data collection processes and their inevitable limitations are taken into account when those data are used.
4 Includes 'Companies', etc.
5 Figures for persons aged 10 to under 18 are included in the totals above.

Source: Justice Statistics Analytical Services in the Ministry of Justice 020 3334 4969

11.6 Offenders found guilty of offences: by age and sex[1,2,3]
England and Wales
Magistrates' courts and the Crown Court

Thousands

		1998	1999	2000	2001	2002	2003	2004	2005	2006	2007	2008[4]
Males												
Indictable offences												
All ages	KEFA	292.9	291.7	276.5	275.5	287.1	283.4	268.4	261.3	258.4	266.9	267.7
10 and under 15 years	KEFB	8.1	8.9	8.7	9.0	8.8	8.0	8.5	8.6	8.3	8.5	7.7
15 and under 18 years	KEFC	35.2	35.1	33.8	34.4	33.7	31.4	31.8	32.0	32.5	35.0	31.9
18 and under 21 years	KEFD	51.8	52.6	49.9	48.2	46.6	43.8	39.9	38.5	39.0	40.6	38.3
21 years and over	KEFE	197.9	195.0	184.0	183.9	198.0	200.2	188.2	182.2	178.7	182.9	189.8
Summary offences												
All ages	KEFF	929.0	886.6	881.0	826.6	866.4	937.1	990.0	931.2	877.7	851.5	778.5
10 and under 15 years	KEFG	3.9	5.1	5.8	6.2	6.1	6.1	6.7	7.2	7.0	7.3	6.3
15 and under 18 years	KEFH	28.5	30.3	32.2	34.5	34.6	35.3	36.4	34.6	32.3	31.9	28.2
18 and under 21 years	KEFI	96.3	94.8	93.0	92.2	94.7	99.9	98.2	89.4	85.1	80.5	76.6
21 years and over	KEFJ	800.3	756.5	750.0	693.6	731.0	795.8	848.8	800.1	753.4	731.8	667.4
Females												
Indictable offences												
All ages	KEFK	47.3	49.0	47.7	47.4	50.0	50.2	48.4	46.1	43.7	45.3	46.4
10 and under 15 years	KEFL	1.4	1.4	1.5	1.6	1.6	1.6	1.7	1.7	1.7	1.8	1.6
15 and under 18 years	KEFM	5.1	5.2	5.2	5.3	5.1	4.9	5.0	5.5	5.1	5.5	4.9
18 and under 21 years	KEFN	7.1	7.6	7.5	7.0	6.9	6.2	5.7	5.3	4.8	4.6	4.7
21 years and over	KEFO	33.7	34.7	33.5	33.5	36.5	37.5	35.9	33.6	32.1	33.4	35.3
Summary offences												
All ages	KEFP	188.3	171.0	208.3	190.2	208.7	210.5	231.2	236.6	233.9	244.2	242.0
10 and under 15 years	KEFQ	0.6	0.8	0.9	0.9	1.1	1.2	1.4	1.6	1.6	1.8	1.7
15 and under 18 years	KEFR	3.8	3.4	3.3	3.6	3.6	4.0	4.6	4.9	5.2	5.7	5.5
18 and under 21 years	KEFS	12.1	10.8	11.8	11.1	11.6	12.6	13.0	13.5	14.2	14.9	16.5
21 years and over	KEFT	171.7	155.9	192.3	174.7	192.4	192.7	212.1	216.6	212.9	221.9	218.3
Companies, etc												
Indictable offences	KEFU	1.5	1.3	1.3	1.3	1.2	1.4	1.1	1.1	1.0	1.1	2.8
Summary offences	KEFV	10.7	8.9	8.8	8.6	7.9	8.6	9.4	8.1	6.6	6.9	25.8

1 See chapter text.
2 These data are on the principal offence basis.
3 Every effort is made to ensure that the figures presented are accurate and complete. However, it is important to note that these data have been extracted from large administrative data systems generated by the courts and police forces. As a consequence, care should be taken to ensure data collection processes and their inevitable limitations are taken into account when those data are used.
4 Excludes data for Cardiff magistrates' court for April, July and August 2008.

Source: Justice Statistics Analytical Services in the Ministry of Justice 020 3334 4969

11.7 Persons cautioned by the police: by age and sex[1,2,3]
England and Wales

Thousands

		1998	1999	2000	2001	2002	2003	2004	2005	2006	2007	2008
Males												
Indictable offences												
All ages	KEGA	142.9	126.1	109.7	103.8	104.4	109.8	110.0	129.9	147.6	148.5	132.8
10 and under 15 years[4]	KEGB	23.7	22.0	20.3	19.7	16.7	16.9	18.7	21.0	21.7	19.7	14.5
15 and under 18 years[4]	KEGC	32.0	28.7	25.0	24.5	23.3	24.1	25.9	28.0	30.2	30.0	24.4
18 and under 21 years	KEGD	25.7	22.7	20.1	18.5	18.9	19.4	16.7	19.8	22.9	23.7	21.6
21 years and over	KEGE	61.5	52.7	44.3	41.2	45.6	49.4	48.7	61.1	72.8	75.1	72.1
Summary offences												
All ages	KEGF	76.9	76.1	69.6	68.0	63.8	70.9	76.0	87.6	112.0	120.2	112.2
10 and under 15 years[4]	KEGG	10.6	11.7	12.0	12.7	10.3	10.9	12.6	15.5	17.9	17.9	12.4
15 and under 18 years[4]	KEGH	16.1	16.1	14.9	15.2	13.3	15.1	17.2	18.6	21.3	21.3	16.8
18 and under 21 years	KEGI	13.2	13.0	11.9	11.0	11.0	12.4	12.3	12.2	15.0	16.4	16.5
21 years and over	KEGJ	37.0	35.3	30.9	29.0	29.2	32.5	33.9	41.2	57.8	64.6	66.5
Females												
Indictable offences												
All ages	KEGK	48.8	44.5	41.2	40.1	38.5	41.0	46.3	53.0	56.2	56.6	47.6
10 and under 15 years[4]	KEGL	11.1	9.8	10.0	10.1	8.4	8.6	10.6	12.2	12.5	12.5	9.0
15 and under 18 years[4]	KEGM	10.3	9.3	9.0	9.3	8.3	9.1	10.7	12.2	12.7	13.0	10.1
18 and under 21 years	KEGN	5.9	5.7	5.2	4.9	4.8	4.9	5.2	5.8	6.2	6.3	5.5
21 years and over	KEGO	21.4	19.6	17.0	15.9	17.0	18.4	19.9	22.8	24.7	24.8	23.0
Summary offences												
All ages	KEGP	19.2	19.4	18.5	18.0	18.6	20.2	23.5	28.5	34.2	37.6	34.3
10 and under 15 years[4]	KEGQ	2.1	2.5	2.8	2.9	2.7	3.0	3.9	5.1	5.6	5.6	4.4
15 and under 18 years[4]	KEGR	3.7	3.9	3.7	3.8	3.6	4.3	5.4	6.2	7.1	7.3	6.2
18 and under 21 years	KEGS	2.6	2.7	2.5	2.3	2.4	2.7	2.9	3.3	4.1	4.7	4.5
21 years and over	KEGT	10.8	10.3	9.6	9.0	9.8	10.2	11.3	13.9	17.4	20.0	19.1

1 See chapter text.
2 These data are on the prinicpal offence basis.
3 Every effort is made to ensure that the figures presented are accurate and complete. However, it is important to note that these data have been extracted from large administrative data systems generated by police forces. As a consequence, care should be taken to ensure data collection processes and their inevitable limitations are taken into account when those data are used.
4 From 1 June 2000 the Crime and Disorder Act 1998 came into force nationally and removed the use of cautions for persons under 18 and replaced them with reprimands and warnings. These are included in the totals.

Source: Justice Statistics Analytical Services in the Ministry of Justice 020 3334 4969

11.8 Sentence or order passed on persons sentenced for indictable offences: by sex[1]
England and Wales
Magistrates' courts and the Crown Court

Percentages and thousands

		1998	1999	2000	2001	2002	2003	2004	2005	2006	2007	2008
Males												
Sentence or order												
Absolute discharge	KEJB	0.7	0.6	0.6	0.6	0.8	0.9	0.8	0.7	0.7	0.7	0.6
Conditional discharge	KEJC	15.3	15.0	14.1	13.4	12.4	13.0	12.2	11.9	11.3	12.2	11.4
Fine	KEJF	28.4	27.7	25.7	24.5	23.9	24.0	20.9	19.4	17.4	16.2	16.0
Community rehabilitation order	KEJD	10.0	10.1	10.1	10.7	10.6	10.1	9.5	5.6	0.8	0.5	0.4
Supervision order	KEJE	2.7	2.7	2.4	2.3	2.1	1.8	2.0	2.1	2.3	2.4	1.9
Community punishment order	KEJG	9.3	9.3	9.5	9.0	8.6	8.3	8.8	6.3	1.2	0.5	0.4
Attendance centre order	KEJH	1.7	1.8	1.5	1.2	0.7	0.6	0.6	0.6	0.6	0.6	0.5
Community punishment and rehabilitation order	KIJW	3.8	3.7	3.6	2.6	2.6	2.6	2.8	2.1	0.5	0.4	0.4
Curfew order	LUJP	0.2	0.3	0.5	0.7	1.1	1.6	2.7	2.3	1.3	1.3	1.4
Reparation order	SNFI	..	..	0.7	1.3	0.8	0.4	0.4	0.5	0.6	0.6	0.6
Action plan order	SNFJ	..	..	0.9	1.7	1.1	0.7	0.8	0.8	0.8	0.8	0.7
Drug treatment and testing order	SNFK	..	..	0.1	1.2	1.4	1.9	2.3	1.6	0.1	–	–
Referral order	SNFL	..	..	..	..	3.0	4.0	4.4	5.2	5.2	5.5	5.0
Community order[2]	GN7P	..	..	..	..	..	..	..	8.7	19.8	20.4	20.7
Suspended sentence order	KEJL	0.7	0.6	0.7	0.6	0.5	0.5	0.6	1.7	6.7	8.6	8.9
Imprisonment												
Sec 90-92	LUJQ	0.2	0.2	0.2	0.2	0.2	0.2	0.2	0.2	0.2	0.1	0.2
Detention and training order	LUJR	–	0.1	1.4	1.9	1.8	1.5	1.6	1.6	1.7	1.5	1.5
Young offender institution	KEJK	6.0	6.2	5.2	4.5	4.2	3.6	3.8	3.7	3.6	3.8	3.6
Unsuspended imprisonment	KEJM	18.2	18.7	19.9	20.0	20.9	20.6	21.5	21.2	20.4	19.9	21.6
Other sentence or order	KEJN	2.6	3.1	3.1	3.4	3.3	3.5	4.1	3.9	4.4	4.0	4.4
Total number of males (thousands) = 100 per cent	KEJA	292.4	291.3	277.1	274.6	285.6	282.3	267.5	259.4	258.4	265.8	266.9
Females												
Sentence or order												
Absolute discharge	KEKB	0.7	0.7	0.6	0.6	0.9	1.0	0.8	0.8	0.7	0.8	0.7
Conditional discharge	KEKC	28.7	26.9	24.9	23.9	22.0	22.5	21.8	20.7	20.1	20.8	20.0
Fine	KEKF	21.3	20.8	20.1	18.6	17.9	18.5	16.7	15.2	12.8	12.1	11.9
Community rehabilitation order	KEKD	19.1	19.4	19.6	19.1	19.2	17.0	15.4	9.0	1.4	0.5	0.4
Supervision order	KEKE	3.1	2.9	2.8	2.7	2.1	2.1	2.1	2.4	2.5	2.6	2.0
Community punishment order	KEKG	6.5	7.1	7.5	7.3	6.8	6.6	7.6	6.1	1.6	0.4	0.2
Attendance centre order	KEKH	0.9	0.9	0.8	0.6	0.4	0.3	0.3	0.3	0.5	0.3	0.3
Community punishment and rehabilitation order	KIJX	3.4	3.3	3.0	2.1	2.1	1.8	1.9	1.5	0.5	0.2	0.2
Curfew order	LUJT	0.1	0.3	0.4	0.6	0.8	1.4	2.2	2.3	1.1	1.1	1.1
Reparation order	SNFX	..	..	0.8	1.6	0.8	0.4	0.5	0.5	0.5	0.6	0.6
Action plan order	SNFZ	..	..	1.0	2.0	1.2	0.8	0.8	1.0	0.9	0.9	0.7
Drug treatment and testing order	SNGA	..	..	0.1	1.4	1.7	2.4	3.2	2.1	0.2	–	–
Referral order	SNGB	..	..	..	..	3.9	5.1	5.6	6.7	6.9	7.0	6.2
Community order[2]	GN7Q	..	..	..	..	..	..	..	9.9	23.3	24.5	25.4
Suspended sentence order	KEKL	1.5	1.3	1.3	1.2	1.1	1.0	1.3	2.5	7.8	9.6	10.1
Imprisonment												
Sec 90-92	LUJU	..	0.1	0.1	0.1	0.1	0.1	0.1	0.1	–	–	
Detention and training order	LUJV	–	–	0.6	0.8	0.8	0.7	0.7	0.8	0.7	0.8	0.7
Young offender institution	KEKK	2.2	2.4	2.2	2.0	1.9	1.7	1.4	1.6	1.6	1.4	1.3
Unsuspended imprisonment	KEKM	10.0	11.0	11.5	12.1	12.7	12.8	13.2	12.6	12.8	12.4	13.5
Other sentence or order	KEKN	2.5	3.0	2.9	3.5	3.4	3.8	4.3	3.8	4.3	3.7	4.7
Total number of females (thousands) = 100 per cent	KEKA	47.2	49.0	47.8	47.3	49.9	50.2	48.3	46.1	43.7	45.4	46.3

1 See chapter text. Every effort is made to ensure that the figures presented are accurate and complete. However, it is important to note that these data have been extracted from large administrative data systems generated by police forces. As a consequence, care should be taken to ensure data collection processes and their inevitable limitations are taken into account when those data are used.

2 The community order was introduced on 4 April 2005 and applies to offences committed on or after that date.

Source: Justice Statistics Analytical Services in the Ministry of Justice 020 3334 5512

11.9 Persons sentenced to life imprisonment or immediate custody: by sex and age
England and Wales

Number of Persons

		1998	1999	2000	2001	2002	2003	2004	2005	2006	2007	2008
Life imprisonment[1]												
Males												
All ages	I28G	380	465	446	484	536	489	548	594	531	471	495
10 - 17 years	I28D	11	26	19	28	21	11	15	27	16	23	24
18 - 20 years	I28E	25	38	9	27	21	47	24	50	46	70	54
21 years and over	I28F	344	401	418	429	494	431	509	517	469	378	417
Females												
All ages	I28K	14	19	21	19	19	24	22	31	16	21	28
10 - 17 years	I28H	1	3	2	1	1	–	1	1	–	3	1
18 - 20 years	I28I	–	2	1	3	2	4	2	4	2	3	2
21 years and over	I28J	13	14	18	15	16	20	19	26	14	15	25
All persons												
All ages	I28O	394	484	467	503	555	513	570	625	547	492	523
10 - 17 years	I28L	12	29	21	29	22	11	16	28	16	26	25
18 - 20 years	I28M	25	40	10	30	23	51	26	54	48	73	56
21 years and over	I28N	357	415	436	444	510	451	528	543	483	393	442
Immediate custody[2]												
Males												
All ages	JF7E	93 619	97 355	97 841	97 728	102 240	98 371	97 020	91 954	86 239	85 285	88 826
10 - 17 years	JF7F	6 870	7 218	6 949	7 119	6 865	5 765	5 866	5 463	5 669	5 277	4 939
18 - 20 years	JF7G	16 127	17 011	17 315	16 855	16 269	14 418	13 793	13 237	12 802	13 126	12 354
21 years and over	JF7H	70 622	73 126	73 577	73 754	79 106	78 188	77 361	73 254	67 768	66 882	71 533
Females												
All ages	JF7I	6 553	7 485	7 879	8 042	8 812	8 786	8 732	8 231	7 783	7 722	8 284
10 - 17 years	JF7J	335	406	444	448	529	424	443	498	453	466	442
18 - 20 years	JF7K	851	961	1 116	1 063	1 071	969	817	875	841	793	782
21 years and over	JF7L	5 367	6 118	6 319	6 531	7 212	7 393	7 472	6 858	6 489	6 463	7 060
All persons												
All ages	JF7M	100 172	104 840	105 720	105 770	111 052	107 157	105 752	100 185	94 022	93 007	97 464
10 - 17 years	JF7N	7 205	7 624	7 393	7 567	7 394	6 189	6 309	5 961	6 122	5 743	5 403
18 - 20 years	JF7O	16 978	17 972	18 431	17 918	17 340	15 387	14 610	14 112	13 643	13 919	13 180
21 years and over	JF7P	75 989	79 244	79 896	80 285	86 318	85 581	84 833	80 112	74 257	73 345	78 881

1 Includes detention under the Powers of Criminal Courts (Sentencing) Act 2000, Secs 90-92 (Childrens and Young Persons Act 1993, Secs 53(1) & (2) prior to Aug 2000) (persons aged 10-17), custody for life under the Powers of Criminal Courts (Sentencing) Act 2000, Secs 93 and 94 (1) (persons aged 18 - 20), mandatory life sentences under the Powers of Criminal Courts (Sentencing) Act 2000

Sec 109 (persons aged 18 and over) and immediate imprisonment (persons aged 21 and over). Indeterminate sentences for public protection under the Criminal Justice Act 2003 are excluded.
2 Excludes life and indeterminate sentences.

Source: Justice Statistics Analytical Services in the Ministry of Justice 020 3334 5512

11.10 Receptions and average population in custody
England and Wales

Numbers[1]

		1997	1998	1999	2000	2001	2002	2003	2004	2005	2006	2007
Receptions												
Type of inmate:												
Untried	KEDA	62 066	64 697	64 572	54 892	53 467	58 708	58 696	54 556	55 455	55 809	55 305
Convicted, unsentenced	KEDB	36 424	43 387	45 893	43 889	46 851	53 301	53 246	50 115	49 104	47 995	43 566
Sentenced	KEDE	87 168	91 282	93 965	93 671	91 978	94 807	93 495	95 161	92 452	90 038	91 736
Immediate custodial sentence	KEDF	80 832	85 908	90 238	91 195	90 523	93 615	92 245	93 326	90 414	88 134	90 261
Young offenders	KEDG	18 743	19 599	21 020	21 333	20 969	20 236	18 179	18 264	17 819	17 985	19 022
Up to 12 months	KEDH	11 867	12 942	14 330	14 639	14 234	12 891	11 850	11 855	11 610	11 526	12 295
12 months up to 4 years	KEDJ	5 949	5 921	5 904	5 877	5 856	6 355	5 412	5 426	5 243	5 317	5 530
4 years up to and including life	KEDL	927	736	786	817	879	990	917	983	966	1 142	1 197
Adults	KFBO	62 089	66 309	69 218	69 862	69 554	73 379	74 066	75 062	72 595	70 149	71 239
Up to 12 months	KEDV	38 702	42 513	45 662	46 759	46 146	47 870	48 962	49 814	48 190	45 768	46 706
12 months up to 4 years	KEDW	17 546	18 100	17 751	17 290	17 116	18 313	17 968	17 988	17 397	16 970	17 233
4 years up to and including life	KEDX	5 841	5 696	5 805	5 813	6 292	7 196	7 136	7 260	7 008	7 411	7 300
Committed in default of payment of a fine	KEDY	6 336	5 374	3 727	2 476	1 455	1 192	1 250	1 835	1 876	1 904	1 475
Young offenders	KEEA	555	568	366	216	138	110	116	155	162	118	92
Adults	KAFQ	5 781	4 806	3 361	2 260	1 317	1 082	1 134	1 680	1 714	1 786	1 383
Non-criminal prisoners	KEDM	3 204	3 290	3 271	3 153	4 630	2 674	3 142	3 669	3 668	4 734	3 888
Immigration Act 1971	KEDN	2 122	2 348	2 443	2 455	4 035	2 093	2 457	3 041	3 093	4 073	3 347
Others	KEDO	1 082	942	828	698	595	581	685	628	575	661	541
Average population												
Total in custody	KEDP	61 114	65 298	64 771	64 602	66 301	70 861	73 038	74 657	75 979	78 150	80 395
Total in prison service establishments	KFBQ	61 114	65 298	64 771	64 602	66 301	70 778	73 038	74 657	75 979	78 127	80 216
Police cells[2]	KFBN	–	–	–	–	–	83	–	–	–	22	179
Untried	KEDQ	8 453	8 157	7 947	7 098	6 924	7 727	7 862	7 735	8 088	8 293	8 273
Convicted, unsentenced	KEDR	3 678	4 411	4 571	4 177	4 314	5 064	5 060	4 750	4 806	4 967	4 560
Sentenced	KEDU	48 413	52 176	51 691	52 685	54 051	57 222	59 007	61 071	61 991	63 504	65 963
Immediate custodial sentence	KFBR	48 272	52 045	51 596	52 620	54 006	57 184	58 959	61 012	61 925	63 429	65 533
Young offenders	KFBS	7 821	8 490	8 336	8 435	8 558	8 777	8 421	8 290	8 239	8 535	9 188
Determinate sentence	I7IJ	7 707	8 363	8 197	8 288	8 408	8 616	8 262	8 123	8 030	8 141	8 502
Indeterminate sentence	I7IL	114	127	139	147	150	161	159	167	209	394	683
Adults	KFCO	40 451	43 556	43 261	44 185	45 448	48 408	50 536	52 721	53 686	54 894	56 776
Determinate sentence	I7IK	36 838	39 733	39 183	39 779	40 768	43 411	45 278	47 264	47 914	47 885	47 850
Indeterminate sentence	I7IM	3 613	3 823	4 078	4 406	4 680	4 997	5 258	5 457	5 772	7 009	8 850
Committed in default of payment of a fine	KFCS	141	131	95	64	45	37	48	59	71	82	79
Young offenders	KFEW	13	15	9	4	6	2	3	4	3	3	3
Adults	KFEX	128	116	86	59	39	35	45	54	68	79	76
Non-criminal prisoners	KEEB	572	554	558	641	1 012	847	1 107	1 100	1 087	1 355	1 420
Immigration Act 1971	KEEC	485	474	485	576	955	777	1 041	1 033	1 022	1 288	1 348
Others	KEED	87	79	73	63	57	69	67	68	65	65	72
Accommodation[3]	I7IQ	56 329	61 253	62 369	63 436	63 757	64 232	66 104	67 576	69 443	70 585	73 618

1 The components do not always add up to the totals as they have been rounded independently.
2 Mostly untried prisoners.
3 In use Certified Normal Accommodation at 30 June every year.

Source: Ministry of Justice: 020 7210 0638

Crime and justice

11.11 Prison population serving sentences: by age and offence[1,2]
England and Wales

				Age in years					
	15 - 17	18 - 20	21 - 24	25 - 29	30 - 39	40 - 49	50 - 59	60 and over	Total
At 30 June 2002									
Offences									
Males									
Total	1 986	5 821	9 722	10 196	15 415	6 630	2 832	1 365	53 967
Violence against the person	336	1 187	1 942	1 937	3 490	1 769	749	267	11 678
Sexual offences	58	167	262	406	1 347	1 241	996	794	5 270
Burglary	396	1 130	2 159	2 331	2 379	448	58	15	8 917
Robbery	503	1 285	1 647	1 390	1 865	443	66	10	7 208
Theft, handling, fraud and forgery	302	570	1 055	1 105	1 416	480	213	62	5 203
Drugs offences	43	431	1 255	1 763	3 142	1 496	495	129	8 754
Other offences	275	875	1 195	1 103	1 555	640	205	73	5 921
Offences not known	72	174	207	162	222	113	50	15	1 016
Females									
Total	103	356	596	662	1 030	439	134	19	3 339
Violence against the person	27	67	73	85	163	84	33	6	538
Sexual offences	-	1	-	1	11	6	3	1	23
Burglary	9	37	58	54	68	12	1	-	239
Robbery	19	63	89	65	60	14	3	1	314
Theft, handling, fraud and forgery	22	56	103	139	168	68	20	4	581
Drugs offences	8	94	206	256	474	216	60	6	1 319
Other offences	12	32	52	50	73	34	9	1	262
Offences not known	6	7	16	13	13	5	4	-	63
At 30 June 2003									
Offences									
Males									
Total	1 724	5 740	10 112	10 441	16 304	7 252	2 975	1 413	55 962
Violence against the person	310	1 257	2 112	2 068	3 733	1 932	780	290	12 482
Sexual offences	42	183	310	390	1 376	1 353	1 023	838	5 514
Burglary	289	919	2 003	2 204	2 555	527	71	11	8 579
Robbery	436	1 370	1 910	1 546	2 022	514	69	12	7 879
Theft, handling, fraud and forgery	291	543	1 020	1 060	1 437	472	201	45	5 069
Drugs offences	43	452	1 256	1 791	3 215	1 579	528	127	8 993
Other offences	271	884	1 329	1 218	1 760	787	263	69	6 581
Offences not known	42	133	172	164	205	89	40	21	865
Females									
Total	57	305	670	702	1 100	492	123	28	3 477
Violence against the person	10	61	91	66	155	82	32	7	506
Sexual offences	-	-	2	1	11	7	3	2	26
Burglary	1	24	64	60	77	12	2	-	240
Robbery	21	60	105	100	93	24	4	-	407
Theft, handling, fraud and forgery	10	56	117	128	199	70	18	11	609
Drugs offences	6	73	226	271	453	253	54	8	1 343
Other offences	7	27	58	66	108	39	6	-	311
Offences not known	2	3	8	10	5	4	4	-	36
At 30 June 2004									
Offences									
Males									
Total	1 706	5 585	10 095	10 738	17 021	7 858	3 013	1 508	57 523
Violence against the person	326	1 353	2 247	2 272	3 965	2 107	799	304	13 373
Sexual offences	55	193	329	424	1 433	1 416	1 030	865	5 747
Burglary	242	855	1 807	2 141	2 662	608	71	11	8 397
Robbery	449	1 254	1 865	1 691	2 127	583	70	17	8 056
Theft, handling, fraud and forgery	272	502	903	1 045	1 479	573	180	63	5 017
Drugs offences	51	471	1 383	1 789	3 258	1 615	537	150	9 256
Other offences	286	848	1 390	1 249	1 895	868	284	87	6 908
Offences not known	25	108	171	126	202	87	41	10	769
Females									
Total	58	300	632	727	1 056	507	152	20	3 453
Violence against the person	15	70	98	89	192	95	36	9	603
Sexual offences	-	-	3	3	8	7	4	2	27
Burglary	6	19	59	83	56	22	3	-	247
Robbery	8	65	93	90	114	20	2	-	392
Theft, handling, fraud and forgery	11	28	100	140	171	67	25	1	543
Drugs offences	6	78	197	245	392	246	65	6	1 235
Other offences	11	37	75	72	108	44	13	2	361
Offences not known	2	3	8	7	15	7	4	-	46

11.11
continued

Prison population serving sentences: by age and offence[1,2]
England and Wales

Numbers

	15 - 17	18 - 20	21 - 24	25 - 29	30 - 39	40 - 49	50 - 59	60 and over	Total
				Age in years					

At 30 June 2005
Offences
Males

	15 - 17	18 - 20	21 - 24	25 - 29	30 - 39	40 - 49	50 - 59	60 and over	Total
Total	1 782	5 595	9 937	10 969	16 843	8 731	3 256	1 594	58 707
Violence against the person	366	1 493	2 553	2 553	4 015	2 402	840	319	14 541
Sexual offences	65	186	397	505	1 436	1 552	1 084	922	6 147
Burglary	285	719	1 559	1 947	2 570	669	78	17	7 844
Robbery	422	1 307	1 819	1 705	2 035	649	83	15	8 035
Theft, handling, fraud and forgery	240	433	858	1 074	1 449	650	238	55	4 997
Drugs offences	76	491	1 332	1 834	3 263	1 741	544	148	9 429
Other offences	310	870	1 306	1 245	1 902	987	360	99	7 079
Offences not known	18	96	113	106	173	81	29	19	635

Females

	15 - 17	18 - 20	21 - 24	25 - 29	30 - 39	40 - 49	50 - 59	60 and over	Total
Total	55	269	614	680	1 073	585	179	24	3 479
Violence against the person	23	68	109	85	190	114	40	9	638
Sexual offences	-	2	3	4	12	8	7	3	39
Burglary	4	18	50	62	79	23	3	-	239
Robbery	16	59	61	82	102	20	3	-	343
Theft, handling, fraud and forgery	4	35	105	119	202	88	27	3	583
Drugs offences	3	54	195	255	366	268	84	9	1 234
Other offences	5	30	84	68	117	56	14	-	374
Offences not known	-	3	7	5	5	8	1	-	29

At 30 June 2006
Offences
Males

	15 - 17	18 - 20	21 - 24	25 - 29	30 - 39	40 - 49	50 - 59	60 and over	Total
Total	1 814	5 716	9 612	11 349	16 828	9 349	3 511	1 719	59 898
Violence against the person	381	1 563	2 616	2 977	4 109	2 609	935	348	15 537
Sexual offences	67	213	452	560	1 497	1 683	1 118	971	6 561
Burglary	275	707	1 363	1 838	2 554	715	97	15	7 563
Robbery	486	1 413	1 739	1 674	1 975	706	91	16	8 100
Theft, handling, fraud and forgery	200	451	830	1 093	1 598	707	214	54	5 147
Drugs offences	68	492	1 232	1 913	3 153	1 829	623	174	9 484
Other offences	327	835	1 326	1 231	1 838	1 040	406	129	7 129
Offences not known	12	43	55	64	105	60	28	10	378

Females

	15 - 17	18 - 20	21 - 24	25 - 29	30 - 39	40 - 49	50 - 59	60 and over	Total
Total	50	271	551	707	1 094	604	189	39	3 506
Violence against the person	11	75	111	101	205	118	48	9	678
Sexual offences	1	3	2	2	8	13	5	3	37
Burglary	7	13	39	63	80	24	2	-	228
Robbery	17	48	67	76	86	18	2	-	315
Theft, handling, fraud and forgery	3	30	97	171	232	106	24	7	671
Drugs offences	4	62	158	217	354	253	88	17	1 163
Other offences	7	36	61	72	120	67	19	3	385
Offences not known	1	5	5	4	9	5	1	-	30

At 30 June 2007
Offences
Males

	15 - 17	18 - 20	21 - 24	25 - 29	30 - 39	40 - 49	50 - 59	60 and over	Total
Total	1 827	6 354	9 860	11 653	16 606	10 092	3 823	1 973	62 188
Violence against the person	402	1 772	2 927	3 183	4 337	2 846	1 063	399	16 929
Sexual offences	73	276	487	675	1 555	1 909	1 202	1 112	7 287
Burglary	281	817	1 334	1 865	2 492	812	109	13	7 723
Robbery	495	1 558	1 855	1 716	1 928	774	96	14	8 437
Theft, handling, fraud and forgery	194	426	677	1 044	1 478	711	246	67	4 844
Drugs offences	71	546	1 285	1 858	3 002	1 908	689	210	9 569
Other offences	294	908	1 237	1 242	1 731	1 087	401	152	7 051
Offences not known	17	51	59	69	83	47	18	5	348

Females

	15 - 17	18 - 20	21 - 24	25 - 29	30 - 39	40 - 49	50 - 59	60 and over	Total
Total	56	280	475	662	1 011	610	202	49	3 345
Violence against the person	20	99	113	111	170	117	47	11	687
Sexual offences	-	1	3	7	16	15	4	2	48
Burglary	2	11	28	56	76	23	1	-	197
Robbery	13	54	53	78	82	27	2	1	311
Theft, handling, fraud and forgery	7	29	68	128	211	111	37	10	601
Drugs offences	3	42	124	201	335	230	90	19	1 044
Other offences	9	45	75	76	115	77	20	6	423
Offences not known	2	-	10	5	6	10	2	-	35

1 The data presented in this table are drawn from administrative IT systems.
Where figures in the table have been rounded to the nearest whole number,
the rounded components do not always add to the totals, which are calculated and rounded independently. Reconciliation exercises with published
Home Office figures may demonstrate differences due to rounded components. A programme of work is currently being undertaken to audit the
quality of the data and to identify priorities for improvements.
2 Excludes persons committed in default of payment of a fine.

Source: Ministry of Justice: 020 7210 8500

Crime and justice

11.12 Expenditure on prisons
England and Wales
Operating cost and total capital employed, years ending 31 March

£ thousand

		2001/02	2002/03	2003/04	2004/05	2005/06	2006/07	2007/08
Expenditure								
Staff costs	KWUV	1 138 400	1 259 502	1 364 193	1 439 882	1 498 446	1 586 126	1 646 757
Accommodation costs	KXCO	193 100	200 000	194 000	185 400	150 270	138 322	144 170
Other operating costs	KXCP	706 100	756 198	653 007	694 618	528 529	498 913	511 688
Depreciation	KXCQ	128 100	132 600	129 600	143 800	7 974	11 044	12 135
Cost of capital	KXCR	284 900	292 700	164 400	170 300	279	905	−610
Total expenditure	KXCS	2 450 600	2 641 000	2 505 200	2 634 000	2 185 498	2 235 310	2 314 140
Income								
Contributions from industries	KXCT	−11 600	−10 100	−11 000	−10 600	−11 154	−7 698	−7 079
Other operating income	KXCU	−13 100	−15 500	−21 000	−38 400	−41 323	−45 411	−43 566
Income from Other Government Departments[1]	GDPM	−180 600	−210 200	−368 000	−381 500	−302 549	−245 917	−205 524
Total income	KXCV	−205 300	−235 800	−400 000	−430 500	−355 026	−299 026	−256 169
Net operating costs	KXCW	2 245 300	2 405 200	2 105 200	2 203 500	1 830 472	1 936 284	2 057 971
Total capital employed	KXCX	4 859 600	4 821 500	5 228 600	5 116 700	5 716	−52 207	−42 577

1 Income from the Youth Justice Board (a non-departmental public body of the Home Office) for the provision of juvenile custody within the Prison Service, Department for Education and Skills for the provision of education services and Department of Health and PCTs for the provision of healthcare.

Source: NOMS Agency: 020 7217 5213

11.13 Crimes and offences recorded by the police: by crime group[1]
Scotland

Thousands

		1999 /00	2000 /01	2001 /02	2002 /03	2003 /04	2004[4] /05	2005 /06	2006 /07	2007 /08	2008 /09
Non-sexual crimes of violence against the person	BEBC	15.8	14.9	15.7	16.1	15.1	14.7	13.8	14.1	12.9	12.6
Serious assault, etc[2]	KAFS	7.3	6.9	7.5	7.6	7.5	7.8	7.2	7.5	6.9	6.6
Robbery	KAFU	4.9	4.3	4.6	4.6	4.2	3.7	3.6	3.6	3.1	3.0
Other	KAFV	3.6	3.6	3.5	3.8	3.5	3.2	3.0	3.0	3.0	3.0
Crimes involving indecency	BEBD	5.8	5.8	6.0	6.6	6.8	7.3	6.6	6.8	6.6	6.3
Rape and attempted rape[1]	OXBQ	0.8	0.7	0.8	0.9	1.0	1.1	1.2	1.1	1.1	1.0
Indecent assault[1]	OXBR	1.1	1.0	1.2	1.4	1.4	1.5	1.5	1.7	1.7	1.6
Lewd and indecent behaviour	KAFY	2.3	2.4	2.4	2.8	2.6	2.8	2.7	2.6	2.6	2.4
Other	KAFZ	1.7	1.6	1.6	1.6	1.7	1.9	1.2	1.4	1.3	1.3
Crimes involving dishonesty	BEBE	275.6	253.3	242.8	224.8	211.0	210.4	187.8	183.7	166.7	167.8
Housebreaking[3]	KAGB	52.9	47.7	45.5	40.6	36.4	35.0	31.3	30.6	25.4	25.5
Theft by opening lockfast places	KAGC	11.6	10.6	8.2	7.8	7.4	7.9	8.3	7.4	6.4	7.0
Theft from a motor vehicle (OLP)	EPI4	38.0	32.0	32.7	30.4	26.8	20.4	16.5	16.1	15.2	13.6
Theft of a motor vehicle	KAGD	28.9	25.6	23.1	20.9	17.6	15.6	14.0	15.0	12.1	11.6
Shoplifting	KAGE	32.1	32.3	31.6	28.3	27.9	28.5	28.2	28.8	29.2	32.0
Other theft	KAGF	81.2	76.6	76.0	73.2	72.5	77.6	72.1	70.2	64.6	64.4
Fraud	KAGG	20.6	20.0	17.4	15.8	15.3	18.3	11.1	9.3	8.4	8.3
Other	KAGH	10.3	8.4	8.4	7.9	7.0	7.1	6.3	6.4	5.3	5.4
Fire-raising, vandalism, etc	BEBF	81.2	85.8	95.0	97.7	103.8	128.5	127.9	129.7	118.0	109.4
Fire-raising	KAGJ	2.3	2.4	2.9	3.8	4.2	4.7	4.9	5.0	4.6	4.7
Vandalism, etc	KAGK	78.9	83.4	92.0	93.8	99.6	123.9	123.0	124.8	113.4	104.8
Other crimes	BEBG	57.1	58.9	66.8	73.2	77.5	77.2	81.9	84.9	81.3	81.3
Crimes against public justice	KAGM	18.4	18.6	20.9	22.7	25.8	25.6	27.7	32.1	31.4	29.5
Handling offensive weapons[2]	KAFT	8.1	8.1	9.0	9.4	9.3	9.5	9.6	10.1	9.0	9.0
Drugs	KAGN	30.4	32.1	36.8	40.9	42.3	41.8	44.2	42.4	40.7	42.5
Other	KAGO	0.1	0.1	0.1	0.2	0.2	0.2	0.3	0.4	0.3	0.3
Total crimes	KAGQ	435.5	418.5	426.2	418.3	414.2	438.1	417.8	419.3	385.5	377.4
Miscellaneous offences	BEBH	151.9	154.8	163.4	169.6	181.0	214.3	219.5	232.4	224.3	226.8
Minor assault	KAGS	54.6	54.1	55.4	55.0	57.4	73.7	72.3	78.2	73.5	74.1
Breach of the peace	KAGT	71.3	70.2	72.7	74.7	77.9	90.0	89.6	93.4	90.3	91.2
Drunkenness	KAGU	7.6	7.8	7.8	7.3	7.5	7.2	7.0	6.7	6.7	6.0
Other	KAGV	18.4	22.8	27.6	32.6	38.2	43.4	50.6	54.2	53.7	55.4
Motor vehicle offences	BEBI	347.5	340.1	362.5	350.1	435.0	424.3	380.5	375.1	347.8	333.5
Dangerous and careless driving	KAGX	13.2	12.0	12.2	12.7	12.0	13.1	13.0	13.6	13.0	11.5
Drunk driving	KAGY	10.9	10.8	10.8	11.5	11.6	11.1	11.3	11.7	10.7	9.8
Speeding	KAGZ	123.4	113.9	126.8	117.2	199.2	210.1	167.7	162.9	137.2	117.3
Unlawful use of a motor vehicle	KAHA	80.7	84.3	94.6	99.5	99.5	76.7	75.1	73.1	73.7	68.6
Vehicle defect offences	KAHB	48.0	46.8	45.5	46.5	37.2	27.0	23.9	21.2	22.3	25.6
Other	KAHC	71.2	73.3	77.9	66.9	75.4	86.3	89.4	92.6	90.8	100.7
Total offences	KAHD	499.4	496.1	532.0	524.1	615.9	638.6	600.0	607.4	572.1	560.3
Total crimes and offences	BEBB	934.9	913.5	952.4	937.8	1 030.1	1 076.7	1 017.7	1 026.6	957.6	937.7

1 See chapter text.
2 Includes murder, attempted murder, culpable homicide and serious assault.
3 Includes dwellings, non-dwellings and other premises.
4 The introduction of the Scottish Crime Recording Standard on 1 April 2004 has increased the number of minor crimes recorded, such as minor crimes of theft, vandalism, petty assault and breach of the peace.

Source: The Scottish Government Justice Department: 0131 244 2635

11.14 Persons with a charge proved: by crime group[1]
Scotland

Numbers

		1998/99	1999/00	2000/01	2001/02	2002/03	2003/04	2004/05	2005/06	2006/07	2007/08	2008[3]/09
Non-sexual crimes of violence	KEHC	2 000	2 003	1 976	2 092	2 381	2 596	2 427	2 455	2 445	2 742	2 637
Homicide	KEHD	92	105	100	103	99	131	143	111	120	135	110
Serious assault, etc	KEHE	1 036	1 053	1 089	1 171	1 360	1 475	1 374	1 560	1 482	1 729	1 692
Robbery	KEHG	652	659	603	627	682	689	610	509	527	542	563
Other violence	KEHH	220	186	184	191	240	301	300	275	316	336	272
Crimes of indecency	KEHI	1 280	790	633	614	562	666	810	853	863	790	944
Rape and attempted rape	HFVU	58	48	52	67	55	58	70	61	58	49	40
Indecent assault	KEHJ	83	84	60	48	65	93	87	84	81	117	107
Lewd and libidinous practices	KEHK	320	302	256	298	273	297	321	319	313	249	333
Other indecency	KEHL	819	356	265	201	169	218	332	389	411	375	464
Crimes of dishonesty	KEHM	24 726	22 652	20 571	21 536	21 700	19 887	19 665	18 045	18 447	17 801	17 426
Housebreaking	KEHN	3 071	2 860	2 676	2 672	2 752	2 508	2 373	2 074	2 025	1 867	1 856
Theft by opening lockfast places	KEHO	1 770	1 614	1 504	1 478	1 448	1 288	1 194	951	911	944	860
Theft of motor vehicle	KEHP	1 882	1 536	1 426	1 386	1 486	1 268	1 099	985	1 028	931	886
Shoplifting	KEHQ	7 559	7 753	7 345	8 366	8 826	8 123	8 427	8 162	8 548	8 457	8 260
Other theft	KEHR	5 796	5 026	4 303	4 234	3 783	3 521	3 551	3 187	3 303	3 150	2 979
Fraud	KEHS	1 920	1 595	1 448	1 479	1 459	1 444	1 355	1 245	1 180	1 165	1 218
Other dishonesty	KEHT	2 728	2 268	1 869	1 921	1 946	1 735	1 666	1 441	1 452	1 287	1 367
Fire-raising, vandalism, etc	KEHU	4 591	3 979	3 942	4 051	4 212	4 759	5 024	4 998	5 437	5 391	4 344
Fire-raising	KEHV	125	102	109	125	147	169	192	192	251	224	242
Vandalism, etc	KEHW	4 466	3 877	3 833	3 926	4 065	4 590	4 832	4 806	5 186	5 167	4 102
Other crime	KEHX	13 698	12 888	12 558	13 823	13 954	15 453	16 800	16 968	19 836	20 245	19 728
Crime against public justice	KFBK	4 776	4 589	4 929	5 257	5 048	5 290	5 767	5 753	7 206	8 038	8 710
Handling offensive weapons	KEHF	2 033	2 118	2 340	2 633	2 771	2 875	3 447	3 500	3 550	3 422	3 529
Drugs offences	KFBL	6 861	6 158	5 279	5 913	6 111	7 258	7 555	7 606	8 877	8 517	7 251
Other	KFBM	28	23	10	20	24	30	31	109	203	268	238
Total crimes	KEHB	46 295	42 312	39 680	42 116	42 809	43 361	44 726	43 319	47 028	46 969	45 079
Miscellaneous offences	KEHZ	35 024	29 505	28 651	30 152	32 062	34 536	37 492	39 679	42 278	41 300	35 671
Common assault	KEIA	11 677	10 749	10 270	10 823	11 745	12 317	13 574	14 427	15 441	15 502	15 105
Breach of the peace	KEIB	17 156	14 023	13 031	13 950	14 384	15 050	16 172	16 901	18 111	17 495	15 962
Drunkenness	KEIC	626	454	430	374	370	418	311	293	261	235	129
Other miscellaneous offences	KEID	5 565	4 279	4 920	5 005	5 563	6 751	7 435	8 058	8 465	8 068	4 475
Motor vehicle offences	KEIE	51 638	51 603	40 264	44 821	47 956	50 622	47 515	45 203	45 065	45 314	44 680
Dangerous and careless driving	KEIF	3 764	3 431	2 561	3 319	3 628	4 118	3 810	3 621	3 773	3 967	3 686
Drunk driving	KEIG	7 290	7 366	6 265	6 538	9 508	8 158	8 001	7 970	8 066	7 820	7 212
Speeding[2]	KEIH	12 971	15 293	9 427	9 988	9 832	12 700	13 546	12 273	13 434	14 185	13 535
Unlawful use of vehicle	KEII	18 662	16 950	15 987	18 553	19 192	19 563	16 696	14 711	13 449	13 621	12 739
Vehicle defect offences	KEIJ	2 470	2 075	1 302	1 252	1 510	1 859	1 791	1 653	1 709	2 320	3 715
Other motor vehicle offences	KEIK	6 481	6 488	4 722	5 171	4 286	4 224	3 671	4 975	4 634	3 401	3 793
Total offences	KEHY	90 879	85 792	73 526	79 482	84 963	90 253	85 007	84 882	87 343	86 614	80 351
Total crimes and offences	KEHA	137 174	128 104	113 206	121 598	127 772	133 614	129 733	128 201	134 371	133 583	125 430

1 See chapter text. Data as at August 2009.
2 Includes motorway and clearway offences.

3 Figures for 2008-09 for some categories dealt with by the High Court - including homicide, rape and major drug cases - may be underestimated slightly due to late recording of disposals on SCRO.

Source: Scottish Government Justice Department: 0131 244 2229

11.15 Persons with a charge proved: by court procedure[1,2]
Scotland

Numbers

		1998/99	1999/00	2000/01	2001/02	2002/03	2003/04	2004/05	2005/06	2006/07	2007/08	2008/09
Court procedure												
High Court[3]	KEIQ	1 043	1 174	1 092	1 125	1 194	1 217	974	882	866	837	784
Sheriff Court	KEIU	74 484	70 541	65 714	72 021	80 117	80 155	80 866	79 956	85 185	85 175	78 200
District Court[4,5]	KEIV	50 784	46 052	38 422	38 484	41 516	47 144	47 891	47 358	48 319	47 569	46 430
Stipendiary Magistrate Court[4]	KEIW	6 646	5 652	3 365	5 455	..	..	..	..	..	..	..
Total called to court[6]	KEIZ	132 957	123 420	108 595	117 089	122 827	128 519	129 733	128 201	134 371	133 583	125 430

1 See chapter text.
2 All figures are now reported as financial years.
3 Including cases remitted to the High Court from the Sheriff Court. Figure for 2007/08 may be an underestimate due to late recording of disposals on the Scottish Criminal History System.

4 District Court figures from 2002/03 include the Stipendiary Magistrate Court.
5 Figure for 2007/08 includes Justice of the Peace courts in Lothian & Borders from 10 March 2008.
6 Includes court type not known.

Source: Scottish Government Justice Department: 0131 244 2229

11.16 Persons with charge proved: by main penalty[1,2]
Scotland

Numbers

Main penalty		1998/99	1999/00	2000/01	2001/02	2002/03	2003/04	2004/05	2005/06	2006/07	2007/08	2008/09
Restriction of liberty order[3]	ZBRE	106	196	152	166	656	879	1 097	1 136	1 179	1 155	1 132
Supervised attendance order[4]	ZBRF	31	37	5	11	13	18	33	99	112	129	197
Drug treatment and testing order[5]	OEWA	..	5	117	286	409	610	713	758	865	822	881
Absolute discharge	KEXA	403	368	364	415	385	435	403	401	411	430	412
Admonition or caution	KEXB	13 442	12 188	11 203	11 702	12 360	12 934	13 744	14 175	15 967	16 083	16 350
Probation	KEXC	6 824	6 542	6 654	7 708	8 451	8 137	8 623	8 785	8 613	9 000	9 858
Remit to children's hearing	KEXD	176	120	116	158	230	196	221	260	313	259	209
Community service order	KEXE	4 811	4 254	4 272	4 323	4 719	4 298	4 849	5 195	5 284	5 599	5 779
Fine	KEXF	91 393	84 255	70 683	76 217	78 541	84 327	83 237	80 723	83 445	82 019	72 571
Compensation order	KEXG	1 238	1 151	1 076	1 142	1 347	1 767	1 695	1 471	1 375	1 325	1 150
Insanity, hospital, guardianship order	KYAN	125	136	116	103	101	129	95	115	65	20	16
Prison	KEXI	10 635	10 609	10 430	11 437	12 427	11 960	12 307	12 153	13 456	13 575	13 851
Young offenders' institution	KEXJ	3 749	3 546	3 394	3 407	3 162	2 801	2 685	2 902	3 241	3 141	3 003
Detention of child	KEXM	24	13	13	14	25	24	20	24	24	26	21
Total persons with charge proved[6]	KEXO	132 957	123 420	108 595	117 089	122 827	128 549	129 733	128 201	134 371	133 583	125 430

1 See chapter text.
2 All figures are now reported as financial years.
3 A community sentence introduced by Section 5 of the Crime and Punishment (Scotland) Act 1995 and available on a pilot basis to 3 Scottish sheriff courts since August 1998. This sentence was made available to High Court, Sheriff Courts and Stipendiary Magistrates court from 1 May 2002.
4 The pilot scheme under the Crime and Punishment (S) Act 1995, where fines for 16 & 17 year olds were replaced by supervised attendance orders, was discontinued in December 1999. The majority of supervised attendance orders recorded from the year 2000-01 onwards were disposals relating to the breach of an existing order.

5 Drug treatment and testing orders are new measures made available on a pilot basis to the High Court and to Sheriff Courts for residents in Glasgow (from October 1999), Fife (from July 2000) and Aberdeen/Aberdeenshire (from December 2001). They are now available to all Sheriff courts and the High Court.
6 Totals from 2002/03 include a small number of cases where penalty is unknown.

Source: Scottish Government Justice Department: 0131 244 2229

11.17 Persons with charge proved[1]: by age and sex
Scotland

Numbers

		1998/99	1999/00	2000/01	2001/02	2002/03	2003/04	2004/05	2005/06	2006/07	2007/08	2008/09
Males	KEWA	114 884	106 654	92 919	100 874	104 312	107 932	108 460	107 801	113 472	112 768	105 908
Under 16	KEWB	112	75	56	80	129	96	107	133	121	156	106
16 to 20	KEWC	27 399	24 671	21 973	23 701	23 948	23 454	23 098	24 051	25 513	24 366	20 349
21 to 30	KEWD	43 599	40 048	35 251	38 441	39 405	40 053	39 336	38 078	40 390	41 216	38 764
Over 30	KEWE	42 857	41 047	34 957	38 362	40 811	44 324	45 913	45 536	47 446	47 030	46 689
Age not known	KEWF	917	813	682	290	19	5	6	3	2	–	–
Females	KEWG	17 405	16 188	15 302	15 871	18 160	20 120	20 775	20 039	20 599	20 560	19 511
Under 16	KEWH	2	5	10	4	5	17	18	8	9	3	18
16 to 20	KEWI	3 252	3 089	2 768	2 742	2 840	2 927	2 891	2 929	3 255	3 302	2 802
21 to 30	KEWJ	6 872	6 219	5 833	6 200	6 843	7 494	7 652	7 387	7 398	7 385	7 281
Over 30	KEWK	6 971	6 614	6 448	6 854	8 468	9 680	10 214	9 715	9 935	9 870	9 410
Age not known	KEWL	308	261	243	71	4	2	–	–	2	–	–
Males and Females	KEWM	132 298	122 858	108 279	116 768	122 484	128 068	129 253	127 848	134 077	133 342	125 419
Under 16	KEWN	114	80	66	84	134	113	125	141	130	159	124
16 to 20	KEWO	30 652	27 761	24 746	26 444	26 790	26 381	25 989	26 981	28 768	27 668	23 151
21 to 30	KEWP	50 473	46 272	41 094	44 652	46 252	47 556	46 993	45 468	47 788	48 606	46 045
Over 30	KEWQ	49 829	47 665	41 437	45 226	49 285	54 011	56 140	55 255	57 387	56 909	56 099
Age not known	KEWR	1 230	1 080	936	363	23	7	6	3	4	–	–
Companies	KEWS	659	562	316	320	343	451	480	353	294	241	11
Total persons with charge proved[2]	KEWT	132 957	123 420	108 595	117 089	122 827	128 519	129 733	128 201	134 363	133 076	125 430

1 See chapter text.
2 Includes sex unknown.

Source: Scottish Government Justice Department: 0131 244 2229

11.18 Penal establishments: average daily population and receptions
Scotland

Numbers

		1999/00	2000/01	2001/02	2002/03	2003/04	2004/05	2005/06	2006/07	2007/08	2008/09
Average daily population											
Male	KEPB	5 765	5 676	5 929	6 193	6 307	6 447	6 523	6 830	7 005	7 422
Female	KEPC	210	207	257	282	314	332	334	353	371	413
Total	KEPA	5 975	5 883	6 186	6 475	6 621	6 779	6 857	7 183	7 376	7 835
Analysis by type of custody											
Remand	KEPD	976	881	1 019	1 247	1 246	1 216	1 242	1 567	1 560	1 678
Untried	JTT6	873	771	898	1 102	1 085	1 031	1 025	1 325	1 305	1 414
Convicted awaiting sentence	JTT7	103	109	120	145	161	185	217	242	255	264
Young offenders	JTT8	270	220	256	272	251	260	284	361	355	334
Adults	JTT9	706	661	763	975	995	956	958	1 206	1 205	1 344
Persons under sentence: total	KEPE	4 997	5 001	5 165	5 226	5 375	5 561	5 614	5 615	5 815	6 156
Adult prisoners	KEPF	4 317	4 346	4 537	4 624	4 802	5 001	4 989	4 970	5 130	4 887
Young offenders	KEPI	679	655	628	601	573	560	625	645	685	659
Young offenders (Fine defaulters)[2]	JTU2	7	9	9	9	7	7	6	5	3	1
Adults (Fine defaulters)[2]	JTU3	49	55	49	53	57	54	48	42	26	10
Persons recalled from supervision/licence[1]	KEPN	100	145	202	250	310	356	400	519	614	599
Others[1]	KEPO	28	36	37	6	6	5	1	–	–	–
Persons sentenced by court martial[1]	KEPP	2	–	–	–	–	1	–	–	–	1
Civil prisoners[1]	KEPQ	1	1	1	2	–	1	1	1	1	–
Receptions to penal establishments											
Remand	KEPR	14 626	14 062	15 725	19 198	18 963	18 892	19 593	23 181	22 491	22 754
Male	KEPS	13 450	13 042	14 402	17 455	17 111	17 085	17 796	21 129	20 256	20 416
Female	KEPT	1 176	1 020	1 323	1 743	1 852	1 807	1 797	2 052	2 235	2 338
Persons under sentence: total	KEPU	20 336	19 136	18 953	20 084	19 357	18 584	19 477	20 403	18 227	16 576
Male	KEPV	19 125	17 953	17 755	18 779	18 013	17 272	18 161	19 018	17 011	15 443
Female	KEPW	1 211	1 183	1 198	1 305	1 344	1 312	1 316	1 385	1 216	1 133
Imprisoned: Adults:											
directly	KEPX	9 217	8 943	9 470	10 571	10 255	10 299	10 746	11 684	11 846	12 381
in default of fine[2]	KEPY	7 030	6 450	5 882	6 081	6 063	5 404	5 442	5 265	3 208	1 321
Sentenced to young offenders' institution:											
directly	KEQA	2 582	2 436	2 312	2 207	1 949	1 908	2 170	2 286	2 359	2 269
in default of fine[2]	KEQB	1 328	1 116	1 109	1 016	825	694	771	698	402	185
Persons recalled from supervision/licence[3]	JYYD	179	191	180	209	265	279	348	470	412	420
Persons sentenced by court martial	KEQH	3	2	2	3	1	5	–	–	1	1
Civil prisoners[2]	KEQI	17	10	8	11	10	7	4	4	11	4

1 Persons recalled from supervision/licence and others are included in persons under sentence. Persons sentenced by court martial and civil prisoners are not included in persons under sentence.

2 Includes in default of compensation orders.
3 Now covers all recalls from supervised release orders.

Source: The Scottish Government Justice Department: 0131 244 8740

11.19 Expenditure on penal establishments[1]
Scotland

Years ended 31 March

£ thousand

		1998/99	1999/00	2000/01	2001/02	2002/03	2003/04	2004/05	2005/06	2006/07	2007/08	2008/09
Departmental Expenditure												
Manpower and Associated Services	KPHC	144 660	170 347	160 242	172 490	168 593	169 784	181 931	200 742	199 854	206 298	214 346
Prisoner and Associated Costs	KPHD	18 891	22 930	23 501	24 652	23 363	51 070	42 767	28 582	41 821	29 408	29 793
Capital Expenditure	KPHE	23 697	28 918	24 283	24 955	36 519	34 617	72 812	70 406	81 818	53 564	100 231
Gross Expenditure	KPHF	187 248	222 195	208 026	222 097	228 475	255 471	297 510	299 730	323 493	289 270	344 370
Less Receipts	KPHG	8 160	6 668	8 380	8 194	3 485	3 298	3 312	2 872	2 178	2 034	2 579
Net Departmental Expenditure	KPHH	179 088	215 527	199 646	213 903	224 990	252 173	294 198	296 858	321 315	287 236	341 791
Plus Annually Managed Expenditure Capital Charges	DSJI	..	..	..	31 341	40 432	41 728	48 497	52 840	41 816	59 498	89 656
Total Net Expenditure	DSNX	179 088	215 527	199 646	245 244	265 422	293 901	342 695	349 698	363 131	346 734	431 447

1 See chapter text.

Source: The Scottish Executive Justice Department: 0131 244 2226

11.20 Recorded crime statistics: by offence group[1]
Northern Ireland

Thousands

| | | Old counting rules | | | New counting rules | | | | | | | | | |
		1996	1997		1999 /00	2000 /01	2001 /02	2002 /03	2003 /04	2004 /05	2005 /06	2006 /07	2007 /08	2008 /09
Violence against the person	RVCP	5.6	5.2	RVCQ	21.4	21.4	26.1	28.5	29.0	29.3	31.0	31.8	29.6	29.5
Sexual offences	RVCR	1.7	1.4	RVCS	1.3	1.2	1.4	1.5	1.8	1.7	1.7	1.8	1.8	1.9
Burglary	RVCT	16.1	14.3	RVCU	16.1	15.8	17.1	18.7	16.4	13.4	12.8	11.6	11.7	12.5
Robbery	RVCV	1.7	1.7	RVCW	1.4	1.8	2.2	2.5	2.0	1.5	1.7	1.6	1.1	1.3
Theft	RVCX	32.8	29.5	RVCY	37.0	36.9	41.7	41.9	35.7	31.1	29.5	27.8	24.7	26.2
Fraud and forgery	RVCZ	4.1	3.8	RVDA	7.9	8.0	8.6	8.8	6.3	5.2	5.1	4.5	2.8	3.6
Criminal damage	RVDB	4.8	4.7	RVDC	31.2	32.3	40.0	36.6	32.4	31.4	34.8	36.3	30.9	28.4
Offences against the state	RVDD	0.4	0.5	RVDE	0.7	0.8	1.2	1.8	1.3	1.2	1.3	1.3	1.1	1.4
Other notifiable offences	RVDF	1.2	1.1	RVDG	2.1	1.7	1.4	2.4	3.2	3.3	5.3	4.5	4.7	5.3
of which drug offences	RVDH	1.1	1.0	RVDI	1.7	1.5	1.1	1.9	2.6	2.6	2.9	2.4	2.7	3.0
Total	RVDR	68.5	62.2	RVDS	119.1	119.9	139.8	142.5	128.0	118.1	123.2	121.1	108.5	110.1

1 See chapter text.

Source: The Police Service of Northern Ireland

11.21 Persons found guilty at all courts: by offence group[1]
Northern Ireland

Numbers

		1996	1997	1998	1999	2000	2001	2002	2003	2004	2005	2006
Violence against the person	KYCT	1 597	1 594	1 596	1 699	1 858	1 621	1 790	1 965	2 012	2 009	2 296
Sexual offences	KEVG	184	130	128	90	130	112	84	108	137	136	161
Burglary	KYBW	801	715	647	703	703	496	595	602	620	557	532
Robbery	KYBX	161	166	134	129	122	121	152	192	159	135	149
Theft	KYBY	2 765	2 596	2 342	1 995	2 111	1 831	1 695	1 803	1 819	1 819	1 728
Fraud and forgery	KYBZ	467	491	426	476	403	398	362	314	359	330	333
Criminal damage	KYCA	1 076	1 163	1 043	931	1 060	917	957	1 034	1 094	1 168	1 295
Offences against the state	KYCB	147	165	198	178	174	158	215	274	252	270	348
Other indictable[2]	KYCC	899	739	936	943	700	495	453	527	636	722	793
Total indictable[3]	KYCD	8 097	7 759	7 450	7 144	7 261	6 149	6 303	6 819	7 088	7 146	7 635
Summary[4]	KYCE	4 402	4 435	4 062	3 598	3 967	3 735	3 453	3 514	3 622	3 575	3 645
Motoring[5]	KYCF	18 177	18 770	15 369	15 782	15 390	14 466	14 344	16 342	17 215	15 534	15 083
All offences	KYCG	30 676	30 964	26 881	26 524	26 618	24 350	24 100	26 675	27 925	26 255	26 363

1 See chapter text.
2 1998 and 1999 figures include 'dangerous driving' (a triable-either-way offence).
3 From 2000, includes 'indictable-only' motoring offences.
4 Excludes motoring offences.
5 Prior to 2000, includes all motoring offences (except for note 2 above). From 2000, includes summary and triable-either-way motoring offences.

Source: Northern Ireland Office: 028 9052 7157

11.22 Juveniles found guilty at all courts:[1] by offence group
Northern Ireland

Numbers

		1996	1997	1998	1999	2000	2001	2002	2003	2004	2005	2006
Violence against the person	KYCH	75	49	97	73	77	66	82	75	78	146	152
Sexual offences	KAHF	4	8	12	12	4	1	6	5	7	9	8
Burglary	KYCI	137	124	108	117	125	73	77	89	66	113	81
Robbery	KYCJ	13	18	4	7	15	8	14	10	6	8	11
Theft	KYCK	338	334	304	227	254	244	212	173	183	291	202
Fraud and forgery	KYCL	14	11	4	10	2	9	3	7	2	6	7
Criminal damage	KYCM	121	136	139	102	143	152	132	162	129	241	240
Offences against the state	KYCN	6	10	11	12	8	10	20	26	18	19	40
Other indictable[2]	KYCO	24	10	20	17	10	12	7	19	22	46	44
Total indictable[3]	KYCP	732	700	699	577	638	575	553	566	511	879	785
Summary[4]	KYCQ	182	198	187	163	180	203	194	174	135	296	258
Motoring[5]	KYCR	58	57	98	97	82	102	89	94	76	280	230
All offences	KYCS	972	955	984	837	900	880	836	834	722	1 455	1 273

1 See chapter text. For the purpose of criminal proceedings, prior to 30 August 2005, a juvenile refers to a person aged 10 years or more but under 17. From 30 August 2005, the youth justice system was extended to include those under the age of 18. The number of juveniles convicted in 2005 and 2006 refers to those aged 10 years or more but under 18.
2 1998 and 1999 figures include 'dangerous driving'.
3 From 2000, includes 'indictable-only' motoring offences.
4 Excludes motoring offences.
5 Prior to 2000 includes all motoring offences (except for note 2 above). From 2000, includes summary and triable-either-way motoring offences.

Source: Northern Ireland Office: 028 9052 7157

11.23 Disposals given to those convicted by court
Northern Ireland

Numbers

Magistrates court - all offences

		1996	1997	1998	1999	2000	2001	2002	2003	2004	2005	2006
Prison[1]	KYAO	1 003	989	996	1 278	1 356	1 048	1 107	1 133	1 101	977	1 018
Custody Probation Order[1]	EOG9	..	..	..	..	..	..	..	7	7	9	12
Young offenders centre	KYAP	443	430	326	243	191	209	288	395	456	416	366
Training school[2]	KYAQ	147	148	136	13	..	..	..	..	..	..	..
Juvenile Justice Centre order[2]	OEUX	..	..	..	22	78	72	58	48	50	50	35
Total immediate custody	KYAR	1 593	1 567	1 458	1 556	1 625	1 329	1 453	1 583	1 614	1 452	1 431
Prison suspended	KYAS	1 722	1 506	1 025	1 080	1 247	1 215	1 278	1 407	1 469	1 584	1 692
YOC suspended	KYAT	444	461	139	104	93	77	100	201	372	375	335
Attendance centre	KYAU	91	66	55	14	20	37	84	91	108	127	132
Probation/supervision[3]	KYAV	1 134	1 155	1 473	1 246	1 096	1 070	1 005	974	991	977	1 045
Community service order	KYAW	591	561	622	678	726	587	643	623	647	628	597
Combination order	OEUZ	..	..	38	7	48	24	36	96	78	106	133
Fine[4]	KYAX	20 614	21 313	17 956	18 076	17 716	16 439	15 968	17 546	18 520	17 231	17 311
Recognizance	KYAY	1 203	1 267	1 134	1 089	1 357	810	912	1 091	913	853	693
Conditional discharge	KYAZ	1 679	1 597	1 538	1 439	1 286	1 559	1 497	1 526	1 524	1 326	1 093
Absolute discharge	KYBA	509	424	303	223	242	209	163	201	183	148	129
Youth conference order[5]	GGL8	..	..	..	..	..	..	..	..	21	74	304
Community responsibility order	GGL9	..	..	..	..	..	..	..	..	1	32	71
Reparation order	J8FR	..	..	..	..	..	..	..	..	..	..	1
Other	KYBC	15	8	123	221	57	61	104	215	190	122	61
Total	KYBD	29 595	29 925	25 864	25 733	25 513	23 417	23 243	25 554	26 631	25 035	25 028

Crown court - all offences

		1996	1997	1998	1999	2000	2001	2002	2003	2004	2005	2006
Prison[1]	KYBE	469	475	520	386	521	407	410	238	259	248	318
Custody Probation Order[1]	EOH2	..	..	..	..	..	..	..	331	332	370	416
Young offenders centre	KYBF	106	111	63	67	32	42	23	51	47	41	38
Training school[2]	KYBG	–	4	2	–	..	..	..	..	..	..	..
Juvenile Justice Centre order[2]	VQEV	..	..	–	–	–	–	2	–	–	–	1
Total immediate custody	KYBH	575	590	585	453	553	449	435	620	638	659	773
Prison suspended	KYBI	253	220	199	185	313	262	220	240	262	260	267
YOC suspended	KYBJ	71	60	49	41	48	37	35	50	72	45	42
Attendance centre	KYBK	–	–	–	–	–	–	1	–	–	–	1
Probation/supervision[3]	KYBL	49	47	70	43	68	48	49	63	93	79	91
Community service order	KYBM	54	37	33	24	29	45	25	27	33	31	32
Combination order	ZAEP	..	..	13	6	7	5	18	34	33	40	22
Fine[4]	KYBN	39	40	25	20	40	38	32	49	108	57	51
Recognizance	KYBO	7	10	7	–	4	11	12	8	6	9	8
Conditional discharge	KYBR	30	31	23	17	38	36	20	24	45	28	33
Absolute discharge	KYBS	–	1	6	–	3	–	6	1	1	6	4
Youth conference order[5]	GGM2	..	..	..	..	..	..	..	..	–	–	5
Community responsibility order	GGM3	..	..	..	..	..	..	..	..	–	–	–
Reparation order	J8FS	..	..	..	..	..	..	..	..	..	..	..
Other	KYBU	3	3	7	2	2	2	4	5	3	6	6
Total	KYBV	1 081	1 039	1 017	791	1 105	933	857	1 121	1 294	1 220	1 335

1 Custody Probation Orders cannot be separately identified from 'prison' sentences from 1998 to 2002. Thus during this timeframe, figures for prison include custody probation orders.
2 The Juvenile Justice Centre order replaced the training school order from 31st January 1999.
3 Supervision orders were abolished with the introduction of the Criminal Justice (Children) Northern Ireland Order 1998.
4 From 2000, fine incorporates 'fine plus disqualification' and 'fine plus penalty points'.
5 Refers to the number of youth conference orders completed.

Source: Northern Ireland Office: 028 9052 7157

11.24 Prisons and Young Offenders Centres
Northern Ireland
Receptions and average population

Numbers

		1997	1998	1999	2000	2001	2002	2003	2004	2005	2006	2007
Receptions:												
Reception of untried prisoners	KEOA	2 188	2 284	2 497	2 197	1 922	2 337	2 439	2 440	2 776	3 193	2 929
Reception of sentenced prisoners:												
Imprisonment under sentence of immediate custody[1]	KEOB	1 062	949	963	1 001	791	916	1 032	975	966	1 075	1 123
Imprisonment in default of payment of a fine	KEOC	1 513	1 530	1 423	1 261	1 090	990	1 143	1 296	1 437	1 569	1 425
Total	KEOD	2 575	2 479	2 386	2 262	1 881	1 906	2 175	2 271	2 403	2 644	2 548
Reception into Young Offender Centres:												
Detention under sentence of immediate custody	KEOE	331	347	346	282	252	315	268	287	222	229	247
Detention in default of payment of a fine	KEOF	366	385	417	389	303	250	310	351	377	382	299
Total	KEOG	697	732	763	671	555	565	578	638	599	611	546
Other receptions[2]	KEOL	42	70	38	56	58	57	117	106	134	24	38
Daily average population:												
Unconvicted[3]	KEON	376	383	377	317	272	347	393	456	450	531	531
Convicted[4]	KEOP	1 256	1 124	867	751	638	679	767	818	851	902	935
Total	KEOM	1 632	1 507	1 244	1 068	910	1 026	1 160	1 274	1 301	1 433	1 466

1 Includes those detained under Section 73 of the Children and Young Persons (NI) Act 1968.

2 Non-criminal prisoners including those imprisoned for non-payment of maintenance, non-payment of debt, contempt of court or are being held under the terms of an Immigration Act.

3 Prisoners on remand or awaiting trial and prisoners committed by civil process.

4 Includes those sentenced to immediate custody and fine defaulters.

Sources: The Northern Ireland Prison Population in 2007;
Northern Ireland Office: 028 9052 7534

Lifestyles

Chapter 12

Lifestyles

Expenditure by the Department for Culture, Media and Sport

(Table 12.1)

The figures in this table are taken from the department's Annual Report and are outturn figures for each of the headings shown (later figures are the estimated outturn). The department's planned expenditure for future years is also shown.

International tourism and holidays abroad

(Tables 12.8 and 12.9)

The figures in these tables are compiled using data from the International Passenger Survey. A holiday abroad is a visit made for holiday purposes. Business trips and visits to friends and relatives are excluded.

Domestic tourism

(Table 12.10)

The figures in this table are compiled using data from the United Kingdom Tourism Survey (UKTS) and represent trips of one or more nights away from home. The UKTS changed survey methodology in 2000 and 2005. Data from 1995 to 1999 were reworked to allow comparisons to be made with 2000–2004 data. Data for 2004 should be used and interpreted with caution. Data for 2005 is not comparable with previous years.

Attendances at leisure and cultural activities

(Table 12.11)

The definitions used in this table differ from those normally used to define regular attendees by the Department for Culture, Media and Sport.

Gambling

(Table 12.12)

The National Lottery figures in this table are the latest figures available at the time of going to press, released by The National Lottery Commission, and represent ticket sales (money staked) for each of the games which comprise the lottery. The figures have been adjusted to real terms using the Retail Prices Index.

The National Lottery commenced on the 19 November 1994, with the first instant ticket being sold in March 1995. Various other games have been started since, the latest shown in the table being the Dream Numbers game. The sum of the individual games may not agree exactly with the figures for total sales. Total sales also include the Easy Play games which commenced in 1998, but were dropped in 1999.

The other gambling figures in this table are obtained from the Gambling Commission (formerly the Gaming Board) and HM Revenue and Customs. The figures have been adjusted to real terms using the Retail Prices Index.

The money staked at bingo clubs refers to licensed clubs only.

12.1 Expenditure by the Department for Culture, Media and Sport[1]

£ million

	Museums, galleries and libraries[2]	The arts (England)	Sports (UK)	Architecture and the Historic Environment (England)	The Royal Parks (UK)	Tourism (UK)	Broadcasting and media (UK)	Administration and research	Gambling and the National Lottery[3]	Commemorative services (Queen's Golden Jubilee)	Regional Cultural Consortiums	Unallocated Provision	Total Resource Budget
	GQIF	KWFP	KWFQ	KWFR	LQYY	KWFS	KWFT	GQIG	SNKA	SNKB	GLZ8	GLZ9	GM22
2001/02	302	254	67	133	42	68	2 337	33	897	–	–	–	4 134
2002/03	424	286	123	142	26	73	2 571	38	698	6	–	–	4 386
2003/04	758	328	67	349	26	52	2 597	42	719	–	–	–	4 937
2004/05	410	367	84	159	27	51	2 677	42	668	–	2	–	4 487
2005/06	506	393	120	150	31	51	2 803	48	848	–	2	5	4 958
2006/07	573	388	136	181	19	55	2 954	55	850	–	2	–	5 213
2007/08	588	404	177	156	21	56	3 121	57	884	–	3	–	5 467
2008/09[4]	618	410	153	174	22	55	3 039	57	899	–	2	–	5 430
2009/10[5]	646	413	185	174	20	51	3 194	53	894	–	–	–	5 630
2010/11[5]	659	430	215	178	20	46	3 357	47	866	..	–	–	5 819

1 Figures are taken from the DCMS Annual Report & Accounts 2009.
2 Includes museums and galleries (England), libraries, (UK), Museums Libraries and Archives Council (UK) and Culture Online.
3 DCMS and Treasury undertook a complete overhaul of the way Lottery expenditure is recorded. For classification of the functions of the government (COFOG) purposes each lottery distrubution body is recorded separately, the exercise offered an opportunity to remove erroneously recorded data.
4 Data was provided for the Public Expenditure Outturn White Paper (PEOWP) estimated outturn.
5 Data are forecasts.

Source: Department for Culture, Media and Sport: 020 7211 6121

12.2 Estimates of Average Issue Readership of National Daily Newspapers
rolling 12 months' periods ending

Thousands

		2007 Mar	2007 Jun	2007 Sep	2007 Dec	2008 Mar	2008 Jun	2008 Sep	2008 Dec	2009 Mar	2009 Jun
The Sun	WSDV	7 840	7 768	7 931	7 980	7 897	8 031	7 949	7 872	7 870	7 860
Daily Mail	WSEI	5 253	5 197	5 239	5 230	5 293	5 347	5 212	5 062	4 949	4 846
Daily Mirror/Daily Record	WSEH	4 937	4 975	4 971	4 895	4 904	4 864	4 758	4 717	4 555	4 608
Daily Mirror	WSEM	3 844	3 880	3 868	3 789	3 748	3 685	3 623	3 600	3 489	3 566
The Daily Telegraph	WSEN	2 177	2 167	2 054	2 075	2 023	2 060	2 048	1 901	1 887	1 843
The Times	WSES	1 730	1 702	1 672	1 666	1 673	1 731	1 764	1 813	1 770	1 801
Daily Express	WSEP	1 742	1 694	1 687	1 678	1 621	1 598	1 605	1 571	1 557	1 624
Daily Star	WSEQ	1 620	1 701	1 690	1 597	1 500	1 484	1 417	1 427	1 451	1 471
The Guardian	WSET	1 239	1 226	1 193	1 121	1 169	1 165	1 240	1 240	1 206	1 205
The Independent	WSEU	767	774	787	745	733	702	722	688	649	679
Financial Times	WSEY	394	398	375	360	362	377	387	418	417	430
Any national morning	WSEZ	21 782	21 702	21 709	21 650	21 536	21 625	21 475	21 203	20 918	20 817

Source: National Readership Surveys Ltd.

Lifestyles

12.3 Employment in creative industries
Great Britain

	Advertising	Architecture	Crafts	Design and designer fashion	Film, video and photography	Music and the visual and performing arts	Publishing	Software computer games and electronic publishing	Television and radio	Art/antiques	All
	EUS8	EUS9	EUT2	EUT3	EUT4	EUT5	EUT6	EUT7	EUT8	EUT9	EUU2
2000	206.0	102.6	111.3	98.5	67.5	224.3	283.9	544.6	109.8	20.9	1 769.4
2001	220.5	103.4	115.1	103.0	75.5	224.6	293.3	567.7	104.1	20.9	1 828.1
2002	215.4	102.9	114.1	115.0	68.9	240.8	286.8	556.7	108.8	21.4	1 830.7
2003	213.8	103.1	108.7	113.2	74.3	245.8	305.2	581.2	110.9	22.5	1 878.8
2004	200.0	102.6	112.9	110.4	65.5	232.3	274.3	593.9	110.6	22.5	1 825.0
2005	223.4	108.2	95.5	115.5	63.8	236.3	253.3	596.8	108.7	22.9	1 824.4
2006	230.3	111.3	99.3	118.7	57.5	257.2	269.7	631.3	109.4	21.7	1 906.3
2007	247.2	120.7	109.7	130.7	65.4	262.8	275.8	640.9	103.4	21.8	1 978.2
2008	248.6	130.1	101.7	107.2	63.5	272.1	242.7	681.6	100.7	23.0	1 971.2

Sources: Creative Industries Economic Estimates Statistical Bulletin;
Department for Culture, Media and Sport

12.4 Cinema statistics[1,2]
United Kingdom

	Sites (numbers)	Screens (numbers)	Total number of admissions[3] (millions)	Gross box office takings[4] (£ million)	Revenue per admission[3] (£)	Revenue per screen (£ thousand)
	JMHX	JMHY	JMHZ	JMIA	JMIB	JMIC
1999	751	2 825	139.1	549.7	3.95	194.6
2000	754	3 017	142.5	572.8	4.02	189.9
2001	766	3 248	155.9	645.0	4.14	198.6
2002	775	3 402	175.9	755.3	4.29	222.0
2003	776	3 433	167.3	742.0	4.44	216.1
2004	773	3 475	171.3	769.6	4.49	221.4
2005	771	3 486	164.7	770.3	4.68	221.0
2006	783	3 569	156.6	762.1	4.87	213.5
2007	775	3 596	162.4	821.0	5.05	228.3
2008	772	3 661	164.2	850.0	5.18	232.2

Source: CAA/Nielsen EDI

1 See chapter text.
2 Includes Isle of Man and the Channel Islands.
3 Admissions are based on all cinemas taking advertising.
4 Box office takings are for UK only.

12.5 Films
United Kingdom

	Production of UK films[1]		Expenditure on feature films (Current prices)		
	Films produced in the UK (numbers)	Production costs (2008 prices)	UK box office	Video rental	Video retail[2]
	KWGD	KWGE	KWHU	KWHV	KWHW
1998	83	389.0	547	437	461
1999	92	507.0	563	408	451
2000	80	578.0	583	444	601
2001	74	379.0	645	465	821
2002	119	550.0	755	476	1 175
2003	164	1 126.0	742	450	1 392
2004	133	811.0	770	461	1 557
2005	163	581.0	770	399	1 399
2006	135	825.0	762	340	1 302
2007	126	753.0	821	297	1 440
2008	111	578.0	850	219	1 454

Source: UK Film Council RSU analysis of Official UK Charts Company and
BVA data:

1 Inward features include inward investment co-productions from 2002.
2 In 2005 the British Video Association changed its methodology for producing market value which has necessitated a change to historical figures quoted.

12.6 Box office top 20 films released in the UK and Republic of Ireland 2004-2007

Rank	2004[1] Film	Box office gross £m	Rank	2005[2] Film	Box office gross £m
1	Shrek 2	48.10	1	Harry Potter and the Goblet of Fire[3]	48.59
2	Harry Potter and the Prisoner of Azkaban	46.08	2	The Chronicles of Narnia: The lion, the witch and the wardrobe[3]	43.64
3	Bridget Jones: The Edge of Reason	36.00	3	Star Wars: Revenge of the Sith	39.43
4	The Incredibles	32.27	4	Charlie and the Chocolate Factory	37.46
5	Spider-Man 2	26.72	5	Wallace & Gromit: The Curse of the Were-Rabbit	32.00
6	The Day After Tomorrow	25.21	6	War of the Worlds	30.65
7	Shark Tale	22.82	7	King Kong[3]	30.04
8	Troy	18.00	8	Meet the Fockers	28.93
9	I, Robot	17.98	9	Madagascar	22.65
10	Scooby-Doo Too	16.49	10	Hitch	17.39
11	Van Helsing	15.15	11	Nanny McPhee	16.49
12	Lemony Snicket's A Series of Unfortunate Events	13.26	12	Batman Begins	16.42
13	Starsky & Hutch	12.60	13	Pride & Prejudice	14.57
14	The Last Samurai	11.90	14	Mr & Mrs Smith	13.59
15	The Bourne Supremacy	11.56	15	Wedding Crashers	13.16
16	The Passion of Christ	11.08	16	Fantastic Four	12.71
17	School of Rock	10.50	17	Ocean's Twelve	12.58
18	The Village	10.31	18	Robots	12.48
19	Lost in Translation	10.06	19	The Hitchhiker's Guide to the Galaxy	10.67
20	Dodge Ball: A True Underdog Story	10.03	20	Valliant	8.52

Rank	2006[4] Film	Box office gross £m	Rank	2007[6] Film	Box office gross £m
1	Casino Royale[5]	55.48	1	Harry Potter and the Order of the Phoenix	49.43
2	Pirates of the Caribbean: Dead Man's Chest	52.52	2	Pirates of the Caribbean: At World's End	40.65
3	The Da Vinci Code	30.42	3	Shrek the Third	38.74
4	Ice Age II	29.60	4	The Simpsons	38.66
5	Borat: Cultural Learnings	24.11	5	Spider-Man 3	33.55
6	Night at the Museum[5]	20.77	6	The Golden Compass[7]	26.00
7	X-Men 3	19.22	7	I Am Legend[7]	25.52
8	Happy Feet[5]	18.86	8	Ratatouille	24.80
9	Cars	16.45	9	The Bourne Ultimatum	23.72
10	Superman Returns	16.12	10	Transformers	23.50
11	Mission: Impossible 3	15.45	11	Mr Bean's Holiday	22.11
12	The Devil Wears Prada	14.02	12	Hot Fuzz	20.99
13	Chicken Little	13.51	13	Enchanted	16.78
14	Over the Hedge	13.22	14	Stardust	15.02
15	The Departed[5]	12.80	15	300	14.22
16	The Holiday	12.34	16	Die Hard 4.0	13.89
17	Flushed Away[5]	11.13	17	Ocean's Thirteen	13.15
18	The Break Up	10.38	18	Hairspray	12.58
19	Walk the Line	10.36	19	Fantastic Four: Rise of the Silver Surfer	12.38
20	Brokeback Mountain	10.08	20	St Trinian's[7]	12.04

1 Box office cumulative total up to 27 February 2005.
2 Box office cumulative total up to 19 February 2006.
3 Films were still being exhibited on 19 February 2006.
4 Box office cumulative total up to 4 March 2007.
5 Films were still being exhibited on 4 March 2007.
6 Box office cumulative total up to 2 March 2008.
7 Films were still being exhibited on 2 March 2008.

Source: Nielsen EDI, RSU

12.7 Activities undertaken by visitors from overseas during visit: by region 2007
Great Britain

Percentages

	London	North East	North West	Yorkshire	West Midlands	East Midlands	East of England	South West	South East	Scotland	Wales
Shopping for clothes/accessories	70	60	60	63	51	52	53	64	60	70	47
Shopping (eg fashion, design, home, antiques)	68	71	57	68	49	50	52	55	62	67	37
Visiting castles, churches, monuments, historic houses	57	35	33	64	37	33	37	61	56	78	54
Going to a pub	49	67	57	60	56	64	52	58	40	67	61
Museums, art galleries	51	24	30	42	26	16	30	44	35	45	34
Visiting parks or gardens	48	20	25	39	30	22	36	37	45	46	32
Socialising with the locals	30	38	61	39	59	57	47	54	47	56	62
Exploring other locations	31	27	34	31	33	31	32	62	49	60	49
Walking in the countryside	12	26	24	37	33	32	27	58	45	52	50
Going to theatre, ballet, opera, concert	25	8	9	5	13	6	15	12	8	12	2
Visiting coastline, countryside	8	20	19	34	22	26	23	52	39	55	40
Sports activities	11	15	18	29	22	30	23	29	22	37	31
Nightclubs	12	39	21	8	16	12	12	7	7	13	6
Learning activites	8	12	10	4	3	4	6	20	17	8	8
Zoos, aquarium, other wildlife	7	1	7	12	12	6	3	10	8	7	4
Watching sport event	3	14	10	5	9	10	6	4	4	7	6
Going to a football match	3	17	6	5	9	5	6	2	1	1	6
Visiting literary, music, tv and film locations	3	4	1	8	2	5	6	5	1	4	2
Visiting a spa/beauty centre	2	1	4	5	3	4	3	6	2	4	1
Researching ancestry	2	3	0	4	2	1	1	1	3	4	5
Playing Golf	0	0	1	5	3	3	3	3	4	7	3
Cycling	1	4	0	2	2	2	3	7	2	2	1

Source: United Kingdom Tourism Survey : 02075781418

Lifestyles

12.8 International tourism[1]

Thousands and £ million

	Visits to the UK by overseas residents (thousands)	Spending in the UK by overseas residents		Visits overseas by UK residents (thousands)	Spending overseas by UK residents	
		Current prices	Constant 1995 prices		Current prices	Constant 1995 prices
	GMAA	GMAK	CQPR	GMAF	GMAM	CQPS
1999	25 394.07	12 498.00	11 133	53 881.16	22 020.00	24 676
2000	25 209.00	12 805.00	11 102	56 837.00	24 251.00	27 281
2001	22 835.00	11 306.00	9 528	58 281.00	25 332.00	27 710
2002	24 180.00	11 737.00	9 641	59 377.00	26 962.00	29 311
2003	24 715.00	11 855.00	9 451	61 424.00	28 550.00	28 677
2004	27 755.00	13 047.00	10 146	64 194.00	30 285.00	30 444
2005	29 970.00	14 248.00	10 714	66 441.00	32 154.00	30 954
2006	32 713.00	16 002.00	11 641	69 536.00	34 411.00	30 904
2007	32 778.00	15 960.00	11 389	69 450.00	35 013.00	32 477
2008	31 888.00	16 323.00	11 276	69 011.00	36 838.00	28 657
2009[2]	29 716.00	16 507.00	10 977	58 433.00	31 757.00	22 765

1 See chapter text.
2 Data for 2009 are provisional.

Sources: International Passenger Survey, Office for National Statistics;
01633 456032

12.9 Holidays abroad:[1] by destination

Percentages

		1981	1991	2001	2002	2003	2004	2005	2006	2007	2008	2009[2]
Spain	JTKC	29.8	21.3	27.9	28.5	29.8	28.4	27.2	27.8	26.5	26.6	26.5
France	JTKD	18.1	25.8	18.3	19.0	18.1	17.3	16.6	15.9	16.7	16.7	18.6
Greece	JTKF	6.6	7.6	7.8	7.0	6.6	5.7	5.1	5.0	5.0	4.2	4.4
United States	JTKE	5.5	6.8	6.3	5.4	5.5	6.1	6.0	5.1	5.2	5.4	5.4
Italy	JTKG	5.0	3.5	4.3	4.6	5.0	5.0	5.4	5.4	5.6	5.2	4.7
Ireland	JTKI	3.7	3.0	4.1	4.1	3.7	3.8	3.8	4.0	3.3	3.2	3.2
Portugal	JTKH	4.0	4.8	3.6	4.0	4.0	3.5	3.6	3.7	4.1	4.8	4.1
Cyprus	JTKL	2.7	2.4	3.5	3.0	2.7	2.6	2.8	2.4	2.4	2.4	2.1
Netherlands	JTKK	2.6	3.5	2.6	2.8	2.6	2.6	2.5	2.7	2.4	2.1	2.2
Turkey	JTKJ	2.3	0.7	2.0	2.2	2.3	2.3	2.7	2.7	2.8	3.7	3.5
Belgium	JTKM	2.2	2.1	2.1	2.0	2.2	1.8	1.9	2.0	2.2	2.0	1.9
Germany	JTKN	1.2	2.7	1.4	1.5	1.2	1.6	1.7	1.7	2.0	1.9	1.7
Austria	JTKP	1.1	2.4	1.1	1.4	1.1	1.4	1.3	1.2	1.2	1.4	1.4
Malta	JTKO	1.0	1.7	1.0	1.0	1.0	1.0	1.1	1.0	0.9	0.9	0.8
Other countries	JTKQ	14.2	11.8	13.8	13.6	14.2	16.8	18.4	20.0	19.6	19.5	19.5

1 See chapter text.
2 Data for 2009 are provisional.

Sources: International Passenger Survey, Office for National Statistics;
01633 456032

12.10 Domestic tourism[1] United Kingdom

	Number of trips (millions)	Number of nights spent (millions)	Expenditure at current prices (£ million)	Average nights spent (numbers)	Average expenditure per trip (£)
	GQGY	GQGZ	GQHA	GQHB	GQHC
1999	173.1	568.6	25 635	3.3	148.1
2000	175.4	576.4	26 133	3.3	149.0
2001	163.1	529.6	26 094	3.2	160.0
2002	167.3	531.9	26 699	3.2	159.6
2003	151.0	490.5	26 482	3.2	175.4
2004[2]	126.6	408.9	24 357	3.2	192.4
2005[3]	138.7	442.3	22 667	3.2	163.4
2006	126.3	400.1	20 965	3.2	165.9
2007	123.5	394.4	21 238	3.2	172.0
2008	117.7	378.4	21 107	3.2	179.3

1 See chapter text.
2 There were concerns that data for 2004 was not truly representative of the United Kingdom population. Data for 2004 should be used and interpreted with caution.

3 The UKTS underwent a methodological change in 2005 and results should not be compared with previous years. The survey did not run between Jan-April 2005, as a result full-year estimates were made using Jan-April 2003 data.

Source: United Kingdom Tourism Survey, Visit England: 020 75781418

12.11 Attendance at leisure and cultural activities[1]
Great Britain
At Spring

Percentages

		1998/99	1999/00	2000/01	2001/02	2002/03	2003/04	2004/05	2005/06	2006/07	2007/08	2008/09
Attendance by men at:												
Cinema	JSPR	57	57	57	57	62	59	64	59	59	64	63
Plays	JSPS	19	21	21	20	22	23	23	25	25	32	29
Art galleries and exhibitions	JSPT	20	21	22	22	23	24	24	27	26	29	28
Classical music	JSPU	10	11	11	12	12	13	12	15	15	18	17
Ballet	JSPV	4	4	4	4	5	5	5	5	5	7	7
Opera	JSPW	6	6	6	5	6	6	6	7	7	8	8
Contemporary dance	JSPX	3	3	3	3	3	5	4	4	5	7	7
Taking part in sporting events - regularly[2]	EU5X	..	50	53	50	51	51	54	54	54	55	58
Watching sporting events	JSPY	86	85	81	76	76	74	77	75	70	65	61
Pop/rock concerts	C3Q8	..	..	..	..	25	26	25	29	30	37	40
Attendance by women at:												
Cinema	JSQA	57	55	54	56	60	62	63	61	61	64	66
Plays	JSQB	24	25	24	26	26	27	27	33	32	37	36
Art galleries and exhibitions	JSQC	22	22	22	23	24	24	25	30	29	30	30
Classical music	JSQD	13	12	12	13	13	14	14	17	17	18	18
Ballet	JSQE	8	8	8	8	9	10	10	12	12	14	14
Opera	JSQF	7	7	7	7	7	8	8	10	9	10	10
Contemporary dance	JSQG	5	5	5	6	6	7	7	9	8	11	10
Taking part in sporting events - regularly[2]	EU5Y	..	38	40	39	41	41	40	43	43	45	46
Watching sporting events	JSQH	66	66	58	56	57	55	62	61	55	47	46
Pop/rock concerts	C3Q9	..	..	..	..	21	23	24	26	28	34	36
Attendance by all persons at:												
Cinema	JSQJ	57	56	55	57	61	65	63	60	61	64	64
Plays	JSQK	22	23	23	23	24	25	25	30	29	35	32
Art galleries and exhibitions	JSQL	21	22	22	22	24	24	25	30	26	30	29
Classical music	JSQM	12	11	12	12	13	13	14	16	16	18	17
Ballet	JSQN	6	6	6	6	7	8	7	9	9	11	10
Opera	JSQO	6	6	6	6	7	7	8	8	8	9	9
Contemporary dance	JSQP	4	4	4	5	5	6	6	7	6	9	9
Taking part in sporting events - regularly[2]	EU5Z	..	44	46	44	46	46	47	48	49	50	52
Watching sporting events	JSQQ	76	75	69	66	66	64	69	68	62	55	53
Pop/rock concerts	C3QA	22	22	22	23	24	25	25	28	29	36	38

1 Percentage of resident population aged 15 and over attending 'these days'. See chapter text.
2 From 2002 the question asked to the respondent was changed.

Source: Target Group Index, (c) Kantar Media UK 2010

12.12 Gambling[1]
United Kingdom

£ million[2] and numbers

		1998/99	1999/00	2000/01	2001/02	2002/03	2003/04	2004/05	2005/06	2006/07	2007/08	2008/09
Money staked on gambling												
National Lottery - Total[3]	C229	5 809	5 450	5 315	5 029	4 670	4 614	4 757	5 000	4 911	4 966	5 149
Lotto including on-line	C3PU	5 064	4 641	4 416	4 038	3 479	3 225	3 225	3 021	2 858	2 752	2 698
Instants[4]	C3PV	744	612	590	606	592	641	729	804	943	1 109	1 221
Thunderball	C3PW	..	197	257	254	287	351	343	355	329	309	297
Lottery Extra[7]	C3PX	..	..	51	131	90	78	77	57	12	–	–
HotPicks	C3PY	..	..	..	..	222	244	219	228	222	210	211
Euromillions	C3Q2	..	..	..	..	..	15	104	427	464	476	618
Daily Play	C3Q3	..	..	..	..	..	45	59	54	49	50	50
Dream Numbers[8]	I67H	..	..	..	..	..	..	..	..	59	59	54
Lotteries (excluding the National Lottery)[5]	C3Q4	179	114	114	114	134	127	141	139	164	170	175
Bingo clubs	C3Q5	1 159	1 179	1 190	1 221	1 256	1 381	1 783	1 826	1 820	1 620	1 694
Football pools	C3Q6	286	221	185	151	124	112	109	90	88	..	..
Off-course betting[6]	C3Q7	7 916	7 996	7 689	9 969	17 985	32 265	44 971	44 437	36 553	..	..
Number operating in GB:												
Casinos and card clubs	JE55	116	118	117	122	126	131	138	140	138	144	145
Bingo clubs	JE56	751	727	705	688	699	696	676	657	634	675	641
Gaming machines	JE57	250 000	250 000	250 000	255 000	255 000	250 000	244 000	235 000	234 000	261 000	248 000
Society Lotteries	JE58	634	646	657	678	651	644	647	660	651	562	542
on-course bookmakers[9]	JE59	..	..	..	..	..	..	..	..	..	579	714
off-course bookmakers[9]	JE5A	..	..	..	..	..	..	..	..	..	801	720
Betting shops[9]	JE5B	..	..	..	..	..	..	..	..	..	8 800	8 862

1 See chapter text.
2 Adjusted to real terms using the Retail Prices Index.
3 Includes Easy Play tickets which are not shown separately.
4 From 2003/04 includes Inter-active games.
5 From 2002/03 includes Hotspot lotteries.
6 From 2001/02 includes Fixed Odds Betting Terminals.

7 Discontinued July 2006.
8 Started July 2006.
9 The Gambling Commission started regulating the betting industry on 1 September 2007, the number of betting shops is an ABB estimate.

Sources: National Lottery Commission;
Gambling Commission: 0121 230 6666;
Department for Culture, Media and Sport: 020 7211 6451

12.13 Most Popular Boy and Girl Baby Names in England and Wales, 2008

Rank	Names Boys	Rank	Names Boys	Rank	Names Girls	Rank	Names Girls
1	Jack	51	Jamie	1	Olivia	51	Lauren
2	Oliver	52	Michael	2	Ruby	52	Georgia
3	Thomas	53	Mason	3	Emily	53	Gracie
4	Harry	54	Toby	4	Grace	54	Eleanor
5	Joshua	55	Aaron	5	Jessica	55	Bethany
6	Alfie	56	Charles	6	Chloe	56	Madison
7	Charlie	57	Ben	7	Sophie	57	Amelie
8	Daniel	58	Theo	8	Lily	58	Isobel
9	James	59	Louis	9	Amelia	59	Paige
10	William	60	Freddie	10	Evie	60	Lacey
11	Samuel	61	Finlay	11	Mia	61	Sienna
12	George	62	Leon	12	Ella	62	Libby
13	Joseph	63	Harley	13	Charlotte	63	Maisie
14	Lewis	64	David	14	Lucy	64	Anna
15	Ethan	65	Mohammad	15	Megan	65	Rebecca
16	Mohammed	66	Reece	16	Ellie	66	Rosie
17	Dylan	67	Kian	17	Isabelle	67	Tia
18	Benjamin	68	Kai	18	Isabella	68	Layla
19	Alexander	69	Kyle	19	Hannah	69	Maya
20	Jacob	70	Brandon	20	Katie	70	Niamh
21	Ryan	71	Hayden	21	Ava	71	Zara
22	Liam	72	Zachary	22	Holly	72	Sarah
23	Jake	73	Kieran	23	Summer	73	Lexi
24	Max	73	Luca	24	Millie	74	Maddison
25	Luke	75	Ashton	25	Daisy	75	Alisha
26	Tyler	76	Bailey	26	Phoebe	76	Sofia
27	Callum	77	Sebastian	27	Freya	77	Skye
28	Matthew	78	Gabriel	28	Abigail	78	Nicole
29	Jayden	79	Sam	29	Poppy	79	Lexie
30	Oscar	80	Evan	30	Erin	80	Faith
31	Archie	81	Bradley	31	Emma	81	Martha
32	Adam	82	Elliot	32	Molly	82	Harriet
33	Riley	83	John	33	Imogen	83	Zoe
34	Harvey	84	Taylor	34	Amy	84	Eve
35	Harrison	85	Joe	35	Jasmine	85	Julia
36	Lucas	86	Corey	36	Isla	86	Aimee
37	Muhammad	87	Reuben	37	Scarlett	87	Hollie
38	Henry	88	Joel	38	Leah	88	Lydia
39	Isaac	89	Robert	39	Sophia	89	Evelyn
40	Leo	90	Ellis	40	Elizabeth	90	Alexandra
41	Connor	91	Blake	41	Eva	91	Maria
42	Edward	92	Aidan	42	Brooke	92	Francesca
43	Finley	93	Louie	43	Matilda	93	Tilly
44	Logan	94	Christopher	44	Caitlin	94	Florence
45	Noah	95	Ewan	45	Keira	95	Alicia
46	Cameron	96	Jay	46	Alice	96	Abbie
47	Alex	97	Morgan	47	Lola	97	Emilia
48	Owen	98	Billy	48	Lilly	98	Courtney
49	Rhys	99	Sean	49	Amber	99	Maryam
50	Nathan	100	Zak	50	Isabel	100	Esme

Source: Office for National Statistics

Environment

Chapter 13

Environment

Environmental Taxes

(Table 13.1)

In 2008, government revenue from environmental taxes was £38.5 billion. As a proportion of Gross Domestic Product (GDP) this amounts to 2.7 per cent, and as a proportion of total taxes and social contributions, environmental taxes were 7.1 per cent in 2008. These proportions are lower than in previous years because growth in the economy and total taxes and social contributions has exceeded that of environmental taxes.

Air emissions

(Table 13.2 to 13.8)

Emissions of air pollutants arise from a wide variety of sources. The National Atmospheric Emissions Inventory (NAEI) is prepared annually for the Government and the devolved administrations by AEA Energy and Environment, with the work being co-ordinated by the Department for Energy and Climate Change (DECC). Information is available for a range of point sources, including the most significant polluters. However, a different approach has to be taken for diffuse sources, such as transport and domestic emissions, where this type of information is not available and estimates for these are derived from statistical information and from research on emission factors for stationary and mobile sources. Although for any given year considerable uncertainties surround the emission estimates for each pollutant, trends over time are likely to be more reliable.

UK national emission estimates are updated annually and any developments in methodology are applied retrospectively to earlier years. Adjustments in the methodology are made to accommodate new technical information and to improve international comparability.

Three different classification systems are used in the tables presented here: a National Accounts basis (Table 13.2); the format required by the Inter-governmental Panel on Climate Change (IPCC) (Table 13.3); and the National Communications (NC) categories (Tables 13.5–13.7).

The NC source categories are detailed below, together with details of the main sources of these emissions:

Energy supply total: power stations, petroleum refining, manufacture of solid fuels and other energy industries, fossil fuel exploration, production, transport and offshore oil – venting and flaring.

Business total: iron and steel combustion, other industrial combustion and miscellaneous industrial and commercial combustion.

Transport total: road transport (passenger cars, light duty vehicles, buses, HGVs, mopeds, motorcycles) and gasoline evaporation from vehicles, tyre and brake wear.

Other transport: civil aviation (domestic cruise, take off and landing cycles); railway locomotives; railway – stationary combustion; shipping; national navigation; fishing vessels; and other mobile sources including agricultural machinery, gardening, construction and aircraft support equipment and mobile industrial equipment powered by diesel or petrol engines.

Residential total: residential plant, household and gardening (mobile).

Agriculture total: stationary combustion, manure liquid systems, manure solid storage and dry lot, other manure management, direct soil emission, and field burning of agricultural wastes.

Industrial process total: industrial process sinter production, iron and steel – flaring, nitric acid production, adipic acid production and metal production.

Solvent and other product use: paint application, degreasing and dry cleaning, chemical products, manufacture and processing wood impregnation, and tyre manufacture.

Land-use change: emissions from managed and unmanaged forests, and forest and grassland conversion.

Waste management total: treatment of domestic, industrial and other waste, including landfill and waste incineration.

Atmospheric emissions on a National Accounts basis

(Table 13.2)

The National Accounts figures in Table 13.2 differ from those on an IPCC basis in that they include estimated emissions from fuels purchased by UK resident households and companies either at home or abroad (including emissions from UK international shipping and aircraft operators), and exclude emissions in the UK resulting from the activities of non-residents. This allows for a more consistent comparison with key National Accounts indicators such as Gross Domestic Product.

Greenhouse gases include carbon dioxide, methane, nitrous oxide, hydro-fluorocarbons, perfluorocarbons and sulphur hexafluoride which are expressed in thousand tonnes of carbon dioxide equivalent.

Acid rain precursors include sulphur dioxide, nitrogen oxides and ammonia which are expressed as thousand tonnes of sulphur dioxide equivalent.

Estimated total emissions of greenhouse gases on an IPCC basis

(Table 13.3)

The IPCC classification is used to report greenhouse gas emissions under the UN Framework Convention on Climate Change (UNFCCC) and includes land use change and all emissions from domestic aviation and shipping, but excludes international marine and aviation bunker fuels. Estimates of the relative contribution to global warming of the main greenhouse gases, or classes of gases, are presented weighted by their global warming potential.

Greenhouse gas emissions bridging table

(Table 13.4)

National Accounts measure to UNFCCC measure

There are a number of formats for the reporting and recording of atmospheric emissions data, including those used by the Department of Energy and Climate Control (DECC) for reporting greenhouse gases under UNFCCC and the Kyoto Protocol, and for reporting air pollutant emissions to the UN Economic Commission for Europe (UNECE), which differ from the National Accounts consistent measure published by the Office for National Statistics (ONS).

Differences between the National Accounts measure and those for reporting under UNFCCC and the Kyoto Protocol, following the guidance of the IPCC, are shown in Table 13.4.

Emissions of carbon dioxide

(Table 13.5)

Carbon dioxide is the main man-made contributor to global warming. The UK contributes about 2 per cent to global man-made emissions which, according to the IPCC, was estimated to be 38 billion tonnes of carbon dioxide in 2004. Carbon

dioxide accounted for about 85 per cent of the UK's man-made greenhouse gas emissions in 2007.

Emissions of methane

(Table 13.6)

Weighted by global warming potential, methane accounted for about 8 per cent of the UK's greenhouse gas emissions in 2007. Methane emissions, excluding those from natural sources, were 53 per cent below 1990 levels. In 2007, the main sources of methane were landfill sites (41 per cent of total) and agriculture (38 per cent). Emissions from landfill have reduced by 59 per cent and emissions from agriculture by 17 per cent since 1990.

Emissions of nitrous oxide

(Table 13.7)

Weighted by global warming potential, nitrous oxide emissions accounted for about 5 per cent of the UK's man-made greenhouse gas emissions in 2007. Nitrous oxide emissions fell by 47 per cent between 1990 and 2007. The largest reductions were in emissions from adipic acid production between 1998 and 1999. This leaves agriculture as the main source, accounting for over two-thirds of emissions, mainly from agricultural soils.

Annual Rainfall

(Table 13.9)

Regional rainfall is derived by the Met Office's National Climate Information Centre for the National Hydrological Monitoring Programme at the Centre for Ecology and Hydrology. These monthly area rainfalls are based initially on a subset of rain gauges (circa 350) but are updated after four to five months with figures using the majority of the UK's rain gauge network.

The regions of England shown in this table correspond to the original nine English regions of the National Rivers Authority (NRA). The NRA became part of the Environment Agency on its creation in April 1996. The figures in this table relate to the country of Wales, not the Environment Agency Welsh Region.

UK Weather Summary

(Table 13.10)

For 2009, initial averages use data available from about 180 observing sites available on 1 January 2010. They represent an initial assessment of the weather that was experienced across the UK during 2009 and how it compares with the 1961 to 1990 average.

For all other years, final averages use quality controlled data from the UK climate network of observing stations. They show the Met Office's best assessment of the weather that was experienced across the UK during the years and how it compares with the 1961 to 1990 average. The columns headed 'Anom' (anomaly) show the difference from, or percentage of, the 1961 to 1990 long-term average.

Biological and chemical quality of rivers and canals

(Table 13.11)

The chemical quality of river and canal waters is monitored in a series of separate national surveys in England, Wales and Northern Ireland. The General Quality Assessment Headline Indicator (GQAHI) and General Quality Assessment (GQA) schemes are used in surveys to provide a rigorous and objective method for assessing the basic chemical quality of rivers and canals. In England the GQAHI survey is based on two determinants, dissolved oxygen and ammoniacal nitrogen. In previous years this assessment included biochemical oxygen demand, however in 2007 this was removed from the assessment and the historic data recalculated. In Wales the GQA assessment is based on three determinants, dissolved oxygen, biochemical oxygen demand and ammoniacal nitrogen. The GQA grades river stretches into six categories (A –F) of chemical quality, and these in turn have been grouped into four broader groups: good (classes A and B), fair (C and D), poor (E) and bad (F)

To provide a more comprehensive picture of the health of rivers and canals, biological testing has also been carried out. The biological grading is based on the monitoring of tiny animals (invertebrates) which live in or on the bed of the river. Research has shown that there is a relationship between species composition and water quality. Using a procedure known as the River Invertebrate Prediction and Classification System, species groups recorded at a site were compared with those which would be expected to be present in the absence of pollution, allowing for the different environmental characteristics in different parts of the country. Two different summary statistics (known as ecological quality indices) were calculated and then the biological quality was assigned to one of six bands based on a combination of these two statistics.

From 2008, Northern Ireland uses a classification system different to that which was previously used. A unit of area known as a waterbody is now the classification unit, rather than discrete stretches of individual rivers.

WFD classifications are based on chemical, physical and ecological parameters (referred to as quality elements). The indicators recorded here are just some of the WFD quality elements that are monitored in river waterbodies.

It should be noted that the monitoring network only covers selected stretches which the Environment Agency are required to monitor. In England and Wales 32,000 km of river network are monitored out of an estimated total river length of 150,000 km. No canals are classified in Northern Ireland.

Biological and chemical quality of rivers and canals Scotland

(Table 13.12)

Scotland's previous classification schemes focused on describing the pollution levels of the water environment. As required by the Water Framework Directive, the new classification scheme for surface waters now assesses:

- the quality of the aquatic ecosystems within rivers, lochs, estuaries and coastal waters

- the extent to which they have been adversely affected by the full range of pressures on the water environment – from water resources and physical habitat to pollution and invasive non-native species

This new scheme which started in 2007 assesses the condition of each river, loch, estuary and coastal water and assigns it a 'status' from high, good, moderate, poor to bad.

The results on the current condition of our rivers, lochs, estuaries, coasts and ground waters are based primarily on monitoring data collected during 2007. However, as the new monitoring programmes have only been in place for one year, the Scottish Environment Protection Agency (SEPA) has supplemented the limited new monitoring data with data from previous assessments (where relevant and available). This is to ensure the classification results reflect the best current understanding of the status of the water environment. As more monitoring data are collected, SEPA expects its confidence in classification to progressively increase over the next five years.

Prior to 2007, river and canal water quality was based on the Scottish River Classification Scheme of 20 June 1997, which combined chemical, biological, nutrient and aesthetic quality using the following classes: excellent (A1), good (A2), fair (B), poor (C) and seriously polluted (D). The figures in the table are rounded to the nearest 10 km and may not sum to totals.

During 2000 a new digitised river network (DRN) was developed, based on 1:50,000 ordnance survey data digitised by the Institute of Hydrology. The DRN ensures consistency between all SEPA areas and includes the Scottish Islands which were not previously covered. Data based on this network were published for the first time in the 2004 edition of *Annual Abstract of Statistics* and are not consistent with data published previously. The DRN includes:

- All mainland and island rivers with a catchment area of 10 km2 or more. This is known as the 'baseline network'

- Mainland and island stream stretches with a catchment of less than 10 km2 which are classified as fair, poor or seriously polluted and have been monitored. These are added to the baseline network to give a 'classification network'

It is intended that future emphasis will be placed on the baseline network, which will be the reportable network for the purposes of the European Commission Water Framework Directive. Efforts to improve the quality of the downgraded smaller streams will continue, but once this has been sustainably achieved, their monitoring may be reduced. Many of these streams are the subject of current attention because of their influence on the quality of larger classification network rivers.

Using the DRN scheme, data for every routine sampling point are automatically applied to an identified river stretch of predetermined length. The loss in total river length in moving to the DRN (that is despite the first time inclusion of island rivers) arises mainly from the exclusion from classification of thousands of small remote headwater streams which were never monitored, but assumed to be of excellent quality. The smaller reduction in length of downgraded waters arises mainly from using 1:50,000 maps for the DRN; in the former system lengths were hand measured from 1:10,000 maps, so more minor channel bends were included.

Reservoir stocks in England and Wales

(Table 13.13)

Data are collected for a network of major reservoirs (or reservoir groups) in England and Wales for the National Hydrological Monitoring Programme at the Centre for Ecology and Hydrology. Figures of usable capacity are supplied by the Water PLCs and the Environment Agency at the start of each month and are aggregated to provide an index of the total reservoir stocks for England and Wales.

Water industry expenditure

(Table 13.14)

The data is taken from the annual regulatory accounts (and the June return submission to Ofwat) of water and sewerage companies and water companies of England and Wales.

Operating expenditure includes: employment costs, power, Environment Agency charges, bulk supply imports, general overheads, customer services, scientific services, local authority rates, local authority sewerage agencies, materials and consumables, charge for bad and doubtful debts, current cost depreciation and the infrastructure renewals charge.

Capital expenditure figures represent all capital additions (both maintenance and enhancement) but exclude infrastructure renewals expenditure. Figures quoted are before deducting grants and contributions, typically received from developers. Adopted assets at nil cost are not included.

All prices are in outturn prices.

Water pollution incidents

(Table 13.15)

The Environment Agency responds to complaints and reported incidents of pollution in England and Wales. Each incident is then logged and categorised according to its severity. The category describes the impact of each incident on water, land and air. The impact of an incident on each medium is considered and reported separately. If no impact has occurred for a particular medium, the incident is reported as a category 4. Before 1999, the reporting system was used only for water pollution incidents; thus the total number of substantiated incidents was lower, as it did not include incidents not relating to the water environment.

Bathing waters

(Table 13.16)

Under the EC Bathing Water Directive 76/160/EEC, 11 physical, chemical and microbiological parameters are measured including total and faecal coliforms which are generally considered to be the most important indicators of the extent to which water is contaminated by sewage. The mandatory value for total coliforms is 10,000 per 100 ml, and for faecal coliforms 2,000 per 100 ml. For a bathing water to comply with the coliform standards, the Directive requires that at least 95 per cent of samples taken for each of these parameters over the bathing season are less than or equal to the mandatory values. In the UK a minimum of 20 samples are

Enviroment

normally taken at each site. In practice this means that where 20 samples are taken, a maximum of only one sample may exceed the mandatory value for the bathing water to comply, and where less than 20 samples are taken none may exceed the mandatory value for the bathing water to comply.

The bathing water season is from mid-May to end-September in England and Wales, but shorter in Scotland and Northern Ireland. Bathing waters which are closed for the season are excluded for that year.

The table shows Environment Agency regions for England and Wales, the boundaries of which are based on river catchment areas and not county borders. In particular, the figures shown for Wales are the Environment Agency Welsh Region, the boundary of which does not coincide with the boundary of Wales.

Surface and groundwater abstractions

(Table 13.17)

Significant changes in the way data is collected and/or reported were made in 1991 (due to the Water Resources Act 1991) and 1999 (commission of National Abstraction Licensing Database). Figures are therefore not strictly comparable with those in previous/intervening years. From 1999, data have been stored and retrieved from one system nationally and are therefore more accurate and reliable. Some regions report licensed and actual abstracts for financial rather than calendar years. As figures represent an average for the whole year expressed as daily amounts, differences between amounts reported for financial and calendar years are small.

Under the Water Act 2003, abstraction of less than 20 m3/day became exempt from the requirement to hold a licence as of 1 April 2005. As a result over 22,000 licences were deregulated, mainly for agricultural or private water supply purposes. However, due to the small volumes involved, this has had a minimal affect on the estimated licensed and actual abstraction totals.

The following changes have occurred in the classification of individual sources:

Spray irrigation: this category includes small amounts of non-agricultural spray irrigation

Mineral washing: from 1999 this was not reported as a separate category; licences for 'Mineral washing' are now contained in 'Other industry'

Private water supply: this was shown as separate category from 1992 and includes private abstractions for domestic use and individual households

Fish farming, cress growing, amenity ponds: includes amenity ponds, but excludes miscellaneous from 1991

Estimates of remaining recoverable oil and gas reserves

(Table 13.18)

Only a small proportion of the estimated remaining recoverable reserves of oil and gas are known with any degree of certainty. The latest oil and gas data for 2008 shows that the upper range of total UK oil reserves was estimated to be around 2.7 billion tonnes, while UK gas reserves were around 1950 billion cubic metres. Of these, proven reserves of oil were 0.4 billion tonnes and proven reserves of gas were 292 billion cubic metres. Compared with a year earlier, proven reserves were 9.7 per cent lower for oil and 14.9per cent lower for gas.

Municipal waste disposal

(Table 13.19)

Municipal waste includes household and non-household waste that is collected and disposed of by local authorities. It includes regular household collections, specific recycling collections, special collections of bulky items, waste received at civic amenity sites, and waste collected from non-household sources that come under the control of local authorities.

Amounts of different materials from household sources collected for recycling

(Table 13.20)

Household recycling includes those materials collected for recycling, composting or reuse by local authorities and those collected from household sources by 'private/voluntary' organisations where this material comes under the possession or control of local authorities. It includes residual waste from the household stream which was diverted for recycling by sorting or further treatment.

'Bring sites' are facilities where members of the public can bring recyclable materials (such as paper, glass, cans, textiles, shoes, etc). These are often located at supermarkets or similar locations, but exclude civic amenity sites.

'Civic Amenity sites' refers to household waste collected at sites provided by local authorities for the disposal of excess household and garden waste free of charge, as required by the Refuse Disposal (Amenity) Act 1978. These are also known as Household Waste Recycling Centres.

Noise incidents

(Table 13.21)

The table shows trends in the number of incidents reported by local authority Environmental Health Officers (EHO). The figures are from those authorities making returns and are calculated per million people based on the population of the authorities making returns. Environmental health has changed from calculating complaints per million of population to incidents per million of the population in 2004/05. The reason for asking about incidents is to better reflect both the local noise environment and investigatory workloads during the reporting year, while avoiding the double counting which occurs with complaints (that is, multiple complaints about the same incident). This change is reflected in the data, which shows a drop in numbers across all categories.

Most complaints about traffic noise are addressed to highways authorities or Department for Transport (DfT) Regional Directors, and will not necessarily be included in the figures. Similarly, complaints about noise from civil aircraft are generally received by aircraft operators, the airport companies, the DfT or Civil Aviation Authority. Complaints about military flying are dealt with either by Station Commanding Officers or by Ministry of Defence headquarters. It is also true that railway noise will be reported elsewhere. Thus the figures in this table will not necessarily include these complaints and are likely to be considerably understated. The information reported to the EHO is therefore considered to give, at best, only a very approximate indication of the trend in noise complaints from these sources.

Over time some of the categories shown in this table have changed. These have included, up until 1996/97, Section 62 of the Control of Pollution Act 1974 which covered noise in the streets; it primarily included the chimes of ice-cream vendors and the use of loudspeakers other than for strictly defined purposes. From 1997/98, all complaints about noise in the street are included with 'vehicles machinery and equipment in streets'. From 1997/98, complaints about roadworks are included with 'vehicles machinery and equipment in streets'.

Material flows

(Table 13.22)

Economy-wide material flow accounts record the total mass of natural resources and products that are used by the UK economy, either directly in the production and distribution of products and services, or indirectly through the movement of materials which are displaced in order for production to take place.

The direct movement of materials into the economy derives primarily from domestic extraction, that is from biomass (agricultural harvest, timber, fish and animal grazing), fossil fuel extraction (such as coal, crude oil and natural gas) and mineral extraction (metal ores, industrial minerals such as pottery clay, and construction material such as crushed rock, sand and gravel). This domestic extraction is supplemented by the imports of products, which may be of raw materials such as unprocessed agricultural products, but can also be of semi-manufactured or finished products. In a similar way the UK produces exports of raw materials, semi-manufactured and finished goods which can be viewed as inputs to the production and consumption of overseas economies.

Indirect flows of natural resources consist of the unused material resulting from domestic extraction, such as mining and quarrying overburden and the soil removed during construction and dredging activities. They also include the movement of used and unused material overseas, which is associated with the production and delivery of imports. Water, except for that included directly in products, is excluded.

There are three main indicators used to measure inputs. The Direct Material Input measures the input of used materials into the economy, that is all materials which are of economic value and are used in production and consumption activities (including the production of exports). Domestic Material Consumption measures the total amount of material directly used in the economy – it includes imports but excludes exports. The Total Material Requirement (TMR) measures the total material basis of the economy, that is the total primary resource requirements of all the production and consumption activities. It includes not only the direct use of resources for producing exports, but also indirect flows from the production of imports and the indirect flows associated with domestic extraction. Although TMR is widely favoured as a resource use indicator, the estimates of indirect flows are less reliable than those for materials directly used by the economy, and the indicator therefore needs to be considered alongside other indicators.

Between 2007 and 2008[1], the quantity of natural resources used by the UK economy, known as domestic material consumption, fell by 67 million tonnes (9.9 per cent) to 613 million tonnes. This is the largest recorded fall since records began in 1970. It follows 10 years where resource use has remained broadly unchanged. This means that, with rising levels of economic activity, UK material productivity has been increasing.

The fall in domestic material consumption mainly reflects decreases in the domestic extraction of minerals, with a decrease of 57 million tonnes (19.3 per cent) driven by a sharp fall in the extraction of primary aggregates – crushed stone, sand and gravel – as demand was impacted by the economic downturn. Imports of minerals also fell in 2008, by 10.9 per cent.

Much of the period 1990 to 2007 had seen strong economic growth in the UK and material productivity increased, with material use falling in relation to the level of economic activity. This in part reflects the increasing importance of the service industries in the UK economy. Gross Domestic Product overall continued to increase in 2008 (by 0.5 per cent) and material use fell. The fall in demand for primary aggregates coincides with the contraction in output of the construction industry in 2008.

1. Figures for 2008 are provisional.

13.1 Government revenues from environmental taxes
United Kingdom

£ million

		1999	2000	2001	2002	2003	2004	2005	2006	2007	2008
Energy											
Duty on hydrocarbon oils	GTAP	22 391	23 041	22 046	22 070	22 476	23 412	23 346	23 448	24 512	24 790
including											
Unleaded petrol[1]	GBHE	11 952	11 481	1 906	–	–	–	–	–	–	–
Leaded petrol/LRP[2]	GBHL	1 630	1 105	650	103	70	67	20	15	13	10
Ultra low sulphur petrol	ZXTK	–	968	10 117	12 624	12 098	12 160	11 688	11 274	11 198	11 077
Diesel[3]	GBHH	1 274	23	65	–	–	–	–	–	–	–
Ultra low sulphur diesel	GBHI	7 338	9 014	8 492	9 029	9 457	10 168	10 829	11 203	12 022	12 244
VAT on duty	CMYA	3 918	4 032	3 858	3 862	3 933	4 097	4 086	4 103	4 290	4 338
Fossil fuel levy	CIQY	104	56	86	32	–	–	–	–	–	–
Gas levy	GTAZ	–	–	–	–	–	–	–	–	–	–
Climate change levy	LSNT	–	–	585	825	828	756	747	711	690	717
Hydro-benefit	LITN	35	42	46	44	44	40	10	–	–	–
Road vehicles											
Vehicle excise duty	CMXZ	4 873	4 606	4 102	4 294	4 720	4 763	4 762	5 010	5 384	5 524
Other environmental taxes											
Air passenger duty	CWAA	884	940	824	814	781	856	896	961	1 883	1 876
Landfill tax	BKOF	430	461	502	541	607	672	733	804	877	954
Aggregates levy	MDUQ	–	–	–	213	340	328	327	321	339	334
Total environmental taxes	JKVW	**32 635**	**33 178**	**32 049**	**32 695**	**33 729**	**34 924**	**34 907**	**35 358**	**37 975**	**38 533**
Environmental taxes as a % of:											
Total taxes and social contributions	JKVX	9.7	9.3	8.6	8.7	8.5	8.3	7.7	7.2	7.4	7.1
Gross domestic product	JKVY	3.5	3.4	3.1	3.0	3.0	2.9	2.8	2.7	2.7	2.7

1 Unleaded petrol includes superunleaded petrol.
2 Lead Replacement Petrol (the alternative to 4-Star leaded petrol introduced in 2000) is lead-free.
3 Duty incentives have concentrated production on ultra low sulphur varieties.

Sources: ONS, Department for Energy and Climate Change; environment.accounts@ons.gsi.gov.uk

13.2 Atmospheric emissions on a National Accounts basis[1], 2007
United Kingdom

	Greenhouse gases[1]	Acid rain precursors[2]	Emissions affecting air quality Thousand Tonnes							Tonnes		
	CO_2 equivalent	SO_2 equivalent	CO_2	PM10[3]	CO	NMVOC[4]	Benzene	Butadiene	Lead	Cadmium	Mercury
Agriculture	49 769	508	6 006	20	45	82	–	–	–	–	–
Mining and quarrying	27 377	86	23 028	13	37	127	–	–	–	–	–
Manufacturing	109 522	384	103 646	30	613	322	2	–	57	2	3
Electricity, gas and water supply	195 810	543	189 690	10	88	45	–	–	3	–	2
Construction	10 785	45	10 190	7	53	62	–	–	–	–	–
Wholesale and retail trade	18 738	48	15 646	4	66	58	–	–	2	–	–
Transport and communication	92 171	707	90 673	46	132	47	3	1	3	1	–
Other business services	7 002	13	6 469	1	30	4	–	–	–	–	–
Public administration	8 862	38	8 679	2	31	4	–	–	1	–	–
Education, health and social work	8 083	11	7 787	1	11	2	–	–	–	–	–
Other services	27 807	35	5 127	1	81	26	2	–	–	–	1
Households	151 181	210	146 158	35	949	248	10	1	5	–	–
Total	707 106	2 629	613 100	169	2 136	1 026	19	2	72	4	7
of which, emissions from road transport	125 093	330	123 673	25	795	89	2	1	2	–	–

1 Carbon dioxide, methane, nitrous oxide, hydro-fluorocarbons, perfluorocarbons and sulphur hexafluoride expressed as thousand tonnes of carbon dioxide equivalent.
2 Sulphur dioxide, nitrogen oxides and ammonia expressed as thousand tonnes of sulphur dioxide equivalent.
3 PM10's are carbon particles in air arising from incomplete combustion.
4 Non-methane volatile organic compounds including benzene and 1,3-butadiene.

Source: AEA Energy & Environment, ONS

Environment

13.3 Greenhouse gas emissions:weighted by global warming potential[1,3,4,5,6]
United Kingdom

Million tonnes (Carbon dioxide equivalent[4])

		1995	1996	1997	1998	1999	2000	2001	2002	2003	2004	2005	2006	2007	2008
Net CO_2 emissions(emissions minus removal)	JZCK	553.1	575.3	551.5	553.6	543.1	551.2	562.6	545.0	556.7	556.3	553.9	551.4	543.6	532.8
Methane(CH_4)	GXDO	91.2	88.8	83.5	79.2	74.0	69.5	63.4	60.4	54.4	52.7	51.5	50.5	49.3	48.7
Nitrous oxide(N_2O)	GXDP	53.5	53.4	54.5	53.9	43.3	42.3	39.8	38.1	37.5	38.0	36.9	35.2	34.7	33.9
Hydrofluorocarbons(HFCs)	JZCN	15.5	16.7	19.0	16.8	10.0	8.7	9.3	9.8	10.5	9.6	10.4	10.8	11.0	11.2
Perfluorocarbons(PFCs)	JZCO	0.5	0.5	0.4	0.4	0.4	0.5	0.4	0.3	0.3	0.3	0.3	0.3	0.2	0.2
Sulphur hexafluoride(SF_6)	JZCP	1.2	1.3	1.2	1.3	1.4	1.8	1.4	1.5	1.3	1.1	1.1	0.9	0.8	0.7
Kyoto greenhouse gas basket[2]	F92X	714.1	735.1	709.6	705.0	672.2	674.1	677.4	655.8	661.2	659.3	655.2	650.0	640.5	628.3

1 Figures for each individual gas include the Land use, Land-Use Change and Forestry sector (LULUCF). These emissions cover the UK and Crown Dependancies, but exclude emissions from UK Overseas Territories.
2 Kyoto basket total differs slightly from sum of individual pollutants above as the basket uses a narrower definition for the LULUCF. This includes emissions from the UK, Crown Dependancies and UK Overseas Territories.
3 Kyoto base year consists of emissions of CO2, CH4, and N2O in 1990 and of HFCs, PFCs and SF6 in 1995. Includes an allowance for net emissions from LULUCF in 1990.

4 The entire time series is revised each year to take account of methodological improvements in the UK emissions inventory.
5 Emissions are presented as carbon dioxide equivalent in line with international reporting and carbon trading. To convert Carbon dioxide into carbon equivalents, divide figures by 44/12.
6 Figures shown do not include any adjustment for the effect of the EU Emissions Trading Scheme (EUETS), which was introduced in 2005.

Source: AEA. Department for Energy and Climate Change: 0300 060 4000

13.4 Greenhouse gas emissions bridging table
Environmental Accounts measure to UNFCCC[1] measure

Thousand tonnes CO2 equivilent

		1990	2000	2001	2002	2003	2004	2005	2006	2007
Greenhouse gases - CO2,CH4,N2O,HFC,PFCs and SF6[2]										
Environmental Accounts measure	JKRU	809 456	733 470	741 756	721 406	729 556	733 455	731 541	719 099	707 106
less										
Bunker emissions[3]	A43J	22 598	36 381	36 324	34 689	35 187	38 777	41 346	42 863	42 282
CO2 from biomass[4]	A43K	2 980	6 573	7 261	7 506	8 366	9 548	10 801	10 882	11 654
Cross boundary adjustment[5]	A43L	12 933	17 191	21 112	23 648	25 480	26 951	26 890	17 671	16 721
plus										
Crown Dependancies[6]	EQ44	1 649	1 907	1 607	1 575	1 485	1 472	1 493	1 540	1 537
Land-use change/forestry (LULUCF)[7]	A43M	2 966	−301	−418	−936	−977	−1 729	−1 881	−1 752	−1 750
Overseas Territories (inc. net emissions from LULUCF)	JTL8	1 552	1 887	1 967	1 960	2 017	2 087	2 107	2 186	2 252
UNFCCC reported in the UK Greenhouse Gas Inventory[8]	A43N	777 118	676 829	680 226	658 171	663 055	660 014	654 230	649 663	638 493
Kyoto Greenhouse Gas Basket	JTL9	772 978	674 743	678 158	656 424	661 134	658 650	652 813	647 949	636 616

1 United Nations Framework Convention on Climate Change.
2 Carbon dioxide, methane, nitrous oxide, hydrofluorocarbons, perfluorocarbon and sulphur hexafluoride expressed as thousand tonnes of carbon dioxide equivalent.
3 Bunker emissions include IPCC memo items International Aviation (source no. 126) and international Shipping (source no. 127).
4 Emissions arising from wood, straw, biogases and poultry litter combustion for energy production.
5 Emissions generated by UK households and businesses transport and travel abroad, net of emissions generated by non-residents travel and transport in the UK.

6 Revisions to the Crown Dependancies are due to a change in their treatment in the National Inventories and their inclusion in the UNFCCC total.
7 Emissions from deforestation, soils and changes in forest and other woody biomass.
8 This is the UK total for the sum of 6 individual pollutants and differs slightly from the Kyoto Greenhouse Gas Basket totals which uses a narrower definition of LULUCF and includes emissions from the UK Overseas Territories (Gibraltar, the Falkland Islands, the Cayman Islands, Montserrat, Bermuda).

Source: AEA Energy & Environment, DECC, ONS

13.5 Estimated emissions[1,2] of carbon dioxide (CO_2)
United Kingdom

Million tonnes as CO_2

		1970	1980	1990	1997	1998	1999	2000	2001	2002	2003	2004	2005	2006	2007	2008
By source NC category																
Energy Supply Total	I6AH	260.3	262.0	243.1	199.0	203.3	192.4	202.7	213.2	210.3	217.5	215.8	216.9	219.8	216.2	209.9
Business Total	I6AI	204.1	131.4	108.5	103.4	102.4	103.4	103.6	103.6	93.4	95.0	93.1	92.4	89.9	88.2	85.5
Transport Total	I6AJ	71.3	90.2	122.6	128.2	127.0	127.8	126.8	126.4	128.5	129.7	130.3	131.9	133.7	134.2	130.3
Public	I6AK	23.7	19.7	13.5	13.8	12.6	12.4	11.7	12.1	10.3	10.1	11.1	10.9	10.4	9.6	10.2
Residential Total	I6AL	96.2	84.4	79.8	85.2	87.2	86.3	86.9	89.1	85.9	86.8	88.4	84.7	81.5	78.2	80.7
Agriculture Total	I6AM	6.2	5.3	5.2	5.3	5.1	5.1	4.8	4.8	4.8	4.8	4.7	4.6	4.4	4.2	4.2
Industrial Process Total	I6AN	21.0	14.2	16.2	15.6	15.5	15.5	14.7	13.4	12.5	13.4	13.8	14.0	13.2	14.6	13.7
Land-use change	I6AO	–	–	2.9	0.6	–	−0.3	−0.4	−0.5	−1.1	−1.1	−1.8	−2.0	−1.9	−2.0	−2.0
Waste Management Total	I6AP	1.4	1.4	1.2	0.5	0.5	0.5	0.5	0.5	0.5	0.5	0.5	0.5	0.4	0.5	0.4
Total	I6AQ	684.3	608.5	592.8	551.5	553.6	543.1	551.2	562.6	545.0	556.7	556.3	553.9	551.4	543.6	532.8

1 The entire time series is revised each year to take account of methodological improvements in the UK emissions inventory.
2 These figures include emissions from the UK and Crown Dependancies, but exclude emissions from Overseas Territories.

Source: AEA. Department for Energy and Climate Change: 0300 060 4000

13.6 Estimated emissions[1] of methane (CH$_4$)[2]
United Kingdom

Thousand tonnes

		1996	1997	1998	1999	2000	2001	2002	2003	2004	2005	2006	2007	2008
By source NC category														
Energy Supply Total	I6AR	1 017.4	968.9	882.6	789.7	724.5	696.1	685.2	547.6	534.5	482.1	450.1	397.8	396.4
Business Total	I6AS	16.3	16.5	16.1	15.9	15.6	14.5	13.3	14.2	13.8	13.6	13.6	13.4	12.5
Transport Total	I6AT	22.7	20.9	19.2	17.6	15.4	13.3	11.9	10.7	9.7	8.7	8.0	7.3	6.5
Public	I6AU	1.5	1.4	1.3	1.2	1.1	1.2	1.0	1.0	1.1	1.1	1.0	0.9	1.0
Residential Total	I6AV	41.9	38.7	40.3	43.0	32.8	29.6	24.6	23.0	22.0	20.0	20.6	22.2	24.0
Agriculture Total	I6AW	1 044.0	1 013.1	1 013.4	1 010.5	968.8	909.9	898.4	898.0	904.7	915.5	898.8	893.1	872.0
Industrial Process	I6AX	11.0	9.5	7.6	6.8	6.3	5.7	5.5	6.7	6.5	5.9	5.8	6.4	6.0
Land Use Change	I6AY	1.0	1.2	0.9	0.8	1.2	1.5	1.3	1.2	1.2	0.9	1.4	1.4	1.3
Waste Management Total	I6AZ	2 072.4	1 908.4	1 791.3	1 640.1	1 541.9	1 349.0	1 235.4	1 088.5	1 016.6	1 004.5	1 005.7	1 003.7	1 000.2
Total	I6B2	4 228.2	3 978.5	3 772.6	3 525.7	3 307.5	3 020.8	2 876.6	2 590.9	2 510.0	2 452.4	2 405.1	2 346.3	2 319.8

1 The entire time series is revised each year to take account of methodological improvements in the UK emissions inventory.
2 These figures include emissions from the UK and Crown Dependancies, but exclude emissions from Overseas Territories.

Source: AEA. Department for Energy and Climate Change: 0300 060 4000

13.7 Estimated emissions[1] of nitrous oxide (N$_2$O)[1,2]
United Kingdom

Thousand tonnes

		1995	1996	1997	1998	1999	2000	2001	2002	2003	2004	2005	2006	2007	2008
By source NC Category															
Energy Supply Total	I6A7	5.6	5.4	4.9	5.1	4.7	5.1	5.4	5.4	5.4	5.2	5.4	5.6	5.2	4.9
Business Total	I6A8	4.7	4.6	4.4	4.3	4.3	4.2	4.2	4.1	4.1	4.2	4.2	4.2	4.2	3.8
Transport Total	I6A9	6.4	6.0	6.1	6.1	6.1	6.1	5.9	5.7	5.6	5.5	5.4	5.4	5.2	4.7
Public Total	I6AA	0.1	0.1	0.1	0.1	0.1	0.1	0.1	–	–	–	–	–	–	–
Residential Total	I6AB	0.7	0.8	0.7	0.7	0.7	0.6	0.6	0.5	0.5	0.5	0.4	0.4	0.4	0.4
Agriculture Total	I6AC	103.5	104.0	107.2	104.2	102.4	98.2	92.6	94.1	91.9	91.4	90.0	86.1	83.7	83.5
Industrial Processes Total	I6AD	48.2	47.9	48.5	49.4	17.5	18.1	15.7	8.8	9.3	11.7	9.2	7.8	9.1	8.0
Waste Management Total	I6AF	3.5	3.6	3.9	4.0	3.8	4.0	4.1	4.1	4.1	4.1	4.1	4.1	4.1	4.2
Total	I6AG	172.7	172.3	175.8	173.9	139.6	136.4	128.5	122.8	120.9	122.7	118.9	113.7	112.0	109.4

1 The entire time series is revised each year to take account of methodological improvements in the UK emissions inventory.
2 These figures include emissions from the UK and Crown Dependancies, but exclude emissions from Overseas Territories.

Source: AEA. Department for Energy and Climate Change: 0300 060 4000

13.8 Road Transport Emissions by Pollutant
United Kingdom

Thousand tonnes

		1996	1997	1998	1999	2000	2001	2002	2003	2004	2005	2006	2007
Pollutant													
Greenhouse gases[1]	I6BZ	118 221	120 403	120 110	121 391	120 563	120 280	122 616	122 368	123 158	123 847	123 841	125 093
of which													
Carbon dioxide	I6C2	116 049	118 243	117 962	119 275	118 509	118 352	120 780	120 638	121 515	121 940	122 354	123 673
Methane	I6C3	499	457	419	380	337	295	260	229	201	178	161	147
Nitrous oxide	I6C4	1 673	1 703	1 729	1 736	1 717	1 633	1 576	1 502	1 442	1 369	1 325	1 273
Acid rain precursors[2]	I6C5	708	682	656	615	566	522	486	449	419	386	359	330
of which													
Sulphur dioxide	I6C6	38	28	23	14	6	3	3	3	3	2	2	2
Nitrogen oxides	I6C7	649	633	612	580	538	497	462	427	398	368	342	316
Ammonia	I6C8	21	21	22	22	22	22	21	20	18	16	14	12
PM10	I6C9	44	42	40	39	33	31	30	29	28	27	26	25
Carbon monoxide	I6CA	4 085	3 721	3 379	3 024	2 505	2 114	1 826	1 559	1 320	1 069	927	795
NMVOCs	I6CB	577	520	450	387	311	255	214	178	146	120	102	89
Benzene	I6CC	27	24	21	18	6	5	5	4	3	3	3	2
1,3-Butadiene	I6CD	7	6	5	5	4	3	3	2	2	2	1	1

1 Greenhouse gases are made up of cardon dioxide, methane & nitrous oxide. Weight in carbon dioxide equivalent.
2 Acid rain precursors are made of sulphur dioxide, nitrogen & ammonia. Weight in sulphur dioxide equivalent.

Sources: AEA Energy & Environment;
Office for National Statistics;
environment.accounts@ons.gsi.gov.uk

Environment

13.9 Annual rainfall: by region
United Kingdom

		Annual rainfall as a percentage of the 1971-2000 average										
		1999	2000	2001	2002	2003	2004	2005	2006	2007	2008	2009[3]
Region[1]	1971 - 2000[4] rainfall average (= 100%) millimetres											
United Kingdom	J8G4	1 084	114	123	97	118	83	112	100	108	110	120	112
North West	J8G5	1 176	111	132	94	121	85	116	96	114	110	126	113
Northumbria	J8G6	831	106	132	106	124	80	120	111	101	105	134	116
Severn Trent	J8G7	759	120	132	104	119	81	110	92	103	123	121	103
Yorkshire	J8G8	814	110	136	99	125	82	114	96	110	115	130	106
Anglian	J8G9	603	113	129	124	118	86	115	89	102	118	116	98
Thames	J8GA	700	111	137	116	128	81	103	79	106	118	115	104
Southern	J8GB	782	105	148	114	129	85	97	79	101	106	108	109
Wessex	J8GC	866	118	136	100	132	83	98	89	100	113	116	109
South West	J8GD	1 208	113	128	92	121	78	99	90	92	110	112	110
England	J8GE	819	113	133	105	123	82	109	91	103	114	120	107
Wales[2]	J8GF	1 373	116	133	98	119	83	108	95	107	108	121	110
Scotland	J8GG	1 440	116	113	91	112	84	117	110	114	109	119	116
Northern Ireland	J8GH	1 111	111	110	81	127	84	98	96	104	99	114	113

1 The regions of England shown in this table correspond to the original nine English regions of the National Rivers Authority (NRA); the NRA became part of the Environment Agency upon its creation in April 1996.
2 The figures in this table relate to the country of Wales, not the Environment Agency Welsh Region.

3 Data from October 2009 are provisional and subject to revision.
4 1971-2000 averages have been derived using Met Office 5km gridded rainfall.

Sources: The Met Office;
Centre for Ecology and Hydrology: 01491 838800

13.10 UK Annual Weather Summary

	Max Temp		Min Temp		Mean Temp		Sunshine		Rainfall	
	Actual (degrees celsius)	Anomaly (degrees celsius)	Actual (degrees celsius)	Anomaly (degrees celsius)	Actual (degrees celsius)	Anomaly (degrees celsius)	Actual (hours/ day)	Anomaly (%)	Actual (mm)	Anomaly (%)
	WLRL	WLRM	WLRO	WLRP	WLRR	WLRS	WLRX	WLRY	WLSH	WLSI
1989	13.1	1.2	5.5	0.7	9.3	1.0	1 563.8	116.9	1 018.5	92.6
1990	13.1	1.2	5.8	0.9	9.4	1.1	1 490.7	111.4	1 172.8	106.7
1991	12.1	0.3	5.1	0.2	8.6	0.3	1 302.0	97.3	998.2	90.8
1992	12.3	0.4	5.2	0.4	8.7	0.4	1 290.8	96.5	1 186.8	107.9
1993	11.8	−0.1	5.0	0.1	8.4	..	1 218.6	91.1	1 121.1	102.0
1994	12.4	0.5	5.5	0.6	8.9	0.6	1 366.9	102.2	1 184.7	107.7
1995	13.0	1.1	5.4	0.6	9.2	0.9	1 588.5	118.7	1 023.7	93.1
1996	11.7	−0.1	4.7	−0.1	8.2	−0.2	1 403.5	104.9	916.6	83.4
1997	13.1	1.3	5.8	1.0	9.4	1.1	1 430.3	106.9	1 024.0	93.1
1998	12.6	0.8	5.8	1.0	9.1	0.8	1 268.4	94.8	1 265.1	115.1
1999	13.0	1.1	5.9	1.0	9.4	1.1	1 419.4	106.1	1 237.2	112.5
2000	12.7	0.8	5.6	0.8	9.1	0.8	1 367.5	102.2	1 335.6	121.5
2001	12.4	0.6	5.3	0.5	8.8	0.5	1 411.9	105.5	1 049.9	95.5
2002	13.0	1.1	6.0	1.2	9.5	1.2	1 304.0	97.5	1 280.5	116.5
2003	13.5	1.6	5.6	0.7	9.5	1.2	1 587.4	118.7	901.5	82.0
2004	13.0	1.2	6.0	1.2	9.5	1.2	1 361.4	101.8	1 210.1	110.1
2005	13.1	1.2	5.9	1.1	9.5	1.1	1 399.2	104.6	1 083.0	98.4
2006	13.4	1.5	6.1	1.3	9.7	1.4	1 495.9	111.8	1 175.9	106.8
2007	13.3	1.4	6.0	1.1	9.6	1.3	1 450.7	108.4	1 197.1	108.8
2008	12.7	0.8	5.5	0.6	9.1	0.7	1 388.8	103.8	1 295.0	117.7
2009[1]	12.8	1.0	5.5	0.7	9.2	0.8	1 487.5	111.2	1 201.3	109.1

1 Data for 2009 are provisional.

Source: Met Office

13.11 Biological[1] and chemical[2] water quality of rivers and canals[3]
England, Wales and Northern Ireland

Percentage of river surveyed (%)

| | | Percentage of river surveyed (%) | | | | | | Percentage of total | |
| | | Good | | Fair | | | | | |
	Years	A	B	C	D	Poor E	Bad F	Good or fair	Poor or bad
Biological quality									
North East	1990	35.8	28.9	12.4	7.3	10.0	5.6	84.4	15.6
	2008	50.1	23.2	12.3	7.3	6.9	0.3	92.9	7.1
North West	1990	14.4	26.2	18.7	6.2	14.1	20.3	65.6	34.4
	2008	21.2	43.1	15.4	9.3	9.4	1.6	88.9	11.1
Midlands	1990	10.6	25.4	27.8	19.4	11.4	5.4	83.2	16.8
	2008	23.2	36.4	25.3	8.0	5.1	2.1	92.9	7.1
Anglian	1990	13.1	37.2	36.5	9.2	2.7	1.3	96.0	4.0
	2008	39.7	42.8	11.7	5.5	-	0.2	99.8	0.2
Thames	1990	25.9	30.2	24.4	9.4	6.7	3.4	89.9	10.1
	2008	33.8	27.9	24.5	8.2	4.7	0.9	94.4	5.6
Southern	1990	37.3	30.1	24.4	6.3	1.8	-	98.2	1.8
	2008	53.6	29.2	13.4	3.3	0.5	-	99.5	0.5
South West	1990	42.4	35.8	14.6	4.0	2.8	0.5	96.7	3.3
	2008	66.4	26.0	6.9	0.6	0.1	-	99.9	0.1
England[4]	1990	25.0	30.4	21.9	9.0	7.7	6.0	86.4	13.6
	2008	39.0	33.0	16.3	6.4	4.3	0.9	94.7	5.3
Wales	1990	37.2	41.3	14.3	5.4	1.6	0.2	98.3	1.7
	2008	35.1	52.9	10.4	0.9	0.7	-	99.3	0.7
Chemical quality									
North East	1990	39.3	29.0	11.5	7.7	10.5	2.0	87.5	12.5
	2008	72.1	12.5	9.2	4.3	1.9	-	98.1	1.9
North West	1990	36.8	21.4	17.3	10.2	10.9	3.5	85.6	14.4
	2008	68.4	13.4	11.4	3.0	3.6	0.2	96.2	3.8
Midlands	1990	19.0	30.0	23.7	14.2	12.8	0.3	86.9	13.1
	2008	45.4	30.9	13.5	6.3	3.9	0.1	96.0	4.0
Anglian	1990	4.1	25.6	38.6	18.8	12.2	0.8	87.0	13.0
	2008	98.0	2.0	98.0	2.0	98.0	2.0	98.0	2.0
Thames	1990	17.6	35.3	21.9	11.3	13.6	0.3	86.1	13.9
	2008	54.1	26.0	11.5	6.4	2.0	-	98.0	2.0
Southern	1990	27.1	29.8	26.3	11.4	5.5	-	94.5	5.5
	2008	32.8	35.8	21.0	7.4	3.1	-	96.9	3.1
South West	1990	46.8	30.8	11.5	7.0	3.9	-	96.1	3.9
	2008	78.4	12.6	6.3	0.9	1.8	-	98.2	1.8
England[4]	1990	25.5	29.7	21.6	11.9	10.4	1.0	88.7	11.3
	2008	55.1	23.4	13.3	5.0	3.2	0.1	96.8	3.2
Wales	1990	51.9	34.4	7.6	3.7	1.6	0.8	97.6	2.4
	2008	76.0	18.8	2.4	0.9	1.8	0.1	98.1	1.9

| Northern Ireland | | | | | | | |
	Years	High	Good	Moderate	Poor	Bad	No Data
Biological[5] quality							
	2008	7.5	33.0	32.5	13.9	3.0	10.1
Chemical[6] quality							
	2008	29.2	28.7	22.1	5.7	1.8	12.5

1 Based on the River invertebrate Prediction and Classification System (RIV-PACS).
2 Based on the General Quality Assessment Headline Indicator (GQAHI) scheme for England, and the General Quality Assessment (GQA) scheme for Wales.
3 See chapter text.

4 Figures for the English regions will not add to the national figure for England because a small amount of river lengths which are located along the border between England and Wales are counted in both the national figures for England and Wales.
5 Based on the River Invertebrate Classification Technique (RICT).
6 Based on WFD classification of Soluble Reactive Phosphorus, pH, Dissolved Oxygen and Ammonia.

Sources: Environment Agency;
Northern Ireland Environment Agency

13.12 Chemical and biological water quality [1]
Scotland

Kilometres and percentages

	Length surveyed							Percentage of total	
	Excellent A1	Good A2	Unclassified assumed good	Fair B	Poor C	Seriously polluted D	Total	Good or fair[2]	Poor or seriously polluted
	DZ38	DZ39	DZ3A	DZ3B	DZ3C	DZ3D	DZ3E	DZ3F	DZ3G
2001	3 870	6 320	11 960	2 340	930	80	25 510	96	4
2002	5 280	8 660	7 990	2 560	900	60	25 440	96	4
2003	6 820	9 540	5 900	2 370	750	50	25 440	97	3
2004	7 660	10 610	3 810	2 590	720	50	25 430	97	3
2005	8 000	12 050	2 130	2 470	720	50	25 430	97	3
2006	7 860	12 330	2 080	2 430	700	40	25 430	97	3

						Ecological potential[3]			
	High	Good	Moderate	Poor	Bad	Good	Moderate	Poor	Bad

River length surveyed (km)

	J8SC	J8SD	J8SF	J8SH	J8SJ	J8SE	J8SG	J8SI	J8SK
2007	1 074	9 077	8 613	3 311	910	1 145	37	533	418

Lake area surveyed (sqkm)

	J8SL	J8SM	J8SO	J8SQ	J8SS	J8SN	J8SP	J8SR	J8ST
2007	173	198	187	52	20	230	11	122	–

Transitional water area surveyed (sqkm)

	JDB5	JDB6	JDB7	JDB8	JDB9
2007	558	202	216	11	6

Coastal water area surveyed (sqkm)

	JDC2	JDC3	JDC4	JDC5	JDC6
2007	33 265	9 396	5 041	7	..

1 See chapter text.
2 Classes A1, A2, B and unclassified.
3 Ecological potential is used to classify artificial and heavily modified water bodies.

Source: Scottish Environment Protection Agency: 01786 457700

13.13 Reservoir stocks in England and Wales:[1] by month

Percentages

		1999	2000	2001	2002	2003	2004	2005	2006	2007	2008	2009
January	JTAS	95.8	95.8	94.8	86.5	95.1	79.9	91.2	85.9	92.2	89.8	92.4
February	JTAT	97.0	95.9	94.4	93.7	95.0	93.8	92.3	88.7	93.7	95.7	95.3
March	JTAU	96.5	97.4	95.0	95.5	92.1	92.1	92.1	91.2	96.7	95.6	93.3
April	JTAV	96.9	95.1	95.5	94.5	92.3	94.4	93.6	96.2	95.2	97.3	94.5
May	JTAW	97.0	97.0	96.7	91.9	88.6	94.7	95.0	93.4	91.9	95.1	92.0
June	JTAX	95.4	95.7	91.9	97.0	93.1	90.5	93.0	94.4	91.1	92.6	93.3
July	JTAY	92.0	93.7	85.1	94.9	87.0	84.8	85.6	88.4	94.4	90.6	88.6
August	JTAZ	82.6	88.5	80.7	91.1	81.1	78.5	77.9	77.2	93.5	92.0	91.0
September	JTBA	76.9	83.2	77.9	85.9	69.9	82.4	71.5	70.7	88.3	92.5	89.7
October	JTBB	79.7	88.0	77.0	77.3	60.4	84.2	67.4	67.8	86.1	90.9	84.0
November	JTBC	81.7	95.1	85.5	82.9	53.0	87.5	77.2	80.0	81.2	93.7	82.0
December	JTBD	84.9	96.7	87.9	91.8	60.9	86.2	83.8	89.8	82.4	93.1	92.6

1 Reservoir stocks are the percentage of useable capacity based on a representative selection of reservoirs; the percentages relate to the beginning of each month.

Sources: Water PLCs;
Environment Agency;
Centre for Ecology and Hydrology: 01491 838800

13.14 Water industry expenditure[1]
England and Wales

£ million

		1998 /99	1999 /00	2000 /01	2001 /02	2002 /03	2003 /04	2004 /05	2005 /06	2006 /07	2007 /08	2008 /09
Operating expenditure												
Water supply	KQQX	2 386.1	2 448.1	2 391.0	2 426.9	2 544.2	2 676.5	2 690.7	2 942.7	3 118.6	3 244.9	3 377.5
Sewerage services	KQQY	1 971.3	2 069.8	2 087.1	2 167.6	2 265.2	2 319.4	2 499.3	2 708.1	2 876.2	3 049.0	3 110.9
Capital expenditure												
Water supply	KQSX	1 299.6	1 285.6	934.7	1 128.6	1 345.8	1 346.5	1 308.6	1 282.5	1 681.7	1 884.5	1 802.9
Sewerage	KQSY	443.3	454.1	322.0	306.5	469.5	590.6	575.5	476.2	585.3	583.5	604.5
Sewage treatment and disposal	KQSZ	1 386.9	1 435.4	1 046.3	999.7	1 068.0	1 235.4	1 185.6	1 046.1	1 289.6	1 542.3	1 467.3

1 See chapter text. All in outturn prices.

Source: Office of Water Services: 0121 625 1300

13.15 Water pollution incidents[1,3]
United Kingdom

Numbers

		1999[2]	2000[2]	2001[2]	2002[2]	2003[2]	2004[2]	2005[2]	2006[2]	2007[2]	2008[2]
Categories 1 to 3											
Environment Agency Regions											
North West	MKDB	1 668	1 757	1 734	1 805	1 534	1 091	1 056	913	932	861
North East	MKDC	1 828	1 822	1 952	1 789	1 971	1 692	1 448	1 132	993	823
Midlands	MKDD	2 804	3 106	2 862	2 843	2 464	1 955	1 890	1 914	1 671	1 532
Anglian	MKDE	1 726	1 369	1 606	1 716	1 616	1 418	1 290	1 223	1 327	1 765
Thames	MKDF	1 208	1 379	1 510	1 630	1 447	1 211	1 203	1 159	1 023	881
Southern	MKDG	1 317	1 540	1 585	1 511	1 543	1 218	955	1 020	887	768
South West	MKDH	2 463	2 294	2 292	1 929	1 882	1 689	1 744	1 539	1 343	1 076
Welsh	MKDI	1 360	1 395	1 475	1 287	1 356	1 309	1 260	1 202	1 193	954
England and Wales	MKDJ	14 374	14 662	15 016	14 510	13 813	11 583	10 846	10 102	9 369	8 660
Scotland	MKDK	2 306	2 345	1 829	1 409	1 708	1 480	1 377	1 641	1 782	..
Northern Ireland	MKDL	1 507	1 705	1 561	1 517	1 552	1 227	1 174	1 133	1 292	1 237
By category in England and Wales											
Category 1	MKDM	90	77	118	82	94	114	99	86	70	74
Category 2	MKDN	863	758	860	784	685	594	562	519	452	368
Category 3	MKDO	13 421	13 827	14 038	13 644	13 034	10 875	10 185	9 497	8 847	8 218
Category 4[3]	MKDP	16 548	21 744	18 706	15 370	15 813	13 613	12 658	11 932	11 339	10 603
Total substantiated incidents[3]	MKDQ	30 922	36 406	33 722	29 880	29 626	25 196	23 504	22 034	20 708	19 263

1 See chapter text. Substantiated incidents to water, unless otherwise specified.
2 From 1999, categories 1-3 do not include all substantiated incidents to water. An additional category (Category 4) was introduced which includes all incidents which were substantiated, but which had no impact on the water environment. Therefore, data are not comparable to previous years.

3 Data for all years refer to financial years.
4 Category 4 and Total substantiated incidents include incidents to other media (air, land), which did not involve the water environment.

Sources: Environment Agency;
Scottish Environment Protection Agency;
Northern Ireland Environment Agency

Environment

13.16 Bathing water:[1] by region
United Kingdom

Numbers and percentages

Compliance with EC Bathing Water Directive coliform standards during the bathing season

		Identified bathing waters (numbers)						Numbers complying						Percentage complying
		2005	2006	2007	2008	2009		2005	2006	2007	2008	2009		2009
Coastal bathing waters														
Environment Agency Regions														
United Kingdom	GPKA	559	561	567	587	587	GPKN	550	559	547	563	573	GPLA	98
North East	GPKB	55	55	55	54	54	GPKO	53	54	52	53	54	GPLB	100
North West	GPKC	34	33	32	33	33	GPKP	32	33	29	30	31	GPLC	94
Anglian	GPKE	39	39	39	38	38	GPKR	39	39	39	38	38	GPLE	100
Thames	GPKF	8	8	8	8	8	GPKS	8	8	8	8	8	GPLF	100
Southern	GPKG	79	78	81	81	81	GPKT	79	78	81	80	81	GPLG	100
South West	GPKH	190	191	190	191	191	GPKU	189	191	187	181	186	GPLH	97
England	GPKI	405	404	405	405	405	GPKV	400	403	396	390	398	GPLI	98
Wales	GPKJ	80	80	80	81	81	GPKW	80	79	78	80	81	GPLJ	100
Scotland	GPKL	58	61	59	77	77	GPKY	55	61	52	70	72	GPLL	94
Northern Ireland	GPKM	16	16	23	24	24	GPKZ	15	16	21	23	22	GPLM	92
Inland bathing waters														
United Kingdom	JTIG	11	11	11	12	12	JTIH	11	10	11	11	12	JTII	100

1 See chapter text.

Sources: Environment Agency;
Scottish Environment Protection Agency;
Northern Ireland Environment Agency (NIEA)

13.17 Estimated abstractions from all surface and groundwater sources: by purpose[1]
England and Wales

Megalitres per day

		1997	1998	1999	2000	2001	2002	2003	2004	2005	2006	2007
Public water supply	JZLA	16 820	16 765	16 255	16 990	16 231	16 938	16 920	17 210	17 370	17 004	16 406
Spray irrigation	JZLB	292	282	325	291	259	248	315	225	226	277	163
Agriculture (excl spray irrigation)[4]	JZLC	108	111	142	152	108	120	132	122	60	48	84
Electricity supply industry[2]	JZLD	33 307	34 587	29 490	31 546	32 263	35 447	31 378	30 568	30 021	32 160	32 380
Other industry[3]	JZLE	4 352	4 964	5 428	5 433	4 772	4 883	6 623	6 585	6 339	6 519	4 910
Mineral washing	JZLF	297	223	..	..	..	..	..	..	..	..	..
Fish farming, cress growing, amenity ponds	JYXG	4 211	5 495	4 867	4 709	4 657	3 215	3 077	4 068	3 654	3 622	3 588
Private water supply	JZLG	162	175	91	102	92	54	61	30	26	37	30
Other	JZLH	408	289	526	559	108	77	86	77	60	86	113
Total	JZLI	59 957	62 891	57 123	59 782	58 489	60 981	58 593	58 885	57 757	59 752	57 674

1 See chapter text.
2 Increased electricity supply abstraction from 2002 due to increased production from power station in Anglian Region and two new licences issued in Southern Region.
3 Three abstraction licences re-assigned to other industry from electricty supply in Midlands Region (2003).
4 Reduction in agricultural abstraction due to deregulation of licences with effect from 1 April 2005.

Source: Environment Agency

13.18 Estimates of remaining recoverable oil and gas reserves
United Kingdom

		1999	2000	2001	2002	2003	2004	2005	2006	2007	2008
Oil (Million tonnes)											
Reserves											
Proven	JKOV	665	630	605	593	571	533	516	479	452	408
Probable	JKOW	455	380	350	327	286	283	300	298	328	361
Proven plus Probable	JKOX	1 120	1 010	955	920	857	816	816	776	780	770
Possible	JKOY	545	480	475	425	410	512	451	478	399	360
Maximum	JKOZ	1 665	1 490	1 430	1 344	1 267	1 328	1 267	1 254	1 179	1 130
Range of undiscovered resources											
Lower	JKNY	250	225	205	272	323	396	346	438	379	454
Upper	JKNZ	2 600	2 300	1 930	1 770	1 826	1 830	1 581	1 637	1 577	1 561
Range of total reserves											
Lower[1]	JKOA	915	855	810	865	894	929	862	917	831	862
Upper[2]	JKOB	4 265	3 790	3 360	3 115	3 093	3 158	2 848	2 892	2 756	2 690
Expected level of reserves[3]											
Opening stocks	JKOC	1 535	1 370	1 235	1 160	1 192	1 180	1 212	1 162	1 215	1 159
Extraction[4]	JKOD	−137	−126	−117	−117	−106	−95	−85	−77	−77	−72
Other volume changes	JKOE	−28	−9	42	149	94	127	35	130	21	136
Closing stocks	JKOF	1 370	1 235	1 160	1 192	1 180	1 212	1 162	1 215	1 159	1 223
Gas (billion cubic metres)											
Reserves											
Proven	JKOH	760	735	695	628	590	531	481	412	343	292
Probable	JKOI	500	460	445	369	315	296	247	272	304	309
Proven plus Probable	JKOJ	1 260	1 195	1 140	998	905	826	728	684	647	601
Possible	JKOK	490	430	395	331	336	343	278	283	293	306
Maximum	JKOL	1 750	1 630	1 535	1 329	1 241	1 169	1 006	967	940	907
Range of undiscovered resources											
Lower	JKOM	355	325	290	238	279	293	226	301	280	319
Upper	JKON	1 465	1 440	1 680	1 386	1 259	1 245	1 035	1 049	1 039	1 043
Range of total reserves											
Lower[1]	JKOO	1 115	1 060	985	866	869	824	707	713	623	611
Upper[2]	JKOP	3 215	3 065	3 215	2 714	2 500	2 415	2 041	2 016	1 979	1 950
Expected level of reserves[3]											
Opening stocks	JKOQ	1 780	1 615	1 520	1 430	1 235	1 184	1 120	954	985	927
Extraction[4]	JKOR	−99	−108	−104	−102	−102	−95	−86	−78	−71	−68
Other volume changes	JKOS	−66	13	14	−93	51	31	−80	109	13	61
Closing stocks	JKOT	1 615	1 520	1 430	1 235	1 184	1 120	954	985	927	920

1 The lower end of the range of total reserves has been calculated as the sum of proven reserves and the lower end of the range of undiscovered reserves.

2 The upper end of the range of total reserves is the sum of proven, probable and possible reserves and the upper end of the range of undiscovered reserves.

3 Expected reserves are the sum of proven reserves, probable reserves and the lower end of the range of undiscovered reserves.

4 Negative extraction is shown here for the purposes of the calculation only. Of itself, extraction should be considered as a positive value.

Sources: Office for National Statistics and Department of Energy and Climate Change;
environment.accounts@ons.gsi.gov.uk

13.19 Municipal waste disposal: by method
United Kingdom

Thousand tonnes

		2000 /01	2001 /02	2002 /03	2003 /04	2004 /05	2005 /06	2006 /07	2007 /08	2008 /09
England										
Household										
Disposed	I6EB	22 270	22 327	22 092	20 927	19 873	18 658	17 799	16 553	15 180
Recycled/composted	I6EC	2 809	3 197	3 740	4 521	5 785	6 796	7 976	8 735	9 146
Total	I6ED	25 079	25 524	25 832	25 448	25 658	25 454	25 775	25 287	24 326
Non Household										
Disposed	I6EE	2 342	2 656	2 730	2 650	2 795	2 289	2 408	2 250	2 072
Recycled/composted	I6EF	636	724	832	1 016	1 167	1 003	961	969	936
Total	I6EG	2 978	3 380	3 562	3 666	3 962	3 292	3 369	3 219	3 007
Total Municipal Waste										
Disposed	I6EH	24 612	24 983	24 822	23 577	22 668	20 947	20 207	18 803	17 252
Recycled/composted	I6EI	3 445	3 921	4 572	5 537	6 952	7 799	8 937	9 703	10 082
Total	I6EJ	28 057	28 905	29 394	29 114	29 619	28 745	29 144	28 506	27 333
Wales										
Household										
Disposed	I6EK	1 314	1 330	1 309	1 271	1 298	1 210	1 153	1 044	938
Recycled/composted	I6EL	90	126	179	252	286	332	419	499	534
Total	I6EM	1 404	1 456	1 488	1 522	1 585	1 542	1 572	1 543	1 472
Non Household										
Disposed	I6EN	223	244	238	227	213	204	132	150	140
Recycled/composted	I6EO	25	18	43	71	131	152	130	100	113
Total	I6EP	248	262	281	298	344	356	262	251	253
Total Municipal Waste										
Disposed	I6EQ	1 537	1 573	1 547	1 498	1 511	1 414	1 285	1 194	1 078
Recycled/composted	I6ER	115	144	222	323	418	484	549	599	646
Total	I6ES	1 652	1 718	1 769	1 820	1 928	1 898	1 834	1 794	1 724
Scotland										
Household										
Disposed	I6ET	2 405	2 472	2 477	2 375	2 276	2 221	2 127	2 022	..
Recycled/composted	I6EU	122	149	206	330	522	665	879	979	..
Total	I6EV	2 527	2 621	2 683	2 705	2 798	2 886	3 006	3 001	..
Non Household										
Disposed	I6EW	662	619	602	545	584	508	332	309	..
Recycled/composted	I6EX	22	27	60	66	125	265	99	103	..
Total	I6EY	684	646	663	611	709	773	431	412	..
Total Municipal Waste										
Disposed	I6EZ	3 067	3 091	3 079	2 920	2 860	2 729	2 459	2 331	..
Recycled/composted	I6F2	145	176	267	397	647	930	978	1 082	..
Total	I6F3	3 211	3 267	3 345	3 317	3 506	3 658	3 437	3 414	..

		2001	2001	2002	2003	2004 /05	2005 /06	2006 /07	2007 /08	2008 /09
Northern Ireland										
Household										
Disposed	I6F4	785	785	813	786	746	708	679	632	579
Recycled/composted	I6F5	94	94	90	112	173	230	260	296	303
Total	I6F6	879	879	902	898	919	937	939	928	880
Non Household										
Disposed	I6F7	..	..	119	116	114	111	108	117	116
Recycled/composted	I6F8	..	..	2	13	18	15	7	15	19
Total	I6F9	135	135	121	129	132	126	125	133	137
Total Municipal Waste										
Disposed	I6FA	..	..	932	902	860	813	792	755	695
Recycled/composted	I6FB	..	..	92	125	191	250	272	306	321
Total	I6FC	1 056	1 056	1 023	1 027	1 051	1 064	1 064	1 061	1 017

Sources: Department for Environment, Food and Rural Affairs 08459 33 55 77;
Welsh Assembly Government 029 2046 6151;
Scottish Environment Protection Agency 01786 457700;
Northern Ireland Environment Agency 028 9056 9427

13.20 Amounts of different materials from household sources collected for recycling by collection method 2008/09[1]

United Kingdom

Thousand tonnes

	Paper & Card	Glass	Compost	Scrap Metal & White Goods	Textiles	Cans	Plastics	Co-Mingled	Other	Total
England[2]										
Kerbside collection	1 032	454	2 381	26	8	66	41	1 787	9	5 803
Bring site collection	185	327	16	2	39	9	21	15	7	621
Civic Amenity site collection	225	58	1 113	526	35	14	17	5	580	2 573
Private/voluntary collection schemes[3]	29	4	5	1	30	2	1	3	184	261
Total	**1 470**	**844**	**3 515**	**555**	**112**	**91**	**79**	**1 812**	**780**	**9 257**
Wales										
Kerbside collection	61	33	107	2	1	8	9	78	0	299
Bring site collection	16	15	4	-	3	1	2	-	-	41
Civic Amenity site collection	15	5	59	37	2	-	3	6	58	184
Private/voluntary collection schemes[3]	-	-	5	-	-	-	-	-	3	9
Total	**93**	**54**	**176**	**39**	**6**	**9**	**14**	**84**	**61**	**534**
Scotland										
Kerbside collection	114	31	187	7	-	4	4	74	20	441
Bring site & Civic Amenity collection	46	44	60	39	12	2	2	14	118	337
Private/voluntary collection schemes[3]	-	-	29	-	-	-	-	-	21	50
Total	**160**	**75**	**276**	**46**	**12**	**6**	**6**	**88**	**159**	**828**
Northern Ireland										
Kerbside collection	78	9	65	-	-	4	10	1	5	172
Bring site collection	1	8	-	-	1	-	-	-	-	10
Civic Amenity site collection	9	7	53	23	2	-	-	-	25	119
Total	**85**	**22**	**118**	**23**	**3**	**4**	**10**	**1**	**30**	**301**

1 See chapter text.
2 Total amount of household waste collected for recycling is greater than that sent for recycling as some material is subsequently rejected during sorting or by the reprocessor.
3 Includes household waste collected from municipal parks, community skips and other methods of capture for recycling/composting and a small quantity of collection rejects.

Sources: Department for Environment Food and Rural Affairs 020 7238 4908;
Welsh Assembly Government 029 20466152;
Scottish Environment Protection Agency 01786 457700;
Northern Ireland Environment Agency 028 9056 9427.

13.21 Noise Incidents[1] received by Environmental Health Officers[2]

England, Wales and Northern Ireland[3]

Number per million people

		2001 /02	2002 /03	2003 /04	2004 /05	2005 /06	2006 /07	2007 /08	2008 /09
Not controlled by the Environmental Protection Act 1990:									
Road traffic	JZLJ	37	36	32	..	..	..	..	..
Aircraft	JZLK	101	104	120	..	..	..	..	..
Railway	JTHH	12	18	21	..	..	..	..	..
Total	JUZR	150	158	173	..	..	..	..	..
Controlled by the Environmental Protection Act 1990:									
Industrial/commercial premises	JZLN	1 273	1 315	1 480	1 260	936	1 021	1 132	1 051
Industrial	EAC3	..	301	284	219	192	176	159	155
Commercial/leisure[4]	EAC4	..	1 014	1 196	1 041	744	845	973	896
Construction/Demolition sites	SNLE	347	325	335	343	220	246	284	203
Domestic premises	JZLP	5 540	5 573	5 973	5 903	4 186	4 329	4 648	4 383
Vehicles, machinery and equipment in streets	JZLQ	372	377	346	330	180	205	211	168
Traffic	I4SR	..	..	..	..	116	154	139	72
Miscellaneous[5]	EAC2	..	..	..	433	267	414	443	268
Total	JZLR	7 532	7 590	8 134	8 269	5 905	6 369	6 857	6 145

1 From 2004/05 Data reported is for incidents per million where previously complaints per million was reported.
2 See chapter text.
3 Before 2005/06 data is for England and Wales only.
4 Includes railway noise and airports (non aircraft).
5 From 2004/05 includes 'traffic' which consists of commercial vehicles, cars motorbikes, fixed-wing aircraft in flight and helicopters in flight. From 2005/06 this data is recorded separately as 'traffic'.

Sources: The Chartered Institute of Environmental Health;
www.cieh.org.uk

13.22 Material flows[1]
United Kingdom

Million tonnes

		1980	1985	1990	1995	2000	2001	2002	2003	2004	2005	2006	2007	2008
Domestic extraction														
Biomass														
Agricultural harvest	JKUN	47	47	46	47	51	46	51	48	49	48	45	43	49
Timber	JKUO	4	5	6	8	8	8	8	8	8	8	8	9	8
Animal grazing	JKUP	49	48	47	45	43	43	43	43	43	43	43	43	43
Fish	JKUQ	1	1	1	1	1	1	1	1	1	1	1	1	1
Total	JKUR	101	100	101	101	103	98	103	100	101	100	98	96	102
Minerals														
Ores	JKUS	1	1	–	–	–	–	–	–	–	–	–	–	–
Clay	JKUT	25	23	21	18	15	14	14	14	15	14	13	13	13
Other industrial minerals	JKUU	11	11	11	10	8	9	8	9	8	8	8	8	8
Sand and gravel	JKUV	110	112	128	106	106	105	98	95	102	99	97	98	67
Crushed stone	JKUW	150	160	212	200	176	183	173	170	175	169	173	176	150
Total	JKUX	297	307	373	334	305	311	293	288	300	290	292	295	238
Fossil fuels														
Coal	JKUY	130	94	94	53	31	32	30	28	25	20	19	17	18
Natural gas	JKUZ	55	37	42	71	108	106	104	103	96	88	80	72	72
Crude oil	JKVA	80	128	92	130	126	117	116	106	95	85	77	77	72
Total	JKVB	266	259	228	254	266	254	250	237	217	193	175	166	162
Total domestic extraction	JKVC	664	666	702	688	673	663	645	626	618	584	565	557	502
Imports														
Biomass	JKVD	30	32	39	41	46	50	50	53	54	54	54	54	52
Minerals	JKVE	24	36	43	53	52	55	56	57	61	59	60	64	57
Fossil fuels	JKVF	76	80	95	82	93	109	105	113	138	148	159	159	152
Other products	JKVG	10	9	10	11	16	17	15	16	18	17	17	17	16
Total	JKVH	141	157	187	188	208	231	226	239	271	278	290	293	278
Exports														
Biomass	JKVI	8	11	14	16	18	14	16	20	19	20	21	21	22
Minerals	JKVJ	26	22	26	39	45	44	42	45	48	49	51	50	48
Fossil fuels	JKVK	63	105	72	111	125	127	130	114	109	99	94	90	89
Other products	JKVL	4	7	5	8	9	9	9	9	9	9	9	9	9
Total	JKVM	101	146	117	173	197	194	197	188	185	177	174	171	168
Domestic Material Consumption	JKVU	704	677	772	704	685	701	675	677	705	686	682	680	613
(domestic extraction + imports - exports)														
of which:														
Biomass	G9A8	123	121	126	126	130	133	137	133	136	134	131	128	132
Minerals	G9A9	296	320	390	348	312	323	306	300	313	301	301	309	247
Fossil fuels	G9AA	279	234	251	225	234	236	225	236	246	243	240	235	225
Indirect flows														
From domestic extraction,[2] excluding soil erosion	JKVN	643	635	703	642	576	583	566	551	548	519	487	493	492
Of which:														
Unused biomass	JKVO	32	36	37	37	41	35	40	38	39	38	36	34	39
Fossil fuels	JKVP	297	281	319	282	234	244	228	212	206	180	151	152	161
Minerals and ores	JKVQ	120	120	144	121	104	103	101	100	104	101	100	105	91
Soil excavation and dredging	JKVR	195	199	203	202	197	200	197	200	199	201	201	202	202
From production of raw materials	JKVS	368	423	457	527	614	711	648	671	692	752	792	763	701
and semi-natural products imported														
Other indicators														
Physical Trade Balance (imports - exports)[3]	DZ76	40	11	70	14	11	37	30	51	86	101	117	122	111
Direct material input														
(Domestic extraction + imports)	JKVT	805	822	889	877	882	895	872	866	890	863	856	851	781
Total material requirement														
(Direct material input + indirect flows)	JKVV	1 816	1 880	2 049	2 046	2 072	2 189	2 086	2 087	2 130	2 134	2 136	2 107	1 974

1 See chapter text. Components may not sum to totals due to rounding.
2 Indirect flows from domestic extraction relate to unused material which is
  moved during extraction, such as overburden from mining and quarrying.
3 A positive physical trade balance indicates a net import of material into the
  UK. This calculation of the PTB differs from the National Accounts formula
  (exports - imports) because flows of materials and products are considered
  the inverse of the flows of money recorded in the National Accounts.

Sources: Office for National Statistics;
environment.accounts@ons.gsi.gov.uk

Housing

Chapter 14

Housing

Permanent dwellings

(Table 14.1, 14.3)

Local housing authorities include the Commission for the New Towns and New Towns Development Corporations, Communities Scotland and the Northern Ireland Housing Executive. The figures shown for housing associations include dwellings provided by housing associations, other than the Communities Scotland and the Northern Ireland Housing Executive, and provided or authorised by government departments for the families of police, prison staff, the Armed Forces and certain other services.

Mortgage possession actions by region

(Table 14.6)

The table shows mortgage possession actions in the county courts of England and Wales and excludes a small number of mortgage actions in the High Court.

A claimant begins an action for an order for possession of a property by issuing a claim in the county court, either by using the Possession Claim Online system or locally through a county court.

In mortgage possession cases, the usual procedure is for the claim being issued to be given a hearing date before a district judge. The court, following a judicial hearing, may grant an order for possession immediately. This entitles the claimants to apply for a warrant to have the defendant evicted. However, even where a warrant for possession is issued, the parties can still negotiate a compromise to prevent eviction.

Frequently, the court grants the claimant possession but suspends the operation of the order. Provided the defendant complies with the terms of suspension, which usually require the defendant to pay the current mortgage instalments plus some of the accrued arrears, the possession order cannot be enforced.

The number of possession claims that lead to an order has replaced the old number of possession orders count. The new measure is more accurate, removing the double-counting of instances where a single claim leads to more than one order. It is also a more meaningful measure of the number of homeowners who are subject to a court repossession order.

The mortgage possession figures do not indicate how many houses have actually been repossessed through the courts. Repossessions can occur without a court order being made while not all court orders result in repossession.

A new mortgage pre-action protocol (MPAP), approved by the Master of the Rolls, was introduced for possession claims in the County Courts with effect from 19 November 2008. The MPAP gives clear guidance on what the courts expect lenders and borrowers to have done prior to a claim being issued.

The introduction of the MPAP coincided with a fall of around 50 per cent in the daily and weekly numbers of new mortgage repossession claims being issued in the courts as evidenced from administrative records. As orders are typically made (where necessary) around 8 weeks after claims are issued, the downward impact on the number of mortgage possession claims leading to an order being made was seen in the first quarter of 2009.

Households in temporary accommodation under homelessness provisions

(Table 14.9)

Comprises households in accommodation arranged by local authorities pending enquiries or after being accepted as owed a main homeless duty under the 1996 Act (includes residual cases awaiting re-housing under the 1985 Act). Excludes 'homeless at home' cases.

14.1 Stock of dwellings: [1,2] by tenure and country

Thousands

		1997	1998	1999	2000	2001	2002	2003	2004	2005	2006	2007
England[3]												
Owner occupied	JUTY	14 111	14 308	14 518	14 701	14 838	14 942	15 088	15 210	15 312	15 390	15 449
Rented	JUUC	6 511	6 470	6 410	6 374	6 369	6 395	6 393	6 426	6 493	6 601	6 739
Local Authority	JUTZ	3 401	3 309	3 178	3 012	2 812	2 706	2 457	2 335	2 166	2 086	1 987
Privately	JUUA	2 125	2 121	2 086	2 089	2 133	2 197	2 285	2 389	2 525	2 673	2 866
Registered Social Landlords	JUUB	985	1 040	1 146	1 273	1 424	1 492	1 651	1 702	1 802	1 842	1 886
All dwellings	JUUD	20 622	20 778	20 927	21 075	21 207	21 337	21 481	21 636	21 805	21 990	22 189
Wales[4]												
Owner occupied	JUUE	891	888	915	903	905	932	925	946	951	955	968
Rented	JUUI	352	363	343	364	370	350	364	352	356	359	356
Local Authority	JUUF	204	201	197	193	188	183	177	162	158	156	154
Privately	JUUG	100	112	94	117	127	110	130	125	133	137	135
Registered Social Landlords	JUUH	48	50	52	54	55	57	57	65	65	66	67
All dwellings	JUUJ	1 243	1 251	1 259	1 267	1 274	1 282	1 290	1 298	1 306	1 314	1 323
Scotland[5]												
Owner occupied	JUUK	1 366	1 400	1 435	1 472	1 446	1 479	1 514	1 544	1 555	1 570	1 587
Rented	JUUO	899	883	869	849	861	853	835	825	833	838	841
Local Authority	JUUL	630	608	583	557	553	531	416	389	374	362	347
Privately	JUUM	154	154	155	155	169	179	180	184	208	225	233
Registered Social Landlords	JUUN	115	121	131	137	139	143	238	251	251	251	261
All dwellings	JUUP	2 266	2 283	2 303	2 322	2 307	2 332	2 349	2 369	2 389	2 408	2 427
Northern Ireland[6]												
Owner occupied	JUUQ	434	446	455	488	–	481	491	501	505	508	523
Rented	JUUU	183	180	180	185	–	187	188	183	193	198	190
Local Authority	JUUR	142	137	131	129	–	120	113	100	102	99	97
Privately	JUUS	26	27	32	37	–	47	54	61	68	76	69
Registered Social Landlords	JUUT	15	16	17	19	–	20	21	22	22	23	24
All dwellings	JUUV	618	626	636	674	–	668	679	684	698	706	713
United Kingdom[7]												
Owner occupied	JUVY	16 751	16 996	17 279	17 494	17 677	17 834	18 018	18 201	18 323	18 423	18 527
Rented	JUWC	7 970	7 915	7 816	7 787	7 785	7 785	7 779	7 785	7 875	7 996	8 126
Local Authority	JUVZ	4 421	4 282	4 120	3 919	3 682	3 540	3 163	2 986	2 800	2 703	2 585
Privately	JUWA	2 402	2 413	2 361	2 393	2 466	2 533	2 649	2 759	2 934	3 111	3 303
Registered Social Landlords	JUWB	1 147	1 220	1 335	1 475	1 637	1 712	1 967	2 040	2 140	2 182	2 238
All dwellings	JUWD	24 721	24 913	25 095	25 281	25 462	25 619	25 799	25 987	26 198	26 418	26 652

1 For detailed definitions of all tenures, see Definitions of housing terms in Housing Statistics home page.
2 April data for census years are based on census output.
3 Series from 1992 to 2001 for England has been adjusted so that 2001 total dwellings estimate matches the 2001 census. Estimates from 2002 are based on local authority and Registered Social Landlord dwelling counts, and the Labour force survey (LFS). Estimates may not be strictky comparable between periods.
4 Information from 1997 onwards uses information from the Labour Force Survey (LFS) Wales.
5 Estimates up to 2000 are based on the 1991 Census. Estimates from 2001 onwards are based on the 2001 General Register Of scotland (GROS) dwelling counts and Scottish Household Survey (SHS) tenure splits are not strictly comparable.

6 To include estimates for vacant dwellings, stock figures in Northern Ireland Statistics 2006/07 table 1.3 have been apportioned according the % of occupied dwellings for each of the tenures given in table 1.4.
7 UK totals from 2002 are derived by summing country totals at 31st March. For 1991-2001 Scotland and Northern Ireland stock levels from the year before is added to the UK total. Data for earlier years are less reliable and definitions may not be consistent throughout the series. Components may not sum to totals due to rounding.

Sources: Communities and Local Government;
Welsh Assembly Government;
Scottish Executive;
Department for Social Development (Northern Ireland)

14.2 Type Of Accommodation by Tenure [1] 2008 Great Britain

Weighted Percentages

	Type of accommodation[2]							
	Detached House	Semi-detached house	Terraced	All Houses	Purpose-built flat or maisonette	Converted flat maisonette/rooms		All flats
Owner-occupied								
Owned outright	39	34	19	92	6	2		8
Owned with mortgage	27	35	30	91	6	2		9
All owners	32	34	25	92	6	2		8
Rented from social sector								
Council[3]	1	24	31	56	42	2		44
Housing association[4]	1	25	30	56	40	4		44
All rented from social sector	1	24	30	56	41	3		44
Rented privately[6]								
Unfurnished[5]	13	21	34	69	18	13		31
Furnished	6	14	35	56	30	14		44
Private renters[6]	12	20	35	66	20	13		34
All Tenures	**24**	**31**	**27**	**82**	**14**	**3**		**18**

1 Results for 2008 include longitudinal data.
2 Tables for type of accommodation exclude households living in caravans.
3 Council includes local authority.
4 Since 1996, housing associations are more correctly described as Registered Social Landlords (RSLs).

5 Unfurnished includes the answer 'partly furnished'.
6 Tenants whose accommodation goes with the job of someone in the household have been allocated to 'rented privately'. Squatters are also included.

Source: General Household Survey, Office for National Statistics

14.3 Permanent dwellings completed:[1] by tenure and country

Numbers

	United Kingdom				England and Wales			
	All dwellings	Local authorities[2]	Private enterprise	Registered Social Landlords[3][4]	All dwellings	Local authorities[2]	Private enterprise	Registered Social Landlords[3][4]
	KAAD	KAAE	KAAF	KAAG	KAAH	KAAI	KAAJ	KAAK
1980	242 000	88 530	131 990	21 480	214 940	78 540	116 180	20 220
1981	206 630	68 330	118 590	19 700	179 790	58 410	104 020	17 360
1982	182 850	40 090	129 020	13 740	159 400	33 540	113 890	11 970
1983	209 030	39 170	153 040	19 700	181 400	31 640	134 900	14 870
1984	220 410	37 570	165 560	17 290	191 110	31 340	145 260	14 510
1985	207 470	30 420	163 400	13 650	178 290	24 360	142 020	11 910
1986	216 540	25 380	178 010	13 160	187 710	20 500	156 060	11 150
1987	226 230	21 830	191 250	13 150	198 740	17 430	169 900	11 410
1988	242 360	21 450	207 420	13 490	214 160	16 920	185 740	11 500
1989	221 460	19 320	187 540	14 600	190 990	15 330	163 340	12 310
1992/93	178 872	4 430	144 420	30 160	152 450	2 710	123 040	26 700
1993/94	185 960	3 590	146 820	36 670	157 810	1 730	122 780	33 310
1994/95	197 169	3 000	156 250	37 600	168 310	990	133 000	34 310
1995/96	198 212	3 040	156 940	38 550	164 580	960	130 900	32 740
1996/97	185 654	1 540	153 450	30 590	156 340	470	128 690	27 180
1997/98	190 748	1 520	160 680	28 550	157 990	320	134 330	23 340
1998/99	178 289	870	154 560	22 870	148 000	210	127 630	20 160
1999/00	183 982	320	160 490	23 170	150 510	60	132 330	18 120
2000/01	175 220	380	152 590	22 250	141 590	230	124 030	17 330
2001/02	173 930	230	153 310	20 400	138 140	130	123 190	14 810
2002/03	183 210	300	164 300	18 610	146 050	210	131 980	13 860
2003/04	190 590	210	172 360	18 020	152 260	210	137 960	14 090
2004/05	206 620	130	184 500	21 990	164 380	130	147 120	17 140
2005/06	214 000	330	189 680	23 990	171 660	330	152 820	18 510
2006/07	219 030	260	192 130	26 650	177 010	250	154 670	22 100
2007/08[5]	216 060	330	187 230	28 500	176 800	310	153 060	23 440
2008/09	172 060	900	139 260	31 890	140 950	570	114 140	26 240

	Scotland				Northern Ireland			
	All dwellings	Local authorities[2]	Private enterprise	Registered Social Landlords[3]	All dwellings	Local authorities[2]	Private enterprise[6]	Registered Social Landlords[3]
	BLFI	BAEZ	BLFK	BLFO	BLGI	BAFA	BLGK	BLGO
1979	23 780	4 760	15 180	3 850	7 250	3 440	3 570	240
1980	20 611	7 488	12 242	881	6 456	2 563	3 568	325
1981	20 011	7 062	11 021	1 928	6 827	3 082	3 557	188
1982	16 423	3 733	11 523	1 167	7 033	3 032	3 606	395
1983	17 929	3 492	13 166	1 271	9 698	4 093	4 971	634
1984	18 838	2 647	14 115	2 076	10 464	3 594	6 177	693
1985	18 411	2 828	14 435	1 148	10 770	3 235	6 940	595
1986	18 637	2 301	14 870	1 466	10 197	2 580	7 082	535
1987	17 707	2 634	13 904	1 169	9 795	1 764	7 451	580
1988	18 272	2 815	14 179	1 278	9 931	1 715	7 511	705
1989	20 190	2 283	16 287	1 620	10 283	1 708	7 911	664
1992/93	19 520	778	15 563	3 179	7 559	992	5 759	808
1993/94	21 256	997	17 407	2 852	7 083	907	5 642	534
1994/95	22 249	1 107	18 195	2 947	7 212	877	5 859	476
1995/96	24 226	709	18 640	4 877	8 990	1 325	6 750	915
1996/97	20 486	106	17 331	3 049	9 166	860	7 373	933
1997/98	22 541	114	17 938	4 489	10 181	1 080	8 371	730
1998/99	20 635	120	18 762	1 753	9 638	538	8 140	960
1999/00	24 196	69	19 024	5 103	10 399	190	9 117	1 092
2000/01	23 434	112	18 004	5 318	11 668	44	10 512	1 112
2001/02	23 598	65	18 054	5 479	13 487	29	12 072	1 386
2002/03	23 361	94	18 572	4 695	14 415	2	13 387	1 026
2003/04	23 749	–	20 079	3 670	14 511	–	13 954	557
2004/05	25 740	–	21 720	4 020	15 760	–	14 940	830
2005/06	25 870	–	21 170	4 700	17 410	–	16 630	780
2006/07	24 060	10	20 830	3 230	17 580	–	16 250	1 330
2007/08	25 740	30	21 620	4 090	12 730	–	11 750	970
2008/09	..	..	..	..	..	..	..	..

1 See chapter text.
2 Including the Commission for the New Towns Development Corporations, Communities Scotland, the Northern Ireland Housing Executive.
3 Dwellings provided by housing associations other than Communities Scotland and the Northern Ireland Housing Trust and provided or authorised by government departments for families of police, prison staff, the armed forces and certain other services.
4 Includes non-registered social landlords.
5 Provisional.
6 Northern Ireland private enterprise completions are statistically adjusted to correct, as far as possible, the proven under recording of private sector completions in NI. This calculation has been revised for 2007/08, as such the figures and not comparable with previous years.

Sources: Communities and Local Government;
Scottish Government;
Welsh Assembly Government;
Department for Social Development, Northern Ireland

14.4 Stock of dwellings: Estimated annual gains and losses
England

Thousands of dwellings

		1997 /98	1998 /99	1999 /00	2000[2] /01	2001 /02	2002 /03	2003 /04	2004 /05	2005 /06	2006 /07	2007 /08
Dwelling stock at start of financial year	GRWM	20 622	20 778	20 927	21 075	21 207	21 337	21 481	21 636	21 805	21 992	22 191
Gains to dwelling stock:												
Housebuilding completions	GRWN	149.6	138.6	141.4	133.1	129.8	137.7	144.0	155.9	163.4	167.6	167.0
Conversions (net gain)[1]	GRWO	2.8	4.2	3.5	2.8	..	..	..	..	..	..	..
Change of use	GRWP	11.6	15.9	13.9	10.1	..	..	..	..	..	..	..
Non-permanent dwellings additions	GRWQ	0.2	0.2	0.3	0.3	..	..	..	..	..	..	..
Losses from dwelling stock:												
Slum clearance (non LA owned dwelling demolished)	GRWR	1.3	1.3	1.4	1.7	..	..	..	..	..	..	..
Other demolitions[1]	GRWS	12.8	13.2	15.8	18.3	..	..	..	..	..	..	..
Change of use	GRWT	0.7	1.4	0.8	0.7	..	..	..	..	..	..	..
Non-permanent dwelling losses	GRWU	0.1	0.2	0.1	0.3	..	..	..	..	..	..	..
New gain in year	GRWV	149.3	143.0	140.9	125.3	130.5	143.7	154.8	169.5	186.6	199.0	207.5
Adjustment[3]	VQDN	6.6	6.6	6.6	6.6	..	..	..	..	..	..	..
Dwelling stock at end of financial year	GRWW	20 778	20 927	21 075	21 207	21 337	21 481	21 636	21 805	21 992	22 191	22 399

1 Conversion figures prior to 1997/98 include change of use.
2 Figures for 2000/01 conversions, change of use and non permanent dwellings are based on reported figures and do not include estimates for missing returns.

3 Series has been adjusted so that the 2000/01 estimates matches the 2001 Census.

Source: Communities and Local Government - 020 7944 4178

14.5 Housebuilding completions: by number of bedrooms

Percentages

		1997 /98	1998 /99	1999 /00	2000 /01	2001[1] /02	2002[1] /03	2003[1] /04	2004[1] /05	2005[1] /06	2006[1] /07	2007[1] /08
England												
1 bedroom	JUWJ	7	7	7	7	7	6	8	10	10	11	11
2 bedrooms	JUWK	27	27	26	27	25	29	33	38	42	42	44
3 bedrooms	JUWL	38	36	35	34	31	30	29	28	27	27	26
4 or more bedrooms	JUWM	28	30	32	32	37	34	30	23	21	20	19
All houses and flats	JUWN	100	100	100	100	100	100	100	100	100	100	100
Wales[2]												
1 bedroom	JUWO	4	3	5	5	4	6	6	7	9	11	10
2 bedrooms	JUWP	24	21	19	18	19	18	20	21	27	28	30
3 bedrooms	JUWQ	46	46	43	42	39	35	37	35	35	33	33
4 or more bedrooms	JUWR	26	30	34	34	38	41	37	37	30	28	27
All houses and flats	JUWS	100	100	100	100	100	100	100	100	100	100	100

1 Figures for 2001/02 onwards for England only are based on just NHBC figures, so there is some degree of variability owing to partial coverage.
2 Figures for all years for Wales are based on the reports of local authority building inspectors and the National House Building Council (NHBC). It does not include information from private approved inspector.

Sources: Communities and Local Government;
Welsh Assembly Government

Housing

14.6 County Court mortgage possession actions:[1] by region

		1999	2000	2001	2002	2003	2004	2005	2006	2007	2008	2009
Claims Issued												
England and Wales	JURS	77.8	70.1	65.5	63.0	65.4	77.0	114.7	131.2	137.7	142.7	93.5
North East	JURT	4.0	4.0	3.5	3.2	3.0	3.4	5.5	7.1	8.1	8.5	5.8
North West	JURU	14.0	12.6	12.0	11.0	9.8	10.4	15.3	19.2	21.7	23.1	15.1
Yorkshire and the Humber	JURV	8.8	7.7	7.0	6.1	5.8	6.6	10.1	12.0	13.8	14.7	10.1
East Midlands	JURW	6.5	5.7	5.2	4.7	4.8	5.7	8.6	10.2	10.8	11.4	7.3
West Midlands	JURX	8.5	8.0	7.4	6.8	7.2	8.6	12.2	14.8	16.2	16.5	10.0
East	JURY	6.8	6.2	5.6	5.4	6.4	7.8	11.2	12.0	12.4	12.8	8.4
London	JURZ	8.7	7.0	7.5	8.6	10.4	13.4	21.1	21.9	20.1	19.5	12.9
South East	JUSA	9.9	9.0	8.4	8.2	9.3	11.4	16.5	17.4	17.0	17.2	11.4
South West	JUSB	5.7	4.9	4.4	4.3	4.5	5.4	7.8	8.5	8.6	9.4	6.3
England	JUSC	72.9	65.1	61.0	58.3	61.2	72.7	108.3	123.0	128.5	133.0	87.3
Wales	JUSD	5.0	5.0	4.6	4.5	4.2	4.3	6.5	8.2	9.2	9.7	6.3
Northern Ireland	JUSE	1.9	1.7	1.6	1.6	1.7	2.2	2.6	2.5	..	..	..
Claims leading to												
Suspended orders made[2,3]												
England and Wales	JUSF	31.5	29.5	28.1	24.3	23.7	25.8	37.0	43.2	41.5	52.1	33.0
North East	JUSG	2.0	2.0	1.7	1.3	1.3	1.2	1.8	2.6	2.5	3.1	2.0
North West	JUSH	5.9	5.5	5.3	4.7	3.9	3.7	5.0	6.5	6.8	8.6	5.3
Yorkshire and the Humber	JUSI	3.8	3.4	3.3	2.5	2.2	2.3	3.4	4.2	4.1	5.4	3.3
East Midlands	JUSJ	2.7	2.4	2.3	1.8	1.8	2.0	2.8	3.3	3.4	4.0	2.4
West Midlands	JUSK	3.5	3.5	3.5	2.8	2.8	3.1	4.2	5.1	5.0	6.4	3.5
East	JUSL	2.7	2.5	2.3	2.1	2.3	2.6	3.7	3.9	3.5	4.6	3.0
London	JUSM	3.1	2.6	2.7	2.7	3.2	3.9	6.3	6.9	5.8	7.0	5.0
South East	JUSN	3.9	3.6	3.3	3.0	3.2	3.7	5.3	5.7	5.1	6.0	4.2
South West	JUSO	2.2	2.0	1.8	1.6	1.6	1.8	2.6	2.8	2.5	3.5	2.1
England	JUSP	29.6	27.4	26.1	22.5	22.1	24.3	35.0	40.6	38.7	48.4	30.7
Wales	JUSQ	2.0	2.1	2.0	1.8	1.7	1.5	2.1	2.6	2.8	3.7	2.3
Northern Ireland	JUSR	0.3	0.2	0.2	0.2	0.3	0.4	0.5	0.4	..	..	..
Claims leading to Outright												
Orders made												
England and Wales	JUSS	22.0	19.0	17.7	16.1	16.1	19.6	31.9	44.8	49.2	59.7	39.3
North East	JUST	1.2	1.1	1.1	0.9	0.8	0.8	1.4	2.4	3.0	3.7	2.8
North West	JUSU	4.1	3.8	3.6	3.1	2.6	2.6	4.0	6.3	7.5	9.8	6.5
Yorkshire and the Humber	JUSV	2.6	2.3	2.2	1.7	1.6	1.7	2.8	4.1	5.0	6.3	4.6
East Midlands	JUSW	2.0	1.5	1.5	1.3	1.2	1.5	2.5	3.7	4.0	5.3	3.2
West Midlands	JUSX	2.2	2.0	2.0	1.7	1.7	2.1	3.2	4.9	5.7	7.1	4.1
East	JUSY	1.9	1.6	1.4	1.3	1.5	2.0	3.2	4.4	4.4	5.4	3.6
London	JUSZ	2.4	1.7	1.8	2.1	2.7	3.7	6.5	8.1	7.7	7.7	4.8
South East	JUTA	2.5	2.1	1.9	1.8	2.1	2.8	4.5	5.6	6.0	6.5	4.6
South West	JUTB	1.7	1.2	1.0	1.0	1.0	1.4	2.2	2.8	3.0	3.8	2.6
England	JUTC	20.5	17.5	16.4	14.9	15.0	18.5	30.2	42.3	46.1	55.6	36.7
Wales	JUTD	1.4	1.5	1.3	1.2	1.0	1.1	1.7	2.7	3.0	4.0	2.6
Northern Ireland	JUTE	0.7	0.6	0.7	0.5	0.6	0.7	0.9	0.9	..	..	..

Note: The mortgage Pre Action Protocol for possession claims relating to mortgage or home purchase arrears was introduced on 19th November 2008. It's introduction has coincided with a substantial fall in the number of new mortgage possession claims in 2008 quarter 4 and subsequently in the number of mortgage possession orders in 2009 quarter 1.

1 Includes all types of mortgage lender.
2 Where the court grants the claimant possession but suspends the operation of the order, provided the defendent complies with the terms of suspension, which usually require the defendent to pay the current mortgage plus some of the accrued arrears, the possession cannot be enforced.
3 Figures have been largely revised due to a change in the methodology as Orders are now recorded as claims leading to an Order.

Sources: Ministry of Justice 020 3334 2747; Northern Ireland Court Service: 028 9032 8594

14.7 Mortgages
United Kingdom

		1999	2000	2001	2002	2003	2004	2005	2006	2007	2008	2009
Mortgages[1] (Thousands)	JUTH	10 987	11 177	11 251	11 368	11 452	11 515	11 608	11 746	11 852	11 667	11 401
Arrears and repossessions[1] (Thousands)												
Loans in arrears at end-period												
By 6-12 months	JUTI	57	48	43	34	31	30	39	35	41	72	92
By over 12 months	JUTJ	30	21	20	17	13	11	15	16	15	30	68
Properties repossessed in period	JUTK	30	23	18	12	9	8	15	21	26	40	48

1 Estimates cover only members of the Council of Mortgage Lenders; these account for 98 per cent of all mortgages outstanding.

Source: Council of Mortgage Lenders

14.8 Sales and transfers of local authority dwellings
Great Britain

Thousands

		1996 /97	1997 /98	1998 /99	1999 /00	2000 /01	2001 /02	2002 /03	2003 /04	2004 /05	2005 /06	2006 /07	2007 /08
Right to buy sales	JUQV	45.0	58.1	56.0	66.8	71.3	66.6	78.5	94.1	74.7	41.6	26.1	19.2
Large scale voluntary transfers[1]	JUQW	29.9	21.1	36.9	88.7	111.4	100.8	102.5	104.6	67.9	81.7	82.7	117.2
Other sales and transfers[2]	JUQX	3.0	3.4	2.7	3.3	2.4	1.6	1.4	0.6	0.5	0.3	3.7	0.3
Total sales and transfers	JUQY	77.9	82.6	95.5	158.8	185.2	168.9	182.4	199.4	143.1	123.6	105.6	136.6

1 Except for 2003 large scale and voluntary transfers are included in other sales and transfers for Wales.
2 Excludes new town and Scottish Homes sales and transfers.

Sources: Communities and Local Government;
Welsh Assembly Government;
Scottish Government

14.9 Households in Temporary Accommodation[1]
Great Britain

As at 31st March of each year

Households

		1998 /99	1999 /00	2000 /01	2001 /02	2002 /03	2003 /04	2004 /05	2005 /06	2006 /07	2007 /08
Bed and breakfast hotels	JUWF	7 062	9 254	11 436	13 404	13 654	8 985	9 100	7 288	6 253	5 731
Hostels/women's refuges	JUWG	11 567	12 068	12 273	11 128	11 707	12 753	12 205	10 979	9 580	8 026
Social sector accommodation[2]	JXVN	20 686	23 510	27 826	30 310	31 719	31 821	31 295	27 758	23 463	24 756
Private sector accommodation and other[3]	JXVO	21 934	25 067	28 533	30 391	38 715	52 456	58 129	61 086	58 586	50 809
All accommodation[4]	JUWI	61 393	70 100	80 334	85 665	96 015	107 146	111 960	108 092	99 436	89 908

1 Households in temporary accommodation arranged by the local authority pending enquiries, or after being accepted as owed a main duty under homelessness legislation. Excludes 'homeless at home' cases who have remained in their existing accommodation after acceptance but have the same rights to suitable alternative housing as those in accommodation arranged directly by authorities.
2 Local authorities' and Registered Social Landlords' own stock.

3 Includes private sector properties leased by social sector landlords, households placed directly with a private sector landlord and other accommodation. From 2002 some self-contained B&B Annexe-style units, previously recorded under B&B have been more appropriately attributed to private sector accommodation.
4 Includes 'homeless at home' for Wales.

Sources: Communities and Local Government;
Welsh Assembly Government;
Scottish Government

Transport and communications

Chapter 15

Transport and communications

Road data

(Tables 15.4, 15.5, 15.6 and 15.7)

The Department for Transport has undertaken significant development work over the last two years to improve its traffic estimates and measurement of traffic flow on particular stretches of the road network. This work has previously been outlined in a number of publications (Road Traffic Statistics: 2001 SB(02)23, Traffic in Great Britain Q4 2002 Data SB(03)5 and Traffic in Great Britain Q1 2003 SB(03)6).

The main point to note is that figures for 1993 to 2004 have been calculated on a different basis from years prior to 1993. Therefore, figures prior to 1993 are not directly comparable with estimates for later years. Estimates on the new basis for 1993 and subsequent years were first published by the Department on 8 May 2003 in Traffic in Great Britain Q1 2003 SB(03)6. A summary of the main methodological changes to take place over the last couple of years appears below.

Traffic estimates are now disaggregated for roads in urban and rural areas rather than between built-up and non built-up roads. Built-up roads were defined as those with a speed limit of 40mph or lower. This created difficulties in producing meaningful disaggregated traffic estimates because an increasing number of clearly rural roads were subject to a 40mph speed limit for safety reasons. The urban/rural split of roads is largely determined by whether roads lie within the boundaries of urban areas with a population of 10,000 or more with adjustments in some cases for major roads at the boundary.

Traffic estimates are based on the results of many 12-hour manual counts in every year, which are grossed up to estimates of annual average daily flows using expansion factors based on data from automatic traffic counters on similar roads. These averages are needed so that traffic in off-peak times, at weekends and in the summer and winter months (when only special counts are undertaken) can be taken into account when assessing the traffic at each site. For this purpose roads are now sorted into 22 groupings (previously there were only seven) and this allows a better match of manual count sites with our automatic count sites. These groupings are based on a detailed analysis of the results from all the individual automatic count sites and take into account regional groupings, road category (that is both the

urban/rural classification of the road and the road class) and traffic flow levels. The groupings range from lightly-trafficked, rural minor roads in holiday areas such as Cornwall and Devon, to major roads in central London.

With the increasing interest in sub-regional statistics, we have undertaken a detailed study of traffic counts on minor roads carried out in the last ten years. This has been done in conjunction with a Geographic Information System to enable us to establish general patterns of minor road traffic in each local authority. As a result of this, we have been able to produce more reliable estimate of traffic levels in each authority in our base year of 1999. This in turn has enabled us to produce better estimates of traffic levels back to 1993, as well as more reliable estimates for 1999 onwards.

The Department created a database for major roads based on a Geographic Information System and Ordnance Survey data. This was checked by local authorities and discussed with Government Regional Offices and the Highways Agency to ensure that good local knowledge supplemented the available technical data.

Road class

(Tables 15.5 and 15.6)

Urban major and minor roads, from 1993 onwards, are defined as being within an urban area with a population of more than 10,000 people, based on the 2001 urban settlements. The definition for urban settlement can be found on the CLG web site at:

www.communities.gov.uk/planningandbuilding/planningbuilding/planningstatistics/urbanrural.

Rural major and minor roads, from 1993 onwards, are defined as being outside an urban settlement.

New vehicle registrations

(Tables 15.9)

Special concession group

Various revisions to the vehicle taxation system were introduced on 1 July 1995 and on 29 November 1995. Separate taxation classes for farmers' goods vehicles were abolished on 1 July 1995; after this date new vehicles of this type were registered as Heavy Goods Vehicles (HGVs). The total includes 5,900 vehicles registered between 1 January and 30 June in the (now abolished) agricultural and special machines group in classes which were not eligible to register in the special concession group. The old agricultural and special machines taxation group was abolished at end June 1995. The group includes agricultural and mowing machines, snow ploughs and gritting vehicles. Electric vehicles are also included in this group and are no longer exempt from Vehicle Excise Duty (VED). Steam propelled vehicles were added to this group from November 1995.

Other licensed vehicles

Includes three wheelers, pedestrian controlled vehicles, general haulage and showmen's tractors and recovery vehicles. Recovery vehicle tax class introduced January 1988.

Special vehicles group

The special vehicles group was created on 1 July 1995 and consists of various vehicle types over 3.5 tonnes gross weight but not required to pay VED as heavy goods vehicles. The group includes mobile cranes, work trucks, digging machines, road rollers and vehicles previously taxed as showman's goods and haulage. Figure shown for 1995 covers period from 1 July to 31 December only.

National Travel Survey data

(Tables 15.1, 15.11)

The National Travel Survey (NTS) is designed to provide a databank of personal travel information for Great Britain. It has been conducted as a continuous survey since July 1988, following ad hoc surveys since the mid-1960s. The survey is designed to identify long-term trends and is not suitable for monitoring short-term trends.

In 2006, a weighting strategy was introduced to the NTS and applied retrospectively to data back to 1995. The weighting methodology adjusts for non-response bias and also adjusts for the drop-off in the number of trips recorded by respondents during the course of the travel week. All results now published for 1995 onwards are based on weighted data, and direct comparisons cannot be made to earlier years or previous publications.

During 2008, over 8,000 households provided details of their personal travel by filling in travel diaries over the course of a week. The drawn sample size from 2002 was nearly trebled compared with previous years following recommendations in a National Statistics Review of the NTS. This enables most results to be presented on a single year basis from 2002.

Travel included in the NTS covers all trips by British residents within Great Britain for personal reasons, including travel in

the course of work. A trip is defined as a one-way course of travel having a single main purpose. It is the basic unit of personal travel defined in the survey. A round trip is split into two trips, with the first ending at a convenient point about half-way round as a notional stopping point for the outward destination and return origin. A stage is that portion of a trip defined by the use of a specific method of transport or of a specific ticket (a new stage being defined if either the mode or ticket changes). The main mode of a trip is that used for the longest stage of the trip. With stages of equal length the mode of the latest stage is used. Walks of less than 50 yards are excluded.

Travel details provided by respondents include trip purpose, method of travel, time of day and trip length. The households also provided personal information, such as their age, sex, working status, driving licence holding, and details of the cars available for their use.

Because estimates made from a sample survey depend on the particular sample chosen, they generally differ from the true values of the population. This is not usually a problem when considering large samples (such as all car trips in Great Britain), but it may give misleading information when considering data from small samples even after weighting.

The most recent editions of all NTS publications are available on the DfT website at: www.dft.gov.uk/transtat/personaltravel. Bulletins of key results are published annually. The most recent bulletin is *National Travel Survey: 2008*.

Households with regular use of cars

(Table 15.12)

The mid-year estimates of the percentage of households with regular use of a car or van are based on combined data from the NTS, the Expenditure and Food Survey (previously the Family Expenditure Survey) and the General Household Survey. The method for calculating these figures was changed slightly in 2006, to incorporate weighted data from the NTS and the GHS. Figures since have also been revised to incorporate weighted data. Results by area type are based on weighted data from the NTS only.

Continuing Survey of Road Goods Transport

(Tables 15.3, 15.18, 15.19)

The estimates are derived from the Continuing Survey of Road Goods Transport (CSRGT) which in 2005 was based on an average weekly returned sample of some 330 HGVs. The samples are drawn from the computerised vehicle licence records held by the Driver and Vehicle Licensing Agency.

Transport and communications

Questionnaires are sent to the registered keepers of the sampled vehicles asking for a description of the vehicle and its activity during the survey week. The estimates are grossed to the vehicle population, and at the overall national level have a 2 per cent margin of error (at 95 per cent confidence level). Further details and results are published in *Road Freight Statistics 2005*, and previously in *Transport of Goods by Road in Great Britain*.

Methodological changes

A key component of National Statistics outputs is a A key component of National Statistics outputs is a programme of quality reviews carried out at least every five years to ensure that such statistics are fit for purpose and that their quality and value continue to improve. A quality review of the Department for Transport's road freight surveys, including the CSRGT, was carried out in 2003. A copy of the report can be accessed at:

www.statistics.gov.uk/nsbase/methods_quality/quality_review/downloads/NSQR30FinalReport.doc

The quality review made a number of recommendations about the CSRGT. The main methodological recommendation was that, to improve the accuracy of survey estimates, the sample strata should be amended to reflect current trends in vehicle type, weight and legislative groups. These new strata are described more fully in Appendix C of the survey report. For practical and administrative reasons, changes were also made to the sample selection methodology (see Appendix B of the report). These changes have resulted in figures from 2004 not being fully comparable with those for 2003 and earlier years. Detailed comparisons should therefore be made with caution.

Railways: permanent way and rolling stock

(Table 15.22)

1. Locomotives - locos owned by Northern Ireland Railways (NIR), does not include those from the Republic of Ireland Railway System..

2. Diesel electric etc rail motor vehicles - powered passenger carrying vehicles, includes diesel electric (DE) power cars and all Construcciones y Auxiliar de Ferocarriles (CAF) vehicles. (Note: only 16 of the CAF sets were delivered to NIR at the time.)

3. Loco hauled coaches - NIR owned De Dietrich plus Gatwick but not including gen van.

4. Rail car trailers - 80 class and 450 class trailers. Not CAF, they are all powered.

5. Rolling stock for maintenance and repair - a 'standalone' figure - may or may not be included in the above totals. Anything listed as 'repair' or 'workshop' in the motive power sheets is included. Also, those CAF vehicles not yet delivered at the time.

6. The information is a 'snapshot' taken from the motive power sheets at end of March, together with any other known information.

Activity at civil aerodromes

(Table 15.27)

Figures exclude Channel Island and Isle of Man airports. Other covers local pleasure flights, scheduled service, positioning flights and non-transport charter flights for reward (for example: aerial survey work, crop dusting and delivery of empty aircraft). Non-commercial covers test and training flights, private, aeroclub, military and official flights, and business aviation, etc.

Postal services and television licences

(Table 15.30)

Letters posted category includes printed papers, newspapers, postcards and sample packets, where airmail includes letters without special charge for air transport..Business reply and freepost is now known as Response Services.

15.1 Trips per person per year: by sex, main mode and trip purpose[1], 2008
Great Britain

Numbers

Males

	Car	Walk	Bus and coach	Rail[2]	Other[3]	All modes
Social/entertainment	148	38	11	5	13	215
Shopping	115	43	13	2	5	177
Other escort	80	7	2	0	1	90
Other personal business	64	21	6	1	4	96
Commuting	124	14	11	17	14	180
Education	19	28	10	2	8	67
Escort education	16	8	0	0	0	25
Business	30	2	1	3	1	37
Holiday/day trip	30	2	1	1	5	40
Other, including just walk	0	42	0	0	0	42
All purpose (=100%) (number)	627	206	55	31	52	970
Base						
Unweighted Base(Trips)	104,731	35,167	8,613	4,473	8,355	161,339

Females

	Car	Walk	Bus and coach	Rail[2]	Other[3]	All modes
Social/entertainment	159	37	13	5	9	223
Shopping	139	47	25	3	5	218
Other escort	85	12	3	0	1	101
Other personal business	71	26	7	1	4	110
Communting	87	19	14	9	5	133
Education	19	23	9	1	5	57
Escort education	35	23	1	0	1	60
Business	18	2	1	2	1	24
Holiday/day trip	33	2	2	1	4	42
Other, including just walk	1	45	0	0	0	46
All purposes (numbers)	646	236	75	23	34	1014
Base						
Unweighted Base(Trips)	114,258	43,580	12,895	3,646	5,841	180,220

All persons

	Car	Walk	Bus and coach	Rail[2]	Other[3]	All modes
Social/entertainment	154	38	12	5	11	219
Shopping	127	45	19	2	5	198
Other escort	83	10	2	0	1	96
Other personal business	67	24	7	1	4	103
Commuting	105	16	13	13	10	156
Education	19	25	10	2	6	62
Escort education	26	16	1	0	0	43
Business	24	2	1	2	1	30
Holiday/daytrip	32	2	2	1	4	41
Other, including just walk	1	43	0	0	0	44
All purposes (numbers)	637	221	65	27	42	992
Base						
Unweighted Base(Trips)	218,989	78,747	21,508	8,119	14,196	341,559

1 Main mode is that used for the longest part of the trip.
2 Includes London Underground.
3 Includes bicycles, two-wheeled motor vehicles, motorcaravans, taxis/ mini-cabs, domestic air travel and other private and public transport.

Source: National Travel Survey, Department for Transport 020 7944 3097

227

Transport and communications

15.2 Retail Prices Index: transport components: 1998-2008
Great Britain

| | All items | Motor vehicles | | | | | Rail fares | Bus fares |
		Purchase	Maintenance	Petrol and oil	Tax and insurance	All motor[1]		
	ENX3	ENX4	ENX5	ZCFV	ENX6	ZCFW	ZCFX	ENX7
1998	100.0	100.0	100.0	100.0	100.0	100.0	100.0	100.0
1999	101.5	95.7	103.9	108.4	108.1	102.4	103.6	103.6
2000	104.5	90.6	108.2	122.7	119.7	106.3	105.4	107.8
2001	106.4	89.3	113.5	116.4	126.0	105.7	109.5	112.4
2002	108.2	87.5	119.4	112.7	127.9	104.9	112.0	115.8
2003	111.3	85.1	126.5	116.8	133.4	106.3	113.9	120.6
2004	114.6	82.4	134.2	123.3	134.1	107.3	118.2	126.8
2005	117.9	78.1	142.3	134.1	132.3	108.0	123.0	135.2
2006	121.6	76.0	151.0	141.5	134.0	109.6	127.9	137.1
2007	126.8	74.0	158.8	145.3	140.1	111.0	134.5	144.9
2008	131.9	68.9	168.1	167.2	144.6	114.4	140.3	153.9

1 The RPI all motor index includes purchase of a vehicle, maintenance, petrol and oil and tax and insurance.

Source: Consumer Prices and Inflation Division, ONS: 020 7944 4442

15.3 Domestic freight transport: by mode
Great Britain

		1998	1999	2000	2001	2002	2003	2004	2005	2006	2007	2008
Goods moved (billion tonnes kilometres)												
Petroleum products												
Road[1]	ZBZP	5.2	5.0	6.4	5.8	5.2	5.5	5.7	5.5	5.6	5.1	6.5
Rail[2]	ZBZQ	1.6	1.5	1.4	1.2	1.2	1.2	1.2	1.2	1.5	1.6	1.5
Water[3]	ZBZR	45.2	48.6	52.7	43.5	51.7	46.9	46.9	47.2	37.8	36.4	36.4
of which: coastwise	ZBZS	36.4	33.3	26.0	23.1	24.2	23.3	26.6	30.3	22.7	25.0	26.5
Pipeline[9]	ZBZT	11.7	11.6	11.4	11.5	10.9	10.5	10.7	10.8	10.8	10.2	10.2
All modes	ZBZU	63.7	66.7	71.9	62.0	69.0	64.1	64.5	64.7	55.8	53.3	54.6
Coal and coke												
Road[1]	ZBZV	2.0	2.2	1.5	2.1	1.5	1.5	1.2	1.5	1.3	1.6	1.0
Rail[2]	ZBZW	4.5	4.8	4.8	6.2	5.7	5.8	6.7	8.3	8.8	7.7	7.9
Water[3]	ZBZX	0.5	0.5	0.2	0.5	0.3	0.5	0.3	0.4	0.5	0.5	0.5
All modes	ZBZY	7.0	7.5	6.5	8.8	7.5	7.9	8.5	10.2	10.4	9.8	9.5
Other traffic												
Road[1]	ZBZZ	153.1	150.5	151.5	150.6	152.7	154.7	155.6	156.4	159.7	166.4	156.0
Rail[2]	ZCAA	11.2	11.9	11.9	12.0	11.7	11.9	12.5	12.2	11.8	11.9	11.2
Water[3]	ZCAB	11.20	9.60	14.60	14.80	15.20	13.50	12.30	13.30	13.49	13.90	12.70
All modes	ZCAC	175.5	172.0	178.0	177.4	179.6	180.0	180.4	181.9	185.0	192.2	179.9
All traffic												
Road[1]	KCTA	160.3	157.7	159.4	158.5	159.4	161.7	162.5	163.4	166.7	173.1	163.5
Rail[2]	KCTB	17.3	18.2	18.1	19.4	18.5	18.9	20.4	21.7	21.9	21.2	20.6
Water[3]	ZCAD	56.90	58.70	67.40	58.80	67.20	60.90	59.45	60.87	51.85	50.80	49.70
Pipeline	KCTE	11.7	11.6	11.4	11.5	10.9	10.5	10.7	10.8	10.8	10.2	10.2
All modes	KCTF	246.2	246.2	256.3	248.2	256.0	252.0	253.0	256.8	251.3	255.3	244.0
Percentage of all traffic												
Road[1]	ZCAE	*65*	*64*	*62*	*64*	*62*	*64*	*64*	*64*	*66*	*68*	*67*
Rail[2]	ZCAF	*7*	*7*	*7*	*8*	*7*	*7*	*8*	*8*	*9*	*8*	*8*
Water[3]	ZCAG	*23*	*24*	*26*	*24*	*26*	*24*	*23*	*24*	*21*	*20*	*20*
Pipeline	ZCAH	*5*	*5*	*4*	*5*	*4*	*4*	*4*	*4*	*4*	*4*	*4*
All modes	ZCAI	*100*	*100*	*100*	*100*	*100*	*100*	*100*	*100*	*100*	*100*	*100*
Goods lifted (million tonnes)												
Petroleum products												
Road[1]	ZCAJ	61	61	75	74	59	64	67	70	69	71	80
Rail[2]	ZCAK	..	..	..	..	..	..	..	..	..	..	..
Water[3]	ZCAL	76	72	72	60	67	64	63	66	57	56	58
of which: coastwise	ZCAM	55	52	40	34	36	35	38	42	34	35	36
Pipeline[9]	ZCAN	153	155	151	151	146	141	158	168	159	146	147
All modes[4]	ZCAO	290	288	298	285	272	269	288	304	285	274	285
Coal and coke												
Road[1]	ZCAP	26	28	22	21	17	22	14	21	17	24	15
Rail[2]	ZCAQ	45	36	35	40	34	35	43	48	49	43	47
Water[3]	ZCAR	3	3	3	3	2	2	1	2	2	2	2
All modes	ZCAS	70	75	60	64	53	59	67	72	68	69	63
Other traffic												
Road[1]	ZCAT	1 640	1 575	1 596	1 587	1 658	1 667	1 782	1 777	1 854	1 906	1 773
Rail[2]	ZCAU	57	61	60	55	53	54	57	58	59	59	56
Water[3]	ZCAV	70	70	62	68	70	67	63	65	66	68	63
All modes	ZCAW	1 767	1 706	1 718	1 710	1 781	1 788	1 902	1 901	1 980	2 032	1 892
All traffic												
Road[1]	KCTG	1 727	1 664	1 693	1 682	1 734	1 753	1 863	1 868	1 940	2 001	1 868
Rail[2]	KCTH	102	97	96	94	87	89	100[6]	105[7]	108[7]	102[8]	103
Water[3]	ZCAX	149.0	144.0	137.0	131.0	139.0	133.0	127.0	133.0	126.0	126.0	123.0
Pipeline	KCTK	153.0	155.0	151.0	151.0	146.0	141.0	158.0	168.0	159.0	146.0	147.0
All modes	KCTL	2 131	2 060	2 077	2 058	2 106	2 116	2 249	2 275	2 333	2 376	2 241
Percentage of all traffic												
Road[1]	ZCAY	*81*	*81*	*82*	*82*	*82*	*83*	*83*	*82*	*83*	*84*	*83*
Rail[2]	ZCAZ	*5*	*5*	*5*	*5*	*4*	*4*	*4*	*5*	*5*	*4*	*5*
Water[3]	ZCBA	*7*	*7*	*7*	*6*	*7*	*6*	*6*	*6*	*5*	*5*	*5*
Pipeline	ZCBB	*7*	*8*	*7*	*7*	*7*	*7*	*7*	*7*	*7*	*6*	*7*
All modes	ZCBC	*100*	*100*	*100*	*100*	*100*	*100*	*100*	*100*	*100*	*100*	*100*

1 All goods vehicles, including those up to 3.5 tonnes gross vehicle weight.
2 Figures for rail are for financial years (e.g 1998 will be 1998/99).
3 Figures for water are for UK traffic.
4 Excludes rail.
5 See footnote 2 Table 4.4 - TSGB publication.
6 See footnote 6 Table 4.1 - TSGB publication.
7 There is a break in the series between 2003-04 and 2004-05, due to a change in the method of data collection.
8 There is a break in the series between 2006-07 and 2007-08 because coal data was not supplied by GB Railfreight prior to 2007-08.
9 Some data for 2008 is based on estmates - this survey is currently under review by DECC to improve data quality.

Sources: Department for Transport;
Rail: 020 7944 4977;
Road 020 7944 4261;
Water: 020 7944 3087;
Pipeline : 020 7215 2718;
Sources - Rail : ORR;
Pipeline : Department for Business Enterprise and Regulatory Reform

Transport and communications

15.4 Passenger transport by mode
Great Britain

		1998	1999	2000	2001	2002	2003	2004	2005	2006	2007	2008
Billion passenger kilometres												
Road												
Buses and coaches	GRXK	45	46	47	47	47	47	48	48	50	50	..
Cars, vans and taxis	GRXG	636	642	640	654	677	673	678	674	682	685	679
Motor cycles	GRXH	4	5	5	5	5	6	6	6	6	6	6
Pedal cycles	GRXI	4	4	4	4	4	5	4	4	5	4	5
All road	GRXJ	689	697	695	710	733	731	736	733	746	749	..
Rail[1]	KCTN	44	46	47	47	48	49	50	52	55	59	51
Air	KCTM	7.0	7.0	8.0	8.0	8.0	9.0	10.0	10.0	10.0	10.0	9.0
All modes[2]	GRXM	740	751	749	765	790	789	796	794	811	817	..
Percentages												
Road												
Buses and coaches	GRXN	6	6	6	6	6	6	6	6	6	6	..
Cars, vans and taxis	GRXO	86	86	85	85	86	85	85	85	85	84	..
Motor cycles	GRXP	1	1	1	1	1	1	1	1	1	1	..
Pedal cycles	GRXQ	1	1	1	1	1	1	–	1	1	1	..
All road	GRXR	93	93	93	93	93	93	92	92	92	92	..
Rail[1]	ZCBJ	6	6	6	6	6	6	6	7	7	7	..
Air	ZCBK	1.0	1.0	1.0	1.0	1.0	1.0	1.0	1.0	1.0	1.0	..
All modes[2]	GRXU	100	100	100	100	100	100	100	100	100	100	..

Note: Bus and coach data not available at time of going to press and rail data for 2008 excludes urban metros.
1 Financial years. National Rail, urban metros and modern trams
2 Excluding travel by water

Sources: Bus & coach: 020 7944 3076;
Car, m/cycle & pedal cycle: 020 7944 3097;
Rail: 020 7944 3076;
Air: 020 7944 3088;
Rail : ORR Air : CAA

15.5 Motor vehicle traffic: by road class: 1996-2006
Great Britain

Billion vehicle kilometres

		1998	1999	2000[1]	2001[2]	2002	2003	2004	2005	2006[6]	2007	2008
Motorways	JSZV	85.7	87.8	88.4	90.8	92.6	93.0	96.6	97.0	99.4	100.6	100.1
Rural 'A' roads[3]												
Trunk[5]	JSZW	63.3	64.7	64.2	65.9	64.6	61.5	59.7	58.0	59.2	58.6	58.6
Principal[5]	JSZX	65.4	66.0	65.8	67.4	71.8	77.7	81.6	83.3	84.4	84.9	84.2
All rural 'A' roads	JSZY	128.7	130.7	130.0	133.3	136.4	139.3	141.3	141.3	143.6	143.5	142.8
Urban 'A' roads[4]												
Trunk[5]	JSZZ	13.8	14.0	14.0	7.6	7.4	6.7	6.0	5.5	5.6	5.4	5.5
Principal[5]	JTAA	67.5	67.9	67.7	74.2	74.8	75.1	76.8	76.2	76.9	75.9	74.6
All urban 'A' roads	JTAB	81.3	81.9	81.7	81.8	82.2	81.7	82.8	81.7	82.5	81.3	80.1
All Major Roads	I45C	295.7	300.4	300.0	305.9	311.2	314.0	320.7	320.1	325.5	325.4	323.0
Minor roads												
Minor rural roads	JTAC	60.4	61.3	61.5	61.6	64.5	64.4	65.9	66.8	69.3	72.0	72.2
Minor urban roads	JTAD	102.4	105.3	105.5	106.9	110.8	111.9	112.0	112.5	112.7	115.5	113.7
All minor roads	JTAE	162.8	166.6	167.0	168.5	175.3	176.4	177.9	179.3	182.0	187.5	185.9
All roads	JTAF	458.5	467.0	467.1	474.4	486.5	490.4	498.6	499.4	507.5	513.0	508.9

1 The decline in the use of cars and taxis in 2000 was due to the fuel dispute.
2 Figures affected by the impact of Foot and Mouth disease during 2001.
3 Rural roads; Major and minor roads, from 1993 onwards, are defined as being outside an urban area. (see definition below).
4 Urban roads; Major and minor roads, from 1993 onwards, are defined as within an urban area with a population of 10,000 or more. These are based on the 2001 urban settlements. The definition for 'urban settlement' is in Urban and Rural area definitions: a user guide which can be found on the Department for Communities and Local Government web site at: http://www.communities.gov.uk/publications/planningandbuilding/urbanrural
5 Figures for trunk and principal 'A' roads in England, from 2001 onwards are affected by the detrunking programme.

Source: Department for Transport: 020 7944 3095

15.6 Public road length:[1] by road type
Great Britain

Kilometres

		1998	1999	2000	2001	2002	2003	2004	2005	2006	2007	2008
Trunk motorway	JSZD	3 376	3 404	3 422	3 431	3 433	3 432	3 478	3 466	3 503	3 518	3 518
Principal motorway	JSZE	44	45	45	45	45	46	46	54	53	41	41
Rural 'A' roads[2]:												
Trunk[3]	JSZF	10 585	10 611	10 627	10 607	9 973	9 027	8 641	8 239	8 277	8 258	8 213
Principal[3]	JSZG	24 783	24 852	24 866	24 915	25 559	26 498	26 889	27 312	27 336	27 346	27 372
All rural 'A' roads	JSZH	35 369	35 463	35 493	35 522	35 532	35 525	35 530	35 550	35 612	35 603	35 586
Urban 'A' roads[4]:												
Trunk[3]	JSZI	1 096	1 087	1 074	762	705	587	506	444	446	425	420
Principal[3]	JSZJ	9 931	10 019	10 040	10 370	10 436	10 539	10 632	10 663	10 696	10 714	10 685
All urban 'A' roads	JSZK	11 027	11 106	11 114	11 132	11 141	11 127	11 138	11 107	11 143	11 139	11 105
Minor rural roads[5]:												
B roads	JSZL	24 586	24 579	24 570	24 562	24 554	24 547	24 640	24 639	24 574	24 795	24 685
C roads	JSZM	73 405	73 500	73 593	73 688	73 783	73 878	73 363	73 581	73 548	73 480	73 582
Unclassified	JSZN	111 132	111 350	111 568	111 787	112 006	112 231	109 561	109 426	115 250	115 365	115 032
All minor rural roads	JSZO	209 123	209 429	209 731	210 037	210 343	210 656	207 565	207 646	213 371	213 641	213 299
Minor urban roads[5]:												
B roads	JSZP	5 622	5 626	5 630	5 633	5 638	5 641	5 538	5 550	5 445	5 470	5 476
C roads	JSZQ	10 986	11 009	11 031	11 054	11 076	11 098	10 859	10 878	10 921	10 942	10 992
Unclassified	JSZR	113 093	113 432	113 772	114 114	114 456	114 816	113 520	113 757	114 355	114 524	114 450
All minor urban roads	JSZS	129 702.0	130 068.0	130 432.0	130 802.0	131 169.0	131 556.0	129 917.0	130 186.0	130 721.0	130 936.0	130 917.0
All major roads	GG5B	49 816	50 018	50 074	50 130	50 152	50 130	50 192	50 176	50 310	50 302	50 250
All minor roads[5]	JSZT	338 825	339 496	340 163	340 838	341 512	342 212	337 482	337 832	344 092	344 577	344 217
All roads	JSZU	388 641	389 515	390 237	390 969	391 663	392 342	387 674	388 008	394 402	394 879	394 467

1 A number of minor revisions have been made to the lengths of major roads from 1993 onwards.
2 Rural roads: Major and minor roads, from 1993 onwards, are defined as being outside an urban area.
3 Figures for trunk and principal 'A' roads in England, from 2001 onwards, are affected by the detrunking programme.

4 Urban roads: Major and minor roads, from 1993 onwards, are defined as within an urban area with a population of 10,000 or more. These are based on the 2001 urban settlements. The definition for 'urban settlement' is in *Urban and rural area definitions : a user guide* which can be found on the Department for Communities and Local Government web site at : http//www.communities.gov.uk/publications/planningandbuilding/urbanrural
5 New information from 2004 and from 2006 has enabled better estimates of minor road lengths to be made.

Sources: National Road Traffic Survey;
Department for Transport 020 7944 3095

15.7 Road traffic: by type of vehicle
Great Britain

Billion vehicle kilometres

		1998	1999	2000[1]	2001[2]	2002	2003	2004	2005	2006	2007[3]	2008
Cars and taxis	JTAH	370.6	377.4	376.8	382.8	392.9	393.1	398.1	397.2	402.6	404.1	401.7
Motor cycles etc.	JTAI	4.1	4.5	4.6	4.8	5.1	5.6	5.2	5.4	5.2	5.6	5.1
Larger buses and coaches	JTAJ	5.2	5.3	5.2	5.2	5.2	5.4	5.2	5.2	5.4	5.5	5.2
Light vans[4]	JTAK	50.8	51.6	52.3	53.7	55.0	57.9	60.8	62.6	65.2	68.4	68.1
Goods vehicles[5]:												
2 axles rigid	JTAL	11.1	11.6	11.7	11.5	11.6	11.7	11.7	11.5	11.3	11.1	10.7
3 axles rigid	JTAM	1.9	1.7	1.7	1.8	1.8	1.8	1.9	1.9	1.9	2.0	2.0
4 or more axles rigid	JTAN	1.6	1.5	1.5	1.5	1.5	1.6	1.6	1.7	1.7	1.8	1.9
3 and 4 axles artic	JTAO	3.0	3.0	2.7	2.5	2.3	2.2	2.2	2.0	1.9	1.8	1.6
5 axles artic	JTAP	7.3	7.2	6.7	6.4	6.4	6.2	6.5	6.4	6.6	6.6	6.5
6 or more axles artic	JTAQ	2.9	3.3	4.1	4.5	4.8	5.0	5.4	5.5	5.7	6.1	6.0
All	JTAR	27.7	28.1	28.2	28.1	28.3	28.5	29.4	29.0	29.1	29.4	28.7
All motor vehicles	JURA	458.5	467.0	467.1	474.4	486.5	490.4	498.6	499.4	507.5	513.0	508.9
Pedal cycles	JURB	4.0	4.1	4.2	4.2	4.4	4.5	4.2	4.4	4.6	4.2	4.7

1 The decline in the use of cars and taxis in 2000 was due to the fuel dispute.
2 Figures affected by the impact of Foot and Mouth disease during 2001.
3 Data for 'Light vans' and 'Larger buses and coaches' for 2007 have been revised.
4 Not exceeding 3,500 kgs gross vehicle weight.
5 Over 3,500 kgs gross vehicle weight.

Sources: National Road Traffic Survey;
Department for Transport 020 7944 3095

15.8 Motor vehicles licensed by tax class: by method of propulsion, 2008
By taxation class

Thousand

	Petrol	Diesel	Gas/petroleum	Gas bi-fuel/Gas diesel	Hybrid-electric	Other[1]	All
Private and light goods	20 140	10 075	30	31	47	-	30 324
ow: body type cars	19 959	6 966	27	21	47	-	27 021
Motorcycles, scooters and mopeds	1 158	1	-	0	0	1	1 160
Bus	1	110	-	0	0	0	111
Goods	1	435	-	0	0	0	436
Special vehicles group	-	53	1	1	-	-	56
Other non-exempt vehicles	12	17	-	0	0	0	29
Exempt vehicles	1 322	727	2	1	-	38	2 091
ow: former Special concessionary group	17	283	-	0	0	8	308
Total All Vehicles	22 634	11 419	34	33	47	39	34 206

1 Other comprises electricity, steam, new fuel technologies, electric diesel and fuel cells.

Source: Department for Transport: 020 7944 3077

15.9 New vehicle registrations by taxation class
Great Britain

Thousands

		1998	1999	2000	2001	2002	2003	2004	2005	2006	2007	2008
Cars	BMAA	2 123.5	2 100.4	2 174.9	2 426.4	2 528.9	2 497.1	2 437.5	2 266.2	2 241.7	2 191.4	1 891.9
Other Vehicles	BMAE	244.5	241.6	254.9	278.0	286.9	323.5	347.2	337.0	338.4	348.0	296.4
Motor Cycles, Scooters and Mopeds	BMAL	143.3	168.4	182.9	177.5	162.3	157.3	133.7	132.1	131.9	143.0	138.4
Goods	BBJY	49.1	48.3	50.4	49.0	44.9	48.4	48.0	51.3	47.9	41.2	47.0
Buses	BBJZ	7.4	8.0	7.5	7.1	7.7	8.4	8.1	8.9	7.6	9.1	8.3
Other Vehicles[1]	I8B3	157.0	174.0	176.0	169.0	192.0	189.0	204.0	218.0	219.0	265.0	..
All Vehicles	BBKD	2 740.3	2 765.8	2 870.9	3 136.6	3 229.5	3 231.9	3 185.3	3 021.4	2 913.6	2 996.9	2 672.2

1 Includes three wheelers, special machines, special concessionary, special vehicles and crown and exempt vehicles.

Source: Department for Transport: 020 7944 3077

15.10 Driving test pass rates: by sex and type of vehicle licence
Great Britain

Percentages

		1989 /90	1991 /92	1998 /99	2001 /02	2002 /03	2003 /04	2004 /05	2005 /06	2006 /07	2007 /08	2008 /09
Males												
Motorcycle	JTRB	72	69	69	67	66	67	66	66	67	68	68
Car	JTRC	58	57	51	47	47	46	46	46	46	47	49
Bus	JTTG	–	–	48	46	44	46	46	43	43	50	51
Lorry	JTTH	–	–	52	50	50	49	47	45	46	46	49
All males	JTTI	–	–	–	50	49	48	47	47	48	49	50
Females												
Motorcycle	JTTJ	68	63	63	55	54	53	53	52	54	56	55
Car	JTTK	47	46	42	40	40	40	39	40	41	41	42
Bus	JTTL	–	–	47	40	40	45	46	47	49	53	55
Lorry	JTTM	–	–	50	47	46	48	45	45	47	48	52
All females	JTTN	–	–	–	41	40	40	40	40	41	42	42
All												
Motorcycle	JTTO	–	–	68	66	65	65	64	64	65	67	66
Car	JTTP	–	–	46	43	43	43	42	42	43	44	45
Bus	JTTQ	–	–	48	45	44	46	44	43	44	50	52
Lorry	JTTR	–	–	52	56	49	49	46	45	46	46	49
All persons	JTTS	–	–	–	46	45	44	43	44	44	45	47

Source: Driving Standards Agency - info.rsis@dsa.gov.uk

15.11 Full car driving licence holders by sex and age[1]
Great Britain

Percentages and millions

	All aged 17+	17-20	21-29	30-39	40-49	50-59	60-69	70 and over	Estimated number of licence holders (millions)
All adults									
1975/76	48	28	59	67	60	50	35	15	19.4
1985/86	57	33	63	74	71	60	47	27	24.3
1989/91	64	43	72	77	78	67	54	32	27.8
1992/94	67	48	75	82	79	72	57	33	29.3
1995/97[2]	69	43	74	81	81	75	63	38	30.3
1998/00	71	41	75	84	83	77	67	39	31.4
	GB9O	C98J	C98K	C98L	C98M	C98N	C98O	C98P	C98Q
2005	72	32	66	82	84	82	74	51	33.3
2006	72	34	67	82	84	82	76	50	33.7
2007	71	38	66	81	83	82	75	52	33.8
2008	72	36	64	82	83	83	78	53	34.5
Males									
1975/76	69	36	78	85	83	75	58	32	13.4
1985/86	74	37	73	86	87	81	72	51	15.1
1989/91	80	52	82	88	89	85	78	58	16.7
1992/94	81	54	83	91	88	88	81	59	17.0
1995/97[2]	81	50	80	88	89	89	83	65	17.2
1998/00	82	44	80	89	91	88	83	65	17.4
	GB9P	C98R	C98S	C98T	C98U	C98V	C98W	C98X	C98Y
2005	81	37	69	86	90	90	88	73	18.1
2006	81	37	71	86	89	91	90	76	18.4
2007	80	41	69	86	88	90	87	75	18.4
2008	81	38	67	87	89	91	90	75	18.7
Females									
1975/76	29	20	43	48	37	24	15	4	6.0
1985/86	41	29	54	62	56	41	24	11	9.2
1989/91	49	35	64	67	66	49	33	15	11.1
1992/94	54	42	68	73	70	57	37	16	12.2
1995/97[2]	57	36	67	74	73	62	45	21	13.1
1998/00	60	38	69	78	76	67	53	22	14.0
	GB9Q	C98Z	C992	C993	C994	C995	C996	C997	C998
2005	63	27	62	77	79	73	61	35	15.2
2006	63	31	63	78	79	74	63	31	15.3
2007	63	34	62	76	78	74	63	36	15.4
2008	65	35	61	78	78	75	67	36	15.8

1 See chapter text.
2 Based on combined survey data sources - Family Expenditure Survey, ONS; General Household Survey, ONS and National Travel Survey, DfT.

Source: National Travel Survey, Department for Transport 020 7944 3097

15.12 Households with regular use of cars[1]
Great Britain

Percentages and millions

	No car	One car	Two cars	Three or more cars	Total (millions)
	ZCGA	ZCGB	ZCGC	ZCGD	ZCGE
1997	30	45	21	5	23.1
1998	28	44	23	5	23.3
1999	28	44	22	5	23.5
2000	27	45	23	5	23.7
2001	26	45	23	5	23.9
2002	26	44	24	5	24.2
2003	26	44	25	5	24.4
2004	25	44	25	5	24.6
2005	25	44	25	5	..
2006	24	44	26	6	25.1
2007	24	44	26	6	..

	No car	One car	Two or more cars	Total
Government Office Regions, 2007[2]				
Great Britain	24	44	32	100
North East	29	44	27	100
North West	26	42	32	100
Yorkshire and The Humber	27	42	30	100
East Midlands	20	45	35	100
West Midlands	21	42	37	100
East	15	45	40	100
London	38	43	18	100
South East	17	43	40	100
South West	17	45	38	100
England	24	43	33	100
Wales	23	46	31	100
Scotland	29	45	26	100
Northern Ireland				100

	No car	One car	Two or more cars	Total
Area type, 2008				
Great Britain	25	43	32	100
London	43	40	17	100
Metropolitan areas	32	41	26	100
Other urban areas with population:				
Over 250,000	23	45	32	100
25,000 - 250,000	24	44	32	100
10,000 - 25,000	23	45	32	100
3,000 - 10,000	16	42	42	100
Rural areas	10	43	47	100

1 Includes cars and light vans normally available to the household.
2 Based on combined survey data sources - Family Expenditure Survey, ONS; General Household Survey, ONS and National Travel Survey, DfT.

Sources: Office for National Statistics; Department for Transport 020 7944 3097

15.13 Vehicles with current licences[1]
Northern Ireland

Numbers

		1998	1999	2000	2001[3]	2002	2003[4]	2004	2005	2006	2007	2008
Private light goods, etc	KNKA	584 706	608 316	615 180	644 968	666 731	711 913	737 198	765 061	800 969	840 621	857 044
Motorcycles, Scooters and mopeds	KNKB	11 663	13 087	14 116	15 205	17 598	23 820	24 533	25 998	27 083	28 150	28 180
Public road passenger vehicles[2]:												
Taxis,buses,coaches	KNKD	..	..	..	..	..	..	..	..	..	..	..
Buses, coaches (9 seats or more)	KNKE	2 175	2 204	2 266	2 315	2 322	2 353	2 378	2 566	2 670	2 865	2 951
Total	KNKC	2 175	2 204	2 266	2 315	2 322	2 353	2 378	2 566	2 670	2 865	2 951
General (HGV) goods vehicles:	KNKF	18 312	17 075	17 864	19 415	20 244	22 100	23 062	23 517	24 806	25 785	25 136
Agricultural tractors and engines, etc[3]	KNKM	5 906	5 505	5 048	4 901	5 731	7 503	8 674	9 584	10 586	12 817	14 326
Other	KNKN	1 193	1 446	1 287	1 366	1 347	1 671	1 794	1 898	2 039	2 125	2 232
Vehicles exempt from duty:												
Government owned	KNKP	3 785	4 032	3 822	6 427	6 383	6 172	6 116	6 367	7 315	9 655	6 902
Other:												
Ambulances	KNKQ	425	417	452	318	299	325	355	355	388	378	390
Fire engines	KNKR	285	286	290	181	174	170	178	179	166	155	142
Other exempt[4]	KNKS	66 981	68 277	70 405	72 209	73 648	76 715	78 973	81 874	82 655	85 738	87 093
Total	KNKO	71 476	73 012	74 969	79 135	80 504	83 382	85 622	88 775	90 524	95 926	94 527
Total	KNKT	695 431	720 645	730 730	767 305	794 477	852 742	883 261	917 399	958 677	1 008 289	1 024 396

1 Licences current at 31 December.
2 Tax class change from 'Hackney' to 'Bus' with effect from July 2005. Only Vehicles with 9 or more seats are included in 'Bus' class. Vehicles with 8 seats or less previously recorded in ' Hackney ' class moved into 'Private Light Goods' class.
3 Taxation classes have been revised
4 New Tax Class 36 introduced.

Source: Driver and Vehicle Agency: 028 7034 6903

15.14 New vehicle registrations
Northern Ireland

Numbers

		1998	1999	2000	2001	2002	2003	2004	2005	2006	2007	2008
Private cars	KNLA	91 141	89 078	84 973	88 592	83 402	87 506	85 190	86 366	91 224	97 346	78 864
Motorcycles	KNLB	4 307	5 310	6 010	5 591	5 596	6 804	4 601	4 648	4 289	4 477	3 985
Public road passenger vehicles	KNLC	486	568	565	451	439	609	467	621	677	629	677
Goods vehicles:												
General haulage vehicles:												
Under 3.5 tonnes	KNLH	10 107	11 054	12 617	13 274	12 007	11 492	11 090	12 300	13 457	13 855	11 451
3.5 tonnes and over	KNLJ	3 572	3 697	3 502	4 534	3 669	4 059	3 987	3 768	4 080	3 676	2 923
Agricultural tractors[1]	KNLM	971	987	1 313	301	1	9	2	2	8	–	1
Vehicles exempt from duty	KNLR	10 718	11 081	10 789	12 126	12 515	11 907	12 881	13 987	13 031	14 083	14 846
General haulage and special types	JTAG	..	..	..	..	15	12	11	16	32	46	16
Total	KNLS	121 302	121 777	119 769	124 869	117 644	122 398	118 229	121 708	126 798	134 112	112 763

1 Agricultural tractors driven on public roads. From April 2001 tractors were exempt.

Source: Driver and Vehicle Agency : 028 7034 6903

15.15 Local bus services: passenger journeys by area: 1998/99-2008/09

Millions

		1998 /99	1999 /00	2000 /01	2001 /02	2002 /03	2003 /04	2004 /05	2005 /06	2006[1] /07	2007[2] /08	2008[2] /09
Great Britain	ZCET	4 350	4 376	4 420	4 455	4 550	4 681	4 737	4 791	5 097	5 163	5 233
London	KILS	1 266	1 294	1 347	1 422	1 527	1 692	1 802	1 881	1 993	2 089	2 149
English Metropolitan Counties	KILT	1 256	1 213	1 203	1 196	1 182	1 162	1 128	1 111	1 141	1 104	1 111
English other areas	KILU	1 286	1 297	1 292	1 263	1 255	1 233	1 210	1 204	1 336	1 328	1 335
All outside London	ZCES	3 084	3 082	3 073	3 033	3 023	2 989	2 935	2 910	3 104	3 074	3 084
England	ZCER	3 808	3 804	3 842	3 881	3 964	4 087	4 140	4 196	4 470	4 522	4 594
Scotland	KILV	424	455	458	466	471	478	479	477	506	517	515
Wales	KILW	118	117	119	108	115	116	118	118	122	124	124

1 There is a break in the series after 2006/07.
2 Provisional data.

Source: Department for Transport 020 7944 3076

Transport and communications

15.16 Local bus services: fare indices: by area:1998/99-2008/09
Current prices

Indices (1995=100)

		1998 /99	1999 /00	2000 /01	2001 /02	2002 /03	2003 /04	2004 /05	2005 /06	2006 /07	2007 /08	2008 /09
Great Britain	KNEU	117.1	121.8	126.4	130.6	134.5	139.2	146.5	157.5	159.0	167.6	176.2
London	KNEP	113.8	117.2	117.3	115.5	114.8	116.9	126.8	139.7	151.5	159.5	160.2
English Metropolitan Counties	KILD	117.9	123.5	128.6	135.5	140.7	146.7	153.3	166.0	168.3	178.3	190.3
English other areas	KILE	117.3	122.6	129.2	136.1	142.4	149.0	155.9	166.2	159.5	168.0	178.6
All outside London	ZCEQ	118.2	123.2	129.0	135.1	140.4	146.0	152.3	162.2	160.7	169.1	180.1
England	ZCEP	116.4	121.4	125.8	130.3	134.3	139.4	147.2	159.4	160.1	169.1	177.4
Scotland	KILF	121.2	124.1	129.1	131.1	133.8	136.1	140.0	143.9	151.0	155.7	166.7
Wales	KILG	116.0	121.9	128.4	135.7	142.3	147.2	153.7	159.9	169.7	177.8	188.1
Retail Prices Index (1995=100)	KNEV	109.9	111.6	114.9	116.6	119.1	122.4	126.2	129.5	134.4	139.9	144.1

Source: Department for Transport 020 7944 4139

15.17 Road accident casualties: by road user type and severity
Great Britain

Numbers

		1998	1999	2000	2001	2002	2003	2004	2005	2006	2007	2008
Child pedestrians[1]:												
Killed	ZCDH	103	107	107	107	79	74	77	63	71	57	57
Killed or seriously injured	KIJS	3 737	3 457	3 226	3 144	2 828	2 381	2 339	2 134	2 025	1 899	1 784
All severities	ZCDI	17 971	16 876	16 184	15 819	14 231	12 544	12 234	11 250	10 131	9 527	8 648
Adult pedestrians[2]:												
Killed	ZCDJ	803	760	750	712	688	695	589	604	602	585	515
Killed or seriously injured	KIJT	6 592	6 221	6 112	5 745	5 644	5 422	5 005	4 847	4 894	4 900	4 724
All severities	ZCDK	25 827	24 806	24 481	23 463	23 258	22 531	21 404	20 725	19 774	19 676	19 013
Child pedal cyclists[1]:												
Killed	ZCDL	32	36	27	25	22	18	25	20	31	13	12
Killed or seriously injured	KIJU	915	950	758	674	594	595	577	527	503	522	417
All severities	ZCDM	6 930	7 290	6 260	5 451	4 809	4 769	4 682	4 286	3 765	3 633	3 306
Adult pedal cyclists[2]:												
Killed	ZCDN	126	135	98	111	107	95	109	127	115	122	103
Killed or seriously injured	KIJV	2 345	2 172	1 954	1 951	1 801	1 776	1 697	1 787	1 898	1 994	2 101
All severities	ZCDO	15 326	14 834	13 630	12 974	11 712	11 643	11 366	11 637	11 911	12 050	12 546
Motorcyclists[3] and passengers:												
Killed	ZCDP	498	547	605	583	609	693	585	569	599	588	493
Killed or seriously injured	ZCDQ	6 442	6 908	7 374	7 305	7 500	7 652	6 648	6 508	6 484	6 737	6 049
All severities	BMDH	24 610	26 192	28 212	28 810	28 353	28 411	25 641	24 824	23 326	23 459	21 550
Car drivers and passengers:												
Killed	ZCDS	1 696	1 687	1 665	1 749	1 747	1 769	1 671	1 675	1 612	1 432	1 257
Killed or seriously injured	ZCDT	21 676	20 368	19 719	19 424	18 728	17 291	16 144	14 617	14 254	12 967	11 968
All severities	ZCDU	210 474	205 735	206 799	202 802	197 425	188 342	183 858	178 302	171 000	161 433	149 188
Bus/coach drivers and passengers:												
Killed	ZCDV	18	11	15	14	19	11	20	9	19	12	6
Killed or seriously injured	KCUZ	631	611	578	562	551	500	488	363	426	455	432
All severities	ZCDW	9 839	10 252	10 088	9 884	9 005	9 068	8 820	7 920	7 253	7 079	6 929
LGV drivers and passengers:												
Killed	ZCDX	67	65	66	64	70	72	62	54	52	58	43
Killed or seriously injured	ZCDY	949	867	813	811	780	765	631	587	564	494	445
All severities	ZCDZ	7 672	7 124	7 007	7 304	7 007	6 897	6 166	6 048	5 914	5 340	4 913
HGV drivers and passengers:												
Killed	ZCEA	60	52	55	54	63	44	47	55	39	52	23
Killed or seriously injured	ZCEB	560	540	571	500	524	429	406	395	383	363	240
All severities	ZCEC	3 444	3 484	3 597	3 388	3 178	3 061	2 883	2 843	2 530	2 476	1 930
All road users[4]:												
Killed	BMDC	3 421	3 423	3 409	3 450	3 431	3 508	3 221	3 201	3 172	2 946	2 538
Killed or seriously injured	ZCEE	44 255	42 545	41 564	40 560	39 407	37 215	34 351	32 155	31 845	30 720	28 572
All severities	BMDA	325 212	320 310	320 283	313 309	302 605	290 607	280 840	271 017	258 404	247 780	230 905

1 Casualities aged 0 - 15.
2 Casualties aged 16 and over.
3 Includes mopeds and scooters.
4 Includes other motor or non-motor vehicle users, and unknown road user
  type and casualty age.

Source: Department for Transport 020 7944 6595

15.18 Freight transport by road: goods moved by goods vehicles over 3.5 tonnes[1]
Great Britain

Billion tonne kilometres

		1998	1999	2000	2001	2002	2003	2004[2]	2005[2]	2006[2]	2007[2]	2008
By mode of working												
Mainly public haulage	KNND	114.3	110.9	113.0	114.7	110.6	114.3	110.8	109.7	112.1	115.6	102.9
Mainly own account	KNNC	37.6	38.3	37.5	34.7	39.2	37.4	41.4	43.0	43.5	45.9	48.9
All modes	KNNB	151.9	149.2	150.5	149.4	149.8	151.7	152.2	152.7	155.6	161.5	151.7
By gross weight of vehicle												
Rigid vehicles:												
Over 3.5 tonnes to 17 tonnes	ZCIL	17.8	17.9	15.8	13.1	11.9	10.1	9.1	8.1	7.2	5.8	5.5
Over 17 tonnes to 25 tonnes	ZCIM	4.2	4.3	4.8	5.7	6.3	6.8	7.9	8.3	8.6	9.5	8.3
Over 25 tonnes	ZCIN	14.7	15.3	15.4	15.6	17.3	18.3	18.9	20.3	20.8	22.5	20.3
All rigids	ZCIO	36.6	37.5	36.0	34.5	35.6	35.2	35.9	36.7	36.6	37.8	34.1
Articulated vehicles:												
Over 3.5 tonnes to 33 tonnes	ZCIP	14.4	14.0	14.0	12.8	9.9	8.8	7.0	6.3	6.1	5.6	5.2
Over 33 tonnes	ZCIQ	100.9	97.7	100.4	102.1	104.4	107.7	109.4	109.7	112.9	118.1	112.5
All articulated vehicles	ZCIR	115.3	111.7	114.4	114.9	114.3	116.5	116.4	116.0	119.0	123.7	117.6
All vehicles												
Over 3.5 tonnes to 25 tonnes	ZCIS	22.5	22.7	21.3	19.3	18.7	17.3	17.3	16.7	16.3	15.7	14.1
Over 25 tonnes	KNNG	129.4	126.5	129.2	130.1	131.1	134.4	134.9	136.0	139.3	145.8	137.6
All weights	ZCIT	151.9	149.2	150.5	149.4	149.8	151.7	152.2	152.7	155.6	161.5	151.7
By commodity												
Food, drink and tobacco	ZCIU	42.5	41.5	44.3	41.4	43.1	42.2	41.7	40.6	42.0	45.1	43.7
Wood, timber and cork	ZCIV	3.6	3.8	3.7	3.9	3.8	4.1	4.5	4.7	4.1	3.3	4.0
Fertiliser	ZCIW	1.2	1.4	1.2	1.2	1.2	1.2	0.8	1.1	0.8	0.9	1.3
Crude minerals	ZCIX	13.3	12.7	12.4	13.0	13.9	13.8	14.1	14.8	15.4	16.0	13.3
Ores	ZCIY	1.1	1.3	1.2	1.2	1.1	1.2	1.4	1.7	1.4	1.8	1.8
Crude materials	ZCIZ	2.6	2.6	2.6	2.3	2.7	2.3	3.3	2.4	2.7	2.6	2.3
Coal and coke	ZCJA	2.0	2.2	1.5	2.1	1.5	1.5	1.2	1.5	1.3	1.6	1.0
Petrol and petroleum products	ZCJB	5.2	5.0	6.4	5.8	5.2	5.5	5.7	5.5	5.7	5.1	6.5
Chemicals	ZCJC	7.9	7.4	6.8	7.2	6.5	6.8	6.3	7.6	6.2	7.0	6.1
Building materials	ZCJD	10.7	10.6	10.6	11.7	10.9	12.0	12.1	10.9	11.5	11.6	11.0
Iron and steel products	ZCJE	7.7	6.8	6.8	5.7	5.3	5.4	5.4	5.2	4.7	6.4	4.1
Other metal products	ZCJF	1.7	1.7	1.7	1.4	1.5	1.5	1.9	2.1	2.1	2.0	1.8
Machinery and transport equipment	ZCJG	9.1	8.7	9.1	8.9	8.5	8.7	8.9	9.3	9.4	9.5	8.9
Miscellaneous manufactures	ZCJH	15.9	15.7	15.1	15.4	16.2	15.8	16.3	15.5	16.3	16.4	12.6
Miscellaneous articles	ZCJI	27.5	27.9	27.1	28.2	28.4	29.5	28.8	29.8	31.7	32.2	33.3
All commodities	ZCJJ	151.9	149.2	150.5	149.4	149.8	151.7	152.2	152.7	155.6	161.5	151.7

1 Rigid vehicles or articulated vehicles (tractive unit and trailer) with gross vehicle weight over 3.5 tonnes.

2 Figures for 2004 onwards are not fully comparable with those for 2003 and earlier years. Detailed comparisons should therefore be made with caution.

Source: Department for Transport 020 7944 3180

15.19 Freight transport by road: goods lifted by goods vehicles over 3.5 tonnes[1]
Great Britain

Million tonnes

		1998	1999	2000	2001	2002	2003	2004[2]	2005[2]	2006[2]	2007[2]	2008
By mode of working												
Mainly public haulage	ZCJK	1 041	991	1 038	1 052	1 019	1 053	1 101	1 079	1 127	1 145	986
Mainly own account	ZCJL	589	576	556	529	608	590	643	667	685	724	748
All modes	ZCJM	1 630	1 567	1 593	1 581	1 627	1 643	1 744	1 746	1 813	1 869	1 734
By gross weight of vehicle												
Rigid vehicles:												
Over 3.5 tonnes to 17 tonnes	ZCJN	268	254	229	203	188	159	160	135	130	109	103
Over 17 tonnes to 25 tonnes	ZCJO	106	86	87	86	90	100	113	118	120	130	122
Over 25 tonnes	ZCJP	401	408	424	443	491	506	539	559	598	629	532
All rigids	ZCJQ	776	748	741	733	768	765	812	812	849	868	757
Articulated vehicles:												
Over 3.5 tonnes to 33 tonnes	ZCJR	125	113	107	97	81	69	60	51	50	50	46
Over 33 tonnes	ZCJS	729	706	746	751	778	809	872	883	914	952	931
All articulated vehicles	ZCJT	854	819	852	848	859	878	932	934	964	1 001	977
All vehicles												
Over 3.5 tonnes to 25 tonnes	ZCJU	382	346	325	294	283	265	277	257	256	245	230
Over 25 tonnes	ZCJV	1 248	1 221	1 268	1 287	1 343	1 378	1 467	1 489	1 557	1 624	1 504
All weights	ZCJW	1 630	1 567	1 593	1 581	1 627	1 643	1 744	1 746	1 813	1 869	1 734
By commodity												
Food, drink and tobacco	ZCJX	346	333	346	321	339	333	351	339	360	373	370
Wood, timber and cork	ZCJY	27	28	26	28	28	32	42	36	30	29	35
Fertiliser	ZCJZ	9	11	10	9	11	12	7	14	7	9	22
Crude minerals	ZCKA	327	297	308	298	333	327	364	370	380	390	317
Ores	ZCKB	18	20	16	16	17	21	22	23	19	22	24
Crude materials	ZCKC	20	20	18	20	21	19	25	22	23	23	20
Coal and coke	ZCKD	26	28	22	21	17	22	14	21	17	24	15
Petrol and petroleum products	ZCKE	61	61	75	74	59	64	67	70	69	71	80
Chemicals	ZCKF	53	47	49	50	41	47	46	53	48	48	45
Building materials	ZCKG	161	159	165	165	167	165	185	169	180	175	177
Iron and steel products	ZCKH	54	48	49	44	39	41	43	42	41	47	33
Other metal products	ZCKI	18	17	16	14	14	16	19	19	21	20	20
Machinery and transport equipment	ZCKJ	73	67	69	70	68	66	70	76	79	83	75
Miscellaneous manufactures	ZCKK	96	91	97	97	105	98	111	109	112	113	95
Miscellaneous articles	ZCKL	342	340	328	353	367	379	378	384	426	440	406
All commodities	ZCKM	1 630	1 567	1 593	1 581	1 627	1 643	1 744	1 746	1 813	1 869	1 734

1 Rigid vehicles or articulated vehicles (tractive unit and trailer) with gross vehicle weight over 3.5 tonnes.

2 Figures for 2004 onwards are not fully comparable with those for 2003 and earlier years. Detailed comparison should therefore be made with caution.

Source: Department for Transport 020 7944 3180

15.20 Rail systems summary

		1998/99	1999/00	2000/01	2001/02	2002/03	2003/04	2004/05	2005/06	2006/07	2007/08	2008/09
Passenger journeys (millions)												
National Rail network[1]	ZCKN	892	931	957	960	976	1 012	1 045	1 082	1 151	1 232	1 274
London Underground	KNOE	866	927	970	953	942	948	976	970	1 040	1 096	1 089
Docklands Light Railway	ZCKO	28	31	38	41	46	48	50	54	64	67	68
Glasgow Underground	ZCKP	15	15	14	14	13	13	13	13	13	14	14
Tyne and Wear Metro[2]	ZCKQ	34	33	33	33	37	38	37	36	38	40	41
Blackpool trams[3]	EL9L	4	4	4	5	4	4	4	4	3	3	2
Manchester Metrolink[4]	ZCKS	13	14	17	18	19	19	20	20	20	20	21
Midland Metro[5]	ZCKR	–	5	5	5	5	5	5	5	5	5	5
Croydon Tramlink[6]	GEOE	–	–	15	18	19	20	22	23	25	27	27
Sheffield Supertram	ZCKT	10	11	11	11	12	12	13	13	14	15	15
Nottingham NET[7]	C3MI	–	–	–	–	–	–	8	10	10	10	10
All rail	ZCKU	1 862	1 971	2 065	2 059	2 072	2 119	2 193	2 229	2 383	2 529	2 566
All light rail	GENZ	104	113	138	146	154	160	172	177	192	201	203
Passenger revenue (£ million at current prices)												
National Rail network	KNDL	3 089	3 368	3 413	3 548	3 663	3 901	4 158	4 493	5 012	5 555	6 004
London Underground	KNOA	977	1 058	1 129	1 151	1 138	1 161	1 241	1 309	1 417	1 525	1 615
Docklands Light Railway	ZCKV	20	22	29	32	36	37	40	46	54	62	63
Glasgow Underground	ZCKW	9	10	10	10	10	10	11	11	13	13	14
Tyne and Wear Metro	ZCKX	23	24	24	25	29	31	33	34	38	32	32
Blackpool trams	EL9M	4	4	4	5	5	4	4	4	5	4	3
Manchester Metrolink	ZCKZ	..	..	18	20	20	21	22	23	24	22	23
Midland Metro	ZCKY	–	..	3	4	5	5	5	6	6	4	5
Croydon Tramlink	GEOF	–	–	12	13	15	16	18	19	20	15	14
Sheffield Supertram	ZCLA	6	7	7	8	10	9	11	10	13	11	12
Nottingham NET	C3MJ	–	–	–	–	–	..	6	7	8	7	8
All rail	ZCLB	3 789	4 493	4 650	4 815	4 931	5 197	5 550	5 963	6 609	7 251	7 792
All light rail	GEOA	69	63	108	117	130	135	151	161	180	171	173
Passenger kilometres (millions)												
National Rail network	KNDZ	36 280	38 472	38 179	39 141	39 678	40 906	41 762	43 211	46 218	49 007	50 698
London Underground	KNOI	6 716	7 171	7 470	7 451	7 367	7 340	7 606	7 586	7 947	8 352	8 646
Docklands Light Railway	ZCLC	144	172	200	207	232	235	245	257	301	326	318
Glasgow Underground	ZCLD	47	47	46	44	43	43	43	42	42	46	45
Tyne and Wear Metro	ZCLE	238	230	229	238	275	284	283	279	295	313	319
Blackpool trams	EL9N	..	13	13	15	14	11	12	11	10	9	7
Manchester Metrolink	ZCLG	117	126	152	161	167	169	204	206	208	210	221
Midland Metro	ZCLF	–	50	56	50	50	54	52	54	51	51	50
Croydon Tramlink	GEOG	–	–	96	99	100	105	112	117	128	141	144
Sheffield Supertram	ZCLH	35	37	38	39	40	42	44	44	42	44	45
Nottingham NET	C3MK	–	–	–	–	–	2	37	42	43	44	42
All rail	ZCLI	43 577	46 318	46 479	47 446	47 965	49 191	50 401	51 849	55 285	58 544	60 535
All light rail	GEOB	581	675	830	854	920	945	1 033	1 052	1 120	1 185	1 191
Route kilometres open for passenger traffic (numbers)												
National Rail network[8]	ZCLJ	15 038	15 038	15 042	15 042	15 042	14 883	14 328	14 356	14 353	14 484	14 494
London Underground	ZCLK	392	408	408	408	408	408	408	408	408	408	408
Docklands Light Railway	ZCLM	22	26	26	26	26	26	26	30	31	32	33
Glasgow Underground	ZCLN	11	11	11	11	11	11	11	10	10	10	10
Tyne and Wear Metro	ZCLO	59	59	59	78	78	78	78	78	78	78	78
Blackpool trams	EL9O	18	18	18	18	18	18	18	18	18	18	18
Manchester Metrolink	ZCLQ	31	39	39	39	39	39	39	39	39	42	39
Midland Metro	ZCLP	–	20	20	20	20	20	20	20	20	20	20
Croydon Tramlink	GEOH	–	–	28	28	28	28	28	28	28	28	28
Sheffield Supertram	ZCLR	29	29	29	29	29	29	29	29	29	29	29
Nottingham NET	C3ML	–	–	–	–	–	14	14	15	14	14	14
All rail	ZCLS	15 600	15 648	15 680	15 699	15 699	15 554	14 999	15 032	15 028	15 186	15 171
All light rail	GEOC	170	202	230	249	249	263	263	268	267	294	269
Stations served (numbers)												
National Rail network	ZCLT	2 499	2 503	2 508	2 508	2 508	2 507	2 508	2 510	2 520	2 516	2 516
London Underground	KNOO	269	274	274	274	274	274	274	274	273	268	270
Docklands Light Railway	ZCLU	29	34	34	34	34	34	34	38	34	39	40
Glasgow Underground	ZCLV	15	15	15	15	15	15	15	15	15	15	15
Tyne and Wear Metro	ZCLW	46	46	46	58	58	58	58	59	59	60	60
Blackpool trams	EL9P	124	124	124	124	124	124	124	124	121	121	121
Manchester Metrolink	ZCLY	26	36	36	36	37	37	37	37	37	37	37
Midland Metro	ZCLX	–	23	23	23	23	23	23	23	23	23	23
Croydon Tramlink	GEOI	–	–	38	38	38	38	38	39	39	38	39
Sheffield Supertram	ZCLZ	47	47	47	48	48	48	48	48	48	48	48
Nottingham NET	C3MM	–	–	–	–	–	23	23	23	23	23	23
All rail	ZCLL	3 055	3 102	3 146	3 145	3 159	3 181	3 182	3 190	3 192	3 188	3 192
All light rail	GSOC	287	325	363	376	377	400	400	406	399	404	406

1 Franchised train operating companies from Feb 1996 after privatisation.
2 Tyne & Wear Metro extension to Sunderland opened in March 2002.
3 Blackpool Trams shown as a self-contained system.
4 Transfer of 20 stations from the rail network to Manchester Metrolink.
5 Midland Metro opened in 1999.
6 Croydon Tramlink opened in 2000.
7 Nottingham Express Transit opened in March 2004.
8 Break in series due to change in methodology.

Sources: Department for Transport: 020 7944 3076/8874;
Network Rail, former Railtrack, ORR, TfL, light rail operators and PTEs

15.21 National railways freight: 1998/99-2008/09
Great Britain

Billion tonne kilometres

		1998[1]/99	1999/00	2000/01	2001/02	2002/03	2003/04	2004/05	2005/06	2006/07	2007/08	2008/09
Freight moved by commodity												
Coal	ZCGG	4.5	4.8	4.8	6.2	5.7	5.8	6.7	8.3	8.6	7.7	7.9
Metals	ZCGH	2.1	2.2	2.1	2.4	2.7	2.6	2.6	2.2	2.0	1.8	1.5
Construction	ZCGI	2.1	2.0	2.4	2.8	2.5	2.7	2.9	2.9	2.7	2.8	2.7
Oil and petroleum	ZCGJ	1.6	1.5	1.4	1.2	1.2	1.2	1.2	1.2	1.5	1.6	1.5
Other traffic	ZCGK	7.1	7.6	7.4	6.7	6.6	6.8	7.0	7.1	7.1	7.2	7.0
All traffic	VOXD	17.3	18.2	18.1	19.4	18.5	18.9	20.4	21.7	21.9	21.2	20.6

Million tonnes

		1998/99	1999[2]/00	2000/01	2001/02	2002/03	2003/04	2004[3]/05	2005[4]/06	2006/07	2007[5]/08	2008/09
Freight lifted by commodity												
Coal	ZCGL	45.3	35.9	35.3	39.5	34.0	35.2	43.3	47.6	48.7	43.3	46.6
Metals	ZCGM	..	..	..	..	..	..	..	..	..	..	..
Construction	ZCGN	..	..	..	..	..	..	..	..	..	..	..
Oil and petroleum	ZCGO	..	..	..	..	..	..	..	..	..	..	..
Other traffic	ZCGP	56.8	60.6	60.3	54.5	53.0	53.7	56.8	57.7	59.5	59.1	56.1
All traffic	VOXE	102.100	96.500	95.600	93.900	87.000	88.900	100.100	105.300	108.211	102.403	102.700

1 There is a break in the series between 1998-99 and 1999-00 due to a change in the source data.
2 Break in series from 1999/2000.
3 Break in series with most of the increase due to changes in the data collection method.
4 Break in the series from 2005/06 as some GB Railfreight tonnes lifted now included.
5 Break in series from 2007/08 as GB Railfreight coal data now included.

Source: Rail :ORR : 020 7944 8874

15.22 Railways: permanent way and rolling stock
Northern Ireland
At end of year

Numbers

		1998	1999	2000	2001	2002	2003	2004	2005	2006	2007	2008
Length of road open for traffic[1] (Km)	KNRA	335	335	356	334	334	334	299	299	299	299	299
Length of track open for traffic (Km)												
Total	KNRB	526	526	547	480	480	480	445	445	445	445	445
Running lines	KNRC	484	484	505	464	464	464	427	427	427	427	427
Sidings (as single track)	KNRD	42	42	42	16	16	16	18	18	18	18	18
Locomotives												
Diesel-electrics	KNRE	5	6	6	6	6	5	6	5	5	5	5
Passenger carrying vehicles												
Total	KNRF	120	105	105	106	100	100	102	124	125	128	130
Rail motor vehicles:												
Diesel-electric, etc	KNRG	28	30	30	29	28	28	28	70	85	84	84
Trailer carriages:												
Total locomotive hauled	KNRH	38	21	21	25	22	22	22	22	22	22	22
Ordinary coaches	KNRI	36	19	19	23	20	20	20	20	20	20	20
Restaurant cars	KNRJ	2	2	2	2	2	2	2	2	2	2	2
Rail car trailers	KNRK	54	54	54	52	50	50	52	32	18	22	24
Rolling stock for maintenance and repair	KNRT	26	18	18	18	18	39	46	48	48	48	48

1 The total length of railroad open for traffic irrespective of the number of tracks comprising the road.

Sources: Department for Regional Development; Northern Ireland: 028 905 40981

15.23 Operating statistics of railways
Northern Ireland

		Unit	1998	1999	2000	2001	2002	2003	2004	2005	2006	2007	2008
Maintenance of way and works													
Material used:													
Ballast	KNSA	Thousand m^2	38.5	40.0	47.0	80.0	40.0	130.0	70.0	90.0	30.0	15.0	10.0
Rails	KNSB	Thousand tonnes	2.5	3.0	3.5	2.5	1.0	4.5	1.0	3.2	1.0	1.0	0.1
Sleepers	KNSC	Thousands	32.0	30.0	40.0	50.0	5.0	40.0	28.0	45.0	2.0	5.0	2.0
Track renewed	KNSD	Km	22.5	7.0	29.0	15.0	5.0	25.8	2.0	29.0	1.0	–	..
New Track laid	KPGD	Km	–	–	21.0	–	–	–	–	–	–	–	..
Engine kilometres													
Total[1]	KNSE	Thousand Km	4 100	4 100	4 100	4 056	4 056	4 170	4 110	3 610	3 900	3 900	3 900
Train kilometres:													
Total	KNSF	"	3 670	3 670	3 670	3 626	3 626	3 704	3 610	3 610	3 900	3 900	3 900
Coaching	KNSG	"	3 666	3 666	3 666	3 622	3 622	3 700	3 610	3 610	3 900	3 900	3 900
Freight	KNSH	"	4	4	4	4	4	4	–	–	–	–	..

1 Including shunting, assisting, light, departmental, maintenance and repair.

Sources: Department for Regional Development;
Northern Ireland: 028 905 40981

15.24 Main output of United Kingdom airlines

Available tonne kilometres (millions)

		1999	2000	2001	2002	2003	2004	2005	2006	2007	2008	2009
All services	KNTA	42 002	43 379	42 370	40 550	42 784	43 883	48 186	50 391	54 181	53 348	49 150
Percentage growth on previous year	KNTB	5.0	3.6	−2.4	−4.3	5.5	2.6	9.8	4.4	7.5	−1.6	−7.9
Scheduled services	KNTC	31 815	32 938	31 866	30 433	31 513	32 422	36 937	38 590	40 971	41 241	39 207
Percentage growth on previous year	KNTD	6.9	3.5	−3.3	−4.5	3.6	2.9	13.9	4.5	6.2	0.7	−5.1
Non-scheduled services	KNTE	10 186	10 440	10 505	10 117	11 271	11 461	11 249	11 801	13 209	12 077	9 944
Percentage growth on previous year	KNTF	−0.7	4.1	0.6	−3.7	11.4	1.7	−1.8	4.3	11.9	−8.6	−17.7

Source: Civil Aviation Authority: 020 7453 6246

15.25 Air traffic between the United Kingdom and abroad[1]

Thousands

		1999	2000	2001	2002	2003	2004	2005	2006	2007	2008	2009
Flights												
United Kingdom airlines												
Scheduled services	KNUA	480.9	520.3	536.7	531.3	517.7	546.5	584.2	596.3	621.9	601.7	550.5
Non-scheduled services	KNUB	212.6	216.2	208.5	218.6	211.0	198.6	200.6	209.6	207.1	193.4	172.6
Overseas airlines[2]												
Scheduled services	KNUC	467.6	467.6	496.8	487.5	487.0	544.2	584.5	629.5	656.9	686.7	700.2
Non-scheduled services	KNUD	31.7	31.7	26.0	36.7	27.1	28.8	33.7	28.4	27.2	24.3	21.9
Total	KNUE	1 192.8	1 235.8	1 268.0	1 274.1	1 242.8	1 318.1	1 403.0	1 463.8	1 513.1	1 506.1	1 445.2
Passengers carried												
United Kingdom airlines												
Scheduled services	KNUF	50 148.5	54 522.8	53 591.7	54 360.0	56 476.7	63 216.1	69 106.2	72 196.4	76 959.9	76 636.5	71 586.9
Non-scheduled services	KNUG	32 603.8	33 185.9	34 009.1	33 935.7	33 385.6	32 195.7	30 179.4	29 725.5	28 524.0	25 906.9	21 774.2
Overseas airlines[2]												
Scheduled services	KNUH	46 628.0	46 627.9	51 107.8	51 317.6	54 504.0	60 278.0	67 634.9	74 670.8	79 820.1	83 176.7	84 321.0
Non-scheduled services	KNUI	4 156.5	4 156.5	3 966.1	3 956.3	3 947.1	4 068.3	4 169.1	4 107.7	3 803.3	3 417.0	3 049.5
Total	KNUJ	133 536.8	138 493.1	142 674.7	143 569.6	148 313.4	159 758.1	171 089.6	180 700.4	189 107.3	189 137.1	180 731.6

1 Excludes travel to and from the Channel Islands.
2 Includes airlines of overseas UK Territories.

Source: Civil Aviation Authority: 020 7453 6246

15.26 Operations and traffic on scheduled services: revenue traffic
United Kingdom airlines[1]

		Unit	1999	2000	2001	2002	2003	2004	2005	2006	2007	2008	2009
All services													
Aircraft stage flights:													
Number	KNFA	Numbers	835 031	878 582	921 556	911 518	895 095	926 498	1 016 354	1 037 729	1 052 799	1 056 298	1 001 504
Average length	KNFB	Kilometres	1 134.0	1 156.0	1 138.0	1 149.0	1 215.0	1 227.0	1 304.0	1 349.0	1 400.0	1 427.9	1 441.3
Aircraft-kilometres flown	KNFC	Millions	947.0	1 016.0	1 049.0	1 047.0	1 088.0	1 137.0	1 325.0	1 400.0	1 474.0	1 508.3	1 443.5
Passengers uplifted	KNFD	"	65.0	70.0	70.0	72.0	76.0	83.0	94.0	98.0	102.0	104.7	102.5
Seat-kilometres used	KNFE	"	160 336.0	170 469.0	158 651.0	156 494.0	164 806.0	173 722.0	200 460.0	213 442.0	227 720.0	232 591.6	230 588.3
Cargo uplifted:[2]	KNFF	Tonnes	860 291.0	897 184.0	742 705.0	768 736.0	800 645.0	842 912.0	921 412.0	946 365.0	941 421.0	979 791.0	900 668.0
Tonne-kilometres used:		Millions											
Passenger	KNFH	"	15 518.0	16 507.0	15 258.0	15 035.0	15 419.0	15 580.0	15 044.0	16 090.0	17 246.0	17 717.7	17 474.4
Freight	KNFI	"	4 925.0	5 160.0	4 548.0	4 941.0	5 187.0	5 297.0	5 998.0	6 213.0	6 199.0	6 283.8	5 863.7
Mail	KNFJ	"	153.0	179.0	102.0	57.0	55.0	75.0	90.0	99.0	112.0	99.0	88.6
Total	KNFG	"	20 596.0	21 846.0	19 908.0	20 032.0	20 660.0	20 952.0	21 133.0	22 402.0	23 557.0	24 100.5	23 426.7
Domestic services													
Aircraft stage flights:													
Number	KNFK	Numbers	354 864	353 525	365 881	359 400	345 954	373 858	394 069	399 438	383 591	369 499	341 207
Average length	KNFL	Kilometres	337.0	344.0	350.0	350.0	357.0	360.0	374.0	371.0	367.0	469.0	360.8
Aircraft-kilometres flown	KNFM	Millions	120.0	121.0	128.0	126.0	123.0	135.0	147.0	148.0	140.0	173.3	123.1
Passengers uplifted	KNFN	"	17.0	18.0	18.0	20.0	21.0	22.0	23.0	23.0	22.0	21.0	19.5
Seat-kilometres used	KNFO	"	7 184.0	7 542.0	7 645.0	8 322.0	8 904.0	9 263.0	9 795.0	9 800.0	9 449.0	8 951.5	8 326.3
Cargo uplifted:[2]	KNFP	Tonnes	25 964	24 644	19 498	16 755	17 248	14 862	10 015	8 498	7 099	6 125	5 202
Tonne-kilometres used:		Millions											
Passenger	KNFR	"	610.0	640.0	649.0	703.0	738.0	757.0	784.0	759.0	733.0	720.2	644.8
Freight	KNFS	"	6.0	6.0	4.0	4.0	3.0	3.0	3.0	2.0	2.0	1.8	1.6
Mail	KNFT	"	4.0	4.0	4.0	3.0	3.0	3.0	–	1.0	1.0	0.1	0.7
Total	KNFQ	"	620.0	650.0	656.0	709.0	744.0	762.0	787.0	762.0	735.0	722.1	647.1
International services													
Aircraft stage flights:													
Number	KNFU	Numbers	480 167	525 057	555 675	552 118	549 141	552 640	622 285	638 291	669 208	686 799	660 027
Average length	KNFV	Kilometres	1 723.0	1 704.0	1 656.0	1 670.0	1 758.0	2 148.0	1 893.0	1 960.0	1 993.0	1 994.4	2 000.5
Aircraft-kilometres flown	KNFW	Millions	827.0	895.0	921.0	921.0	965.0	1 002.0	1 178.0	1 251.0	1 333.0	1 371.0	1 320.4
Passengers uplifted	KNFX	"	48.0	52.0	52.0	52.0	56.0	61.0	71.0	75.0	80.0	83.8	82.9
Seat-kilometres used	KNFY	"	153 153.0	162 927.0	151 006.0	148 172.0	155 903.0	164 459.0	190 666.0	203 642.0	218 271.0	223 640.1	222 262.0
Cargo uplifted:[2]	KNFZ	Tonnes	834 327	872 540	723 206	751 975	783 397	828 051	911 398	937 868	934 323	973 665	895 466
Tonne-kilometres used:		Millions											
Passenger	KNJX	"	14 908.0	15 867.0	14 610.0	14 332.0	14 681.0	14 824.0	14 260.0	15 331.0	16 513.0	16 997.5	16 829.6
Freight	KNJY	"	4 919.0	5 154.0	4 544.0	4 937.0	5 184.0	5 294.0	5 995.0	6 383.0	6 197.0	6 282.0	5 862.1
Mail	KNJZ	"	149.0	176.0	98.0	54.0	51.0	72.0	90.0	99.0	111.0	98.9	88.6
Total	KNJW	"	19 976.0	21 197.0	19 252.0	19 322.0	19 916.0	20 190.0	20 345.0	21 813.0	22 822.0	23 378.4	22 780.3

1 Includes services of British Airways and other UK private companies.
2 Cargo has re-defined as freight and mail.

Source: Civil Aviation Authority: 020 7453 6246

15.27 Activity at civil aerodromes
United Kingdom[1]

Thousands and tonnes

		2000	2001	2002	2003	2004	2005	2006	2007	2008	2009
Movement of civil aircraft (thousands)											
Commercial											
Transport	KNQC	2 045	2 095	2 094	2 160	2 277	2 406	2 451	2 494	2 407	2 195
Other[2]	KNQD	159	150	120	117	116	120	129	124	113	96
Total	KNQB	2 204	2 245	2 214	2 277	2 393	2 526	2 580	2 609	2 520	2 291
Non-commercial[3]	KNQE	1 186	1 207	1 100	1 186	1 135	1 129	1 059	1 033	964	912
Total	KNQA	3 390	3 452	3 314	3 463	3 528	3 655	3 639	3 637	3 484	3 203
Passengers handled											
Terminal	KNQG	179 885	181 231	188 761	199 950	215 681	228 214	235 139	240 722	235 359	218 126
Transit	KNQH	1 167	1 087	1 054	990	950	984	1 016	963	735	519
Total	KNQF	181 052	182 318	189 815	200 940	216 631	229 198	236 155	241 685	236 094	218 645
Commercial freight handled[4] (tonnes)											
Set down	KNQJ	1 174 635	1 093 142	1 124 026	1 172 552	1 267 411	1 282 724	1 277 177	1 316 359	1 274 539	1 120 886
Picked up	KNQK	1 139 292	1 052 379	1 071 407	1 035 680	1 103 539	1 080 620	1 038 261	1 009 414	1 007 616	926 974
Total	KNQI	2 313 927	2 145 521	2 195 433	2 208 232	2 370 950	2 363 344	2 315 438	2 325 773	2 282 155	2 047 860
Mail handled											
Set down	KNQM	101 743	98 690	90 738	86 415	108 481	102 344	91 535	102 027	111 002	96 183
Picked up	KNQN	123 352	117 389	99 747	93 096	112 424	110 576	98 391	105 755	123 014	112 001
Total	KNQL	225 095	216 079	190 485	179 511	220 905	212 920	189 926	207 790	234 016	208 184

1 Figures exclude Channel Island and Isle of Man Airports.
2 Local pleasure flights for reward (eg aerial survey work, crop dusting and delivery of empty aircraft) and empty positioning flights.
3 Test and Training flights, Other flights by Air Transport Operators, Aero-club, Private, Official, Military & Business Aviation.

4 With effect from 2001, passengers, freight and mail handled exclude traffic carried on air taxi operations.

Source: Civil Aviation Authority: 020 7453 6258

15.28 Household digital television[1]: by type of service[2,3]
United Kingdom[1]

Percentages

	Total digital television	Digital satellite	Digital terrestrial	Digital cable
	IM6S	IM6T	IM6U	IM6V
2000	15.5	17.6	2.8	13.6
2001	30.9	22.4	4.5	14.8
2002	38.5	25.0	5.2	14.5
2003	43.2	28.6	5.9	13.4
2004	53.0	29.1	14.1	13.5
2005	61.9	31.3	20.3	13.2
2006	69.7	33.1	25.3	13.2
2007	79.6	35.7	33.0	13.0
2008	87.1	36.6	37.9	12.5
2009	89.2	36.8	38.5	12.9

1 Multichannel take-up on main sets.
2 Data are at the end of the first quarter in each year.
3 GfK research from Q1 2007 onwards, previous years use platform operator data, research and Ofcom estimates.

Source: Ofcom: 020 7981 3000

15.29 Telephones and The Internet

	Call Revenue (All Operators)							
	Business call revenue (£s millions)				Residential call revenue (£s millions)			
	UK Geographic calls	International calls	Calls to mobiles	Other calls[1]	UK Geographic calls	International calls	Calls to mobiles	Other calls[1]
	IM6A	IM6B	IM6C	IM6D	IM6E	IM6F	IM6G	IM6H
2007	581	256	670	256	863	308	966	897
2008	498	254	591	219	868	300	943	814
2008 Q3	122	60	148	52	215	74	231	196
Q4	115	61	140	52	220	73	227	199
2009 Q1	120	62	149	53	221	71	216	183
Q2	115	60	142	54	220	69	217	201
Q3	112	58	141	52	223	70	218	193

	Call Volumes (All Operators)							
	Business call volumes (millions of minutes)				Residential call volumes (millions of minutes)			
	UK Geographic calls	International calls	Calls to mobiles	Other calls[1]	UK Geographic calls	International calls	Calls to mobiles	Other calls[1]
	IM6I	IM6J	IM6K	IM6L	IM6M	IM6N	IM6O	IM6P
2007	29 442	2 724	6 829	11 076	66 651	3 166	7 536	33 513
2008	26 145	2 382	6 512	9 283	65 747	3 790	6 765	23 179
2008 Q3	6 489	589	1 638	2 344	15 935	933	1 662	5 589
Q4	6 148	560	1 555	2 219	16 402	964	1 604	5 129
2009 Q1	6 239	564	1 599	2 220	16 719	1 001	1 551	5 014
Q2	5 839	524	1 516	2 122	15 849	1 021	1 550	4 726
Q3	5 755	490	1 514	2 137	15 949	1 057	1 568	4 711

	Selected lines with Carrier Pre-Selection (000's)		Exchange line numbers (All operators)	
	CPS lines[2]	WLR lines[3]	Business (000's)	Residential (000's)
	IM6W	IM6X	IM6Q	IM6R
2007	24 026	17 406	11 667	25 996
2008	..	..	10 482	24 099
2008 Q3	..	..	11 059	24 118
Q4	..	..	10 482	24 099
2009 Q1	..	..	10 622	24 285
Q2	..	..	10 001	23 147
Q3	..	..	9 896	23 284

Data taken from the Telecommunications Market Data Update Q4 2007.

Source: Ofcom Tel: 020 7981 3000

1 Includes freephone, special services, premium rate, directory enquiries and all other call types.
2 Allows usage of any service provide through a BT line.
3 Service which any other operator takes control of all connections made through a telephone line and connects subscription fee from the subscribers.

15.29 Telephones and The Internet

continued

Percentages

Selected uses of the Internet, United Kingdom: by age, 2009

	16-24	25-44	45-54	55-64	65 plus	All
Sending/receiving emails	94	92	88	86	82	90
Finding information about goods or services	64	83	80	81	75	78
Using services related to travel and accommodation	53	75	72	72	65	69
Internet banking	50	61	55	48	43	54
Reading or downloading online news, magazines	46	58	52	47	44	52
Playing or downloading games, images, films or music	70	46	35	26	16	44
Listening to web radio or watching web TV	53	46	35	34	25	42
Seeking health-related information	31	45	47	44	38	42
Posting messages to chat sites, blogs etc	71	45	25	19	..	40
Consulting the Internet with the purpose of learning	41	39	38	32	26	37
Looking for information - education, training, courses	53	38	36	21	15	36
Downloading software	46	39	31	25	25	36

Internet purchases by adults, United Kingdom

	2006	2007	2008	2009
Films, music	53	51	41	50
Clothes or sports goods	37	38	42	49
Household goods	24	39	40	47
Travel, accommodation or holidays	51	46	48	42
Books, magazines or newspapers	37	35	37	41
Tickets for events	35	33	37	37
Electronic equipment	25	20	26	28
Food and groceries	20	20	19	22
Computer software and upgrades	29	21	22	20
Shares, financial services or insurance	24	9	11	17
Computer hardware	22	17	12	14
Lotteries or betting	7	6	10	-
Other goods and services	11	8	8	5

Households with access to the Internet, Great Britain and United Kingdom, 2002 to 2009[1]

	Great Britain				United Kingdom		
Year	Per cent	Number of Households	Percentage change on previous year	Year	Per cent	Number of Households	Percentage change on previous year
2002	46	11.02m	-	2002	-	-	-
2003	50	11.88m	8	2003	-	-	-
2004	51	12.16m	2	2004	-	-	-
2005	55	13.26m	9	2005	-	-	-
2006	57	13.93m	5	2006	57	14.26m	-
2007	61	14.94m	7	2007	61	15.23m	7
2008	65	16.05m	7	2008	65	16.46m	8
2008	-	-	-	2008	70	18.31	11

1 The survey is conducted in the first quarter of each year but should not be confused with being quarterly figures as they relate to use at a point in time.

Sources: Office for National Statistics; Omnibus survey, Internet Access 2008;
01633 456769

Transport and communications

15.30 Postal services and television licences[1]
United Kingdom

	Price of first class stamp (p)	Volume of first class stamped mail delivered (million items)	Total first class mail delivered (million items)	Price of second class stamp (p)	Volume of second class stamped mail delivered (million items)	Total second class mail delivered (million items)	Domestic parcels (million)	International parcels (million)
	IM7A	IM7B	IM7C	IM7D	IM7E	IM7F	IM7G	IM7H
2005 Q4	30	516	1 499	21	536	2 413	10.2	0.8
2006 Q1	30	399	1 280	21	284	2 059	8.6	0.5
Q2	32	396	1 292	23	267	1 978	9.0	0.6
Q3	32	340	1 217	23	242	1 811	9.0	0.5
Q4	32	479	1 377	23	507	2 146	11.8	0.8
2007 Q1	32	365	1 189	23	272	1 786	9.6	0.6
Q2	34	342	1 185	24	244	1 696	11.1	0.6
Q3	34	320	1 118	24	229	1 560	9.8	0.6
Q4	34	412	1 250	24	457	1 852	12.4	0.8
2008 Q1	34	373	1 195	24	282	1 664	10.5	0.7
Q2	36	317	1 092	27	238	1 490	10.8	0.7
Q3	36	259	997	27	205	1 362	9.7	0.9
Q4	36	351	1 092	27	433	1 580	12.1	1.0
2009 Q1	36	295	974	27	250	1 399	10.4	0.9
Q2	39	291	965	30	223	1 285	11.5	0.3
Q3	39	232	856	30	183	1 118	10.6	0.3

		1998	1999	2000	2001	2002[3]	2003	2004	2005	2006	2007	2008[3]
Letters, etc posted (millions)	KMRA	18 350	18 878	19 711	20 076	20 648	21 979	22 837	24 341	24 880	24 089	23 705
of which:												
Registered and insured	KMRB	28.7	31.6	30.2	32.3	36.1	38.5	41.4	45.3	45.3	44.7	46.6
Airmail (Commonwealth and foreign)	KMRC	658.4	693.2	672.3	659.2	600.7	541.6	512.0	457.9	502.2	541.0	470.3
Business reply and freepost items	KMRD	524.7	503.6	475.3	487.4	486.2	434.4	397.7	401.1	402.3	373.7	349.1
Postal orders												
Total issued (thousands)[2]	KMRH	31 907	30 289	30 153	30 931	29 150	28 666	28 888	29 344	20 489	19 714	16 650
Television licences (thousands)												
In force on 31 March	KMQL	21 723	22 240	22 625	22 839	23 157	23 486	23 899	24 162	24 419	24 546	24 740
of which:												
Colour	KMQM	21 344	21 944	22 413	22 684	23 040	23 392	23 824	24 103	24 370	24 505	24 706

1 See chapter text.
2 Excluding those issued on HM ships, in many British possessions and in other places abroad. Up to 1998 includes Postal Orders issued Overseas and by Ministry of Defence.
3 53 week year rather than 52 week standard

Sources: Royal Mail Group : 0207 2502890;
Capita Business Services Limited: 0117 302 1088;
Post Office Limited: 0207 3207424

National accounts

Chapter 16

National accounts

National accounts

(Tables 16.1 to 16.22)

The tables which follow are based on those in the *Blue Book* 2009 Edition. Some of the figures are provisional and may be revised later; this applies particularly to the figures for 2007 and 2008. The accounts are based on the European System of Accounts 1995 (ESA95). The *Blue Book* contains an introduction to the system of the UK accounts outlining some of the main concepts and principles of measurement used. It explains how key economic indicators are derived from the sequence of accounts and how the figures describing the whole economy are broken-down by sector and by industry. A detailed description of the structure for the accounts is provided in a separate Office for National Statistics publication *United Kingdom National Accounts: Concepts, Sources and Methods* (TSO 1998). Further information on the financial accounts is given in the *Financial Statistics Explanatory Handbook*.

In the tables in this chapter on national income, analyses by industry are based, as far as possible, on the Standard Industrial Classification Revised 2003. The principal aggregate measured in these tables is the Gross Domestic Product (GDP). This is a concept of the value of the total economic activity taking place in UK territory. It can be viewed as incomes earned, as expenditures incurred, or as production. Adding all primary incomes received from the rest of the world and deducting all primary incomes payable to non-residents produces Gross National Income (GNI) (previously known as Gross National Product). This is a concept of the value of all incomes earned by UK residents.

ESA95, the internationally compatible accounting framework, provides a systematic and detailed description of the UK economy. It includes the sector accounts which provide, by institutional sector, a description of the different stages of the economic process from production through income generation, distribution and use of income to capital accumulation and financing; and the input–output framework, which describes the production process in more detail. It contains all the elements required to compile such aggregate measures as GDP, GNI and saving.

Gross Domestic Product and Gross National Income

(Tables 16.1, 16.2, 16.3)

Table 16.1 shows the main national accounts aggregates, both at current prices and chained volume measures.

Table 16.2 shows the various money flows which generate the GDP and GNI. The output approach to GDP shows the total output of goods and services, the use of goods and services in the production process (intermediate consumption) and taxes and subsidies on products. The expenditure approach to GDP shows consumption expenditure by households and government, gross capital formation and expenditure on UK exports by overseas purchasers. The sum of these items overstates the amount of income generated in the UK by the value of imports of goods and services. This item is therefore subtracted to produce GDP at market prices.

The income approach to GDP shows gross operating surplus, mixed income and compensation of employees (previously known as income from employment). Taxes are added and subsidies are deducted to produce the total of the income based components at market prices.

Table 16.2 also shows the primary incomes received from the rest of the world, which are added to GDP, and primary incomes payable to non-residents, which are deducted from GDP, to arrive at GNI. Primary income comprises compensation of employees, taxes less subsidies on production, and property and entrepreneurial income.

Table 16.3 shows the expenditure approach to the chained volume measure of GDP. When looking at the change in the economy over time the main concern is usually whether more goods and services are actually being produced now than at some time in the past. Over time changes in current price GDP show changes in the monetary value of the components of GDP and, as these changes in value can reflect changes in both price and volume, it is difficult to establish how much of an increase in the series is due either to increased activity in the economy or to an increase in the price level. As a result, when looking at the real growth in the economy over time, it is useful to look at volume estimates of GDP. In chained volume series, volume measures for each year are produced in prices of the previous year. These volume measures are then 'chain-linked' together to produce a continuous time series.

Industrial analysis

(Tables 16.4, 16.5)

The analysis of gross value added by industry at current prices shown in Table 16.4 reflects the estimates based on the

Standard Industrial Classification, revised 2003 (SIC2003). The table is based on current price data reconciled through the input–output process for 1992 to 2007. The estimates are valued at basic prices, that is, the only taxes included in the price will be taxes paid as part of the production process, such as business rates, and not any taxes specifically levied on the production of a unit of output, for example VAT.

Table 16.5 shows chained volume measures of gross value added at basic prices by industry. Chained volume measures of gross value added (output approach) provides the lead indicator of economic change in the short term. The output analysis of gross value added is estimated in terms of change and expressed in index number form. It is therefore inappropriate to show as a statistical adjustment any divergence of an output measure of GDP derived from other measures of GDP. Such an adjustment does, however, exist implicitly.

Sector analysis – Distribution of income accounts and capital account

(Tables 16.6 to 16.13)

The National Accounts accounting framework includes the sector accounts which provide, by institutional sector, a description of the different stages of the economic process, from production through income generation, distribution and use of income to capital accumulation and financing. Tables 16.6 to 16.12 show the allocation of primary income account and the secondary distribution of income account for the non-financial corporations, financial corporations, government and households sectors. Additionally, Table 16.12 shows the use of income account for the households sector and Table 16.13 provides a summary of the capital account. The full sequence of accounts is shown in the *Blue Book*.

The allocation of primary income account shows the resident units and institutional sectors as recipients rather than producers of primary income. It demonstrates the extent to which operating surpluses are distributed to the owners of the enterprises. The resources side of the allocation of primary income accounts includes the components of the income approach to measurement of GDP. The balance of this account is the gross balance of primary income (B.5g) for each sector, and if the gross balance is aggregated across all sectors of the economy the result is *Gross National Income*.

The secondary distribution of income account describes how the balance of income for each sector is allocated by redistribution; through transfers such as taxes on income, social contributions and benefits and other current transfers. The balancing item of this account is Gross Disposable Income

(GDI) (B.6g). For the households sector, the chained volume measure of GDI is shown as real household disposable income.

Table 16.12 shows, for the households sector, the use of disposable income where the balancing item is saving (B.8g). For the non-financial corporations sector the balancing item of the secondary distribution of income account, gross disposable income (B.6g) is equal to saving (B.8g).

The summary capital account (Table 16.13) brings together the saving and investment of the several sectors of the economy. It shows saving, capital transfers, gross capital formation and net acquisition of non-financial assets for each of the four sectors.

Household and non-profit institutions serving households consumption expenditure at current market prices and chained volume measures

(Tables 16.14 to 16.17)

Household and non-profit institutions serving households (NPISH) consumption expenditure is a major component of the expenditure measure of GDP, both at current prices (Table 16.2) and chained volume measures (Table 16.3). Household final consumption expenditure includes the value of income-in-kind and imputed rent of owner-occupied dwellings, but excludes business expenditure allowed as deductions in computing income for tax purposes. It includes expenditure on durable goods, for instance motor cars, which from the point of view of the individual might more appropriately be treated as capital expenditure. The only exceptions are the purchase of land and dwellings and costs incurred in connection with the transfer of their ownership and expenditure on major improvements by occupiers, which are treated as personal capital expenditure. The estimates of household consumption expenditure include purchases of second-hand as well as new goods, less the proceeds of sales of used goods. The most detailed figures are published quarterly in *Consumer Trends* (available as a web-only publication on the Office for National Statistics website: www.statistics.gov.uk).

Change in inventories (previously known as value of physical increase in stocks and work in progress)

(Table 16.18)

This table gives a broad analysis by industry and, for manufacturing industry, by asset, of the value of entries less withdrawals and losses of inventories (stocks).

Gross fixed capital formation

(Table 16.19 to 16.22)

Gross fixed capital formation comprises expenditure on the replacement of, and additions to, fixed capital assets located in the UK, including all ships and aircraft of UK ownership.

16.1 United Kingdom national and domestic product[1]
Main aggregates
At current prices and chained volume measures, reference year 2005

Indices (2005=100) and £ million

		2001	2002	2003	2004	2005	2006	2007	2008	2009
INDICES (2005=100)										
VALUES AT CURRENT PRICES										
Gross domestic product at current market prices ("money GDP")	YBEU	81.5	85.8	90.9	95.9	100.0	105.7	111.5	115.5	111.3
Gross value added at current basic prices	YBEX	81.3	85.7	90.9	95.9	100.0	105.8	111.6	116.3	112.9
CHAINED VOLUME MEASURES										
Gross domestic product at market prices	YBEZ	90.6	92.5	95.1	97.9	100.0	102.9	105.5	106.1	100.8
Gross national disposable income at market prices	YBFP	89.8	92.9	95.6	98.4	100.0	101.7	105.4	106.9	101.3
Gross value added at basic prices	CGCE	90.7	92.3	94.9	97.7	100.0	103.0	105.7	106.2	101.3
PRICES										
Implied deflator of GDP at market prices	YBGB	90.0	92.7	95.6	98.0	100.0	102.8	105.7	108.9	110.4
VALUES AT CURRENT PRICES (£ million)										
Gross measures (before deduction of fixed capital consumption) at current market prices										
Gross Domestic Product ("money GDP")	YBHA	1 021 828	1 075 564	1 139 746	1 202 956	1 254 058	1 325 795	1 398 882	1 448 391	1 395 872
Employment, property and entrepreneurial income from the rest of the world (receipts *less* payments)	YBGG	9 425	18 286	17 523	17 845	21 855	9 573	20 775	26 940	..
Subsidies (receipts) *less* taxes (payments) on products from/to the rest of the world	-QZOZ	−3 920	−2 890	−2 596	−1 234	−4 260	−4 496	−4 731	−4 906	..
Other subsidies on production from/to the rest of the world	-IBJL	298	519	..	..	..	..	..	..	..
Gross National Income (GNI)	ABMX	1 027 915	1 091 479	1 155 265	1 220 159	1 275 061	1 334 091	1 417 878	1 476 869	1 423 812
Current transfers from the rest of the world (receipts *less* payments)	-YBGF	−3 182	−6 500	−7 843	−9 645	−11 052	−10 617	−11 796	−11 814	..
Gross National Disposable Income	NQCO	1 024 733	1 084 979	1 147 422	1 210 514	1 264 009	1 323 474	1 406 082	1 464 654	1 409 872
Adjustment to current basic prices										
Gross Domestic Product (at current market prices)	YBHA	1 021 828	1 075 564	1 139 746	1 202 956	1 254 058	1 325 795	1 398 882	1 448 391	1 395 872
Adjustment to current basic prices (*less* taxes *plus* subsidies on products)	-NQBU	−114 234	−118 470	−124 738	−132 005	−137 410	−144 654	−153 147	−149 781	−135 212
Gross Value Added (at current basic prices)	ABML	907 594	957 094	1 015 008	1 070 951	1 116 648	1 181 141	1 245 735	1 298 795	1 260 660
Net measures (after deduction of fixed capital consumption) at current market prices	-NQAE	−115 347	−121 448	−124 999	−133 804	−137 843	−147 461	−154 276	−151 273	..
Net domestic product	NHRK	906 032	953 650	1 014 143	1 067 889	1 115 786	1 178 252	1 241 498	1 283 841	..
Net national income	NSRX	912 119	969 565	1 029 662	1 085 092	1 136 789	1 186 548	1 260 494	1 308 983	..
Net national disposable income	NQCP	908 937	963 065	1 021 819	1 075 447	1 125 737	1 175 931	1 248 698	1 297 169	..
CHAINED VOLUME MEASURES (Reference year 2005, £ million)										
Gross measures (before deduction of fixed capital consumption) at market prices										
Gross Domestic Product	ABMI	1 135 823	1 159 641	1 192 206	1 227 387	1 254 058	1 289 833	1 322 842	1 330 088	1 264 646
Terms of trade effect ("Trading gain or loss")	YBGJ	−4 007	3 980	8 094	9 005	−	−1 941	2 132	6 909	..
Real gross domestic income	YBGL	1 131 816	1 163 621	1 200 300	1 236 392	1 254 058	1 287 892	1 324 974	1 339 561	..
Real employment, property and entrepreneurial income from the rest of the world (receipts *less* payments)	YBGI	10 414	19 769	18 445	18 340	21 855	9 294	19 692	24 922	..
Subsidies (receipts) *less* taxes (payments) on production from/to the rest of the world	-QZPB	−4 334	−3 126	−2 734	−1 268	−4 260	−4 365	−4 484	−4 538	..
Other subsidies on production from/to the rest of the world	-IBJN	643	561	623	608	3 408	3 125	2 798	2 875	..
Gross National Income (GNI)	YBGM	1 138 515	1 180 825	1 216 632	1 254 069	1 275 061	1 295 946	1 342 980	1 362 820	..
Real current transfers from the rest of the world (receipts *less* payments)	-YBGP	−3 516	−7 027	−8 256	−9 913	−11 052	−10 309	−11 181	−10 929	..
Gross National Disposable Income	YBGO	1 135 008	1 173 799	1 208 376	1 244 156	1 264 009	1 285 638	1 331 799	1 351 379	1 280 225
Adjustment to basic prices										
Gross Domestic Product (at market prices)	ABMI	1 135 823	1 159 641	1 192 206	1 227 387	1 254 058	1 289 833	1 322 842	1 330 088	1 264 646
Adjustment to basic prices (*less* taxes *plus* subsidies on products)	-NTAQ	−123 376	−128 776	−132 043	−136 609	−137 410	−139 992	−142 684	−142 935	..
Gross Value Added (at basic prices)	ABMM	1 012 564	1 030 892	1 060 186	1 090 812	1 116 648	1 149 841	1 180 158	1 185 413	1 130 607
Net measures (after deduction of fixed capital consumption) at market prices	-CIHA	−121 383	−126 830	−128 992	−136 211	−137 842	−144 769	−148 761	−145 429	..
Net national income at market prices	YBET	1 017 722	1 054 214	1 087 183	1 116 527	1 136 789	1 151 866	1 195 057	1 207 080	..
Net national disposable income at market prices	YBEY	1 014 250	1 047 201	1 078 932	1 106 615	1 125 737	1 141 556	1 183 876	1 196 151	..

1 See chapter text.

Source: Office for National Statistics: 020 7014 2083

16.2 United Kingdom gross domestic product and national income[1]
Current prices

£ million

		2001	2002	2003	2004	2005	2006	2007	2008	2009
Gross domestic product: Output										
Gross value added, at basic prices										
Output of goods and services	NQAF	1 861 011	1 939 534	2 040 175	2 140 893	2 257 761	2 389 308	2 512 632	..	..
less intermediate consumption	-NQAJ	-953 417	-982 440	-1 025 167	-1 069 942	-1 141 113	-1 208 167	-1 266 897	..	..
Total Gross Value Added	ABML	907 594	957 094	1 015 008	1 070 951	1 116 648	1 181 141	1 245 735	1 298 795	1 260 660
Value added taxes (VAT) on products	QYRC	67 097	71 059	77 335	81 540	83 382	87 679	92 000	..	..
Other taxes on products	NSUI	52 845	53 945	54 813	58 307	59 167	62 869	66 721	63 300	..
less subsidies on products	-NZHC	-5 708	-6 534	-7 410	-7 846	-5 182	-5 973	-5 591	-5 516	..
Gross Domestic Product at market prices	YBHA	1 021 828	1 075 564	1 139 746	1 202 956	1 254 058	1 325 795	1 398 882	1 448 391	1 395 872
Gross domestic product: Expenditure										
Final consumption expenditure										
Actual individual consumption										
Household final consumption expenditure	ABPB	647 778	680 964	714 608	749 867	784 140	817 036	859 268	891 371	875 234
Final consumption expenditure of NPISH	ABNV	25 111	26 422	27 668	29 197	30 824	32 439	33 722	37 129	35 334
Individual government final consumption expenditure	NNAQ	118 458	130 816	143 954	148 789	160 199	172 856	182 035	194 461	206 608
Total actual individual consumption	NQEO	791 347	838 202	886 230	927 853	975 163	1 022 331	1 075 025	1 122 961	1 117 176
Collective government final consumption expenditure	NQEP	76 126	81 761	88 865	102 325	107 889	112 331	112 678	119 101	120 858
Total final consumption expenditure	ABKW	867 473	919 963	975 095	1 030 178	1 083 052	1 134 662	1 187 703	1 242 062	1 238 034
Households and NPISH	NSSG	672 889	707 386	742 276	779 064	814 964	849 475	892 990	928 500	910 568
Central government	NMBJ	118 778	130 348	142 658	152 274	161 329	173 428	177 779	190 146	199 920
Local government	NMMT	75 806	82 229	90 161	98 840	106 759	111 759	116 934	123 416	127 546
Gross capital formation										
Gross fixed capital formation	NPQX	171 782	180 551	186 700	200 415	209 758	227 370	248 766	242 822	207 918
Changes in inventories	ABMP	6 189	2 909	3 983	4 886	4 472	5 008	6 986	1 432	-14 694
Acquisitions less disposals of valuables	NPJO	396	214	-37	-37	-376	285	374	614	581
Total gross capital formation	NQFM	178 367	183 674	190 646	205 264	213 854	232 663	256 126	244 868	193 808
Exports of goods and services	KTMW	276 866	280 536	290 677	303 796	330 794	377 879	371 503	422 401	388 838
less imports of goods and services	-KTMX	-300 878	-308 609	-316 672	-336 282	-373 641	-419 409	-416 450	-460 640	-421 315
External balance of goods and services	KTMY	-24 012	-28 073	-25 995	-32 486	-42 847	-41 530	-44 947	-38 239	-32 477
Statistical discrepancy between expenditure components and GDP	RVFD	–	–	–	–	–	–	–	-299	-3 492
Gross Domestic Product at market prices	YBHA	1 021 828	1 075 564	1 139 746	1 202 956	1 254 058	1 325 795	1 398 882	1 448 391	1 395 872
Gross domestic product: Income										
Operating surplus, gross										
Non-financial corporations										
Public non-financial corporations	NRJT	6 879	6 586	7 200	6 927	8 661	9 562	10 167	8 281	9 263
Private non-financial corporations	NRJK	183 157	188 444	201 091	216 746	225 040	247 013	254 243	265 021	241 026
Financial corporations	NQNV	12 965	27 125	33 218	32 879	33 135	38 847	46 377	63 695	66 938
Adjustment for financial services	-NSRV	-33 648	-41 136	-45 370	-50 165	-51 922	-53 065	-57 536	..	..
General government	NMXV	9 796	10 289	10 807	11 312	11 927	12 647	13 171	13 859	14 701
Households and non-profit institutions serving households	QWLS	53 000	55 647	60 984	65 755	67 497	70 116	77 874	75 173	60 359
Total operating surplus, gross	ABNF	265 797	288 091	313 300	333 619	346 260	378 185	401 832	426 029	392 287
Mixed income	QWLT	61 282	64 967	68 324	74 282	79 061	80 023	82 398	83 573	84 283
Compensation of employees	HAEA	564 194	587 396	616 893	646 351	677 478	708 414	746 384	771 539	767 571
Taxes on production and imports	NZGX	137 507	143 117	150 665	158 587	162 059	171 518	180 262	..	..
less subsidies	-AAXJ	-6 952	-8 007	-9 436	-10 000	-11 039	-12 285	-12 013	-12 069	..
Statistical discrepancy between income components and GDP	RVFC	–	–	–	–	–	–	–	1 003	-816
Gross Domestic Product at market prices	YBHA	1 021 828	1 075 564	1 139 746	1 202 956	1 254 058	1 325 795	1 398 882	1 448 391	1 395 872

16.2

United Kingdom gross domestic product and national income[1]
Current prices
continued

		2001	2002	2003	2004	2005	2006	2007	2008	2009
Gross Domestic Product at market prices	YBHA	1 021 828	1 075 564	1 139 746	1 202 956	1 254 058	1 325 795	1 398 882	1 448 391	1 395 872
Compensation of employees										
receipts from the rest of the world	KTMN	1 087	1 121	1 116	931	974	938	981	1 045	916
less payments to the rest of the world	-KTMO	−1 021	−1 054	−1 057	−1 425	−1 584	−1 896	−1 715	−1 759	−1 604
Total	KTMP	66	67	59	−494	−610	−958	−734	−714	−688
less Taxes on products paid to the rest of the world										
plus Subsidies received from the rest of the world	-QZOZ	−3 920	−2 890	−2 596	−1 234	−4 260	−4 496	−4 731	−4 906	..
Other subsidies on production	-IBJL	298	519	..	..	..	..	..	..	..
Property and entrepreneurial income										
receipts from the rest of the world	HMBN	137 447	120 543	122 069	137 380	185 766	236 684	290 321	260 022	174 655
less payments to the rest of the world	-HMBO	−128 088	−102 324	−104 605	−119 041	−163 301	−226 153	−268 812	−229 015	−145 311
Total	HMBM	9 359	18 219	17 464	18 339	22 465	10 531	21 509	31 007	29 344
Gross National Income at market prices	ABMX	1 027 915	1 091 479	1 155 265	1 220 159	1 275 061	1 334 091	1 417 878	1 476 869	1 423 812

1 See chapter text.

Source: Office for National Statistics: 020 7014 2083

16.3

United Kingdom gross domestic product[1]
Chained volume measures, reference year 2005

£ million

		2001	2002	2003	2004	2005	2006	2007	2008	2009
Gross domestic product: expenditure approach										
Final consumption expenditure										
Actual individual consumption										
Household final consumption expenditure	ABPF	694 810	720 417	742 755	766 856	784 140	795 595	815 157	822 086	795 847
Final consumption expenditure of non-profit institutions serving households	ABNU	30 752	30 761	30 865	30 827	30 824	31 868	30 040	30 832	29 628
Individual government final consumption expenditure	NSZK	114 159	117 238	120 288	..	..	..	..	..	..
Total actual individual consumption	YBIO	868 304	899 025	926 191	955 004	975 163	990 185	1 010 718	1 025 495	..
Collective government final consumption expenditure	NSZL	88 420	91 435	95 103	105 567	107 889	109 549	109 967	113 440	..
Total final consumption expenditure	ABKX	963 758	997 754	1 028 666	1 060 572	1 083 052	1 099 734	1 120 685	1 138 935	..
Gross capital formation										
Gross fixed capital formation	NPQR	185 952	192 734	194 819	204 756	209 758	223 305	240 613	232 202	197 592
Changes in inventories	ABMQ	5 760	2 364	4 112	4 843	4 472	4 789	6 646	866	−15 185
Acquisitions less disposals of valuables	NPJP	−376	−217	6	−39	−377	304	562	1 295	1 233
Total gross capital formation	NPQU	191 982	195 012	198 418	209 599	213 853	228 398	247 821	236 254	..
Gross domestic final expenditure	YBIK	1 155 830	1 192 759	1 227 030	1 270 171	1 296 905	1 328 132	1 368 506	1 369 962	1 297 934
Exports of goods and services	KTMZ	283 840	286 679	291 946	306 582	330 794	368 076	357 677	361 535	323 256
Gross final expenditure	ABME	1 439 784	1 479 170	1 518 564	1 576 494	1 627 699	1 696 207	1 726 183	1 731 497	1 621 190
less imports of goods and services	-KTNB	−304 476	−319 408	−326 301	−348 894	−373 641	−406 374	−403 341	−401 136	−353 383
Statistical discrepancy between expenditure components and GDP	GIXS	−	−	−	−	−	−	−	−271	−3 161
Gross Domestic Product at market prices	ABMI	1 135 823	1 159 641	1 192 206	1 227 387	1 254 058	1 289 833	1 322 842	1 330 088	1 264 646
of which External balance of goods and services	KTNC	−20 636	−32 729	−34 355	−42 312	−42 847	−38 298	−45 664	−39 601	−30 127

1 See chapter text.

Source: Office for National Statistics: 020 7014 2083

16.4 Gross value added at current basic prices: by industry[1,2]
United Kingdom

£ million

		2001	2002	2003	2004	2005	2006	2007	2008	2009
Agriculture, hunting, forestry and fishing	EWSH	8 333	9 007	9 806	10 670	7 530	7 911	9 302	..	..
Production										
Mining and quarrying										
Mining and quarrying of energy producing materials										
Mining of coal	QTOQ	545	538	472	380	343	346	379	..	..
Extraction of mineral oil and natural gas	QTOR	20 825	19 911	19 451	20 657	24 995	29 631	29 127	..	..
Other mining and quarrying	QTOS	1 750	1 469	1 520	1 848	2 115	2 330	2 690	..	..
Total mining and quarrying	EWSL	23 120	21 918	21 442	22 885	27 453	32 307	32 196	..	..
Manufacturing										
Food; beverages and tobacco	QTOU	20 655	20 834	21 408	22 101	22 019	22 133	22 587	..	..
Textiles and textile products	QTOV	5 343	4 818	4 282	4 071	3 888	3 985	4 031	..	..
Leather and leather products	QTOW	645	590	462	398	391	344	333	..	..
Wood and wood products	QTOX	2 332	2 479	2 655	2 744	2 759	2 863	3 016	..	..
Pulp, paper and paper products; publishing and printing	QTOY	20 129	20 008	19 780	19 784	19 479	20 082	19 831	..	..
Coke, petroleum products and nuclear fuel	QTOZ	2 488	2 435	2 377	2 396	2 492	2 258	2 708	..	..
Chemicals, chemical products and man-made fibres	QTPA	16 077	16 083	16 149	15 644	16 771	18 553	19 508	..	..
Rubber and plastic products	QTPB	7 656	7 569	7 516	7 545	7 400	7 077	7 188	..	..
Other non-metal mineral products	QTPC	5 033	5 296	5 417	5 253	5 298	5 379	5 700	..	..
Basic metals and fabricated metal products	QTPD	15 525	14 897	14 774	15 075	16 093	16 381	17 064	..	..
Machinery and equipment not elsewhere classified	QTPE	12 256	12 085	12 146	12 373	12 245	12 958	12 693	..	..
Electrical and optical equipment	QTPF	18 347	16 468	15 545	15 651	16 493	16 876	17 358	..	..
Transport equipment	QTPG	16 091	16 178	15 903	16 110	16 216	16 526	15 770	..	..
Manufacturing not elsewhere classified	QTPH	6 643	6 567	6 429	6 546	6 569	6 646	7 131	..	..
Total manufacturing	EWSP	149 223	146 308	144 845	145 691	148 111	152 060	154 919	..	..
Electricity, gas and water supply	EWST	15 660	16 052	16 405	16 106	16 685	20 005	21 086	..	..
Total production	QTPK	188 000	184 277	182 690	184 682	192 251	204 373	208 200	..	..
Construction	EWSX	50 526	54 684	59 522	66 029	69 868	74 509	80 148	..	..
Service industries										
Wholesale and retail trade (including motor trade); repair of motor vehicles, personal and household goods	QTPM	110 250	113 776	120 520	127 366	129 811	134 525	140 904	..	..
Hotels and restaurants	QTPN	26 927	28 638	30 120	31 870	32 901	34 275	35 289	..	..
Transport, storage and communication										
Transport and storage	QTPO	43 184	44 501	47 022	48 703	50 203	51 845	54 303	..	..
Communication	QTPP	27 317	28 562	29 566	30 317	30 684	30 928	32 551	..	..
Total	EWTF	70 502	73 064	76 587	79 020	80 889	82 773	86 854	..	..
Financial intermediation	QTPR	48 202	63 368	71 530	75 117	79 554	90 790	103 646	..	..
Adjustment for financial services (FISIM)	-NSRV	-33 648	-41 136	-45 370	-50 165	-51 922	-53 065	-57 536	..	..
Real estate, renting and business activities										
Letting of dwellings including imputed rent of owner occupiers	QTPS	61 352	64 249	69 298	74 249	76 817	80 222	88 248	..	..
Other real estate, renting and business activities	QTPT	142 689	150 599	162 909	174 427	183 299	195 669	205 958	..	..
Total	QTPU	204 041	214 848	232 207	248 676	260 116	275 891	294 206	..	..
Public administration and defence (PAD)	EWTN	45 025	47 528	51 302	55 393	60 096	63 033	..	..	..
Education	QTPW	51 675	55 099	58 328	61 934	65 739	68 993	73 477	..	..
Health and social work	QTPX	59 549	64 493	70 592	75 154	79 965	84 715	88 170	..	..
Other social and personal services, private households with employees and extra-territorial organisations	EWTV	44 561	48 312	51 804	54 947	57 961	60 125	62 455	..	..
Total service industries	QTPZ	660 729	709 122	762 988	809 569	847 001	894 348	948 085	..	..
All industries	ABML	907 594	957 094	1 015 008	1 070 951	1 116 648	1 181 141	1 245 735	1 298 795	1 260 660

1 See chapter text. Components may not sum to totals as a result of rounding.

2 Because of differences in the annual and monthly production inquiries, estimates of current price output and value added by industry derived from the current price input-output supply-use balances are not consistent with the equivalent measures of constant price growth given in Table 16.5. These differences do not affect GDP totals. For further information see "Experimental Constant Price Input-Output Supply-Use Balances: An approach to improving the quality of the national accounts" Nadim Ahmad, *Economic Trends*, July 1999 (No. 548).

Source: Office for National Statistics: 020 7014 2083

16.5 Gross value added at basic prices: by industry[1,2,3,4]
Chained volume indices
United Kingdom

Indices (2005=100)

	Weight per 1000[1]		2001	2002	2003	2004	2005	2006	2007	2008	2009
	2003										
Agriculture, hunting, forestry and fishing	9.9	GDQA	84.7	94.6	93.0	92.9	100.0	100.7	95.9	96.1	91.9
Production											
Mining and quarrying											
Mining and quarrying of energy producing materials											
Mining of coal	0.6	CKZP	167.9	157.5	148.7	129.5	100.0	97.2	85.5	88.8	83.1
Extraction of mineral oil and natural gas	25.1	CKZO	129.9	128.3	121.3	111.4	100.0	90.9	88.9	84.6	78.1
Other mining and quarrying	2.0	CKZQ	72.4	87.7	88.8	91.1	100.0	106.1	113.2	87.5	51.4
Total mining and quarrying	27.7	CKYX	124.6	125.0	118.7	109.7	100.0	92.1	90.7	84.8	..
Manufacturing											
Food; beverages and tobacco	23.8	CKZA	95.4	98.1	96.5	98.0	100.0	99.3	99.4	97.7	95.6
Textiles and textile products	6.3	CKZB	117.4	110.6	111.1	101.5	100.0	99.4	97.3	98.2	89.5
Leather and leather products	0.7	CKZC	191.2	173.8	149.1	109.6	100.0	104.5	107.0	102.1	95.5
Wood and wood products	2.7	CKZD	96.7	97.5	98.8	104.0	100.0	97.7	101.8	94.1	79.2
Pulp, paper and paper products; publishing and printing	23.2	CKZE	106.9	107.1	105.2	104.0	100.0	99.5	99.7	97.6	89.3
Coke, petroleum products and nuclear fuel	2.9	CKZF	96.3	98.4	90.1	101.3	100.0	94.5	95.7	97.8	93.6
Chemicals, chemical products and man-made fibres	18.4	CKZG	92.3	93.1	93.9	97.4	100.0	103.1	101.8	101.4	96.7
Rubber and plastic products	9.0	CKZH	106.2	102.0	102.9	101.2	100.0	104.2	103.3	98.2	85.3
Other non-metallic mineral products	5.8	CKZI	91.2	90.2	94.2	99.8	100.0	102.7	103.2	97.5	84.7
Basic metals and fabricated metal products	17.8	CKZJ	96.7	97.8	96.6	99.1	100.0	101.5	103.1	99.1	80.5
Machinery and equipment not elsewhere classified	13.9	CKZK	95.5	90.3	91.5	96.9	100.0	106.4	111.1	109.8	87.3
Electrical and optical equipment	21.3	CKZL	122.0	106.0	102.0	103.9	100.0	99.7	99.2	93.7	83.7
Transport equipment	18.1	CKZM	93.6	90.7	95.1	100.4	100.0	104.6	105.1	102.1	88.6
Manufacturing not elsewhere classified	7.6	CKZN	98.3	99.4	99.3	98.6	100.0	101.0	104.0	97.8	90.0
Total manufacturing	171.6	CKYY	100.5	98.3	98.0	100.2	100.0	101.6	102.2	99.2	88.8
Electricity, gas and water supply	18.2	CKYZ	97.1	97.6	99.3	100.3	100.0	99.5	99.7	99.9	92.0
Total production	217.6	CKYW	102.5	100.9	100.2	101.3	100.0	100.0	100.3	97.2	87.3
Construction	56.7	GDQB	87.7	91.1	95.8	99.0	100.0	101.1	103.8	103.0	92.0
Service industries											
Wholesale and retail trade (including motor trade); repair of motor vehicles, personal and household goods	125.5	GDQC	84.9	89.7	92.8	98.6	100.0	103.2	106.4	105.0	100.8
Hotels and restaurants	33.3	GDQD	91.3	93.9	96.6	98.3	100.0	104.2	107.5	107.4	101.1
Transport, storage and communication											
Transport and storage	49.8	GDQF	91.9	93.1	92.0	96.8	100.0	102.4	105.0	106.4	97.8
Communication	31.3	GDQG	87.1	86.2	92.3	95.7	100.0	102.3	107.6	110.1	109.4
Total	81.0	GDQH	89.9	90.3	92.1	96.4	100.0	102.4	106.0	107.8	102.2
Financial intermediation	48.5	GDQI	81.8	85.5	91.5	95.4	100.0	107.2	114.9	121.6	116.4
Adjustment for financial services (FISIM)	−38.1	GDQJ	86.3	89.2	100.0	113.0	123.3	138.8	162.8	..	..
Real estate, renting and business activities											
Letting of dwellings, including imputed rent of owner occupiers	77.8	GDQL	97.5	98.3	100.1	99.4	100.0	101.8	102.2	102.8	104.1
Other real estate, renting and business activities	160.4	GDQK	83.5	83.7	87.7	93.3	100.0	107.3	114.7	116.6	108.4
Total	238.3	GDQM	87.4	87.8	91.1	95.0	100.0	105.7	111.0	112.5	107.0
Public administration and defence (PAD)[4]	55.6	GDQO	90.7	93.3	98.1	99.2	100.0	100.6	100.4	99.0	100.1
Education	58.7	GDQP	97.2	99.2	100.1	99.4	100.0	100.0	99.5	100.2	100.7
Health and social work[4]	62.3	GDQQ	87.0	90.6	94.1	97.2	100.0	102.8	105.5	108.9	111.8
Other social and personal services, private households with employees and extra-territorial organisations	51.0	GDQR	97.4	99.5	100.3	99.2	100.0	99.9	101.4	103.5	94.8
Total service industries	715.8	GDQS	88.4	90.5	93.7	97.0	100.0	103.6	107.2	108.7	104.9
All industries	1 000.0	CGCE	90.7	92.3	94.9	97.7	100.0	103.0	105.7	106.2	101.3

1 See chapter text. The weights are in proportion to total gross value added (GVA) in 2003 and are used to combine the industry output indices to calculate the totals for 2004 and 2005. For 2003 and earlier, totals are calculated using the equivalent weight for the previous year (eg totals for 2002 use 2001 weights).

2 As GVA is expressed in index number form, it is inappropriate to show as a statistical adjustment any divergence from the other measures of GDP. Such an adjustment does, however, exist implicitly.

3 See footnote 2 to Table 16.4.

4 The GVA for PAD, education and Health and social work in this table follows the SIC(92) and differs from that used in Table 2.3 in *United Kingdom National Accounts* (the *Blue Book*) which is based on Input-Output groups. The administration costs of the NHS are included in PAD in this table but are included in Health and social work in Table 2.3.

Source: Office for National Statistics: 020 7014 2083

16.6 Non-financial corporations[1]
Allocation of primary income account[2]
United Kingdom. ESA95 sector S.11

£ million

		2001	2002	2003	2004	2005	2006	2007	2008	2009
Resources										
Operating surplus, gross	NQBE	190 036	195 030	208 291	223 673	233 701	256 575	264 410	273 302	250 289
Property income, received										
Interest	EABC	13 177	9 330	9 727	14 141	17 380	24 385	29 468	22 648	4 243
Distributed income of corporations	EABD	36 868	32 210	..	..	..	..	..	..	..
Reinvested earnings on direct foreign investment	HDVR	22 950	26 893	12 492	22 713	33 199	36 511	49 474	34 398	27 861
Attributed property income of insurance policy-holders	FAOF	280	302	..	..	..	..	..	..	..
Rent	FAOG	117	118	..	..	..	..	..	..	..
Total	FAKY	74 102	67 229	73 070	80 463	98 125	105 667	118 840	105 702	89 002
Total resources	FBXJ	264 138	262 259	281 361	304 136	331 826	362 242	383 250	379 004	339 291
Uses										
Property income, paid										
Interest	EABG	30 661	29 045	29 592	34 961	39 356	44 949	54 970	48 912	28 737
Distributed income of corporations	NVCS	100 810	91 868	..	..	..	..	..	..	..
Reinvested earnings on direct foreign investment	HDVB	1 699	1 614	3 955	6 325	4 983	15 452	15 331	3 923	2 486
Rent	FBXO	1 896	1 853	..	..	..	..	..	..	..
Total	FBXK	137 950	119 879	128 885	136 773	152 133	170 586	177 416	169 503	140 526
Balance of primary incomes, gross	NQBG	126 188	142 380	152 476	167 363	179 693	191 656	205 834	209 501	198 765
Total uses	FBXJ	264 138	262 259	281 361	304 136	331 826	362 242	383 250	379 004	339 291
After deduction of fixed capital consumption	-DBGF	-68 362	-70 547	-72 598	-75 559	-77 277	-80 329	-83 485	-86 765	..
Balance of primary incomes, net	FBXQ	57 826	71 833	79 878	91 804	102 416	111 327	122 349	116 417	..

1 See chapter text.
2 Before deduction of fixed capital formation.

Source: Office for National Statistics: 020 7014 2014

16.7 Non-financial corporations[1]
Secondary distribution of income account
United Kingdom. ESA95 sector S.11

£ million

		2001	2002	2003	2004	2005	2006	2007	2008	2009
Resources										
Balance of primary incomes, gross	NQBG	126 188	142 380	152 476	167 363	179 693	191 656	205 834	209 501	198 765
Social contributions										
Imputed social contributions	NSTJ	4 357	4 575	4 229	3 838	4 124	4 192	4 346	4 148	4 712
Current transfers other than taxes, social contributions and benefits										
Non-life insurance claims	FCBP	4 565	7 789	..	..	..	..	..	..	..
Miscellaneous transfers	NRJY	619	616	..	..	..	..	..	..	..
Total	NRJB	3 836	5 543	6 124	6 550	7 261	7 819	4 220	5 682	5 203
Total resources	FCBR	134 381	152 498	162 829	177 751	191 078	203 667	214 400	219 331	208 680
Uses										
Current taxes on income, wealth etc.										
Taxes on income	FCBS	23 177	24 038	23 702	27 366	33 618	37 211	38 358	41 795	34 353
Social benefits other than social transfers in kind	NSTJ	4 357	4 575	4 229	3 838	4 124	4 192	4 346	4 148	4 712
Current transfers other than taxes, social contributions and benefits										
Net non-life insurance premiums	FCBY	4 565	7 789	..	..	..	..	..	..	..
Miscellaneous current transfers	FDBI	411	422	434	446	..	..	..	..	..
Total, other current transfers	FCBX	4 220	5 876	6 462	6 973	7 749	8 296	4 708	6 170	5 691
Gross Disposable Income	NRJD	102 627	118 009	128 436	139 574	145 587	153 968	166 988	167 218	163 924
Total uses	FCBR	134 381	152 498	162 829	177 751	191 078	203 667	214 400	219 331	208 680
After deduction of fixed capital consumption	-DBGF	-68 362	-70 547	-72 598	-75 559	-77 277	-80 329	-83 485	-86 765	..
Disposable income, net	FCCF	34 265	47 462	55 838	64 015	68 310	73 639	83 503	74 663	..

1 See chapter text.

Source: Office for National Statistics: 020 7014 2014

16.8

General government[1]
Allocation of primary income account

United Kingdom. ESA95 sector S.13 Unconsolidated

£ million

		2001	2002	2003	2004	2005	2006	2007	2008	2009
Resources										
Operating surplus, gross	NMXV	9 796	10 289	10 807	11 312	11 927	12 647	13 171	13 859	14 701
Taxes on production and imports, received										
Taxes on products										
Value added tax (VAT)	NZGF	63 525	68 258	74 603	79 755	81 426	85 591	89 698	89 732	77 908
Taxes and duties on imports excluding VAT										
Import duties	NMXZ	–	–	–	–	–	–	–	–	..
Taxes on imports excluding VAT and import duties	NMBT	–	–	–	–	..	..	..	..	..
Taxes on products excluding VAT and import duties	NMYB	50 745	52 001	52 858	56 137	56 906	60 540	64 309	60 666	60 349
Total taxes on products	NVCC	114 267	120 252	127 453	135 892	138 332	146 131	154 007	150 348	137 262
Other taxes on production	NMYD	17 565	18 113	18 517	18 853	19 706	20 831	21 543	22 618	24 248
Total taxes on production and imports, received	NMYE	131 832	138 365	145 970	154 745	158 038	166 962	175 550	173 391	161 510
less Subsidies, paid										
Subsidies on products	-NMYF	−3 953	−4 672	−5 311	−5 121	−5 182	−5 973	−5 591	−5 658	−6 288
Other subsidies on production	-LIUF	−662	−954	−1 434	−1 562	−2 449	−3 093	−3 470	−3 445	−3 391
Total	-NMRL	−4 615	−5 626	−6 745	−6 683	−7 631	−9 066	−9 061	−8 959	−9 679
Property income, received										
Total Interest	NMYL	7 359	6 683	7 131	6 838	6 471	7 137	8 109	8 780	6 515
Distributed income of corporations	NMYM	4 710	3 290	3 027	2 794	2 900	2 570	3 153	3 149	1 968
Property income attributed to insurance policy holders	NMYO	24	22	19	19	27	25	20	16	20
Rent										
from sectors other than general government	NMYR	1 919	1 901	1 565	1 182	1 229	1 226	1 233	1 162	1 172
Total	NMYU	14 012	11 892	11 742	10 833	10 627	10 958	12 515	13 114	9 675
Total resources	NMYV	151 025	154 920	161 774	170 207	172 961	181 501	192 175	191 405	176 207
Uses										
Property income, paid										
Total interest	NRKB	27 911	25 410	26 913	26 973	29 376	30 485	34 171	36 422	..
Total	NMYY	27 911	25 410	26 913	26 973	29 376	30 485	34 171	36 418	29 865
Balance of primary incomes, gross	NMZH	123 114	129 510	134 861	143 234	143 585	151 016	158 004	154 987	146 342
Total uses	NMYV	151 025	154 920	161 774	170 207	172 961	181 501	192 175	191 405	176 207
After deduction of fixed capital consumption	-NMXO	−9 796	−10 289	−10 807	−11 312	−11 927	−12 647	−13 171	−13 859	−14 701
Balance of primary incomes,net	NMZI	113 318	119 221	124 054	131 922	131 658	138 369	144 833	140 113	..

1 See chapter text.

Source: Office for National Statistics: 020 7014 2122

16.9 General government[1]
Secondary distribution of income account
United Kingdom. ESA95 sector S.13 Unconsolidated

£ million

		2001	2002	2003	2004	2005	2006	2007	2008	2009
Resources										
Balance of primary incomes, gross	NMZH	123 114	129 510	134 861	143 234	143 585	151 016	158 004	154 987	146 342
Current taxes on income, wealth etc.										
Taxes on income	NMZJ	147 264	142 842	144 234	154 127	172 498	192 812	200 213	207 619	182 907
Other current taxes	NVCM	22 068	23 664	26 016	28 001	29 443	30 908	32 719	34 102	35 059
Total	NMZL	169 332	166 506	170 250	182 128	201 941	223 720	232 932	241 721	217 966
Social contributions										
Actual social contributions										
Employers' actual social contributions	NMZM	38 460	38 780	45 067	49 490	52 852	56 000	58 723	65 051	63 436
Employees' social contributions	NMZN	28 725	29 568	34 376	39 062	41 836	44 360	45 587	45 767	44 339
Social contributions by self- and non-employed persons	NMZO	2 183	2 318	2 595	2 727	2 825	2 930	3 013	3 092	3 112
Total	NMZP	69 368	70 666	82 038	91 279	97 513	103 290	107 323	113 910	110 887
Imputed social contributions	NMZQ	7 577	8 348	6 456	6 219	7 383	7 289	7 933	7 918	8 961
Total	NMZR	76 945	79 014	88 494	97 498	104 896	110 579	115 256	121 828	119 848
Other current transfers										
Non-life insurance claims	NMZS	353	400	296	338	328	366	277	299	340
Current transfers within general government	NMZT	72 522	77 592	85 224	94 720	101 369	110 407	113 210	117 933	125 017
Current international cooperation	NMZU	4 568	3 112	3 570	3 673	3 726	3 674	3 676	4 966	5 528
Miscellaneous current transfers										
from sectors other than general government	NMZX	460	502	562	721	728	606	556	573	460
Other current transfers	NNAA	77 815	81 526	89 632	99 452	106 151	115 053	117 719	123 846	131 345
Total resources	NNAB	447 206	456 556	483 237	522 312	556 573	600 368	623 911	642 382	615 501
Uses										
Social benefits other than social transfers in kind	NNAD	129 591	136 801	146 066	154 314	161 422	167 052	178 379	190 084	210 483
Other current transfers										
Net non-life insurance premiums	NNAE	353	400	296	338	328	366	277	299	340
Current transfers within general government	NNAF	72 522	77 592	85 224	94 720	101 369	110 407	113 210	117 933	125 017
Current international cooperation	NNAG	2 190	2 362	2 433	3 080	3 255	3 632	3 930	4 292	4 694
Miscellaneous current transfers										
to sectors other than general government	NNAI	22 131	27 351	30 275	31 178	34 355	34 695	35 878	36 966	40 848
Of which: GNP based fourth own resource	NMFH	3 858	5 335	6 772	7 549	8 732	8 521	8 323	8 423	10 555
Other current transfers	NNAN	97 108	107 625	118 208	129 316	139 307	149 100	153 295	159 565	170 899
Gross Disposable Income	NNAO	219 605	211 254	218 121	237 758	254 822	283 141	291 126	291 586	232 930
Total uses	NNAB	447 206	456 556	483 237	522 312	556 573	600 368	623 911	642 382	615 501
After deduction of fixed capital consumption	-NMXO	–9 796	–10 289	–10 807	–11 312	–11 927	–12 647	–13 171	–13 859	–14 701
Disposable income, net	NNAP	209 809	200 965	207 314	226 446	242 895	270 494	277 955	276 511	..

1 See chapter text.

Source: Office for National Statistics: 020 7014 2122

16.10 Households and non-profit institutions serving households[1]
Allocation of primary income account
United Kingdom. ESA95 sectors S.14 and S.15

£ million

		2001	2002	2003	2004	2005	2006	2007	2008	2009
Resources										
Operating surplus, gross	QWLS	53 000	55 647	60 984	65 755	67 497	70 116	77 874	75 173	60 359
Mixed income, gross	QWLT	61 282	64 967	68 324	74 282	79 061	80 023	82 398	83 573	84 283
Compensation of employees										
Wages and salarles	QWLW	491 044	508 681	527 689	549 501	569 861	592 857	629 100	651 910	645 706
Employers' social contributions	QWLX	73 216	78 782	89 263	96 356	107 007	114 599	116 550	118 915	121 177
Total	QWLY	564 260	587 463	616 952	645 857	676 868	707 456	745 650	770 825	766 883
Property income										
Interest	QWLZ	31 957	26 658	27 251	34 805	40 332	42 856	53 975	47 034	8 933
Distributed income of corporations	QWMA	49 894	43 787	45 248	46 705	50 397	51 249	50 087	51 062	54 623
Attributed property income of insurance policy holders	QWMC	53 277	52 104	55 008	54 623	64 028	66 649	71 684	75 123	69 123
Rent	QWMD	105	106	108	110	110	110	110	115	115
Total	QWME	135 233	122 655	127 615	136 243	154 867	160 864	175 856	173 334	132 794
Total resources	QWMF	813 775	830 732	873 875	922 137	978 293	1 018 459	1 081 778	1 102 905	1 044 319
Uses										
Property income										
Interest	QWMG	33 752	30 512	32 001	43 846	50 309	54 117	72 829	64 306	4 545
Rent	QWMH	215	216	220	224	224	222	234	239	239
Total	QWMI	33 967	30 728	32 221	44 070	50 533	54 339	73 063	64 545	4 784
Balance of primary incomes, gross	QWMJ	779 808	800 004	841 654	878 067	927 760	964 120	1 008 715	1 038 360	1 039 535
Total uses	QWMF	813 775	830 732	873 875	922 137	978 293	1 018 459	1 081 778	1 102 905	1 044 319
After deduction of										
fixed capital consumption	-QWLL	-32 726	-35 852	-36 704	-42 241	-43 165	-48 592	-51 912	-44 922	..
Balance of primary incomes, net	QWMK	746 900	763 961	804 751	835 558	884 503	915 497	954 086	983 824	..

1 See chapter text.

Source: Office for National Statistics: 020 7014 2131

16.11 Households and non-profit institutions serving households[1]
Secondary distribution of income account
United Kingdom. ESA95 sectors S.14 and S.15

£ million

		2001	2002	2003	2004	2005	2006	2007	2008	2009
Resources										
Balance of primary incomes, gross	QWMJ	779 808	800 004	841 654	878 067	927 760	964 120	1 008 715	1 038 360	1 039 535
Imputed social contributions	RVFH	502	530	505	499	506	514	518	524	524
Social benefits other than social transfers in kind	QWML	171 814	182 673	193 596	198 691	212 272	226 629	227 520	250 336	275 456
Other current transfers										
Non-life insurance claims	QWMM	11 723	17 327	13 890	17 479	17 199	20 713	14 842	20 024	18 283
Miscellaneous current transfers	QWMN	29 080	33 041	34 687	34 845	37 840	38 729	40 518	40 321	42 130
Total	QWMO	40 803	50 368	48 577	52 324	55 039	59 442	55 360	60 345	60 413
Total resources	QWMP	992 927	1 033 575	1 084 332	1 129 581	1 195 577	1 250 705	1 292 113	1 349 565	1 375 928
Uses										
Current taxes on income, wealth etc										
Taxes on income	QWMQ	111 888	112 171	113 087	119 591	130 200	139 897	151 891	155 315	143 735
Other current taxes	NVCO	21 166	22 788	25 174	27 077	28 421	29 833	31 608	32 955	33 870
Total	QWMS	133 054	134 959	138 261	146 668	158 621	169 730	183 499	188 270	177 605
Social contributions										
Actual social contributions										
Employers' actual social contributions	QWMT	60 296	64 805	77 571	85 297	94 487	102 093	103 239	105 805	106 460
Employees' social contributions	QWMU	60 599	62 458	66 490	70 264	77 929	83 170	84 907	89 380	83 629
Social contributions by self and non-employed	QWMV	2 183	2 318	2 595	2 727	2 825	2 930	3 013	3 092	3 112
Total	QWMW	123 078	129 581	146 656	158 288	175 241	188 193	191 159	197 319	..
Imputed social contributions	QWMX	12 920	13 977	11 692	11 059	12 520	12 506	13 311	13 110	14 717
Total	QWMY	135 998	143 558	158 348	169 347	187 761	200 699	204 470	211 387	207 918
Social benefits other than social transfers in kind	QWMZ	977	1 006	987	988	1 000	1 010	1 014	1 020	1 020
Other current transfers										
Net non-life insurance premiums	QWNA	11 723	17 327	13 890	17 479	17 199	20 713	14 842	20 024	18 283
Miscellaneous current transfers	QWNB	11 081	11 458	11 930	12 462	13 442	13 286	14 405	13 838	14 009
Total	QWNC	22 804	28 785	25 820	29 941	30 641	33 999	29 247	33 862	32 292
Gross Disposable Income[2]	QWND	700 094	725 267	760 916	782 637	817 554	845 267	873 883	915 026	957 093
Total uses	QWMP	992 927	1 033 575	1 084 332	1 129 581	1 195 577	1 250 705	1 292 113	1 349 565	1 375 928
After deduction of fixed capital consumption	-QWLL	−32 726	−35 852	−36 704	−42 241	−43 165	−48 592	−51 912	−44 922	..
Disposable income, net	QWNE	667 186	689 224	724 013	740 128	774 297	796 644	819 254	858 464	..

1 See chapter text.
2 Gross household disposable income revalued by the implied households and NPISH's final consumption expenditure deflator. For more details see table 6.1.4 on page 217 in *United Kingdom National Accounts* (the *Blue book*).

Source: Office for National Statistics: 020 7014 2131

16.12 Households and non-profit institutions serving households[1]
Use of disposable income account
United Kingdom. ESA95 sectors S.14 and S.15

£ million and percentages

		2001	2002	2003	2004	2005	2006	2007	2008	2009
Resources										
Disposable income, gross	QWND	700 094	725 267	760 916	782 637	817 554	845 267	873 883	915 026	957 093
Adjustment for the change in net equity of households in pension funds	NSSE	16 038	17 784	21 377	26 386	30 881	29 339	38 766	27 844	21 555
Total resources	NSSF	716 132	743 051	782 293	809 023	848 435	874 606	912 649	942 870	978 648
Uses										
Final consumption expenditure										
Individual consumption expenditure	NSSG	672 889	707 386	742 276	779 064	814 964	849 475	892 990	928 500	910 568
Saving, gross	NSSH	43 243	35 665	40 017	29 959	33 471	25 131	19 659	14 370	68 080
Total uses	NSSF	716 132	743 051	782 293	809 023	848 435	874 606	912 649	942 870	978 648
Saving ratio (percentages)	RVGL	6.0	4.8	5.1	3.7	3.9	2.9	2.2	1.5	7.0

1 See chapter text.

Source: Office for National Statistics: 020 7014 2131

16.13 The sector accounts: key economic indicators[1]
United Kingdom

£ million and indices (2005=100)

		2001	2002	2003	2004	2005	2006	2007	2008	2009
Net lending/borrowing by:										
Non-financial corporations	EABO	−6 366	10 549	22 971	32 464	27 110	34 530	31 499	38 700	75 836
Financial corporations	NHCQ	−22 123	4 386	13 451	18 702	9 017	3 124	27 249	59 214	36 099
General government	NNBK	7 660	−20 183	−41 173	−41 889	−40 156	−34 722	−36 947	−70 285	−156 537
Households and NPISH's	NSSZ	1 044	−12 477	−12 091	−32 130	−27 310	−45 799	−56 945	−47 665	27 119
Rest of the world	NHRB	19 784	17 725	16 841	22 853	31 338	42 867	35 144	18 734	14 806
Private non-financial corporations										
Gross trading profits										
Continental shelf profits	CAGJ	20 397	18 742	..	..	..	..	..	..	..
Others	CAED	151 364	160 068	173 584	185 842	190 286	207 737	217 179	218 382	207 237
Rental of buildings	FCBW	12 394	12 904	13 891	14 796	15 819	16 095	16 592	17 511	17 389
less Holding gains of inventories	-DLQZ	438	−2 856	−4 266	−2 906	−4 378	−4 426	−6 399	−7 964	−4 822
Gross operating surplus	NRJK	183 157	188 444	201 091	216 746	225 040	247 013	254 243	265 021	241 026
Households and NPISH										
Household gross disposable income	QWND	700 094	725 267	760 916	782 637	817 554	845 267	873 883	915 026	957 093
Implied deflator of household and NPISH individual consumption expenditure indicies (2003=100)	YBFS	92.8	94.2	96.0	97.7	100.0	102.7	105.7	108.9	110.3
Real household disposable income:										
Chained volume measures (Reference year 2003)	RVGK	754 606	770 013	792 958	801 321	817 554	823 364	827 113	840 543	867 652
Indices (2003=100)	OSXR	92.3	94.2	97.0	98.0	100.0	100.7	101.2	102.8	106.1
Gross saving	NSSH	43 243	35 665	40 017	29 959	33 471	25 131	19 659	14 370	68 080
Households total resources	NSSJ	834 590	873 867	926 247	957 812	1 008 634	1 047 462	1 094 684	1 137 331	1 185 256
Saving ratio (percentages)	RVGL	6.0	4.8	5.1	3.7	3.9	2.9	2.2	1.5	7.0

1 See chapter text.

Source: Office for National Statistics: 020 7014 2083

16.14 Household final consumption expenditure: by purpose[1]
Current market prices
United Kingdom

£ million

		2001	2002	2003	2004	2005	2006	2007	2008	2009
Durable goods										
Furnishings, household equipment and routine maintenance of the house	LLIJ	19 275	20 470	21 595	21 909	22 363	22 616	23 284	23 266	22 241
Health	LLIK	2 109	2 411	2 604	2 512	2 400	2 674	2 765	2 830	2 805
Transport	LLIL	35 864	36 574	38 016	38 443	38 562	39 020	42 169	39 973	40 895
Communication	LLIM	636	644	810	890	950	990	969	1 025	1 047
Recreation and culture	LLIN	15 970	16 471	17 752	18 859	19 954	21 006	21 372	21 105	20 653
Miscellaneous goods and services	LLIO	3 750	4 204	4 284	4 815	4 622	5 102	4 795	4 921	4 753
Total durable goods	UTIA	77 604	80 774	85 061	87 428	88 851	91 408	95 354	93 120	92 394
Semi-durable goods										
Clothing and footwear	LLJL	36 092	38 351	40 389	41 639	42 767	43 639	44 643	45 134	45 950
Furnishings, household equipment and routine maintenance of the house	LLJM	12 400	13 361	13 932	14 009	14 166	14 894	15 594	15 318	15 168
Transport	LLJN	2 783	3 112	3 423	3 323	3 789	3 769	3 700	3 855	3 907
Recreation and culture	LLJO	21 606	23 910	26 009	26 811	25 953	26 476	28 412	28 992	28 237
Miscellaneous goods and services	LLJP	2 427	2 886	3 356	3 421	3 290	3 452	3 641	3 303	3 484
Total semi-durable goods	UTIQ	75 308	81 620	87 109	89 203	89 965	92 230	95 990	96 602	96 746
Non-durable goods										
Food & drink	ABZV	59 804	61 310	63 174	65 156	67 138	69 510	72 313	78 520	80 893
Alcohol & tobacco	ADFL	25 158	25 966	27 297	28 579	28 853	29 261	29 845	30 289	30 507
Housing, water, electricity, gas and other fuels	LLIX	23 076	23 444	24 241	28 324	32 195	36 546	37 175	43 047	44 048
Furnishings, household equipment and routine maintenance of the house	LLIY	2 972	3 169	3 338	3 748	3 805	3 847	3 856	3 783	4 005
Health	LLIZ	3 613	3 855	3 938	4 264	4 370	4 475	4 723	5 059	5 018
Transport	LLJA	19 391	19 129	20 072	22 583	24 729	25 525	28 080	31 450	27 639
Recreation and culture	LLJB	13 107	13 392	13 507	14 235	14 444	15 097	15 480	15 828	15 497
Miscellaneous goods and services	LLJC	9 884	11 272	12 602	12 966	13 266	13 804	14 746	15 193	14 963
Total non-durable goods	UTII	157 005	161 537	168 169	179 855	188 800	198 065	206 218	223 169	222 570
Total goods	UTIE	309 917	323 931	340 339	356 486	367 616	381 703	397 562	412 891	411 710
Services										
Clothing and footwear	LLJD	730	741	766	700	765	852	954	945	932
Housing, water, electricity, gas and other fuels	LLJE	92 829	97 794	104 810	110 792	117 114	124 286	134 582	141 438	152 346
Furnishings, household equipment and routine maintenance of the house	LLJF	3 327	3 448	3 601	3 826	4 141	3 860	3 478	3 522	3 366
Health	LLJG	4 254	4 512	4 793	5 105	5 413	5 611	6 287	6 004	5 597
Transport	LLJH	38 397	41 332	43 058	45 123	49 106	51 606	56 514	60 046	55 779
Communication	LLJI	13 521	14 031	14 844	16 327	16 989	17 275	17 527	17 730	17 510
Recreation and culture	LLJJ	22 769	25 349	27 118	28 542	29 779	31 053	33 796	36 075	33 932
Education	ADIE	9 409	9 381	9 610	10 763	11 050	11 765	12 443	12 641	12 458
Restaurants and hotels	ADIF	71 620	76 426	78 902	82 886	85 473	87 595	90 816	94 267	91 883
Miscellaneous goods and services	LLJK	71 481	73 456	74 609	77 377	84 735	90 043	93 100	92 324	81 313
Total services	UTIM	328 337	346 470	362 111	381 441	404 565	423 946	449 497	464 992	455 116
Final consumption expenditure in the UK by resident and non-resident households (domestic concept)	ABQI	638 254	670 401	702 450	737 927	772 181	805 649	847 059	877 883	866 826
Final consumption expenditure outside the UK by UK resident households	ABTA	22 907	24 435	26 314	27 550	29 028	30 389	31 701	33 286	27 901
less Final consumption expenditure in the UK by households resident in the rest of the world	CDFD	−13 383	−13 872	−14 156	−15 610	−17 069	−19 002	−19 492	−19 798	−19 493
Final consumption expenditure by UK resident households in the UK and abroad (national concept)	ABPB	647 778	680 964	714 608	749 867	784 140	817 036	859 268	891 371	875 234

1 See chapter text. Additional detail is published in *Consumer Trends* and table A7 of *UK Economic Accounts*, available from the National Statistics website *www.statistics.gov.uk/statbase/Product.asp?vlnk=1904*.

Source: *Office for National Statistics: 01633 456660*

16.15 Household final consumption expenditure: by purpose[1]
Chained volume measures, reference year 2005

United Kingdom

£ million

		2001	2002	2003	2004	2005	2006	2007	2008	2009
Durable goods										
Furnishings, household equipment and routine maintenance of the house	LLME	19 656	20 724	21 721	22 219	22 363	22 377	22 241	21 360	19 480
Health	LLMF	2 968	3 075	3 307	2 543	2 400	2 689	2 731	2 754	2 776
Transport	LLMG	34 837	35 788	37 732	36 995	38 562	40 162	43 191	42 030	42 411
Communication	LLMH	578	636	805	810	950	1 065	1 272	1 602	1 893
Recreation and culture	LLMI	10 399	11 620	13 834	16 503	19 954	23 586	27 747	32 353	34 802
Miscellaneous goods and services	LLMJ	4 012	4 449	4 371	4 856	4 622	4 805	4 304	4 110	3 705
Total durable goods	UTIC	70 727	74 782	80 698	83 597	88 851	94 684	101 486	104 209	105 067
Semi-durable goods										
Clothing and footwear	LLNG	32 009	35 822	38 349	40 644	42 767	44 056	45 511	47 885	51 066
Furnishings, household equipment and routine maintenance of the house	LLNH	12 810	13 853	14 604	13 750	14 166	14 986	15 512	15 066	14 485
Transport	LLNI	3 114	3 430	3 701	3 421	3 789	3 646	3 529	3 558	3 423
Recreation and culture	LLNJ	18 646	21 121	23 844	26 302	25 953	26 880	28 757	29 691	28 959
Miscellaneous goods and services	LLNK	2 510	3 007	3 455	3 522	3 290	3 393	3 464	2 952	3 011
Total semi-durable goods	UTIS	68 764	76 927	83 702	87 631	89 965	92 961	96 773	99 152	100 944
Non-durable goods										
Food & drink	ADIP	61 833	62 942	63 986	66 130	67 138	67 916	67 557	67 341	65 777
Alcohol & tobacco	ADIS	27 083	27 478	27 901	28 925	28 853	28 844	28 745	27 981	26 732
Housing, water, electricity, gas and other fuels	LLMS	28 162	28 071	28 494	31 098	32 195	31 071	29 259	29 258	27 881
Furnishings, household equipment and routine maintenance of the house	LLMT	2 770	2 984	3 213	3 747	3 805	3 719	3 649	3 479	3 424
Health	LLMU	3 475	3 672	3 713	4 225	4 370	4 493	4 675	4 919	4 796
Transport	LLMV	22 372	22 687	22 970	24 473	24 729	24 245	25 929	25 204	24 130
Recreation and culture	LLMW	13 721	13 867	13 690	14 307	14 444	14 739	14 903	14 651	13 688
Miscellaneous goods and services	LLMX	9 385	10 891	12 338	12 842	13 266	14 277	14 825	15 155	14 114
Total non-durable goods	UTIK	168 526	172 603	176 472	185 778	188 800	189 304	189 542	187 988	180 542
Total goods	UTIG	306 591	323 594	340 776	356 809	367 616	376 949	387 801	391 349	386 553
Services										
Clothing and footwear	LLMY	813	798	788	736	765	815	871	833	801
Housing, water, electricity, gas and other fuels	LLMZ	114 405	115 883	116 667	115 936	117 114	119 324	121 576	121 414	122 560
Furnishings, household equipment and routine maintenance of the house	LLNA	4 126	4 045	3 996	4 032	4 141	3 696	3 182	3 069	2 877
Health	LLNB	4 576	4 558	4 683	5 215	5 413	5 414	5 866	5 555	5 004
Transport	LLNC	43 920	45 677	46 156	47 213	49 106	49 689	52 462	53 416	48 515
Communication	LLND	13 674	13 951	14 626	15 987	16 989	17 288	18 091	18 678	18 357
Recreation and culture	LLNE	27 342	27 612	28 562	29 638	29 779	29 640	31 086	32 184	29 390
Education	ADMJ	11 662	11 007	10 482	11 285	11 050	11 140	10 966	10 429	9 715
Restaurants and hotels	ADMK	80 627	82 599	83 231	85 932	85 473	84 422	84 469	84 198	80 170
Miscellaneous goods and services	LLNF	79 210	80 413	81 487	81 028	84 735	85 871	85 886	87 998	86 098
Total services	UTIO	379 784	386 085	390 363	396 976	404 565	407 299	414 455	417 774	403 487
Final consumption expenditure in the UK by resident and non-resident households (domestic concept)	ABQJ	684 173	708 436	730 668	753 705	772 181	784 248	802 256	809 123	790 040
Final consumption expenditure outside the UK by UK resident households	ABTC	26 043	27 590	27 526	29 363	29 028	29 739	31 151	30 847	23 085
less Final consumption expenditure in the UK by households resident in the rest of the world	CCHX	−14 968	−15 104	−14 960	−16 164	−17 069	−18 392	−18 250	−17 884	−17 278
Final consumption expenditure by UK resident households in the UK and abroad (national concept)	ABPF	694 810	720 417	742 755	766 856	784 140	795 595	815 157	822 086	795 847

1 See chapter text. Additional detail is published in *Consumer Trends* and table A7 of *UK Economic Accounts*, available from the National Statistics website *www.statistics.gov.uk/statbase/Product.asp?vlnk=1904*.

Source: Office for National Statistics: 01633 456660

263

16.16 Individual consumption expenditure: by households, NPISHs and general government[1] Current market prices

United Kingdom. Classified by function (COICOP/COPNI/COFOG)[2]

£ million

		2001	2002	2003	2004	2005	2006	2007	2008	2009
FINAL CONSUMPTION EXPENDITURE OF HOUSEHOLDS										
Food and non-alcoholic beverages	ABZV	59 804	61 310	63 174	65 156	67 138	69 510	72 313	78 520	80 893
Food	ABZW	52 742	53 984	55 507	57 059	58 822	60 729	63 455	69 530	71 455
Non-alcoholic beverages	ADFK	7 062	7 326	7 667	8 097	8 316	8 781	8 858	8 990	9 438
Alcoholic beverages and tobacco	ADFL	25 158	25 966	27 297	28 579	28 853	29 261	29 845	30 289	30 507
Alcoholic beverages	ADFM	10 700	11 344	12 027	13 274	13 476	13 540	13 931	14 307	14 250
Tobacco	ADFN	14 458	14 622	15 270	15 305	15 377	15 721	15 914	15 982	16 257
Clothing and footwear	ADFP	36 822	39 092	41 155	42 339	43 532	44 491	45 597	46 079	46 882
Clothing	ADFQ	32 103	33 927	35 689	36 490	37 529	38 117	39 111	39 281	40 081
Footwear	ADFR	4 719	5 165	5 466	5 849	6 003	6 374	6 486	6 798	6 801
Housing, water, electricity, gas and other fuels	ADFS	115 905	121 238	129 051	139 116	149 309	160 832	171 757	184 485	196 394
Actual rentals for housing	ADFT	25 302	25 828	27 610	28 648	29 547	32 217	36 192	38 460	41 717
Imputed rentals for housing	ADFU	59 581	63 279	68 458	72 850	77 339	80 979	86 363	91 301	99 334
Maintenance and repair of the dwelling	ADFV	11 340	12 306	12 615	14 235	14 509	14 214	14 933	14 465	13 785
Water supply and miscellaneous dwelling services	ADFW	5 059	5 222	5 438	5 773	6 428	6 904	7 277	7 779	8 093
Electricity, gas and other fuels	ADFX	14 623	14 603	14 930	17 610	21 486	26 518	26 992	32 480	33 465
Furnishings, household equipment and routine maintenance of the house	ADFY	37 974	40 448	42 466	43 492	44 475	45 217	46 212	45 889	44 780
Furniture, furnishings, carpets and other floor coverings	ADFZ	14 362	15 591	16 789	16 806	16 816	17 027	17 679	17 226	16 689
Household textiles	ADGG	4 636	5 086	5 452	5 455	5 248	5 599	5 933	5 832	5 864
Household appliances	ADGL	5 758	5 715	5 578	6 104	6 414	6 446	6 359	6 277	5 862
Glassware, tableware and household utensils	ADGM	4 609	4 710	4 701	4 010	4 415	4 454	4 468	4 534	4 377
Tools and equipment for house and garden	ADGN	2 977	3 355	3 589	4 141	4 244	4 589	5 070	5 208	5 154
Goods and services for routine household maintenance	ADGO	5 632	5 991	6 357	6 976	7 338	7 102	6 703	6 812	6 834
Health	ADGP	9 976	10 778	11 335	11 881	12 183	12 760	13 775	13 893	13 420
Medical products, appliances and equipment	ADGQ	5 722	6 266	6 542	6 776	6 770	7 149	7 488	7 889	7 823
Out-patient services	ADGR	2 344	2 422	2 553	2 747	2 909	2 984	3 575	3 211	2 673
Hospital services	ADGS	1 910	2 090	2 240	2 358	2 504	2 627	2 712	2 793	2 924
Transport	ADGT	96 435	100 147	104 569	109 472	116 186	119 920	130 463	135 324	128 220
Purchase of vehicles	ADGU	35 864	36 574	38 016	38 443	38 562	39 020	42 169	39 973	40 895
Operation of personal transport equipment	ADGV	37 028	38 816	40 507	44 081	48 685	50 170	55 048	59 633	54 462
Transport services	ADGW	23 543	24 757	26 046	26 948	28 939	30 730	33 246	35 718	32 863
Communication	ADGX	14 157	14 675	15 654	17 217	17 939	18 265	18 496	18 755	18 557
Postal services	CDEF	870	878	890	961	1 016	1 059	1 060	972	848
Telephone & telefax equipment	ADWO	636	644	810	890	950	990	969	1 025	1 047
Telephone & telefax services	ADWP	12 651	13 153	13 954	15 366	15 973	16 216	16 467	16 758	16 662
Recreation and culture	ADGY	73 452	79 122	84 386	88 447	90 130	93 632	99 060	102 000	98 319
Audio-visual, photographic and information processing equipment	ADGZ	17 580	18 051	19 408	20 564	20 919	21 084	20 906	19 978	18 818
Other major durables for recreation and culture	ADHL	4 325	4 672	5 126	5 381	5 835	6 127	6 306	6 662	7 120
Other recreational items and equipment; flowers, garden and pets	ADHZ	20 216	22 475	23 894	24 224	24 144	25 261	28 004	29 484	29 295
Recreational and cultural services	ADIA	21 034	23 555	25 278	26 572	27 365	28 769	31 068	33 563	31 187
Newspapers, books and stationery	ADIC	10 297	10 369	10 680	11 706	11 867	12 391	12 776	12 313	11 899
Package holidays[3]	ADID	–	–	–	–	–	–	–	–	–
Education										
Education services	ADIE	9 409	9 381	9 610	10 763	11 050	11 765	12 443	12 641	12 458
Restaurants and hotels	ADIF	71 620	76 426	78 902	82 886	85 473	87 595	90 816	94 267	91 883
Catering services	ADIG	62 449	66 701	68 839	72 667	74 642	75 923	78 167	80 777	78 749
Accommodation services	ADIH	9 171	9 725	10 063	10 219	10 831	11 672	12 649	13 490	13 134
Miscellaneous goods and services	ADII	87 542	91 818	94 851	98 579	105 913	112 401	116 282	115 741	104 513
Personal care	ADIJ	14 626	16 444	18 181	19 083	19 392	19 973	21 019	21 329	21 301
Personal effects not elsewhere classified	ADIK	5 455	6 140	6 462	6 838	6 656	7 494	7 228	7 388	7 239
Social protection	ADIL	8 963	9 219	9 501	8 805	9 131	9 866	9 936	10 529	10 821
Insurance	ADIM	25 423	25 456	24 373	25 119	26 397	26 733	27 326	26 981	24 587
Financial services not elsewhere classified	ADIN	26 990	28 384	29 977	31 843	36 794	40 772	42 763	41 802	33 393
Other services not elsewhere classified	ADIO	6 085	6 175	6 357	6 891	7 543	7 563	8 010	7 712	7 172
Final consumption expenditure in the UK by resident and non-resident households (domestic concept)	ABQI	638 254	670 401	702 450	737 927	772 181	805 649	847 059	877 883	866 826
Final consumption expenditure outside the UK by UK resident households	ABTA	22 907	24 435	26 314	27 550	29 028	30 389	31 701	33 286	27 901
less Final consumption expenditure in the UK by households resident in the rest of the world	CDFD	–13 383	–13 872	–14 156	–15 610	–17 069	–19 002	–19 492	–19 798	–19 493
Final consumption expenditure by UK resident households in the UK and abroad (national concept)	ABPB	647 778	680 964	714 608	749 867	784 140	817 036	859 268	891 371	875 234

16.16
continued

Individual consumption expenditure: by households, NPISHs and general government[1] Current market prices

United Kingdom. Classified by function (COICOP/COPNI/COFOG)[2]

£ million

		2001	2002	2003	2004	2005	2006	2007	2008	2009
FINAL CONSUMPTION EXPENDITURE OF UK RESIDENT HOUSEHOLDS										
Final consumption expenditure of UK resident households in the UK and abroad	ABPB	647 778	680 964	714 608	749 867	784 140	817 036	859 268	891 371	875 234
FINAL INDIVIDUAL CONSUMPTION EXPENDITURE OF NPISH										
Final individual consumption expenditure of NPISH	ABNV	25 111	26 422	27 668	29 197	30 824	32 439	33 722	37 129	35 334
FINAL INDIVIDUAL CONSUMPTION EXPENDITURE OF OF GENERAL GOVERNMENT										
Health	QYOT	57 248	63 134	69 433	76 429	82 315	90 032	94 797	101 348	..
Recreation and culture	QYSU	4 049	4 335	4 513	4 272	..	..	..	..	..
Education	QYSE	34 057	37 624	40 394	43 483	46 765	49 754	52 861	55 915	..
Social protection	QYSP	19 441	22 464	25 517	28 028	..	..	..	..	..
Housing	QYXO	–	–	..	..	..	..	..	..	..
Final individual consumption expenditure of general government	NNAQ	118 458	130 816	143 954	148 789	160 199	172 856	182 035	194 461	206 608
Total, individual consumption expenditure/ actual individual consumption	NQEO	791 347	838 202	886 230	927 853	975 163	1 022 331	1 075 025	1 122 961	1 117 176

1 See chapter text.
2 "Purpose" or "function" classifications are designed to indicate the "socioeconomic objectives" that institutional units aim to achieve through various kinds of outlays. COICOP is the Classification of Individual Consumption by Purpose and applies to households. COPNI is the Classification of the Purposes of Non-Profit Institutions Serving Households and COFOG the Classification of the Functions of Government. The introduction of ESA95 coincides with the redefinition of these classifications and data will be available on a consistent basis for all European Union member states.
3 Package holidays data are dispersed between components (transport etc).

Source: Office for National Statistics: 01633 456660

16.17 Individual consumption expenditure: by households, NPISHs and general government[1] Chained volume measures, reference year 2005

United Kingdom. Classified by function (COICOP/COPNI/COFOG)[2]

£ million

		2001	2002	2003	2004	2005	2006	2007	2008	2009
FINAL CONSUMPTION EXPENDITURE OF HOUSEHOLDS										
Food and non-alcoholic beverages	ADIP	61 833	62 942	63 986	66 130	67 138	67 916	67 557	67 341	65 777
Food	ADIQ	54 775	55 630	56 312	58 006	58 822	59 452	59 344	59 229	57 649
Non-alcoholic beverages	ADIR	7 073	7 322	7 677	8 125	8 316	8 464	8 213	8 112	8 128
Alcoholic beverages and tobacco	ADIS	27 083	27 478	27 901	28 925	28 853	28 844	28 745	27 981	26 732
Alcoholic beverages	ADIT	10 532	11 198	11 695	13 070	13 476	13 772	14 136	13 731	12 819
Tobacco	ADIU	16 796	16 436	16 319	15 879	15 377	15 072	14 609	14 250	13 913
Clothing and footwear	ADIW	32 788	36 604	39 129	41 379	43 532	44 871	46 382	48 718	51 867
Clothing	ADIX	28 428	31 753	34 015	35 672	37 529	38 405	39 881	41 873	45 035
Footwear	ADIY	4 365	4 856	5 119	5 707	6 003	6 466	6 501	6 845	6 832
Housing, water, electricity, gas and other fuels	ADIZ	142 716	144 101	145 308	147 062	149 309	150 395	150 835	150 672	150 441
Actual rentals for housing	ADJA	29 890	29 526	30 100	29 861	29 547	31 245	32 920	33 805	34 490
Imputed rentals for housing	ADJB	74 341	75 880	76 535	76 138	77 339	77 575	77 851	77 666	78 711
Maintenance and repair of the dwelling	ADJC	13 304	13 920	13 825	14 648	14 509	13 802	13 834	12 721	11 631
Water supply and miscellaneous dwelling services	ADJD	6 418	6 472	6 489	6 342	6 428	6 464	6 414	6 441	6 368
Electricity, gas and other fuels	ADJE	18 566	18 097	18 144	19 974	21 486	21 309	19 816	20 039	19 241
Furnishings, household equipment and routine maintenance of the house	ADJF	39 215	41 509	43 469	43 743	44 475	44 778	44 584	42 974	40 266
Furniture, furnishings, carpets and other floor coverings	ADJG	15 212	16 273	17 187	17 278	16 816	16 644	16 633	15 394	14 323
Household textiles	ADJH	4 819	5 360	5 793	5 333	5 248	5 719	6 114	6 026	5 896
Household appliances	ADJI	5 293	5 309	5 321	6 009	6 414	6 612	6 369	6 199	5 422
Glassware, tableware and household utensils	ADJJ	4 655	4 717	4 701	3 925	4 415	4 464	4 343	4 289	3 972
Tools and equipment for house and garden	ADJK	3 109	3 524	3 907	4 071	4 244	4 519	4 900	4 969	4 833
Goods and services for routine household maintenance	ADJL	6 031	6 270	6 544	7 157	7 338	6 820	6 225	6 097	5 820
Health	ADJM	10 843	11 130	11 490	11 982	12 183	12 596	13 272	13 228	12 576
Medical products, appliances and equipment	ADJN	6 282	6 590	6 826	6 765	6 770	7 182	7 406	7 673	7 572
Out-patient services	ADJO	2 358	2 295	2 352	2 792	2 909	2 861	3 304	2 959	2 403
Hospital services	ADJP	2 229	2 283	2 353	2 424	2 504	2 553	2 562	2 596	2 601
Transport	ADJQ	104 246	107 565	110 686	112 060	116 186	117 742	125 111	124 208	118 479
Purchase of vehicles	ADJR	34 837	35 788	37 732	36 995	38 562	40 162	43 191	42 030	42 411
Operation of personal transport equipment	ADJS	44 354	45 985	45 803	47 331	48 685	47 528	50 120	49 267	46 248
Transport services	ADJT	25 145	25 925	27 047	27 763	28 939	30 052	31 800	32 911	29 820
Communication	ADJU	14 241	14 580	15 425	16 791	17 939	18 353	19 363	20 280	20 250
Postal services	CCGZ	890	896	880	918	1 016	1 160	1 288	1 345	1 395
Telephone & telefax equipment	ADQF	582	640	810	810	950	1 065	1 272	1 602	1 893
Telephone & telefax services	ADQG	12 788	13 060	13 750	15 070	15 973	16 128	16 803	17 333	16 962
Recreation and culture	ADJV	68 015	72 745	79 109	86 360	90 130	94 845	102 493	108 879	106 839
Audio-visual, photographic and information processing equipment	ADJW	11 277	12 514	14 899	17 919	20 919	23 726	27 206	31 431	33 849
Other major durables for recreation and culture	ADJX	4 771	5 039	5 363	5 445	5 835	6 098	6 315	6 575	6 775
Other recreational items and equipment; flowers, gardens and pets	ADJY	17 659	20 136	22 231	23 985	24 144	25 615	28 338	29 802	28 840
Recreational and cultural services	ADJZ	25 240	25 538	26 530	27 568	27 365	27 450	28 585	29 988	27 049
Newspapers, books and stationery	ADKM	11 166	11 007	10 930	11 799	11 867	11 956	12 049	11 083	10 326
Package holidays[3]	ADMI	–	–	–	–	–	–	–	–	–
Education										
Education services	ADMJ	11 662	11 007	10 482	11 285	11 050	11 140	10 966	10 429	9 715
Restaurants and Hotels	ADMK	80 627	82 599	83 231	85 932	85 473	84 422	84 469	84 198	80 170
Catering services	ADML	70 634	72 375	72 774	75 178	74 642	73 301	72 837	72 087	68 259
Accommodation services	ADMM	9 994	10 225	10 454	10 752	10 831	11 121	11 632	12 111	11 911
Miscellaneous goods and services	ADMN	94 696	98 547	101 591	102 270	105 913	108 346	108 479	110 215	106 928
Personal care	ADMO	14 804	16 622	18 286	19 229	19 392	20 236	20 669	20 559	19 570
Personal effects not elsewhere classified	ADMP	5 727	6 423	6 600	6 918	6 656	7 166	6 628	6 395	5 950
Social protection	ADMQ	11 304	10 969	10 678	9 363	9 131	9 292	9 004	9 161	8 959
Insurance	ADMR	27 353	26 715	26 157	26 291	26 397	25 738	25 622	26 010	24 399
Financial services not elsewhere classified	ADMS	27 698	30 011	32 092	32 927	36 794	38 925	39 563	41 809	42 400
Other services not elsewhere classified	ADMT	7 757	7 425	7 222	7 316	7 543	6 989	6 993	6 281	5 650
Final consumption expenditure in the UK by resident and non-resident households (domestic concept)	ABQJ	684 173	708 436	730 668	753 705	772 181	784 248	802 256	809 123	790 040
Final consumption expenditure outside the UK by UK resident households	ABTC	26 043	27 590	27 526	29 363	29 028	29 739	31 151	30 847	23 085
less Final consumption expenditure in the UK by households resident in the rest of the world	CCHX	−14 968	−15 104	−14 960	−16 164	−17 069	−18 392	−18 250	−17 884	−17 278
Final consumption expenditure by UK resident households in the UK and abroad (national concept)	ABPF	694 810	720 417	742 755	766 856	784 140	795 595	815 157	822 086	795 847

16.17
continued

Individual consumption expenditure: by households, NPISHs and general government[1] Chained volume measures, reference year 2005
United Kingdom. Classified by function (COICOP/COPNI/COFOG)[2]

£ million

		2001	2002	2003	2004	2005	2006	2007	2008	2009
FINAL CONSUMPTION EXPENDITURE OF UK RESIDENT HOUSEHOLDS										
Final consumption expenditure of UK resident households in the UK and abroad	ABPF	694 810	720 417	742 755	766 856	784 140	795 595	815 157	822 086	795 847
FINAL INDIVIDUAL CONSUMPTION EXPENDITURE OF NPISH										
Final individual consumption expenditure of NPISH	ABNU	30 752	30 761	30 865	30 827	30 824	31 868	30 040	30 832	29 628
FINAL INDIVIDUAL CONSUMPTION EXPENDITURE OF GENERAL GOVERNMENT										
Health	EMOA	61 019	63 272	65 611	68 758	..	..	..	..	..
Recreation and culture	QYXK	3 968	4 470	4 717	..	..	..	..	..	..
Education	EMOB	37 100	37 535	37 732	37 944	..	..	..	..	..
Social protection	QYXM	26 235	27 587	28 673	29 645	29 614	29 612	29 154	29 526	..
Housing	QYXN	–	–	–	..	..	..	..	..	..
Final individual consumption expenditure of general government	NSZK	114 159	117 238	120 288	..	..	..	..	..	..
Total, individual consumption expenditure/ actual individual consumption	YBIO	868 304	899 025	926 191	955 004	975 163	990 185	1 010 718	1 025 495	..

1 See chapter text.
2 "Purpose" or "function" classifications are designed to indicate the "socio-economic objectives" that institutional units aim to achieve through various kinds of outlays. COICOP is the Classification of Individual Consumption by Purpose and applies to households. COPNI is the Classification of the Purposes of Non-Profit Institutions Serving Households (NPISH) and COFOG the Classification of the Functions of Government. The introduction of ESA95 coincides with the redefinition of these classifications and data will be available on a consistent basis for all European Union member states.
3 Package holidays data are dispersed between components (transport etc).

Source: Office for National Statistics: 01633 456660

16.18

Change in inventories[1,2]
Chained volume measures, reference year 2005
United Kingdom

Reference year 2005, £ million

	Mining and quarrying	Manufacturing industries				Electricity, gas and water supply	Distributive trades		Other industries[4]	Change in inventories
		Materials and fuel	Work in progress	Finished goods	Total		Wholesale[3]	Retail[3]		
	FADO	FBID	FBIE	FBIF	DHBH	FADP	FAJM	FBYH	DLWV	ABMQ
2000	−224	592	307	356	1 526	226	2 003	1 606	−297	4 800
2001	74	−559	317	136	20	18	916	1 208	3 629	5 760
2002	−32	−541	−129	−317	−1 178	−148	814	1 861	1 018	2 364
2003	−56	−215	−558	−118	−1 143	−14	421	1 347	3 566	4 112
2004	−40	294	−541	−106	−345	2	300	995	3 769	4 843
2005	−16	385	938	357	1 679	656	931	−447	1 668	4 472
2006	−22	293	1 319	567	2 179	380	947	685	620	4 789
2007	−97	374	−357	402	419	−284	−70	1 724	4 954	6 646
2008	−47	−864	−723	−378	−1 965	936	967	−223	1 198	866
2009	−66	−1 455	−146	−2 262	−3 863	−69	−4 198	1 052	−8 042	−15 185

1 See chapter text. Estimates are given to the nearest £ million but cannot be regarded as accurate to this degree.
2 Components may not sum to totals due to rounding.
3 Wholesaling and retailing estimates exclude the motor trades.
4 Quarterly alignment adjustment included in this series.

Source: Office for National Statistics 020 7014 2083

16.19 Gross fixed capital formation at current purchasers' prices: by broad sector and type of asset[1,2]

United Kingdom. Total economy

£ million

		2001	2002	2003	2004	2005	2006	2007	2008	2009
Private sector										
New dwellings, excluding land	DFDF	27 085	31 455	34 804	40 926	43 844	49 273	51 860	46 310	35 475
Other buildings and structures	EQBU	32 730	33 580	35 366	33 171	35 714	37 797	44 604	50 055	..
Transport equipment	EQBV	13 897	15 637	14 708	13 135	13 819	14 201	14 714	14 096	..
Other machinery and equipment and cultivated assets	EQBW	58 062	53 498	50 228	54 938	55 446	58 037	64 960	63 301	..
Intangible fixed assets	EQBX	4 285	4 674	4 894	5 258	5 594	..	..	..	..
Costs associated with the transfer of ownership of non-produced assets	EQBY	12 697	15 399	16 385	20 739	19 940	24 611	26 400	13 706	8 231
Total	EQBZ	148 756	154 243	156 385	170 025	177 123	..	..	..	..
Public non-financial corporations										
New dwellings, excluding land	DEER	2 387	2 837	3 509	3 235	3 574	4 049	3 899	3 967	4 065
Other buildings and structures	DEES	1 854	2 304	2 236	1 493	2 111	1 830	1 710	1 212	..
Transport equipment	DEEP	171	110	126	193	334	181	154	298	..
Other machinery and equipment and cultivated assets	DEEQ	628	787	1 037	1 042	16 478	986	1 241	2 108	..
Intangible fixed assets	DLXJ	397	556	623	737	753	769	802	840	..
Costs associated with the transfer of ownership of non-produced assets	DLXQ	−2 254	−2 764	−5 674	−5 440	−2 675	−2 375	−2 032	−1 106	−262
Total	FCCJ	3 183	3 830	1 857	1 260	20 575	5 440	5 774	6 953	8 182
General government										
New dwellings, excluding land	DFHW	334	207	149	137	71	9	3	14	..
Other buildings and structures	EQCH	10 348	11 678	14 693	15 866	18 884	20 930	22 177	28 036	..
Transport equipment	EQCI	588	567	758	1 011	610	500	524	403	..
Other machinery and equipment and cultivated assets	EQCJ	2 239	2 867	3 176	3 652	−12 438	2 480	2 822	3 466	..
Intangible fixed assets	EQCK	334	358	384	400	304	418	331	216	..
Costs associated with the transfer of ownership of non-produced assets	EQCL	−310	−225	1 349	2 153	−340	−670	−315	1 174	..
Total	NNBF	13 533	15 452	20 509	23 219	7 091	23 667	25 542	32 966	37 438
Total gross fixed capital formation	NPQX	171 782	180 551	186 700	200 415	209 758	227 370	248 766	242 822	207 918

1 See chapter text.
2 Components may not sum to totals due to rounding.

Source: Office for National Statistics: 020 7014 2083

16.20 Gross fixed capital formation at current purchasers' prices: by type of asset[1,2]

United Kingdom. Total economy

£ million

		2001	2002	2003	2004	2005	2006	2007	2008	2009
Tangible fixed assets										
New dwellings, excluding land	DFDK	29 806	34 499	38 462	44 298	47 489	53 331	55 762	50 292	39 539
Other buildings and structures	DLWS	44 932	47 562	52 295	50 530	56 709	60 557	68 491	79 303	..
Transport equipment	DLWZ	14 656	16 314	15 592	14 339	14 763	14 882	15 392	14 845	12 289
Other machinery and equipment and cultivated assets	DLXI	60 929	57 152	54 441	59 632	59 486	61 503	69 023	69 069	56 547
Total	EQCQ	150 323	155 527	160 790	168 799	178 447	190 273	208 668	213 388	..
Intangible fixed assets	DLXP	11 326	12 614	13 850	14 164	14 386	15 531	16 045	16 736	17 782
Costs associated with the transfer of ownership of non-produced assets	DFBH	10 132	12 410	12 059	17 452	16 925	21 566	24 053	13 992	..
Total gross fixed capital formation	NPQX	171 782	180 551	186 700	200 415	209 758	227 370	248 766	242 822	207 918

1 See chapter text.
2 Components may not sum to totals due to rounding.

Source: Office for National Statistics: 020 7014 2083

16.21 Gross fixed capital formation: by broad sector and type of asset[1,2,3]
Chained volume measures, reference year 2005

United Kingdom. Total economy

£ million

		2001	2002	2003	2004	2005	2006	2007	2008	2009
Private sector										
New dwellings, excluding land	DFDP	35 578	38 340	39 542	43 527	43 844	47 514	49 113	43 486	34 912
Other buildings and structures	EQCU	34 421	34 577	36 607	33 276	35 714	37 650	44 373	49 707	..
Transport equipment	EQCV	14 109	15 987	14 966	13 301	13 819	14 034	14 534	13 224	..
Other machinery and equipment and cultivated assets	EQCW	51 006	49 372	47 321	53 651	55 446	58 873	66 679	64 096	..
Intangible fixed assets	EQCX	11 445	11 908	13 094	13 278	13 329	14 141	14 393	14 922	..
Costs associated with the transfer of ownership of non-produced assets	EQCY	18 900	20 294	19 145	23 332	19 940	22 610	21 612	11 044	7 491
Total	EQCZ	166 510	170 382	170 413	179 931	182 092	194 821	210 704	196 468	..
Public non-financial corporations										
New dwellings, excluding land	DEEW	2 632	3 023	3 662	3 299	3 574	3 974	3 633	3 571	3 830
Other buildings and structures	DEEX	2 156	2 573	2 455	1 566	2 111	1 738	1 532	1 027	..
Transport equipment	DEEU	180	114	123	191	334	179	153	298	..
Other machinery and equipment and cultivated assets	DEEV	545	710	960	993	16 478	1 076	1 257	2 053	..
Intangible fixed assets	EQDE	445	613	667	759	753	746	743	752	..
Costs associated with the transfer of ownership of non-produced assets	EQDF	−3 046	−3 332	−6 112	−6 103	−2 675	−2 221	−1 760	−934	−226
Total	EQDG	1 129	1 405	866	1 224	20 575	5 493	5 558	6 890	..
General government										
New dwellings, excluding land	DFID	354	213	149	138	71	9	3	12	..
Other buildings and structures	EQDI	12 550	13 686	16 597	17 068	18 884	19 758	20 110	24 907	..
Transport equipment	EQDJ	516	449	582	610	610	641	597	541	..
Other machinery and equipment and cultivated assets	EQDK	1 855	2 518	2 850	3 370	−12 438	2 788	3 320	3 762	..
Intangible fixed assets	EQDL	204	219	401	410	304	412	316	202	..
Costs associated with the transfer of ownership of non-produced assets	EQDM	4 731	2 253	−11 645	3 340	−340	−617	6	1 064	..
Total	EQDN	14 981	16 866	21 973	23 799	7 091	22 991	24 351	29 735	34 345
Total gross fixed capital formation	NPQR	185 952	192 734	194 819	204 756	209 758	223 305	240 613	232 202	197 592

1 See chapter text.
2 For the years before 2003, the total differs from the sum of their components.
3 Components may not sum to totals due to rounding.

Source: Office for National Statistics: 020 7014 2083

16.22 Gross fixed capital formation: by type of asset[1,2,3]
Chained volume measures, reference year 2005

United Kingdom. Total economy

£ million

		2001	2002	2003	2004	2005	2006	2007	2008	2009
Tangible fixed assets										
New dwellings, excluding land	DFDV	38 555	41 565	43 396	46 958	47 489	51 497	52 749	47 070	38 741
Other buildings and structures	EQDP	49 560	51 165	55 845	51 942	56 709	59 146	66 015	75 641	..
Transport equipment	DLWJ	14 746	16 470	15 645	14 116	14 763	14 854	15 284	13 940	10 534
Other machinery and equipment and cultivated assets	DLWM	53 366	52 605	51 166	58 035	59 486	62 737	71 255	69 854	54 251
Total	EQDS	157 158	161 982	165 621	171 062	178 447	188 234	205 304	206 591	..
Intangible fixed assets	EQDT	12 011	12 654	14 165	14 446	14 386	15 299	15 452	15 805	16 378
Costs associated with the transfer of ownership of non-produced assets	DFDW	15 782	17 169	14 689	19 535	16 925	19 772	19 857	11 379	..
Total gross fixed capital formation	NPQR	185 952	192 734	194 819	204 756	209 758	223 305	240 613	232 202	197 592

1 See chapter text.
2 For the years before 2003, the total differs from the sum of their components.
3 Components may not sum to totals due to rounding.

Source: Office for National Statistics: 020 7014 2083

Prices

Chapter 17

Prices

Producer price index numbers

(Tables 17.1 and 17.2)

The producer price indices (PPIs) were published for the first time in August 1983, replacing the former wholesale price indices. Full details of the differences between the two indices were given in an article published in *British Business*, 15 April 1983. The producer price indices are calculated using the same general methodology as that used by the wholesale price indices.

The high level index numbers in Tables 17.1 and 17.2 are constructed on a net sector basis. That is to say, they are intended to measure only transactions between the sector concerned and other sectors. Within sector transactions are excluded. Index numbers for the whole of manufacturing are thus not weighted averages of sector index numbers.

The index numbers for selected industries in Tables 17.1 and 17.2 are constructed on a gross sector basis, that is, all transactions are included in deriving the weighting patterns, including sales within the same industry.

All the index numbers are compiled exclusive of Value Added Tax (VAT). Excise duties on cigarettes, manufactured tobacco and alcoholic liquor are included, as is the duty on hydrocarbon oils.

The indices relate to the average prices for a year. The movement in these prices are weighted to reflect the relative importance of the composite products in a chosen year (known as the base year), currently 2005.

Since July 1995, PPIs have been published fully reclassified to the 1992 version of the Standard Industrial Classification (SIC).

Further details are available from the Office for National Statistics website: www.statistics.gov.uk/ppi.

Purchasing power of the pound

(Table 17.3)

Changes in the internal purchasing power of a currency may be defined as the 'inverse' of changes in the levels of prices; when prices go up, the amount which can be purchased with a given sum of money goes down. Movements in the internal purchasing power of the pound are based on the consumers' expenditure deflator (CED) prior to 1962 and on the General index of retail prices (RPI) from January 1962 onwards. The

CED shows the movement in prices implied by the national accounts estimates of consumers' expenditure valued at current and at constant prices, while the RPI is constructed directly by weighting together monthly movements in prices according to a given pattern of household expenditure derived from the Expenditure and Food Survey. If the purchasing power of the pound is taken to be 100p in a particular month (quarter, year), the comparable purchasing power in a subsequent month (quarter, year) is:

$$100 \quad \times \quad \frac{\text{earlier period price index}}{\text{later period price index}}$$

where the price index used is the CED for years 1946–1961 and the RPI for periods after 1961.

Consumer prices index

(Table 17.4)

The Consumer Prices Index (CPI) is the main UK domestic measure of inflation for macro-economic purposes. Like the RPI (see below) it measures the average change from month to month in the prices of consumer goods and services purchased in the UK, but there are differences in coverage and methodology. A detailed description of these differences is given in the paper entitled 'The New Inflation Target: the Statistical Perspective'. This paper is available at: www. statistics.gov.uk/StatBase/Product.asp?vlnk=10913.

Since 10 December 2003, the Government inflation target for the UK has been defined in terms of the CPI measure of inflation. Prior to that the CPI had been published in the UK as the Harmonised Index of Consumer Prices (HICP); the two shall remain one and the same index.

The HICPs are calculated in each member state of the European Union (EU), according to rules specified in a series of European regulations developed by the EU statistical office in conjunction with the EU Member States. The HICPs are used to compare inflation rate across the EU. Since January 1999 it has also been used by the European Central Bank (ECB) as the measure of price stability across the euro area. Additional information on HICPs is available at: www.statistics.gov.uk/ hicp

Further details on the CPI are available at: www.statistics.gov.uk/cpi

Retail prices index

(Table 17.5)

The Retail Prices Index (RPI) is the most familiar general purpose measure of inflation in the UK, measuring the percentage changes month by month in the average level of prices of the goods and services purchased by the great majority of households in the UK. The uses of the RPI include indexation of pensions, state benefits and index-linked gilts. The expenditure pattern on which the index is based is revised each year using information from the Expenditure and Food Survey. The expenditure of certain higher income households and households of retired people dependent mainly on social security benefits is excluded.

The index covers a large and representative selection of more than 650 separate goods and services, for which price movements are regularly measured in around 150 locations throughout the country. Around 120,000 separate price quotations are used in compiling the index.

Further details are available at: www.statistics.gov.uk/rpi

Tax and price index (TPI)

(Table 17.6)

The purpose and methodology of the TPI were described in an article in the August 1979 issue (No. 310) of *Economic Trends*. The TPI measures the change in gross taxable income needed for taxpayers to maintain their purchasing power, allowing for changes in retail prices. The TPI thus takes account of the changes to direct taxes (and employees' National Insurance (NI) contributions) facing representative cross-section of taxpayers as well as changes in the RPI.

When direct taxation or employees' NI contributions change, the TPI will rise by less than or more than the RPI according to the type of changes made. Between Budgets, the monthly increase in the TPI is normally slightly larger than that in the RPI, since all the extra income needed to offset any rise in retail prices is fully taxed.

Index numbers of agricultural prices

(Tables 17.7 and 17.8)

The indices of producer prices of agricultural products are currently based on the calendar year 2000. They are designed to provide short-term and medium-term indications of movements in these prices. All annual series are base-weighted Laspeyres type, using value weights derived from the *Economic Accounts for Agriculture* prepared for the Statistical Office of the European Union. Prices are measured exclusive of VAT. For Table 17.7, it has generally been necessary to measure the prices of materials (inputs) ex-supplier. For Table 17.8, it has generally been necessary to measure the prices received by producers (outputs) at the first marketing stage. The construction of the indices enables them to be combined with similar indices for other member countries of the EU to provide an overall indication of trends within the Union which appears in the Union's Eurostat series of publications.

Index numbers at a more detailed level and for earlier based series are available from the Department for Environment, Food and Rural Affairs, SSP, Room 146 Foss House, Kingspool 1–2 Peasholme Green, York, YO1 7PX, tel: +44 (0)1904 455249.

Prices

17.1 Producer price index of materials and fuels purchased: by all manufacturing and selected industries SIC(92)[1]

United Kingdom: Annual averages

Indices (2005=100)

			2002	2003	2004	2005	2006	2007	2008	2009
Net sector										
Materials and fuel purchased by manufacturing industry[2]	RNNK	6292000050	88.0	88.5	90.5	100.0	109.5	112.8	137.2	132.3p
Materials	PLKX	6292000010	90.1	90.6r	92.3	100.0	107.5	111.8	135.0	128.9p
Fuels[2]	RNNL	6292000060	67.6	66.6	71.9	100.0	130.7	122.7	159.5	168.1
Materials and fuels purchased by manufacturing industry-seasonally adjusted[2]	RNPE	6292008950	94.4	95.7	99.5	111.0	121.8	125.7	..	..
Materials and fuels purchased by manufacturing industry other than food, beverages, petroleum and tobacco[2]	RNNQ	6292990050	94.6	93.3	93.8	100.0	106.9	109.3	127.3	129.6p
Materials	RWCJ	6292990010	97.6	96.1	96.1	100.0	104.5	108.0	124.1	125.7
Fuel[2]	RNNS	6292990060	67.8	66.7	72.0	100.0	130.8	123.2	159.8	168.6
Materials and fuels purchased by manufacturing industries other than food, beverages, petroleum and tobacco-seasonally adjusted[2]	RNPF	6292998950	94.7	93.3	93.9	100.0	107.0	109.4	127.4	129.6p
Gross sector[3]										
All manufacturing	RBBO	6192000000	92.6	93.3	95.1	100.0	105.8	109.2	122.1	121.1
Other mining and quarrying products[4]	RABE	6112140000	93.2	95.9	95.2	100.0	105.3	106.5	121.7	131.7p
Manufacture of food products	RBBQ	6192151600	94.6	96.6	98.9	100.0	104.2	109.1	126.6	128.1p
Food products and beverages	RABF	6112150000	96.0	96.7	97.7	100.0	103.1	106.6	121.7	126.8p
Tobacco products	RABG	6112160000	92.5	96.5	99.8	100.0	105.3	111.1	129.3	129.2
Manufacture of textiles	RBBR	6192171800	96.6	96.8	96.7	100.0	103.4	104.0	112.0	115.4p
Textiles	RABH	6112170000	95.4	95.7	95.5	100.0	104.1	104.1	112.6	116.9p
Wearing apparel	RABI	6112180000	98.7	98.4	98.8	100.0	102.2	103.8	111.0	113.0p
Manufacture of leather	RBBS	6192190000	97.5	97.9	97.8	100.0	103.2	104.6	114.4	118.8p
Manufacture of wood and wood products	RBBT	6192200000	94.2	93.8	96.1	100.0	104.7	113.3	121.0	121.5p
Manufacture of pulp, paper, publishing and printing	RBBU	6192212200	97.7	97.1	97.4	100.0	104.7	106.6	114.3	118.6
Pulp and paper products	RABL	6112210000	99.1	97.2	96.9	100.0	106.2	108.2	117.8	122.7p
Printed matter and recording material	RABM	6112220000	96.9	97.2	97.7	100.0	103.7	105.5	111.8	115.8
Manufacture of coke	RBBV	6192230000	58.5	62.4	71.5	100.0	117.4	121.4	171.3	131.3p
Manufacture of chemical products	RBBW	6192240000	91.5	93.4	94.5	100.0	106.7	107.7	121.6	127.9p
Manufacture of rubber products	RBBX	6192250000	88.5	89.7	92.3	100.0	106.5	108.5	119.7	120.3p
Manufacture of other non-metallic mineral products	RBBY	6192260000	90.8	90.9	92.1	100.0	107.9	108.4	125.1	130.1p
Manufacture of basic metals	RBBZ	6192272800	82.0	84.3	92.9	100.0	111.8	120.3	134.9	127.0p
Basic metals	RABV	6112270000	79.1	82.2	92.2	100.0	115.2	124.4	144.1	133.5
Fabricated metal products	RABW	6112280000	83.6	84.8	91.6	100.0	110.6	117.0	129.0	125.6p
Manufacture of machinery and equipment not elsewhere classified	RBCA	6192290000	92.9	92.8	95.2	100.0	105.3	108.7	118.6	120.9p
Manufacture of electrical and optical equipment	RBCB	6192303300	111.8	104.4	99.5	100.0	103.2	102.7	107.6	111.8p
Office machinery and computers	RABY	6112300000	121.9	109.2	101.5	100.0	101.0	97.4	100.7	104.8
Electrical machinery and apparatus not elsewhere classified	RACB	6112310000	100.9	97.8	96.9	100.0	106.2	108.5	115.3	118.0p
Radio, television and communication equipment	RACC	6112320000	112.8	106.2	100.5	100.0	102.0	101.4	105.4	110.3p
Medical, precision, optical instruments and clocks	RACD	6112330000	112.6	105.3	99.5	100.0	103.0	102.2	107.5	112.8p
Manufacture of transport equipment	RBCC	6192343500	95.6	96.0	96.7	100.0	104.1	107.1	113.8	116.7p
Motor vehicles, trailers and semi-trailers	RACE	6112340000	95.5	96.0	96.7	100.0	103.7	106.8	113.8	116.7p
Other transport equipment	RACF	6112350000	95.9	95.8	96.7	100.0	105.1	108.0	113.4	116.2p
Manufacturing not elsewhere classified	RBCD	6192363700	92.3	93.4	95.7	100.0	105.8	109.8	118.3	119.7p
Electricity including Climate Change Levy	RCVR	7167850000	72.5	70.0	74.7	100.0	135.9	138.2	166.2	193.5
Gas including Climate Change Levy	RCVW	7167860000	58.9	61.0	67.1	100.0	123.8	99.8	149.7	129.0
Collected and purified water	PQNB	7167870000	79.5	82.2	87.1	100.0	110.1	118.2	126.2	133.2

1 See chapter text.
2 These indices include the Climate Change Levy which was introduced in April 2001.
3 The Climate Change Levy is excluded from the detailed industry input index.
4 These indices include the Aggregates Levy which was introduced in April 2002.

Source: Office for National Statistics: 01633 815783

17.2 Producer price index of output: by all manufacturing and selected industries SIC(92)[1]

United Kingdom: Annual averages

Indices (2005=100)

			2002	2003	2004	2005	2006	2007	2008	2009
Net sector										
Output of manufactured products	PLLU	7209200000	95.8	96.8	98.2	100.0	102.2	104.8	112.5	113.9p
All manufacturing excluding duty	PVNP	7209200010	96.1	97.1	98.3	100.0	102.2	104.6	112.3	113.1p
All manufacturing excluding duty - seasonally adjusted	PVNQ	7209200890	99.8	101.2	103.7	106.8	109.7	113.0	..	..
Products of manufacturing industries other than the food, beverages, petroleum and tobacco manufacturing industries - not seasonally adjusted	PLLV	7209299000	98.0	98.6	99.1	100.0	101.8	103.7	108.6	110.8p
All manufacturing excluding food, beverages, tobacco and petroleum - seasonally adjusted	PLLW	7209299890	99.3	100.6	102.5	104.7	107.1	109.6	..	..
Gross sector										
Manufactured products excluding duty	POKE	7109200000	92.1	93.6	96.2	100.0	103.3	106.7	117.2	115.6
Manufactured products excluding food, drink, tobacco and petroleum	POKF	7109299000	95.0	96.0	97.8	100.0	102.7	105.9	111.7	113.6
Other mining and quarrying products[2]	ROFV	7112148000	96.8	99.6	99.7	100.0	101.9	105.5	120.7	127.6
Food products, beverages and tobacco excluding duty	POKH	7111151600	96.4	97.6	99.4	100.0	101.8	106.4	117.2	120.9
Food products, beverages and tobacco including duty	RBGA	7111151680	95.9	97.1	99.1	100.0	101.9	106.4	116.6	121.0
Food products and beverages including duty	RPUN	7112150080	96.6	97.6	99.5	100.0	101.6	106.1	116.9	121.1
Food products excluding beverages	RBGD	7112159900	96.8	97.8	99.6	100.0	101.5	106.1	117.9	121.4
Alcoholic beverages including duty	RPUX	7113159080	95.5	..	..	100.0	101.9	104.9	..	..
Tobacco products including duty	RPUS	7112160080	90.0	92.8	96.2	100.0	104.1	109.1	113.9	120.4
Textiles and textile products	POKI	7111171800	99.2	98.8	98.5	100.0	101.1	102.0	103.6	105.6
Textiles	POKZ	7112170000	98.5	98.3	98.0	100.0	101.3	102.5	104.4	106.7
Wearing apparel: Furs	POLA	7112180000	100.9	100.0	99.5	100.0	100.7	101.1	101.8	102.7
Leather and leather products	POKJ	7111190000	98.6	98.8	98.7	100.0	101.7	102.7	103.3	103.7
Wood and wood products	POKK	7111200000	92.7	93.9	96.1	100.0	102.5	111.4	116.2	118.6
Pulp, paper and paper products, recorded media and printing services	POKL	7111212200	96.3	98.0	99.1	100.0	101.7	103.6	106.7	109.4
Pulp, paper and paper products	POLD	7112210000	102.4	102.2	101.5	100.0	101.6	105.0	108.6	110.6
Printed matter and recorded media	POLE	7112220000	94.3	96.6	98.3	100.0	101.8	103.2	106.1	109.4
Chemicals, chemical, products and manmade fibres	POKN	7111240000	94.6	96.9	98.0	100.0	103.4	105.7	117.1	121.9
Rubber and plastic products	POKO	7111250000	95.8	95.8	96.3	100.0	103.0	104.3	109.1	110.9
Other non-metallic mineral products	POKP	7111260000	93.2	95.5	96.9	100.0	103.4	108.5	114.0	118.3
Base metals and fabricated metal products	POKQ	7111272800	87.3	88.4	93.5	100.0	105.4	111.1	118.7	116.8
Base metals	POLJ	7112270000	78.9	99.2	113.1	126.6	141.5	154.9	..	..
Fabricated metal products, except machinery and equipment	POLK	7112280000	90.4	91.3	94.4	100.0	102.6	106.8	113.1	114.4
Machinery and equipment not elsewhere classified	POKR	7111290000	96.4	96.4	97.5	100.0	102.0	105.5	109.1	112.9
Electrical and optical equipment	POKS	7111343500	106.1	103.0	100.5	100.0	101.2	101.1	102.9	104.1
Office machinery and computers	POLM	7112300000	142.5	127.0	108.9	100.0	95.0	87.8	85.1	84.6
Electrical machinery and apparatus not elsewhere classified	POLN	7112310000	96.1	96.2	97.5	100.0	104.4	107.7	111.4	112.6
Radio, television and communication equipment and apparatus	POLO	7112320000	117.7	110.6	104.8	100.0	98.5	94.2	91.2	93.0
Medical precision and optical instruments, watches and clocks	POLP	7112330000	98.4	99.3	99.4	100.0	100.7	100.8	103.8	105.2
Transport equipment	POKT	7111343500	96.9	97.3	98.2	100.0	101.5	102.5	106.8	112.8
Motor vehicles, trailers and semi-trailers	POLQ	7112340000	98.7	98.3	98.7	100.0	100.9	101.0	105.1	110.4
Other transport	POLR	7112350000	93.3	95.3	97.2	100.0	102.5	105.3	110.1	117.7
Furniture: other manufactured goods not elsewhere classified	POLS	7112360000	97.9	100.5	100.3	100.0	100.9	102.9	106.4	110.1

1 See chapter text.
2 These indices include the Aggregates Levy which was introduced in April 2002. These indices do not feed into Net Sector output (PLLU).

Source: Office for National Statistics: 01633 815783

17.3 Internal purchasing power of the pound[1,2]
United Kingdom

Pence

	1989	1990	1991	1992	1993	1994	1995	1996	1997	1998	1999	2000	2001	2002	2003	2004	2005	2006	2007	2008
	BAMV	BAMW	BASX	CZVM	CBXX	DOFX	DOHR	DOLM	DTUL	CDQG	JKZZ	ZMHO	IKHI	FAUI	SEZH	C687	E9AO	GB4Y	HT4R	J5TL
1990	91	100	106	110	112	114	118	121	125	129	131	135	137	140	144	148	152	157	164	170
1991	86	94	100	104	105	108	112	114	118	122	124	128	130	132	136	140	144	148	155	161
1992	83	91	96	100	102	104	108	110	114	118	119	123	125	127	131	135	139	143	149	155
1993	82	90	95	98	100	102	106	109	112	116	118	121	123	125	129	133	136	141	147	153
1994	80	88	93	96	98	100	103	106	109	113	115	118	120	122	126	130	133	137	143	149
1995	77	85	90	93	94	97	100	102	106	109	111	114	116	118	122	125	129	133	139	144
1996	75	83	87	91	92	94	98	100	103	107	108	112	113	115	119	122	126	130	135	141
1997	73	80	85	88	89	92	95	97	100	103	105	108	110	112	115	119	122	126	131	136
1998	71	77	82	85	86	88	92	94	97	100	102	105	106	108	111	115	118	122	127	132
1999	70	76	81	84	85	87	90	92	95	98	100	103	105	107	110	113	116	120	125	130
2000	68	74	78	81	83	85	88	90	92	96	97	100	102	103	106	110	113	116	121	126
2001	66	73	77	80	81	83	86	88	91	94	95	98	100	102	105	108	111	114	119	124
2002	65	72	76	79	80	82	85	87	89	92	94	97	98	100	103	106	109	112	117	122
2003	64	70	74	76	78	79	82	84	87	90	91	94	96	97	100	103	106	109	114	118
2004	62	68	72	74	75	77	80	82	84	87	89	91	93	94	97	100	103	106	111	115
2005	60	66	70	72	73	75	78	80	82	85	86	89	90	92	94	97	100	103	108	112
2006	58	64	67	70	71	73	75	77	80	82	83	86	87	89	92	94	97	100	104	108
2007	56	61	65	67	68	70	72	74	76	79	80	82	84	85	88	90	93	96	100	104
2008	54	59	62	64	65	67	69	71	73	76	77	79	81	82	84	87	89	92	96	100
2009	54	59	62	65	66	67	70	71	74	76	77	80	81	82	85	87	90	93	97	101

1 See chapter text. These figures are calculated by taking the inverse ratio of the respective annual averages of the Retail Prices Index (RPI).

2 To find the purchasing power of the pound in 1995, given that it was 100 pence in 1990, select the column headed 1990 and look at the 1995 row. The result is 85 pence.

Source: Office for National Statistics: 020 7533 5874

17.4 Consumer Prices Index:[1] detailed figures by division
United Kingdom

Indices (2005=100)

	Food and non-alcoholic beverages	Alcoholic beverages and tobacco	Clothing and footwear	Housing, water, electricity, gas & other fuels	Furniture, household equipment & routine mainte-nance	Health	Transport	Commun-ication	Recreation and culture	Education	Restaur-ants and hotels	Miscell-aneous goods and services	CPI (overall index)
COICOP Division	01	02	03	04	05	06	07	08	09	10	11	12	
Weights 2006	102	44	65	108	73	24	155	25	147	17	134	106	1000
	D7BU	D7BV	D7BW	D7BX	D7BY	D7BZ	D7C2	D7C3	D7C4	D7C5	D7C6	D7C7	D7BT
2007 Sep	107.4	107.1	92.5	114.0	102.1	107.1	105.7	96.6	97.6	122.9	107.6	105.8	104.8
Oct	109.1	106.8	92.5	114.3	100.8	107.5	106.6	96.2	97.7	133.2	107.9	106.4	105.3
Nov	110.1	106.4	92.9	114.6	101.6	107.3	107.0	96.3	97.6	133.2	108.0	106.6	105.6
Dec	111.1	105.7	92.2	114.7	104.2	107.6	108.7	96.2	98.0	133.2	108.3	106.8	106.2
2008 Jan	110.8	106.9	87.5	115.4	100.0	108.1	108.6	95.8	97.0	133.2	108.3	106.8	105.5
Feb	111.3	108.1	87.6	119.1	101.3	108.2	109.1	94.3	97.2	133.2	108.7	107.1	106.3
Mar	111.8	108.2	87.9	119.5	103.5	108.4	110.3	94.2	96.8	133.2	109.2	107.5	106.7
Apr	113.2	111.5	87.8	122.0	102.1	108.9	110.8	94.4	97.3	133.2	110.4	108.3	107.6
May	115.1	112.0	87.8	122.3	103.5	109.0	112.7	94.3	97.3	133.2	110.8	108.5	108.3
Jun	117.5	111.9	86.5	122.5	105.9	109.3	114.6	94.9	97.6	133.2	111.1	108.6	109.0
Jul	118.4	111.4	83.8	123.0	102.6	110.1	116.6	94.1	96.9	133.2	111.6	109.0	109.0
Aug	120.0	111.8	84.9	125.6	103.4	110.3	116.5	94.3	97.3	133.2	111.7	109.2	109.7
Sep	119.6	111.7	86.8	131.1	105.1	110.2	113.8	94.1	97.8	136.2	112.2	109.4	110.3
Oct	120.1	111.4	86.3	131.6	104.0	110.4	111.3	94.1	97.4	144.6	112.5	109.6	110.0
Nov	121.8	110.6	86.3	131.5	104.7	111.0	108.4	94.8	97.6	144.6	112.5	110.1	109.9
Dec	122.7	110.4	82.7	131.1	105.0	109.9	108.9	92.9	96.8	144.6	112.2	109.6	109.5
2009 Jan	122.0	112.5	78.8	131.1	102.1	110.5	106.5	93.8	96.5	144.6	112.2	110.0	108.7
Feb	124.0	114.2	79.4	131.1	104.6	110.8	107.6	93.7	97.5	144.6	112.6	110.5	109.6
Mar	123.5	114.6	80.3	129.8	106.9	111.0	108.1	93.4	97.6	144.6	112.9	110.8	109.8
Apr	122.9	114.6	80.4	129.5	105.7	111.8	109.8	95.5	97.8	144.6	113.2	110.8	110.1
May	124.1	116.4	80.7	129.0	106.8	111.9	111.5	95.5	98.1	144.6	113.6	110.9	110.7
Jun	123.8	115.6	79.5	129.2	107.9	112.1	113.1	95.5	98.7	144.6	113.8	110.9	111.0
Jul	123.3	116.0	77.0	129.4	105.0	112.9	115.0	95.5	98.9	144.6	113.9	111.3	110.9
Aug	122.6	116.4	77.9	129.6	106.5	113.4	116.8	95.5	99.0	144.6	114.0	111.4	111.4
Sep	121.4	116.4	80.7	129.6	108.2	113.7	115.1	95.1	99.2	147.3	114.0	111.6	111.5
Oct	122.7	116.2	80.4	129.8	107.4	114.2	115.2	96.6	99.4	152.6	114.3	111.1	111.7
Nov	123.4	115.5	80.9	129.9	108.3	113.9	115.9	96.3	99.6	152.2	114.3	111.2	112.0
Dec	124.6	115.3	79.8	130.1	110.7	113.4	118.4	96.4	99.6	152.2	114.3	111.6	112.6

Percentage change on a year earlier

	D7G8	D7G9	D7GA	D7GB	D7GC	D7GD	D7GE	D7GF	D7GG	D7GH	D7GI	D7GJ	D7G7
2007 Nov	4.8	2.9	−4.4	0.8	1.7	3.1	5.8	−4.0	−1.1	13.2	3.4	1.6	2.1
Dec	5.4	2.7	−3.9	0.2	0.9	3.3	5.8	−3.8	−1.3	13.2	3.4	1.9	2.1
2008 Jan	6.1	2.2	−4.9	0.4	1.7	3.1	6.4	−3.2	−1.4	13.2	3.3	1.5	2.2
Feb	5.6	2.9	−4.7	3.5	1.7	3.1	6.2	−3.9	−1.2	13.2	3.3	1.2	2.5
Mar	5.5	2.5	−5.3	3.9	0.5	3.5	7.0	−4.0	−1.5	13.2	3.3	1.2	2.5
Apr	6.6	4.2	−6.3	5.4	1.4	3.3	6.1	−2.9	−1.0	13.2	3.8	2.3	3.0
May	7.8	4.9	−6.3	6.3	1.7	3.0	6.2	−2.4	−0.8	13.2	3.9	2.6	3.3
Jun	9.5	4.5	−7.5	7.0	1.8	3.0	7.3	−1.3	−	13.2	3.9	2.7	3.8
Jul	12.3	4.3	−6.7	7.6	2.8	3.3	8.0	−0.7	−0.1	13.2	4.1	2.8	4.4
Aug	13.0	4.4	−6.7	10.1	3.2	3.2	7.3	−3.0	−0.2	13.2	4.0	3.4	4.7
Sep	11.3	4.3	−6.2	15.0	2.9	2.9	7.6	−2.7	0.2	10.8	4.3	3.4	5.2
Oct	10.1	4.4	−6.7	15.2	3.1	2.6	4.3	−2.2	−0.2	8.6	4.2	3.0	4.5
Nov	10.6	4.0	−7.1	14.8	3.0	3.5	1.3	−1.5	−	8.6	4.1	3.3	4.1
Dec	10.4	4.4	−10.3	14.3	0.8	2.1	0.1	−3.4	−1.2	8.6	3.6	2.6	3.1
2009 Jan	10.2	5.3	−10.0	13.6	2.2	2.2	−1.9	−2.0	−0.5	8.6	3.6	3.0	3.0
Feb	11.5	5.7	−9.3	10.0	3.2	2.4	−1.4	−0.7	0.3	8.6	3.6	3.2	3.2
Mar	10.5	5.9	−8.7	8.6	3.3	2.3	−2.0	−0.8	0.8	8.6	3.4	3.1	2.9
Apr	8.6	2.8	−8.4	6.1	3.5	2.7	−0.9	1.2	0.5	8.6	2.5	2.4	2.3
May	7.8	3.9	−8.1	5.5	3.2	2.6	−1.1	1.3	0.8	8.6	2.5	2.3	2.2
Jun	5.4	3.3	−8.1	5.5	1.9	2.6	−1.3	0.7	1.2	8.6	2.4	2.1	1.8
Jul	4.1	4.1	−8.1	5.2	2.4	2.5	−1.4	1.5	2.0	8.6	2.0	2.1	1.8
Aug	2.2	4.1	−8.2	3.3	3.0	2.9	0.3	1.2	1.8	8.6	2.0	2.0	1.6
Sep	1.6	4.2	−6.9	−1.1	3.0	3.2	1.2	1.1	1.4	8.2	1.6	2.0	1.1
Oct	2.2	4.3	−6.8	−1.3	3.3	3.4	3.5	2.6	2.0	5.2	1.6	1.3	1.5
Nov	1.3	4.5	−6.3	−1.2	3.5	2.6	6.9	1.6	2.0	5.2	1.6	1.0	1.9
Dec	1.6	4.4	−3.5	−0.8	5.4	3.1	8.7	3.8	2.9	5.2	1.8	1.8	2.9
2010 Jan	1.9	6.2	−4.5	−0.3	5.1	3.7	11.0	4.1	3.6	5.2	2.2	2.0	3.5
Feb	1.3	4.2	−3.3	−1.0	3.7	3.4	10.6	4.6	2.4	5.2	2.4	1.6	3.0

1 See chapter text. Prior to 10 December 2003, the consumer prices index (CPI) was published in the UK as the harmonised index of consumer prices (HICP).

Source: Office for National Statistics: 020 7533 5874

Prices

17.5 Retail Prices Index[1]
United Kingdom

Indices (13 January 1987=100)

	All items (RPI)	All items excluding mortgage interest payments (RPIX)	mortgage interest payments and depreciation	housing	food	seasonal food[2]	Food and catering	Alcohol and tobacco	Housing and household expenditure	Personal expenditure	Travel and leisure	Consumer durables	All items excluding mortgage interest payments & indirect taxes (RPIY)[3]
Weights													
	CZGU	CZGY	DOGZ	CZGX	CZGV	CZGW	CBVV	CBVW	CBVX	CBVY	CBVZ	CBWA	
2001	1 000	954	914	795	884	982	169	97	362	96	276	125	
2002	1 000	964	924	801	886	980	166	99	363	94	278	126	
2003	1 000	961	919	797	891	983	160	98	365	92	285	126	
2004	1 000	961	914	791	889	981	160	97	367	93	283	121	
2005	1 000	950	901	776	890	981	159	96	387	89	269	122	
2006	1 000	950	906	778	895	983	155	96	392	90	267	117	
2007	1 000	945	895	762	895	981	152	95	408	83	262	109	
2008	1 000	940	885	746	889	980	158	86	417	83	256	104	
2009	1 000	959	909	764	882	979	168	90	416	80	246	106	
Annual averages													
	CHAW	CHMK	CHON	CHAZ	CHAY	CHAX	CHBS	CHBT	CHBU	CHBV	CHBW	CHBY	CBZW
2001	173.3	171.3	169.5	163.7	178.0	174.3	162.2	216.9	180.0	135.7	172.0	105.0	163.7
2002	176.2	175.1	172.5	166.0	181.1	177.2	164.8	222.3	184.6	133.2	174.2	101.9	167.5
2003	181.3	180.0	176.2	168.9	186.7	182.4	167.9	228.0	194.3	133.2	177.0	99.8	172.0
2004	186.7	184.0	179.1	170.9	192.8	187.9	170.0	233.6	207.4	131.5	178.1	97.7	175.5
2005	192.0	188.2	182.6	173.7	198.7	193.3	172.9	239.8	219.4	131.0	179.2	95.3	179.4
2006	198.1	193.7	187.8	178.3	205.2	199.5	176.9	247.1	231.8	131.7	181.1	94.0	184.8
2007	206.6	199.9	193.3	183.2	213.9	207.9	184.3	256.2	248.1	132.9	183.8	93.3	190.8
2008	214.8	208.5	201.9	191.3	221.2	216.0	198.5	266.7	258.6	132.4	189.0	91.6	199.2
2009	213.7	212.6	207.2	196.3	218.3	214.6	207.6	276.7	247.4	131.4	191.2	90.7	204.8
Monthly figures													
2006 Dec	202.7	197.4	191.2	181.7	210.1	204.1	180.6	249.4	242.7	132.9	181.0	96.7	188.6
2007 Jan	201.6	196.1	189.8	180.0	208.9	203.0	180.0	251.3	240.6	130.1	180.8	91.1	187.3
Feb	203.1	197.1	190.7	181.1	210.4	204.4	181.2	252.4	243.0	131.3	181.4	92.1	188.4
Mar	204.4	198.3	191.9	182.4	211.7	205.7	182.1	253.8	245.3	132.5	181.6	95.1	189.5
Apr	205.4	199.3	192.9	182.7	212.8	206.8	182.7	256.8	245.7	133.8	183.1	93.5	190.0
May	206.2	200.0	193.6	183.4	213.6	207.5	183.6	257.0	246.5	134.0	184.3	94.4	190.7
Jun	207.3	200.7	194.1	184.0	214.7	208.6	184.5	257.5	248.9	133.9	184.5	95.8	191.4
Jul	206.1	199.4	192.7	182.2	213.7	207.6	182.7	257.6	247.2	131.2	184.7	91.0	190.1
Aug	207.3	200.1	193.3	182.9	215.0	208.7	183.5	257.9	249.4	132.2	185.2	91.9	190.9
Sep	208.0	200.8	193.8	183.5	215.5	209.4	185.2	258.2	251.3	133.7	183.7	93.7	191.6
Oct	208.9	201.6	194.6	184.3	216.2	210.2	187.3	257.7	251.9	134.1	184.7	92.8	192.3
Nov	209.7	202.4	195.4	185.1	216.9	211.0	188.8	257.3	253.0	134.3	185.4	93.2	193.2
Dec	210.9	203.5	196.6	186.3	218.0	212.2	190.2	256.9	254.8	134.0	186.8	94.8	194.4
2008 Jan	209.8	202.7	195.7	185.2	216.8	211.1	190.2	258.0	252.6	130.7	186.7	89.8	193.5
Feb	211.4	204.3	197.3	187.0	218.5	212.8	191.0	260.2	255.5	132.0	187.2	91.2	195.2
Mar	212.1	205.3	198.5	188.2	219.2	213.5	191.7	261.2	256.0	133.0	188.0	92.6	196.3
Apr	214.0	207.2	200.4	189.6	221.1	215.3	193.7	267.9	258.0	133.4	188.9	91.7	197.5
May	215.1	208.7	201.9	191.2	221.9	216.3	196.0	268.9	258.3	133.5	190.7	92.7	199.0
Jun	216.8	210.4	203.7	193.2	223.3	218.0	199.2	269.1	260.2	132.8	192.9	94.4	200.8
Jul	216.5	210.0	203.3	192.8	222.7	217.7	200.6	268.7	258.3	130.9	194.1	90.2	200.4
Aug	217.2	210.6	204.0	193.5	223.2	218.4	202.4	269.2	260.2	132.1	192.6	90.8	201.2
Sep	218.4	211.8	205.4	194.8	224.7	219.7	202.3	269.6	264.3	133.7	191.0	92.6	202.4
Oct	217.7	211.1	204.8	194.0	223.8	218.9	203.1	269.7	264.2	133.3	188.5	91.3	201.7
Nov	216.0	210.2	204.1	193.2	221.3	217.0	205.5	268.8	261.6	133.6	184.3	91.6	200.8
Dec	212.9	209.2	203.3	192.4	217.5	213.7	206.2	268.7	254.5	130.1	183.1	90.8	201.9
2009 Jan	210.1	207.5	201.8	190.6	214.4	210.9	205.5	270.9	249.4	127.6	180.6	86.7	200.0
Feb	211.4	209.5	203.9	193.0	215.5	212.1	208.3	273.4	248.6	129.8	182.9	88.8	202.1
Mar	211.3	209.9	204.5	193.7	215.4	212.1	207.7	274.2	247.0	131.2	183.9	90.7	202.5
Apr	211.5	210.7	205.5	194.4	215.8	212.4	207.2	274.8	245.2	131.7	186.8	90.3	202.9
May	212.8	212.0	207.0	195.9	217.1	213.6	208.4	278.2	245.6	132.0	189.3	91.1	204.1
Jun	213.4	212.6	207.5	196.6	217.8	214.2	208.2	277.7	245.9	131.4	191.3	91.7	204.7
Jul	213.4	212.6	207.5	196.4	218.0	214.4	207.7	278.1	245.1	129.6	193.5	88.9	204.7
Aug	214.4	213.6	208.3	197.3	219.3	215.5	206.9	278.8	246.4	130.8	195.2	90.2	205.8
Sep	215.3	214.5	209.2	198.3	220.5	216.5	206.0	278.7	247.6	133.1	196.2	92.4	206.5
Oct	216.0	215.1	209.7	198.8	221.0	217.1	207.5	278.8	248.4	133.3	196.5	91.5	207.3
Nov	216.6	215.8	210.3	199.5	221.7	217.6	208.0	278.2	249.0	133.7	197.9	92.3	207.9
Dec	218.0	217.2	211.7	201.0	223.1	219.0	209.4	278.3	250.8	132.9	200.1	93.7	209.5

1 See chapter text.
2 Seasonal food is defined as items of food the prices of which show significant seasonal variations. These are fresh fruit and vegetables, fresh fish, eggs and home-killed lamb.

3 There are no weights available for RPIY.

Source: Office for National Statistics: 020 7533 5874

17.6 Tax and Price Index[1]
United Kingdom

Tax and Price Index: (January 1988=100)

DQAB

	1995	1996	1997	1998	1999	2000	2001	2002	2003	2004	2005	2006	2007	2008	2009
January	137.2	141.6	143.6	147.1	150.5	152.7	156.7	156.5	161.4	166.9	172.1	175.9	183.3	190.7	188.6
February	138.2	142.3	144.2	147.9	150.8	153.7	157.6	157.0	162.3	167.6	172.8	176.7	184.8	192.3	189.8
March	138.8	143.0	144.6	148.4	151.2	154.6	157.8	157.7	163.0	168.4	173.7	177.4	186.1	192.9	189.7
April	140.3	141.7	143.8	149.7	151.2	155.7	156.3	158.6	164.9	168.9	174.1	178.3	186.3	192.2	188.5
May	141.0	142.0	144.4	150.6	151.7	156.3	157.4	159.1	165.2	169.7	174.5	179.5	187.1	193.4	189.7
June	141.2	142.1	145.0	150.5	151.7	156.7	157.6	159.1	165.0	170.0	174.7	180.3	188.2	195.1	190.2
July	140.4	141.5	145.0	150.1	151.1	156.1	156.5	158.8	165.0	170.0	174.7	180.3	187.0	194.8	190.2
August	141.3	142.2	146.0	150.8	151.5	156.1	157.2	159.3	165.4	170.6	175.1	181.0	188.2	195.5	191.3
September	142.0	143.0	146.9	151.5	152.3	157.3	157.8	160.6	166.3	171.3	175.6	181.9	188.9	196.7	192.2
October	141.2	143.0	147.1	151.6	152.6	157.2	157.5	160.9	166.4	171.8	175.8	182.2	189.8	196.0	192.9
November	141.2	143.1	147.2	151.5	152.8	157.7	156.8	161.2	166.5	172.2	176.1	182.8	190.6	194.3	193.4
December	142.1	143.6	147.6	151.5	153.4	157.8	156.6	161.5	167.3	173.1	176.6	184.4	191.8	191.2	194.8

Retail Prices Index: (January 1988=100)

CHAW

	1995	1996	1997	1998	1999	2000	2001	2002	2003	2004	2005	2006	2007	2008	2009
January	146.0	150.2	154.4	159.5	163.4	166.6	171.1	173.3	178.4	183.1	188.9	193.4	201.6	209.8	210.1
February	146.9	150.9	155.0	160.3	163.7	167.5	172.0	173.8	179.3	183.8	189.6	194.2	203.1	211.4	211.4
March	147.5	151.5	155.4	160.8	164.1	168.4	172.2	174.5	179.9	184.6	190.5	195.0	204.4	212.1	211.3
April	149.0	152.6	156.3	162.6	165.2	170.1	173.1	175.7	181.2	185.7	191.6	196.5	205.4	214.0	211.5
May	149.6	152.9	156.9	163.5	165.6	170.7	174.2	176.2	181.5	186.5	192.0	197.7	206.2	215.1	212.8
June	149.8	153.0	157.5	163.4	165.6	171.1	174.4	176.2	181.3	186.8	192.2	198.5	207.3	216.8	213.4
July	149.1	152.4	157.5	163.0	165.1	170.5	173.3	175.9	181.3	186.8	192.2	198.5	206.1	216.5	213.4
August	149.9	153.1	158.5	163.7	165.5	170.5	174.0	176.4	181.6	187.4	192.6	199.2	207.3	217.2	214.4
September	150.6	153.8	159.3	164.4	166.2	171.7	174.6	177.6	182.5	188.1	193.1	200.1	208.0	218.4	215.3
October	149.8	153.8	159.5	164.5	166.5	171.6	174.3	177.9	182.6	188.6	193.3	200.4	208.9	217.7	216.0
November	149.8	153.9	159.6	164.4	166.7	172.1	173.6	178.2	182.7	189.0	193.6	201.1	209.7	216.0	216.6
December	150.7	154.4	160.0	164.4	167.3	172.2	173.4	178.5	183.5	189.9	194.1	202.7	210.9	212.9	218.0

Percentage changes on one year earlier[1]

	1995	1996	1997	1998	1999	2000	2001	2002	2003	2004	2005	2006	2007	2008	2009
Tax and Price Index[1]															
January		3.9	3.2	1.4	2.4	2.3	1.5	2.6	−0.1	3.1	3.4	3.1	2.2	4.2	4.0	−1.1
February		4.0	3.0	1.3	2.6	2.0	1.9	2.5	−0.4	3.4	3.3	3.1	2.3	4.6	4.1	−1.3
March		4.0	3.0	1.1	2.6	1.9	2.2	2.1	−0.1	3.4	3.3	3.1	2.1	4.9	3.7	−1.7
April		3.7	1.0	1.5	4.1	1.0	3.0	0.4	1.5	4.0	2.4	3.1	2.4	4.5	3.2	−1.9
May		3.8	0.7	1.7	4.3	0.7	3.0	0.7	1.1	3.8	2.7	2.8	2.9	4.2	3.4	−1.9
June		4.0	0.6	2.0	3.8	0.8	3.3	0.6	1.0	3.7	3.0	2.8	3.2	4.4	3.7	−2.5
July		3.9	0.8	2.5	3.5	0.7	3.3	0.3	1.5	3.9	3.0	2.8	3.2	3.7	4.2	−2.4
August		4.1	0.6	2.7	3.3	0.5	3.0	0.7	1.3	3.8	3.1	2.6	3.4	4.0	3.9	−2.1
September		4.3	0.7	2.7	3.1	0.5	3.3	0.3	1.8	3.5	3.0	2.5	3.6	3.8	4.1	−2.3
October		3.5	1.3	2.9	3.1	0.7	3.0	0.2	2.2	3.4	3.2	2.3	3.6	4.2	3.3	−1.6
November		3.4	1.3	2.9	2.9	0.9	3.2	−0.6	2.8	3.3	3.4	2.3	3.8	4.3	1.9	−0.5
December		3.6	1.1	2.8	2.6	1.3	2.9	−0.8	3.1	3.6	3.5	2.0	4.4	4.0	−0.3	1.9
Retail Prices Index															
January		3.3	2.9	2.8	3.3	2.4	2.0	2.7	1.3	2.9	2.6	3.2	2.4	4.2	4.1	0.1
February		3.4	2.7	2.7	3.4	2.1	2.3	2.7	1.0	3.2	2.5	3.2	2.4	4.6	4.1	0.0
March		3.5	2.7	2.6	3.5	2.1	2.6	2.3	1.3	3.1	2.6	3.2	2.4	4.8	3.8	−0.4
April		3.3	2.4	2.4	4.0	1.6	3.0	1.8	1.5	3.1	2.5	3.2	2.6	4.5	4.2	−1.2
May		3.4	2.2	2.6	4.2	1.3	3.1	2.1	1.1	3.0	2.8	2.9	3.0	4.3	4.3	−1.1
June		3.5	2.1	2.9	3.7	1.3	3.3	1.9	1.0	2.9	3.0	2.9	3.3	4.4	4.6	−1.6
July		3.5	2.2	3.3	3.5	1.3	3.3	1.6	1.5	3.1	3.0	2.9	3.3	3.8	5.0	−1.4
August		3.6	2.1	3.5	3.3	1.1	3.0	2.1	1.4	2.9	3.2	2.8	3.4	4.1	4.8	−1.3
September		3.9	2.1	3.6	3.2	1.1	3.3	1.7	1.7	2.8	3.1	2.7	3.6	3.9	5.0	−1.4
October		3.2	2.7	3.7	3.1	1.2	3.1	1.6	2.1	2.6	3.3	2.5	3.7	4.2	4.2	−0.8
November		3.1	2.7	3.7	3.0	1.4	3.2	0.9	2.6	2.5	3.4	2.4	3.9	4.3	3.0	0.3
December		3.2	2.5	3.6	2.8	1.8	2.9	0.7	2.9	2.8	3.5	2.2	4.4	4.0	0.9	2.4

1 See chapter text.

Source: Office for National Statistics: 020 7533 5874

Prices

17.7 Index of purchase prices of the means of agricultural production[1]
United Kingdom
Annual averages

Indices (2005=100)

		2002	2003	2004	2005	2006	2007	2008	2009
Goods and services currently consumed[2]	C3FU	103.7	93.7	100.3	100.0	103.8	115.3	145.5	136.8
Seeds	C3FV	105.5	110.4	130.3	100.0	90.5	100.3	110.4	109.4
Energy, lubricants	C3FW	92.4	73.9	79.8	100.0	112.2	117.9	158.2	132.9
Fuels for heating	C3FX	87.2	65.8	74.5	100.0	116.5	127.9	173.1	139.0
Motor fuel	C3FY	91.6	71.1	77.7	100.0	109.5	111.1	160.4	123.3
Electricity	C3FZ	96.2	87.2	89.3	100.0	119.2	135.6	143.4	161.9
Fertilisers and soil improvers	C3G3	110.3	79.3	88.3	100.0	107.4	113.3	229.4	233.9
Straight nitrogen	C3G4	120.2	87.4	94.1	100.0	100.0	147.3	390.1	220.1
Compound fertilisers	C3G5	103.0	84.8	91.8	100.0	103.9	122.7	302.6	221.0
Other fertiliser (mainly lime and chalk)	C3G6	104.0	94.1	97.3	100.0	101.8	103.7	105.8	105.2
Fungicides	JT6Q	..	88.0	88.2	100.0	106.2	111.1	113.3	126.7
Insecticides	JT6R	..	92.1	95.9	100.0	103.3	104.8	107.0	107.4
Herbicides	JT6S	..	96.9	99.9	100.0	100.1	101.4	103.2	99.9
Plant protection products	C3G7	95.8	96.9	99.9	100.0	99.6	101.6	103.7	99.9
Feed wheat	C3G9	97.3	109.1	122.2	100.0	114.7	160.0	215.8	159.5
Feed barley	JT6U	..	106.5	114.6	100.0	111.5	161.8	194.6	134.0
Feed oats	JT6V	..	89.4	99.2	100.0	108.2	130.9	164.7	116.5
Soya bean meal	JT6W	..	107.7	112.2	100.0	95.8	116.4	174.7	193.8
White fish meal	C3GE	134.7	102.0	95.0	100.0	144.2	137.2	174.7	174.8
Field beans	JT6X	..	103.3	114.9	100.0	94.9	167.9	207.1	160.0
Field Peas	JT6Y	..	99.5	99.5	99.5	99.5	99.5	99.5	99.5
Dried Sugar Beet Pulp	JT6Z	..	100.0	100.0	100.0	100.0	100.0	100.0	100.0
All straight feedstuffs	C3GG	101.3	104.9	112.2	100.0	106.4	142.9	184.0	156.1
Compound feedstuffs for:	C3GI	104.9	99.7	106.1	100.0	103.2	119.7	154.6	151.8
Cattle and calves	C3GJ	105.9	98.6	104.2	100.0	101.4	116.4	151.6	149.1
Pigs	C3GK	103.3	101.0	107.3	100.0	105.5	122.7	151.6	149.4
Poultry	C3GL	104.5	100.6	108.0	100.0	104.9	123.6	162.2	158.1
Sheep	C3GM	106.2	98.1	104.6	100.0	99.8	112.2	141.9	143.5
Maintenance and repair of plant	C3GN	109.4	89.1	94.0	100.0	105.8	109.9	116.3	121.5
Maintenance and repair of buildings	C3GO	105.1	91.4	95.9	100.0	106.3	114.1	122.3	121.9
Veterinary services	C3GP	97.8	97.9	100.7	100.0	106.9	108.4	103.9	104.6
Other goods and services	C3GQ	105.5	91.4	96.2	100.0	102.6	107.9	113.6	116.1
Goods and services contributing to investment in agriculture	C3GR	100.0	93.5	96.1	100.0	103.0	106.7	111.0	115.2
Machinery and other equipment	C3GT	95.7	91.6	92.5	100.0	104.5	110.3	117.6	121.9
Machinery and plant for cultivation	C3GU	98.6	90.2	94.8	100.0	101.4	106.3	113.8	115.7
Machinery and plant for harvesting	C3GV	88.8	90.1	89.2	100.0	107.7	115.8	125.1	130.7
Farm machinery and installations	C3GW	108.2	97.0	97.2	100.0	100.9	102.8	104.6	109.3
Tractors	C3GX	98.4	91.8	96.1	100.0	101.2	101.2	103.8	113.7
Other vehicles	C3GY	96.7	106.9	104.5	100.0	97.8	95.7	90.8	91.7
Buildings	C3GZ	107.8	90.7	95.5	100.0	105.9	113.0	120.3	120.5
Engineering and soil improvement operations	C3H2	107.2	93.6	96.4	100.0	102.1	107.3	112.0	116.6
All means of Agricultural Production	JT72	..	93.6	99.6	100.0	103.6	113.8	139.6	133.1

1 See chapter text.
2 The sum of the percentages of categories included does not add up to 100% due to the exclusion of some minor categories.

Source: Department for Environment, Food and Rural Affairs: 01904 456561

17.8 Index of producer prices of agricultural products[1]
United Kingdom
Annual averages

		2002	2003	2004	2005	2006	2007	2008	2009
Wheat for:									
breadmaking	C3H9	101.4	109.5	117.0	100.0	106.7	176.6	210.3	162.1
other milling	C3HA	92.9	112.3	121.5	100.0	113.6	188.5	206.9	152.8
feeding	C3HB	96.7	108.4	122.9	100.0	114.3	158.2	216.2	159.8
Barley for:									
feeding	C3HC	89.1	106.6	112.7	100.0	111.3	162.7	189.9	133.1
malting	C3HD	96.5	105.8	98.4	100.0	109.5	187.6	205.7	128.9
Oats for:									
milling	C3HE	89.0	87.1	92.7	100.0	111.7	141.6	167.3	125.0
feeding	C3HF	91.2	88.6	98.8	100.0	108.4	129.7	167.8	116.4
Potatoes									
early	C3HH	73.0	107.6	116.8	100.0	111.8	166.7	207.1	106.8
Main crop	C3HI	90.6	91.8	127.3	100.0	134.5	104.2	142.1	124.5
Industrial crops	C3HJ	114.4	108.6	106.8	100.0	106.7	108.2	152.4	132.5
Oilseed rape (non set-aside)	C3HK	121.2	123.7	117.1	100.0	119.8	143.9	232.9	183.2
Sugar beet	C3HL	114.8	94.1	131.0	100.0	130.9	149.1	155.0	83.2
Fresh vegetables	C3HM	112.7	104.1	95.6	100.0	108.2	122.1	117.5	114.0
Cauliflowers	C3HN	117.7	97.3	82.6	100.0	105.1	130.7	107.7	116.6
Lettuce	C3HO	128.6	108.4	93.9	100.0	109.4	107.1	119.1	108.1
Tomatoes	C3HP	107.6	116.4	89.3	100.0	109.9	110.8	117.7	103.8
Carrots	C3HQ	150.4	90.3	83.7	100.0	107.6	123.4	128.2	130.3
Cabbage	C3HR	109.8	95.5	92.0	100.0	103.8	139.6	124.6	124.5
Beans	C3HS	118.0	100.8	109.1	100.0	137.5	153.7	138.9	123.5
Onions	C3HT	126.7	118.7	115.3	100.0	129.3	165.4	131.2	132.5
Mushrooms	C3HU	95.9	119.2	112.5	100.0	95.7	84.5	84.6	84.6
Fresh fruit	C3HV	113.9	111.9	98.4	100.0	104.1	107.4	126.4	124.6
Dessert apples	C3HW	111.3	110.7	104.4	100.0	105.7	121.5	130.9	130.9
Dessert pears	C3HX	124.8	102.7	102.2	100.0	108.6	106.0	134.0	150.4
Cooking apples	C3HY	109.4	135.8	121.3	100.0	111.5	122.9	155.1	128.2
Strawberries	C3HZ	121.7	111.3	87.8	100.0	96.5	101.5	112.9	122.1
Raspberries	C3I2	128.9	101.8	96.6	100.0	111.5	100.5	119.6	120.9
Seeds (excluding cereal seeds)	C3I3	95.7	73.8	80.4	100.0	100.2	118.3	126.4	126.4
Flowers and plants	C3I4	106.8	101.9	99.9	100.0	103.4	110.1	115.1	115.7
Other crop products	C3I5	98.9	81.6	86.2	100.0	100.5	113.3	119.4	119.4
Crop Products	JT6M	..	102.8	107.0	100.0	109.4	133.6	153.7	131.2
Animals and animal products	C3I6	102.7	98.6	101.2	100.0	101.0	108.5	136.0	138.4
Animals for slaughter	C3I7	103.2	98.6	101.2	100.0	103.5	105.5	133.2	144.7
Calves	C3I8	120.2	135.3	137.1	100.0	117.0	132.6	155.0	194.1
Clean cattle	C3I9	103.8	93.1	99.0	100.0	108.3	109.9	141.7	151.1
Clean pigs	C3IA	98.7	99.3	99.6	100.0	101.0	104.1	121.7	140.3
Sows and boars	C3IB	94.0	83.1	99.1	100.0	101.5	80.9	126.4	152.2
Sheep	JT6O	..	108.0	107.1	100.0	102.0	90.6	116.0	143.4
Ewes and rams	C3ID	149.6	127.1	125.1	100.0	106.6	104.2	120.5	182.5
All poultry	C3IE	97.2	98.4	100.7	100.0	98.6	107.1	134.6	134.8
Chickens	C3IF	99.5	98.2	101.3	100.0	98.1	106.0	130.8	132.8
Turkeys	C3IG	89.5	103.7	101.0	100.0	99.4	114.6	157.6	157.8
Cows' milk	C3IH	101.0	97.6	100.0	100.0	97.2	112.2	140.4	127.9
Eggs	C3II	109.5	104.7	109.9	100.0	104.0	118.3	140.4	144.0
Wool (clip)	C3IK	96.4	117.5	116.3	100.0	36.4	77.7	78.9	71.0
Total of all products	JT6P	..	100.3	103.6	100.0	104.5	118.8	143.3	135.4

1 See chapter text.
2 The sum of the percentages of all the categories does not add up to 100%
  due to the exclusion of some minor categories.

Source: Department for Environment, Food and Rural Affairs: 01904 455249

Prices

17.9 Harmonised Indices of Consumer Prices (HICPs) International comparisons: EU countries
percentage change over 12 months

Per cent

		2007	2008	2009	2009 Jan	2009 Feb	2009 Mar	2009 Apr	2009 May	2009 Jun	2009 Jul	2009 Aug	2009 Sep	2009 Oct	2009 Nov	2009 Dec	2010 Jan
European Union countries																	
United Kingdom[1]	D7G7	2.3	3.6	2.2	3.0	3.2	2.9	2.3	2.2	1.8	1.8	1.6	1.1	1.5	1.9	2.9	3.5
Austria	D7SK	2.2	3.2	0.4p	1.2	1.4	0.6	0.5	0.1	−0.3	−0.4	0.2	–	0.1	0.6	1.1	1.2
Belgium	D7SL	1.8	4.5	–	2.1	1.9	0.6	0.7	−0.2	−1.0	−1.7	−0.7	−1.0	−0.9	–	0.3	0.8
Bulgaria	GHY8	7.6	12.0	2.5	6.0	5.4	4.0	3.8	3.0	2.6	1.0	1.3	0.2	0.3	0.9	1.6	1.8
Cyprus	D7RO	2.2	4.4	0.2	0.9	0.6	0.9	0.6	0.5	0.1	−0.8	−0.9	−1.2	−1.0	1.0	1.6	2.5
Czech Republic	D7RP	3.0	6.3	0.6	1.4	1.3	1.7	1.3	0.9	0.8	−0.1	–	−0.3	−0.6	0.2	0.5	0.4
Denmark	D7SM	1.7	3.6	1.1	1.7	1.7	1.6	1.1	1.1	0.9	0.7	0.7	0.5	0.6	0.9	1.2	1.9
Estonia	D7RQ	6.7	10.6	0.2	4.7	3.9	2.5	0.9	0.3	−0.5	−0.4	−0.7	−1.7	−2.1	−2.1	−1.9	−1.0
Finland	D7SN	1.6	3.9	1.6	2.5	2.7	2.0	2.1	1.5	1.6	1.2	1.3	1.1	0.6	1.3	1.8	1.6
France	D7SO	1.6	3.2	0.1	0.8	1.0	0.4	0.1	−0.3	−0.6	−0.8	−0.2	−0.4	−0.2	0.5	1.0	1.2
Germany	D7SP	2.3	2.8	0.2	0.9	1.0	0.4	0.8	–	–	−0.7	−0.1	−0.5	−0.1	0.3	0.8	0.8
Greece	D7SQ	3.0	4.2	1.3	2.0	1.8	1.5	1.1	0.7	0.7	0.7	1.0	0.7	1.2	2.1	2.6	2.3
Hungary	D7RR	7.9	6.0	4.0	2.4	2.9	2.8	3.2	3.8	3.7	4.9	5.0	4.8	4.2	5.2	5.4	6.2
Ireland	D7SS	2.9	3.1	−1.7	1.1	0.1	−0.7	−0.7	−1.7	−2.2	−2.6	−2.4	−3.0	−2.8	−2.8	−2.6	−2.4
Italy	D7ST	2.0	3.5	0.8	1.4	1.5	1.1	1.2	0.8	0.6	−0.1	0.1	0.4	0.3	0.8	1.1	1.3
Latvia	D7RS	10.1	15.3	3.3	9.7	9.4	7.9	5.9	4.4	3.1	2.1	1.5	0.1	−1.2	−1.4	−1.4	−3.3
Lithuania	D7RT	5.8	11.1	4.2	9.5	8.5	7.4	5.9	4.9	3.9	2.6	2.2	2.3	1.0	1.3	1.2	−0.3
Luxembourg	D7SU	2.7	4.1	–	–	0.7	−0.3	−0.3	−0.9	−1.0	−1.5	−0.2	−0.4	−0.2	1.7	2.5	3.0
Malta	D7RU	0.7	4.7	1.8	3.1	3.5	3.9	4.0	3.4	2.8	0.8	1.0	0.8	−0.5	−0.1	−0.4	1.2
Netherlands	D7SV	1.6	2.2	1.0p	1.7	1.9	1.8	1.8	1.5	1.4	−0.1	−0.1	–	0.4	0.7	0.7	0.4
Poland	D7RV	2.6	4.2	4.0	3.2	3.6	4.0	4.3	4.2	4.2	4.5	4.3	4.0	3.8	3.8	3.8	3.9
Portugal	D7SX	2.4	2.7	−0.9	0.1	0.1	−0.6	−0.6	−1.2	−1.6	−1.4	−1.2	−1.8	−1.6	−0.8	−0.1	0.1
Romania	GHY7	4.9	7.9	5.6	6.8	6.9	6.7	6.5	5.9	5.9	5.0	4.9	4.9	4.3	4.6	4.7	5.2
Slovakia	D7RW	1.9	3.9	0.9	2.7	2.4	1.8	1.4	1.1	0.7	0.6	0.5	–	−0.1	–	–	−0.2
Slovenia	D7RX	3.8	5.5	0.9	1.4	2.1	1.6	1.1	0.5	0.2	−0.6	0.1	–	0.2	1.8	2.1	1.8
Spain	D7SY	2.8	4.1	−0.3	0.8	0.7	−0.1	−0.2	−0.9	−1.0	−1.4	−0.8	−1.0	−0.6	0.4	0.9	1.1
Sweden	D7SZ	1.7	3.3	1.9	2.0	2.2	1.9	1.8	1.7	1.6	1.8	1.9	1.4	1.8	2.4	2.8	2.7
EICP[2] EU 27 average[3]	GJ2E	2.4	3.7	1.0	1.8	1.8	1.3	1.3	0.8	0.6	0.2	0.6	0.3	0.5	1.0	1.5	1.7

Note: Further information on HICP is available from the National Statistics Website: www.statistics.gov.uk/hicp.

1 Published as the Consumer Prices Index (CPI) in the UK. (UK 2005=100, others 1996=100)
2 The EICP (European Index of Consumer Prices)is the official EU aggregate. It covers 15 member states until April 2004, 25 member states from May 2004, and 27 members from Jan 2007, the new member states being integrated using a chain index formula. The EU 25 annual average for 2004 is calculated from the EU 15 average from January to April and the EU 25 average from May to December.
3 The coverage of the European Union was extended to include Cyprus, Czech Republic, Estonia, Hungary, Latvia, Lithuania, Malta, Poland, Slovakia and Slovenia from 1 May 2004 and Bulgaria and Romania from 1 Jan 2007.
4 P = Provisional

Sources: Statistical Office of the European Communities (Eurostat); Office for National Statistics: 01633 456900

Government finance

Chapter 18

Government finance

Public sector

(Tables 18.1 to 18.3 and 18.5)

In Table 18.1 the term public sector describes the consolidation of central government, local government and public corporations. General government is the consolidated total of central government and local government. The table shows details of the key public sector finances' indicators, consistent with the European System of Accounts 1995 (ESA95), by sub-sector.

The concepts in Table 18.1 are consistent with the format for public finances in the Economic and Fiscal Strategy Report (EFSR), published by HM Treasury on 11 June 1998, and the Budget. The public sector current budget is equivalent to net saving in national accounts plus capital tax receipts. Net investment is gross capital formation, plus payments less receipts of investment grants, less depreciation. Net borrowing is net investment less current budget. Net borrowing differs from the net cash requirement (see below) in that it is measured on an accruals basis whereas the net cash requirement is mainly a cash measure which includes some financial transactions. Table 18.2 shows the public sector key fiscal balances. The table shows the component detail of the public sector key fiscal balance by economic category. The tables are consistent with the Budget.

Table 18.3 shows public sector net debt. Public sector net debt consists of the public sector's financial liabilities at face value, minus its liquid assets – mainly foreign currency exchange reserves and bank deposits. General government gross debt (consolidated) in Table 18.3 is consistent with the definition of general government gross debt reported to the European Commission under the requirements of the Maastricht Treaty.

More information on the concepts in Table 18.1, 18.2 and 18.3 can be found in a guide to monthly public sector finance statistics, *GSS Methodology Series* No 12, the ONS Statistical Bulletin *Public Sector Finances and Financial Statistics Explanatory Handbook*.

Table 18.6 shows the taxes and National Insurance contributions paid to central government, local government, and to the institutions of the European Union. The table is the same as Table 11.1 of the *National Accounts Blue Book*. More information on the data and concepts in the table can be found in Chapter 11 of the *Blue Book*.

Consolidated Fund and National Loans Fund

(Tables 18.4, 18.5 and 18.7)

The central government embraces all bodies for whose activities a Minister of the Crown, or other responsible person, is accountable to Parliament. It includes, in addition to the ordinary government departments, a number of bodies administering public policy, but without the substantial degree of financial independence which characterises the public corporations. It also includes certain extra-budgetary funds and accounts controlled by departments.

The government's financial transactions are handled through a number of statutory funds or accounts. The most important of these is the Consolidated Fund, which is the government's main account with the Bank of England. Up to 31 March 1968 the Consolidated Fund was virtually synonymous with the term 'Exchequer', which was then the government's central cash account. From 1 April 1968 the National Loans Fund, with a separate account at the Bank of England, was set up by the National Loans Act 1968. The general effect of this Act was to remove from the Consolidated Fund most of the government's domestic lending and the whole of the government's borrowing transactions, and to provide for them to be brought to account in the National Loans Fund.

Revenue from taxation and miscellaneous receipts, including interest and dividends on loans made from votes, continue to be paid into the Consolidated Fund.

After meeting the ordinary expenditure on Supply Services and the Consolidated Fund Standing Services, the surplus or deficit of the Consolidated Fund (Table 18.4), is payable into or met by the National Loans Fund. Table 18.4 also provides a summary of the transactions of the National Loans Fund. The service of the National Debt, previously borne by the Consolidated Fund, is now met from the National Loans Fund which receives:

(a) interest payable on loans to the nationalised industries, local authorities and other bodies, whether the loans were made before or after 1 April 1968, and

(b) the profits of the Issue Department of the Bank of England, mainly derived from interest on government securities, which were formerly paid into the Exchange Equalisation Account. The net cost of servicing the National Debt after applying these interest receipts and similar items is a charge on the Consolidated Fund as part of the standing services. Details of National Loans Fund loans outstanding are shown in Table 18.5. Details of borrowing and repayments of debt, other than loans from the National Loans Fund, are shown in Table 18.7.

Income tax

(Table 18.11, 18. 12)

Following the introduction of Independent Taxation from 1990/91, the Married Couple's Allowance was introduced. It is payable in addition to the Personal Allowance and between 1990/91 and 1992/93 went to the husband unless the transfer condition was met. The condition was that the husband was unable to make full use of the allowance himself and in that case he could transfer part or all of the Married Couple's Allowance to his wife. In 1993/94 all or half of the allowance could be transferred to the wife if the couple had agreed beforehand. The wife has the right to claim half the allowance. The Married Couple's Allowance, and allowances linked to it, were restricted to 20 per cent in 1994/95 and to 15 per cent from 1995/96. From 2000/01 only people born before 6 April 1935 are entitled to Married Couple's Allowance.

The age allowance replaces the single allowance, provided the taxpayer's income is below the limits shown in the table. From 1989/90, for incomes in excess of the limits, the allowance is reduced by £1 for each additional £2 of income until the ordinary limit is reached (before it was £2 for each £3 of additional income). The relief is due where the taxpayer is aged 65 and over in the year of assessment.

The additional Personal Allowance could be claimed by a single parent (or by a married man if his wife was totally incapacitated) who maintained a resident child at his or her own expense. Widow's Bereavement Allowance was due to a widow in the year of her husband's death and in the following year provided the widow had not remarried before the beginning of that year. Both the additional Personal Allowance and the Widow's Bereavement Allowance were abolished from April 2000.

The Blind Person's Allowance may be claimed by blind persons (in England and Wales, registered as blind by a local authority) and surplus Blind Person's Allowance may be transferred to a husband or wife. Relief on life assurance premiums is given by deduction from the premium payable. From 1984/85 it is confined to policies taken out before 14 March 1984.

From 1993/94 until 1998/99 a number of taxpayers with taxable income in excess of the lower rate limit only paid tax at the lower rate. This was because it was only their dividend income and (from 1996/97) their savings income which took their taxable income above the lower rate limit but below the basic rate limit, and such income was chargeable to tax at the lower rate and not the basic rate.

In 1999/2000 the 10 per cent starting rate replaced the lower rate and taxpayers with savings or dividend income at the basic rate of tax are taxed at 20 per cent and 10 per cent respectively. Before 1999/2000 these people would have been classified as lower rate taxpayers. The 10 per cent starting rate was abolished in 2009/10.

Rateable values

(Table 18.14)

Major changes to local government finance in England and Wales took effect from 1 April 1990. These included the abolition of domestic rating (replaced by the Community Charge, then replaced in 1993 by the Council Tax), the revaluation of all non-domestic properties, and the introduction of the Uniform Business Rate. Also in 1990, a new classification scheme was introduced which has resulted in differences in coverage. Further differences are caused by legislative changes which have changed the treatment of certain types of property. There was little change in the total rateable value of non-domestic properties when all these properties were revalued in April 1995. Rateable values for offices fell and there was a rise for all other property types shown in the table.

With effect from 1 April 2000, all non-domestic properties were revalued. Overall there was an increase in rateable values of over 25 per cent compared to the last year of the 1995 list. The largest proportionate increase was for offices and cinemas, with all property types given in the table showing rises.

The latest revaluation affecting all non-domestic properties took effect from 1 April 2005. In this revaluation the overall increase in rateable values between 1 April of the first year of the new list and the same day on the last year of the 2000 list was 17 per cent. The largest proportionate increase was for theatres and music halls with again all property types in the table showing rises.

Local authority capital expenditure and receipts

(Table 18.17)

Authorities finance capital spending in a number of ways, including use of their own revenue funds, borrowing or grants, and contributions from elsewhere. Until 31 March 2004, the capital finance system laid down in Part 4 of the Local Government and Housing Act 1989 (the '1989 Act') provided the framework within which authorities were permitted to finance capital spending from sources other than revenue – that is by the use of borrowing, long-term credit or capital receipts.

Government finance

Until 31 March 2004, capital spending could be financed by:

- revenue resources – either the General Fund Revenue Account, the Housing Revenue Account (HRA) or the Major Repairs Reserve – but an authority could not charge council tenants for spending on general services, or spending on council houses to local taxpayers

- borrowing or long-term credit as authorised by the credit approvals issued by central government. Credit approvals were normally accompanied by an element of Revenue Support Grant (RSG) covering most of the costs of borrowing

- grants received from central government

- contributions or grants from elsewhere – including the National Lottery; NDPBs such as Sport England, English Heritage and Natural England; private sector partners; capital receipts (that is, proceeds from the sale of land, buildings or other fixed assets); and sums set aside as Provision for Credit Liabilities (PCL). This required the use of a credit approval, unless the authority was debt-free

From 1 April 2004, capital spending can be financed in the same ways, except that central government no longer issues credit approvals to allow authorities to finance capital spending by borrowing. However, it continues to provide financial support in the usual way, via RSG or HRA subsidy, towards some capital spending financed by borrowing that is Supported Capital Expenditure (Revenue). Authorities are now free to finance capital spending by self-financed borrowing within limits of affordability set, having regard to the 2003 Act and the CIPFA Prudential Code. The concept of PCL has not been carried forward into the new system, although authorities which were debt-free and had a negative credit ceiling at the end of the old system could still spend amounts of PCL built up under the old rules.

In 2008/09 capital receipts fell to £1.4 billion, a year-on-year decrease of 66 per cent. This fall reflects the effect of the economic climate over that period on local authority sales of assets.

In 2008/09 capital expenditure of almost £4.2 billion (about 21 per cent) was financed by self-financed borrowing, an increase of 33 per cent from the amount financed in 2007/08.

In 2008/09, government grants accounted for 28 per cent of the total financing. Financing by government grant in 2007/08 was affected by the grant of £1.7 billion paid by the Department for Transport to the Greater London Authority (GLA) in respect of Metronet liabilities; this caused government grants to account for 34 per cent of the total financing for 2007/08.

Local authority financing for capital expenditure

(Table 18.18)

Capital spending by local authorities is mainly for buying, constructing or improving physical assets such as:

- buildings – schools, houses, libraries and museums, police and fire stations

- land – for development, roads, playing fields

- vehicles, plant and machinery – including street lighting and road signs

It also includes grants and advances made to the private sector or the rest of the public sector for capital purposes, such as advances to Registered Social Landlords. Local authority capital expenditure more than doubled between 2001/02 and 2007/08.

The underlying trend in capital expenditure (excluding an exceptional event in 2007/08) shows an increase of 9 per cent from 2007/08 to 2008/09. The exceptional event was the payment by the Greater London Authority (Transport for London) of £1.7 billion to Metronet in 2007/08.

New construction, conversion and renovation forms the major part of capital spending. The largest increases in capital expenditure in 2008/09 were in police (44 per cent), and education (22 per cent). Capital expenditure on transport increased by 14 per cent, allowing for the Greater London Authority's grant payment via TfL in respect of Metronet in 2007/08. Between 2004/05 and 2008/09 capital expenditure on transport has risen from 20 per cent to 24 per cent of the total, while capital expenditure on housing has fallen from 28 per cent to 25 per cent of the total.

18.1 Sector analysis of key fiscal balances[1]
United Kingdom
Not seasonally adjusted

£ million[2]

		1999/00	2000/01	2001/02	2002/03	2003/04	2004/05	2005/06	2006/07	2007/08	2008/09	2009/10
Surplus on current budget[3]												
Central Government	ANLV	24 401	26 756	13 812	−8 121	−17 559	−17 757	−13 495	−5 795	−5 824	−47 675	..
Local government	NMMX	−4 507	−3 790	−3 909	−4 960	−3 245	−3 135	−5 094	−3 016	−2 849	−4 363	..
General Government	ANLW	20 878	21 996	10 861	−11 103	−19 005	..	−18 657	−8 292	−12 103	−53 658	..
Public corporations	IL6M	983	808	1 311	541	1 694	2 003	4 573	3 685	3 640	2 494	..
Public sector	ANMU	20 995	23 432	12 144	−11 323	−17 418	−19 249	−13 943	−4 919	−4 846	−49 638	..
Net investment[4]												
Central government	-ANNS	9 493	8 947	14 234	18 231	19 570	20 798	20 000	26 834	32 882	44 106	..
Local government	-ANNT	−832	−1 882	−1 824	−3 595	−682	1 756	419	−121	−3 779	1 250	..
General Government	-ANNV	6 461	6 574	10 951	12 487	16 371	..	19 721	25 955	29 980	46 916	..
Public corporations	-JSH6	−2 737	−2 180	−1 435	−1 761	−2 493	−653	3 163	−645	−1 035	−7 459	..
Public sector	-ANNW	5 501	5 125	11 901	13 805	15 623	20 574	23 466	25 917	29 176	36 664	..
Net borrowing[5]												
Central government	-NMFJ	−14 908	−17 809	422	26 352	37 129	38 555	33 495	32 629	38 706	91 781	..
Local government	-NMOE	3 134	2 490	2 081	1 078	99	3 924	5 324	2 537	−9	4 474	..
General Government	-NNBK	−11 797	−17 269	3 178	26 863	38 417	43 045	38 216	34 933	38 122	96 385	..
Public corporations	-IL6E	−3 720	−2 988	−2 746	−2 302	−4 187	−2 656	−1 410	−4 330	−4 675	−9 953	..
Public sector	-ANNX	−15 494	−18 307	−243	25 128	33 041	39 823	37 409	30 836	34 022	86 302	..
Net cash requirement												
Central government[6]	RUUX	−10 664	−37 251	3 366	24 214	42 717	37 454	35 908	36 891	29 621	162 513	..
Local government	ABEG	979	−611	−423	−2 715	−2 712	1 270	4 153	58	−723	4 401	..
General Government	RUUS	−9 685	−37 862	2 943	21 499	40 005	38 724	40 061	36 949	28 898	166 914	..
Public corporations	IL6F	1 622	1 324	1 135	3 063	−1 557	−303	335	−1 839	−7 377	−107 358	..
Public sector	RURQ	−8 063	−36 538	4 078	24 562	38 448	38 421	40 396	35 110	21 521	59 556	..
Public sector debt												
Public sector net debt	BKQK	344 352	311 143	314 257	346 034	381 502	422 065	461 671	497 806	621 588	742 317	889 988
Public sector net debt (£ billion)	RUTN	344.4	311.1	314.3	346.0	381.5	422.1	461.7	497.8	621.6	742.8	..
Public sector net debt as a percentage of GDP	RUTO	35.6	30.7	29.7	30.8	32.1	34.0	35.3	36.0	43.0	52.9	62.0
Excluding financial interventions												
Net debt	HF6W	344.4	311.1	314.3	346.0	381.5	422.1	461.7	497.8	527.2	617.1	..
Net debt as a % GDP	HF6X	35.6	30.7	29.7	30.8	32.1	34.0	35.3	36.0	36.5	43.8	..

1 National accounts entities as defined under the European System of Accounts 1995 (ESA95) consistent with the latest national accounts. See chapter text.
2 Unless otherwise stated.
3 Net saving *plus* capital taxes.
4 Gross capital formation *plus* payments *less* receipts of investment grants *less* depreciation.

5 Net investment *less* surplus on current budget. A version of General government net borrowing is reported to the European Commision under the requirements of the Maastricht Treaty.
6 Central government net cash requirement (own account).

Source: Office for National Statistics: 020 7014 2124

18.2 Public sector transactions and fiscal balances[1]
United Kingdom

£ million

		1998 /99	1999 /00	2000 /01	2001 /02	2002 /03	2003 /04	2004 /05	2005 /06	2006 /07	2007 /08	2008 /09
Current receipts												
Taxes on income and wealth	ANSO	123 875	133 720	144 157	145 122	143 228	145 475	160 400	179 716	194 206	207 937	199 738
Taxes on production	NMYE	115 227	125 099	129 273	133 043	139 827	148 832	155 131	159 450	170 126	176 034	167 736
Other current taxes[2]	MJBC	17 688	18 916	19 696	21 569	23 194	25 794	27 422	28 808	30 315	31 931	33 092
Taxes on capital	NMGI	1 804	2 054	2 236	2 383	2 370	2 521	2 941	3 276	3 618	3 890	23 783
Social contributions	ANBO	54 746	56 935	62 068	63 162	63 529	75 148	80 923	85 559	90 818	95 234	96 951
Gross operating surplus	ANBP	16 822	16 949	16 669	16 907	17 106	18 393	18 611	21 574	22 647	22 912	22 649
Interest and dividends from private sector and Rest of World	ANBQ	5 283	4 368	6 226	4 898	4 606	4 662	6 079	6 729	6 230	8 242	6 623
Rent and other current transfers[3]	ANBS	891	1 037	2 036	2 427	2 470	2 036	1 964	1 969	1 864	1 762	1 761
Total current receipts	ANBT	336 336	359 078	382 361	389 511	396 330	422 861	453 471	487 081	519 824	547 968	530 971
Current expenditure												
Current expenditure on goods and services[4]	GZSN	159 443	172 299	185 875	198 935	217 512	236 606	255 961	273 737	287 767	300 117	315 724
Subsidies	NMRL	4 164	4 215	4 412	4 504	6 043	6 787	7 461	8 140	8 843	9 565	8 589
Social benefits	ANLY	106 585	105 555	108 010	118 269	122 636	130 799	136 848	142 370	147 429	157 821	171 833
Net current grants abroad[5]	GZSI	−1 018	−461	−380	−2 075	−824	−1 352	−637	−64	108	−72	−1 322
Other current grants	NNAI	15 199	19 106	21 676	23 932	27 555	30 369	32 502	34 079	34 886	37 110	37 089
Interest and dividends paid to private sector and Rest of World	ANLO	29 289	25 297	26 400	22 495	21 453	22 822	24 955	26 816	28 800	31 389	31 570
Total current expenditure	ANLT	313 662	326 011	345 993	366 060	394 375	426 010	457 029	485 014	507 765	535 803	563 711
Saving, gross plus capital taxes	ANSP	22 674	33 067	36 368	23 451	1 955	−3 149	−3 558	2 067	12 059	12 165	−32 740
Depreciation	-ANNZ	−12 436	−12 764	−13 107	−13 572	−14 459	−14 942	−15 608	−16 437	−17 277	−18 009	−18 932
Surplus on current budget	ANMU	10 423	20 995	23 432	12 144	−11 323	−17 418	−19 249	−13 943	−4 919	−4 846	−49 638
Net investment												
Gross fixed capital formation[6]	ANSQ	14 061	14 150	13 283	17 308	20 125	21 079	25 644	27 857	28 971	32 726	41 438
Less depreciation	-ANNZ	−12 436	−12 764	−13 107	−13 572	−14 459	−14 942	−15 608	−16 437	−17 277	−18 009	−18 932
Increase in inventories and valuables	ANSR	231	−472	−126	−10	−74	2 011	−234	−118	−141	−153	−18
Capital grants to private sector and Rest of World	ANSS	4 942	4 371	3 875	7 958	7 564	10 142	11 046	12 451	15 335	14 776	41 300
Capital grants from private sector and Rest of World	-ANST	−367	−427	−756	−989	−1 091	−1 352	−972	−1 202	−1 413	−1 089	−26 900
Total net investment	-ANNW	5 955	5 501	5 125	11 901	13 805	15 623	20 574	23 466	25 917	29 176	36 664
Net borrowing[7]	-ANNX	−4 468	−15 494	−18 307	−243	25 128	33 041	39 823	37 409	30 836	34 022	86 302
Financial transactions determining net cash requirement												
Net lending to private sector and Rest of World	ANSU	171	2 212	3 174	2 674	2 736	2 641	925	874	435	4 214	5 452
Net acquisition of UK company securities	ANSV	704	−310	949	−394	765	355	521	655	−2 270	−2 104	−3 770
Accounts receivable/payable	ANSW	803	8 393	−17 163	2 210	−2 779	9 031	2 453	2 370	9 105	−8 988	33 784
Adjustment for interest on gilts	ANSX	−2 446	−1 294	−2 630	−361	−1 444	−1 187	−2 304	−2 749	−1 279	−4 619	−4 608
Other financial transcations[8]	ANSY	−909	−1 570	−2 561	192	156	−5 433	−2 997	1 837	−1 717	−1 004	−57 604
Public sector net cash requirement	RURQ	−6 145	−8 063	−36 538	4 078	24 562	38 448	38 421	40 396	35 110	21 521	59 556

1 See chapter text.
2 Includes domestic rates, council tax, community charge, motor vehicle duty paid by household and some licence fees.
3 ESA95 transactions D44, D45, D74, D75 and D72-D71: includes rent of land, oil royalties, other property income and fines.
4 Includes non-trading capital consumption.

5 Net of current grants received from abroad.
6 Including net acquisition of land.
7 Net investment *less* surplus on current budget.
8 Includes statistical discrepancy, finance leasing and similar borrowing, insurance technical reserves and some other minor adjustments.

Source: Office for National Statistics: 020 7014 2124

18.3 Public sector net debt[1]
United Kingdom

£ million

		2001 /02	2002 /03	2003 /04	2004 /05	2005 /06	2006 /07	2007 /08	2008 /09	2009 /10
Central government sterling gross debt:										
British government stock										
Conventional gilts	BKPK	200 833	206 119	232 877	261 373	287 481	306 489	320 622	426 107	608 511
Index linked gilts	BKPL	70 417	75 966	78 982	86 749	98 654	113 090	132 404	154 038	178 170
Total	BKPM	271 250	282 085	311 859	348 122	386 135	419 579	453 026	580 145	786 681
Sterling Treasury bills	BKPJ	9 700	15 000	19 300	20 350	19 100	15 600	17 569	43 748	62 866
National savings	ACUA	62 275	63 087	66 522	68 504	73 365	78 885	84 768	97 202	98 719
Tax instruments	ACRV	478	376	407	350	308	353	428	1 121	819
Other sterling debt[2]	BKSK	28 276	32 711	35 032	32 279	36 481	41 261	39 373	57 702	40 037
Central government sterling gross debt total	BKSL	371 979	393 259	433 120	469 605	515 389	555 678	595 164	779 918	989 122
Central government foreign currency gross debt:										
US$ bonds	BKPG	2 107	–	1 632	1 587	1 730	1 530	1 509	–	–
ECU bonds	EYSJ	–	–	–	–	–	–	–	–	–
ECU/Euro Treasury notes	EYSV	1 225	–	–	–	–	–	–	–	–
Other foreign currency debt	BKPH	243	172	105	57	1	–	–	–	–
Central government foreign currency gross debt total	BKPI	3 575	172	1 738	1 644	1 731	1 530	1 509	–	–
Central government gross debt total	BKPW	375 554	393 431	434 858	471 249	517 120	557 208	596 673	779 918	989 122
Local government gross debt total	EYKP	52 566	51 353	50 547	53 300	60 114	62 425	66 371	67 301	68 151
less										
Central government holdings of local government debt	-EYKZ	–47 530	–44 836	–41 540	–42 339	–46 664	–47 956	–50 364	–50 508	–50 882
Local government holdings of central government debt	-EYLA	–29	–184	–510	–62	–62	–	–81	–2 960	–2 706
General government gross debt (consolidated)	BKPX	380 561	399 764	443 355	482 148	530 508	571 677	612 599	793 751	1 003 685
Public corporations gross debt	EYYD	8 859	18 660	13 895	14 875	14 687	14 430	13 753	13 560	10 579
less:										
Central government holdings of public corporations debt	-EYXY	–4 308	–4 171	–5 188	–5 740	–5 631	–4 984	–5 092	–4 879	–5 617
Local government holdings of public corporations debt	-EYXZ	–122	–121	–120	–121	–112	–103	–104	–107	–176
Public corporations holdings of central government debt	-BKPZ	–4 638	–4 928	–4 780	–5 080	–2 822	–2 255	–4 119	–3 947	–3 292
Public corporations holdings of local government debt	-EYXV	–60	–50	–84	–138	–79	–198	–39	–33	–52
Public sector gross debt (consolidated)	BKQA	380 292	409 154	447 078	485 944	536 551	578 567	616 998	798 345	1 005 127
Public sector liquid assets:										
Official reserves	AIPD	28 055	26 387	25 266	25 813	27 835	26 631	29 561	31 527	..
Central government deposits[3]	BKSM	2 802	2 900	3 879	3 868	5 212	6 171	5 439	5 242	4 318
Other central government	BKSN	10 743	8 141	7 077	3 044	8 498	11 369	14 834	37 352	45 822
Local government deposits[3]	BKSO	13 698	14 797	16 797	18 718	20 993	23 740	28 327	21 781	18 277
Other local government short term assets	BKQG	5 990	6 061	5 573	5 057	5 381	4 709	4 946	4 142	4 244
Public corporations deposits[3]	BKSP	2 336	2 133	2 813	3 411	2 375	3 746	2 366	1 781	2 122
Other public corporations short term assets	BKSQ	1 180	1 586	2 845	2 457	2 453	2 378	2 254	2 166	2 284
Public sector liquid assets total	BKQJ	64 804	62 005	64 250	62 368	72 747	78 744	87 727	103 991	121 719
Public sector net debt	BKQK	314 257	346 034	381 502	422 065	461 671	497 806	621 588	742 317	889 988
as percentage of GDP[4]	RUTO	*29.7*	*30.8*	*32.1*	*34.0*	*35.3*	*36.0*	*43.0*	*52.9*	*62.0*

1 See chapter text.
2 Including overdraft with Bank of England.
3 Bank and building society deposits.
4 Gross domestic product at market prices from 12 months centred on the
 end of the month.

Source: Office for National Statistics: 020 7014 2124

18.4 Central government surplus on current budget and net borrowing
United Kingdom

£ million

	Current receipts									
	Taxes on production	of which	Taxes on income and wealth				Compulsory social contributions	Interest and dividends	Other receipts[3]	Total
	Total	VAT	Total	Income and capital gains tax[1]	Other[2]	Other taxes				
	NMBY	NZGF	NMCU	LIBR	LIBP	LIQR	AIIH	LIQP	LIQQ	ANBV
2004	154 582	79 755	154 127	120 725	33 402	10 862	79 224	7 739	7 247	413 781
2005	157 869	81 426	172 498	131 689	40 809	11 481	84 459	7 662	7 517	441 486
2006	166 719	85 591	192 600	141 714	50 886	12 262	89 550	7 941	7 527	476 599
2007	175 325	89 698	200 039	153 477	46 562	13 213	93 210	9 370	7 702	498 859
2008	173 135	89 732	207 539	156 997	50 542	12 892	98 580	10 162	7 916	510 224
2009	161 166	77 908	182 907	145 167	37 740	12 197	95 565	7 225	8 192	467 252
2003/04	148 753	76 633	145 487	115 233	30 254	10 309	75 148	7 795	7 166	394 658
2004/05	154 962	79 979	160 490	124 477	36 013	10 950	80 923	7 495	7 302	422 122
2005/06	159 281	81 505	179 960	134 918	45 042	11 760	85 559	7 768	7 529	451 857
2006/07	169 874	87 739	194 198	146 478	47 720	12 520	90 916	7 996	7 543	483 047
2007/08	175 806	89 891	208 122	158 781	49 341	13 264	95 437	9 986	7 714	510 329
2008/09	167 483	85 350	200 815	153 744	47 071	12 651	96 961	9 639	8 035	495 584
2003 Q2	36 502	18 852	29 393	23 166	6 227	2 464	17 670	1 657	1 784	89 470
Q3	36 547	18 479	36 155	28 114	8 041	2 613	18 245	1 851	1 781	97 192
Q4	38 806	20 000	32 347	23 702	8 645	2 597	18 403	1 940	1 788	95 881
2004 Q1	36 898	19 302	47 592	40 251	7 341	2 635	20 830	2 347	1 813	112 115
Q2	38 433	19 732	31 440	23 846	7 594	2 657	18 829	1 640	1 802	94 801
Q3	38 806	19 859	39 043	30 295	8 748	2 834	19 275	1 852	1 810	103 620
Q4	40 445	20 862	36 052	26 333	9 719	2 736	20 290	1 900	1 822	103 245
2005 Q1	37 278	19 526	53 955	44 003	9 952	2 723	22 529	2 103	1 868	120 456
Q2	39 227	20 146	35 024	26 726	8 298	2 865	20 289	1 713	1 899	101 017
Q3	40 454	20 736	43 615	32 760	10 855	3 175	20 546	1 963	1 854	111 607
Q4	40 910	21 018	39 904	28 200	11 704	2 718	21 095	1 883	1 896	108 406
2006 Q1	38 690	19 605	61 417	47 232	14 185	3 002	23 629	2 209	1 880	130 827
Q2	41 563	21 299	37 343	28 779	8 564	3 116	21 613	1 831	1 887	107 353
Q3	42 710	22 155	49 653	35 611	14 042	3 073	21 624	1 773	1 862	120 695
Q4	43 756	22 532	44 187	30 092	14 095	3 071	22 684	2 128	1 898	117 724
2007 Q1	41 845	21 753	63 015	51 996	11 019	3 260	24 995	2 264	1 896	137 275
Q2	43 911	22 369	39 276	30 688	8 588	3 311	22 354	2 129	1 959	112 940
Q3	44 757	22 848	51 160	37 952	13 208	3 438	22 560	2 164	1 914	125 993
Q4	44 812	22 728	46 588	32 841	13 747	3 204	23 301	2 813	1 933	122 651
2008 Q1	42 326	21 946	71 098	57 300	13 798	3 311	27 222	2 880	1 908	148 745
Q2	45 525	24 235	39 467	30 346	9 121	3 299	23 871	2 365	1 959	116 486
Q3	43 251	22 533	53 087	38 696	14 391	3 278	23 684	2 580	2 041	127 921
Q4	42 033	21 018	43 887	30 655	13 232	3 004	23 803	2 337	2 008	117 072
2009 Q1	36 674	17 564	64 374	54 047	10 327	3 070	25 603	2 357	2 027	134 105
Q2	40 078	18 960	35 313	28 268	7 045	3 027	23 408	1 944	2 033	105 803
Q3	41 565	19 957	42 834	34 428	8 406	3 206	22 762	1 496	2 002	113 865
Q4	42 849	21 427	40 386	28 424	11 962	2 894	23 792	1 428	2 130	113 479
2008 Aug	14 059	7 208	13 087	11 961	1 126	1 032	7 756	764	682	37 380
Sep	14 429	7 632	13 632	10 510	3 122	1 078	8 010	1 044	679	38 872
Oct	14 480	7 334	20 204	10 289	9 915	1 151	7 840	848	669	45 192
Nov	14 442	7 254	10 333	9 512	821	949	7 673	740	670	34 807
Dec	13 111	6 430	13 350	10 854	2 496	904	8 290	749	669	37 073
2009 Jan	12 191	5 952	32 083	24 062	8 021	972	8 132	615	677	54 670
Feb	11 685	5 296	18 920	17 561	1 359	931	8 269	591	676	41 072
Mar	12 798	6 316	13 371	12 424	947	1 167	9 202	1 151	674	38 363
Apr	13 190	6 085	14 880	10 014	4 866	1 058	7 723	826	677	38 354
May	12 986	6 090	9 169	8 301	868	955	7 637	540	678	31 965
Jun	13 902	6 785	11 264	9 953	1 311	1 014	8 048	578	678	35 484
Jul	14 094	6 912	20 590	14 232	6 358	1 053	7 576	453	667	44 433
Aug	13 560	6 429	11 457	10 727	730	991	7 587	372	667	34 634
Sep	13 911	6 616	10 787	9 469	1 318	1 162	7 599	671	668	34 798
Oct	14 773	7 443	16 779	9 411	7 368	1 017	7 766	549	710	41 594
Nov	14 161	7 110	10 783	9 263	1 520	925	7 818	482	709	34 878
Dec	13 915	6 874	12 824	9 750	3 074	952	8 208	397	711	37 007
2010 Jan	13 560	7 650	26 898	19 447	7 451	936	8 014	341	702	50 451
Feb	..	6 879	..	..	..	..	..	..	..	..

18.4 Central government surplus on current budget and net borrowing
continued   United Kingdom

| | Current expenditure | | | | Saving, gross plus capital taxes | Depreciation | Surplus on current budget | Net investment | Net borrowing |
	Interest	Net Social Benefits	Other	Total					
	NMFX	GZSJ	LIQS	ANLP	ANPM	NSRN	ANLV	-ANNS	-NMFJ
2004	22 955	122 033	281 640	426 628	−12 847	5 495	−18 342	18 955	37 297
2005	25 640	126 132	301 017	452 789	−11 303	5 711	−17 014	20 409	37 423
2006	26 666	130 115	323 791	480 572	−3 973	5 860	−9 833	25 292	35 125
2007	30 287	139 097	332 671	502 055	−3 196	6 071	−9 267	27 801	37 068
2008	32 247	148 805	349 958	531 010	−20 786	6 399	−27 205	39 469	66 674
2009	25 863	164 482	368 123	558 468	−91 216	6 637	−100 462	55 765	156 227
2003/04	22 281	116 926	267 496	406 703	−12 045	5 514	−17 559	19 570	37 129
2004/05	23 936	122 624	287 806	434 366	−12 244	5 513	−17 757	20 798	38 555
2005/06	25 808	127 304	306 506	459 618	−7 761	5 734	−13 495	20 000	33 495
2006/07	27 580	131 346	324 035	482 961	86	5 881	−5 795	26 834	32 629
2007/08	29 957	140 725	339 346	510 028	301	6 125	−5 824	32 882	38 706
2008/09	30 507	153 588	352 699	536 794	−41 210	6 530	−47 675	44 106	91 781
2003 Q2	5 681	27 835	67 149	100 665	−11 195	1 374	−12 569	4 108	16 677
Q3	5 268	28 921	64 769	98 958	−1 766	1 363	−3 129	4 491	7 620
Q4	6 028	31 080	66 676	103 784	−7 903	1 375	−9 278	4 166	13 444
2004 Q1	5 304	29 090	68 902	103 296	8 819	1 402	7 417	6 805	−612
Q2	5 515	29 988	70 342	105 845	−11 044	1 360	−12 404	4 121	16 525
Q3	5 644	30 431	70 667	106 742	−3 122	1 355	−4 477	4 002	8 479
Q4	6 492	32 524	71 729	110 745	−7 500	1 378	−8 878	4 027	12 905
2005 Q1	6 285	29 681	75 068	111 034	9 422	1 420	8 002	8 648	646
Q2	6 259	30 201	75 127	111 587	−10 570	1 436	−12 006	−163	11 843
Q3	6 206	31 101	75 274	112 581	−974	1 407	−2 381	4 925	7 306
Q4	6 890	35 149	75 548	117 587	−9 181	1 448	−10 629	6 999	17 628
2006 Q1	6 453	30 853	80 557	117 863	12 964	1 443	11 521	8 239	−3 282
Q2	6 334	31 795	82 844	120 973	−13 620	1 454	−15 074	6 054	21 128
Q3	6 433	32 899	80 410	119 742	953	1 458	−505	5 208	5 713
Q4	7 446	34 568	79 980	121 994	−4 270	1 505	−5 775	5 791	11 566
2007 Q1	7 367	32 084	80 801	120 252	17 023	1 464	15 559	9 781	−5 778
Q2	7 412	34 238	84 821	126 471	−13 531	1 525	−15 056	4 313	19 369
Q3	7 016	35 249	83 717	125 982	11	1 530	−1 519	6 266	7 785
Q4	8 492	37 526	83 332	129 350	−6 699	1 552	−8 251	7 441	15 692
2008 Q1	7 037	33 712	87 476	128 225	20 520	1 518	19 002	14 862	−4 140
Q2	8 542	36 908	89 760	135 210	−18 724	1 607	−20 344	5 820	26 164
Q3	7 989	37 838	85 494	131 321	−3 400	1 630	−5 044	9 305	14 349
Q4	8 679	40 347	87 228	136 254	−19 182	1 644	−20 819	9 482	30 301
2009 Q1	5 297	38 495	90 217	134 009	96	1 649	−1 468	19 499	20 967
Q2	7 025	40 566	95 526	143 117	−37 314	1 669	−39 182	12 097	51 279
Q3	4 438	41 509	91 613	137 560	−23 695	1 618	−25 450	9 218	34 668
Q4	9 103	43 912	90 767	143 782	−30 303	1 701	−34 362	14 951	49 313
2008 Jul	3 283	12 689	27 507	43 479	8 190	543	7 641	1 899	−5 742
Aug	3 385	12 617	28 314	44 316	−6 936	543	−7 488	1 553	9 041
Sep	1 321	12 532	29 673	43 526	−4 654	544	−5 197	5 853	11 050
Oct	3 511	12 558	28 095	44 164	1 028	548	476	2 008	1 532
Nov	3 273	14 742	29 207	47 222	−12 415	548	−12 982	1 975	14 957
Dec	1 895	13 047	29 926	44 868	−7 795	548	−8 313	5 499	13 812
2009 Jan	2 759	13 574	28 782	45 115	9 555	550	9 037	6 276	−2 761
Feb	2 394	12 104	27 989	42 487	−1 415	550	−1 937	5 203	7 140
Mar	144	12 817	33 446	46 407	−8 044	549	−8 568	8 020	16 588
Apr	3 085	13 388	33 259	49 732	−11 378	556	−12 391	1 585	13 976
May	3 324	13 599	30 837	47 760	−15 795	556	−16 086	3 449	19 535
Jun	616	13 579	31 430	45 625	−10 141	557	−10 705	7 063	17 768
Jul	2 723	14 310	30 072	47 105	−2 672	539	−3 342	2 572	5 914
Aug	1 526	13 476	30 023	45 025	−10 391	539	−11 158	2 565	13 723
Sep	189	13 723	31 518	45 430	−10 632	540	−10 950	4 081	15 031
Oct	3 858	13 796	30 072	47 726	−6 132	567	−6 627	2 778	9 405
Nov	3 506	15 996	29 769	49 271	−14 393	567	−15 892	3 044	18 936
Dec	1 739	14 120	30 926	46 785	−9 778	567	−11 843	9 129	20 972
2010 Jan	4 267	13 994	31 231	49 492	959	560	..	..	..

1 Includes capital gains tax paid by households. Includes income tax and capital gains tax paid by corporations.

2 Mainly comprises corporation tax and petroleum revenue tax.
3 Includes receipts from the spectrum.

Source: Office for National Statistics; HM Treasury

18.5 National Loans Fund: assets and liabilities[1]
United Kingdom
At 31 March each year

£ million

		2001	2002	2003	2004	2005	2006	2007	2008	2009
NATIONAL LOANS FUND[2]										
Total assets	KQKD	425 955.6	434 544.6	448 006.3	108 243.1	94 226.5	83 227.6	82 872.1	89 765.2	394 715.0
Total National Loans Fund loans outstanding[3]	KQKE	51 037.6	50 251.4	47 719.0	2 963.1	2 910.2	2 964.2	3 022.1	2 970.5	2 853.4
Loans to Public Corporations:										
Royal Mail Group plc	KQKF	500.0	500.0	550.0	500.0	500.0	500.0	500.0	500.0	500.0
Civil Aviation Authority	KQKQ	92.5	9.8	8.8	8.2	7.6	11.0	10.1	9.1	8.0
British Railways Board	KQKS	481.3	..	..	..	..	..	..	..	..
British Waterways Board	KQKU	16.7	16.3	14.7	14.7	14.7	10.6	9.9	7.9	6.8
New Towns - Development										
Royal Mint	KQLP	5.0	14.8	11.3	15.7	18.1	22.5	14.9	8.1	7.4
Harbour Authorities	KQLV	0.1	0.1	0.1	0.1	0.1	0.1	0.1	0.1	0.1
Ordnance Survey	GPVF	13.9	12.3	11.0	9.9	8.9	8.0	7.3	6.7	6.2
Registers of Scotland	KZBB	4.0	3.7	3.6	3.5	3.3	3.2	3.1	3.0	3.0
East of Scotland Water Authority	KZBC	268.0	258.0	248.0	238.0	223.0	213.0	203.0	203.0	201.0
North of Scotland Water Authority	KZBD	236.5	236.5	231.5	231.5	226.5	226.5	226.5	226.5	226.5
West of Scotland Water Authority	KZBE	412.4	412.4	412.4	402.4	402.4	402.4	377.4	357.4	352.4
Loans to local authorities	KQLY	47 239.1	47 093.4	44 640.3	41 468.3	42 102.9	47 123.7	48 111.0	50 753.0	–
Loans to private sector:										
Housing associations	KGVS	0.5	..	..	..	..	..	..	..	..
Loans within central government:										
New Towns - Development										
Corporations and Commission	KQLD	8.0	8.0	7.9	7.9	7.9	7.9	7.9	7.9	7.9
Scottish Homes	KQLF	161.6	149.7	138.1	100.6	–	..	..	..	..
Housing Corporation (England)	KQLH	3.0	2.0	2.0	1.2	1.4	1.4	1.4	1.4	–
Welsh Development Agency	KQLN	0.3	0.2	0.1	..	..	..	..	..	..
Development Board for Rural Wales	KQLO	4.0	4.0	4.0	4.0	4.0	4.0	3.9	3.9	3.9
Northern Ireland Exchequer	KGVW	1 533.1	1 473.9	1 380.4	1 372.0	1 440.5	1 503.5	1 608.3	1 589.1	1 485.8
Married quarters for Armed Forces	KGVX	57.7	56.4	54.9	53.4	51.8	50.1	48.3	46.4	44.4
Other assets:										
Exchange Equalisation Account - Advances o/s	KGVZ	5 680.0	831.0	30.0	670.0	910.0	2 005.0	1 805.0	1 330.0	760.0
Subscriptions and contributions to international financial organisations:										
International Monetary Fund	KGXE	9 496.6	9 494.5	9 293.8	8 696.8	8 615.9	8 813.5	8 271.3	8 880.8	11 195.9
Borrowing included in public sector net debt but not brought to account by 31 March	KGXF	405.9	417.5	467.1	..	..	..	..	..	..
Other NLF Assets	GLX9	..	..	..	18 545.9	18 792.0	20 735.2	20 859.0	25 180.0	36 261.4
Debt Management Account -advances outstanding	GPVG	35 000.0	35 000.0	28 000.0	35 000.0	20 000.0	–	..	–	292 000.0
Consolidated Fund liability	KCYI	324 335.5	338 550.2	362 496.5	395 161.4	436 345.0	483 836.2	519 312.1	571 228.4	730 371.4
Total liabilities										
National Loans Fund - Gross liabilities outstanding	KCYJ	425 955.59	434 544.59	448 006.31	503 404.50	530 571.50	567 063.81	602 184.19	660 993.56	11 250 856.00

1 See Chapter text.
2 From 2003-04 the NLF Account has been prepared on an Accruals basis. The figures from 2004 onwards reflect this accounting change.
3 Restated from 2004 onward. PWLB advances no longer included with NLF loans.

Source: HM Treasury: 020 7270 4761

18.6 Taxes paid by UK residents to general government and the European Union[1]
Total economy sector S.1

£ million

		1999 /00	2000 /01	2001 /02	2002 /03	2003 /04	2004 /05	2005 /06	2006 /07	2007 /08	2008 /09
Generation of income											
Uses											
Taxes on production and imports											
Taxes on products and imports											
Value added tax (VAT)											
Paid to central government	NZGF	58 688	60 746	64 735	69 087	76 633	79 979	81 505	87 739	89 891	85 350
Paid to the European Union	FJKM	3 451	4 172	3 592	2 518	2 574	1 905	1 964	2 288	2 571	2 455
Total	QYRC	62 127	64 908	68 322	71 599	79 201	81 869	83 421	89 855	92 433	..
Taxes and duties on imports excluding VAT											
Paid to EU: import duties	FJWE	2 049	2 103	2 024	1 893	1 957	2 207	2 264	2 332	2 462	2 667
Taxes on products excluding VAT and import duties											
Paid to central government											
Customs and Excise revenue											
Beer	GTAM	2 848	2 798	2 907	2 952	3 084	3 099	3 092	3 068	3 034	..
Wines, cider, perry & spirits	GTAN	3 652	3 814	4 068	4 430	4 526	4 790	4 784	4 846	5 181	..
Tobacco	GTAO	7 796	7 638	7 639	8 046	8 092	8 113	7 952	8 146	8 006	..
Hydrocarbon oils	GTAP	22 510	22 630	21 916	22 147	22 780	23 313	23 438	23 585	24 905	..
Betting, gaming & lottery	CJQY	1 500	1 517	1 317	977	898	876	884	958	961	..
Air passenger duty	CWAA	882	956	802	804	799	872	906	1 114	1 949	..
Insurance premium tax	CWAD	1 511	1 751	1 921	2 189	2 313	2 353	2 349	2 317	2 314	..
Landfill tax	BKOF	456	475	501	545	639	673	754	837	898	..
Other	ACDN	–	–	–	–	–	–	–	–	–	..
Fossil fuel levy	CIQY	84	52	92	9	–	–	–	–	–	–
Gas levy	GTAZ	–	–	–	–	–	–	–	–	–	–
Stamp duties	GTBC	6 898	8 165	6 983	7 549	7 544	8 966	10 918	13 386	14 123	..
Camelot payments to National Lottery											
Distribution Fund	LIYH	1 593	1 542	1 520	1 382	1 311	1 354	1 397	1 366	1 349	..
Hydro-benefit	LITN	38	44	44	44	43	40	–	–	–	–
Aggregates Levy	MDUQ	–	–	–	293	341	326	323	327	340	..
Climate change levy	LSNT	–	–	822	813	816	750	741	711	705	..
Renewable energy obligations	EP89	–	–	–	265	375	368	381	389	..	..
Other taxes and levies	GCSP	–	–	–	–	–	–	–	–	–	..
Total paid to central government	NMBV	49 768	51 382	50 551	52 486	53 664	56 183	57 965	61 268	64 434	58 989
Paid to the European Union											
Sugar levy	GTBA	46	43	27	25	19	24	24	–	–	–
Total paid to the European Union	FJWG	46	43	27	25	19	24	24	–	–	–
Total taxes on products excluding VAT & import duties	QYRA	49 814	51 425	50 578	52 511	53 643	55 989	57 945	61 050	64 415	..
Total taxes on products and imports	NZGW	113 990	118 436	120 924	126 003	134 801	140 065	143 630	153 236	159 313	..
Production taxes other than on products											
Paid to central government											
Consumer Credit Act fees	CUDB	156	171	157	200	211	223	189	234	328	..
National non-domestic rates	CUKY	14 353	15 154	16 252	16 728	16 902	17 206	18 147	19 168	19 584	21 072
Old style non-domestic rates	NSEZ	123	132	131	136	140	146	193	326	372	..
Levies paid to CG levy-funded bodies	LITK	234	213	215	190	194	218	239	244	256	..
Motor vehicle duties paid by businesses	EKED	1 559	1 230	751	736	787	802	850	869	880	..
Regulator fees	GCSQ	86	105	95	94	101	88	74	71	75	..
Total	NMBX	16 511	17 005	17 601	18 084	18 360	18 802	19 793	20 912	21 484	22 990
Paid to local government											
Old style non-domestic rates	NMYH	144	150	161	176	181	167	187	207	229	245
Total production taxes other than on products	NMYD	16 655	17 155	17 762	18 260	18 541	18 969	19 980	21 119	21 713	23 440
Total taxes on production and imports, paid											
Paid to central government	NMBY	124 727	129 536	133 199	140 152	148 753	154 962	159 281	169 874	175 806	167 483
Paid to local government	NMYH	144	150	161	176	181	167	187	207	229	245
Paid to the European Union	FJWB	5 546	6 318	5 643	4 436	4 550	4 136	4 252	4 620	5 033	5 122
Total	NZGX	130 645	135 591	138 686	144 263	153 367	159 094	163 486	174 793	181 032	..

18.6 Taxes paid by UK residents to general government and the European Union[1]
Total economy sector S.1
continued

£ million

		1999/00	2000/01	2001/02	2002/03	2003/04	2004/05	2005/06	2006/07	2007/08	2008/09
Secondary distribution of income											
Uses											
Current taxes on income, wealth etc											
Taxes on income											
Paid to central government											
Household income taxes	DRWH	96 977	106 866	108 526	110 407	112 356	121 273	130 555	141 226	152 194	144 443
Petroleum revenue tax	DBHA	853	1 518	1 310	958	1 179	1 284	2 016	2 155	1 680	2 567
Windfall tax	EYNK	–	–	–	–	–	–	–	–	–	–
Other corporate taxes	BMNX	1 842	3 458	3 302	2 657	3 974	4 445	5 539	7 006	8 029	..
Total	NMCU	133 994	144 263	145 185	143 256	145 487	160 490	179 960	194 198	208 122	200 815
Other current taxes											
Paid to central government											
Motor vehicle duty paid by households	CDDZ	3 296	3 039	3 540	3 600	3 902	3 935	4 100	4 270	4 513	4 684
Old style domestic rates	NSFA	117	108	109	104	129	227	235	247	272	284
Licences	NSNP	8	2	–	–	–	–	–	–	–	–
National non-domestic rates paid by non-market sectors	BMNY	1 002	997	1 065	1 013	1 008	1 093	1 221	1 274	1 313	1 362
Passport fees	E8A6	89	113	139	153	198	237	285	346	..	..
Television licence fee	DH7A	2 286	2 064	2 183	2 287	2 391	2 508	2 623	2 734	..	..
Total	NMCV	6 798	6 323	7 036	7 157	7 633	8 019	8 484	8 902	9 374	9 519
Paid to local government											
Old style domestic rates	NMHK	68	76	80	85	92	111	149	157	173	..
Council tax	NMHM	12 918	14 155	15 371	16 809	18 911	20 190	21 227	22 299	23 398	..
Total	NMIS	12 986	14 231	15 451	16 894	19 016	20 335	21 375	22 497	23 677	24 729
Total	NVCM	19 784	20 554	22 487	24 051	26 649	28 354	29 859	31 399	33 051	34 446
Total current taxes on income, wealth etc											
Paid to central government	NMCP	140 792	150 586	152 215	150 447	153 191	168 509	188 444	203 400	217 662	210 532
Paid to local government	NMIS	12 986	14 231	15 451	16 894	19 016	20 335	21 375	22 497	23 677	24 729
Total	NMZL	153 778	164 817	167 666	167 341	172 207	188 844	209 819	225 897	241 339	235 261
Social contributions											
Actual social contributions											
Paid to central government											
(National Insurance Contributions)											
Employers' compulsory contributions	CEAN	31 705	35 212	35 816	35 476	41 459	44 864	47 425	50 356	54 030	55 952
Employees' compulsory contributions	GCSE	23 289	24 772	25 130	25 701	31 013	33 088	35 181	37 426	39 250	..
Self- and non-employed persons' compulsory contributions	NMDE	1 941	2 084	2 216	2 352	2 676	2 744	2 852	2 956	3 032	3 112
Total	AIIH	56 935	62 068	63 162	63 529	75 148	80 923	85 559	90 916	95 437	96 961
Capital account											
Changes in liabilities and net worth											
Other capital taxes											
Paid to central government											
Inheritance tax	GILF	2 016	2 181	2 346	2 323	2 486	2 874	3 226	3 508	3 814	..
Tax on other capital transfers	GILG	38	55	37	47	35	48	50	50	50	..
Development land tax and other	GCSV	–	–	–	–	–	–	–	–	–	..
Total	NMGI	2 054	2 236	2 383	2 370	2 521	2 941	3 276	3 618	3 890	23 783
Total taxes and compulsory social contributions											
Paid to central government	GCSS	324 736	344 015	350 642	355 995	379 465	406 928	436 107	467 323	492 501	..
Paid to local government	GCST	13 130	14 381	15 612	17 070	19 195	20 498	21 563	22 663	23 800	..
Paid to the European Union	FJWB	5 546	6 318	5 643	4 436	4 550	4 136	4 252	4 620	5 033	5 122
Total	GCSU	343 412	364 714	371 897	377 501	403 258	431 975	462 356	495 079	520 614	504 909
Total taxes and social contributions as percentage of GDP	GDWM	36.3	36.8	36.0	34.5	34.8	35.5	36.4	36.8	36.6	..

1 See chapter text.

Sources: HM Treasury;
Office for National Statistics: 020 7014 2129

18.7 Borrowing and repayment of debt[1]
United Kingdom
Years ending 31 March

£ million

		1999/00	2000/01	2001/02	2002/03	2003/04	2004/05	2005/06	2006/07	2007/08	2008/09
Borrowing											
Government securities: new issues	KQGA	26 426.5	25 789.8	43 433.4	54 068.9	53 220.9	57 290.5	80 668.9	66 233.4	64 197.4	276 504.4
National savings securities:											
National savings certificates	KQGB	1 962.7	3 086.2	2 580.7	2 434.3	1 940.4	1 696.4	1 206.8	1 464.7	2 524.9	3 390.9
Capital bonds	KQGC	35.40	29.00	40.90	107.30	65.00	25.20	34.30	20.70	31.60	0.03
Income bonds	KQGD	653.4	760.5	625.6	484.8	415.3	426.6	567.5	593.5	1 502.6	3 213.2
Deposit bonds	KQGE	..	..	..	..	–	..	..	..	..	..
British savings bonds	KQGF	..	..	..	..	–	..	..	..	..	..
Premium savings bonds	KQGG	3 449.4	3 296.0	3 859.6	4 604.5	7 530.1	5 737.8	7 817.5	8 432.5	6 573.2	8 472.2
Residual Account	JT3F	..	..	..	..	..	..	..	..	..	343.3
Save As You Earn	KQGH	5.0	0.3	..	..	–	..	..	..	..	..
Yearly plan	KQGI	..	..	..	..	–	..	..	..	..	..
National savings stamps and gift tokens	KQGJ	..	..	..	..	–	..	..	..	..	..
National Savings Bank Investments	KQGK	901.6	955.3	864.9	1 012.4	809.9	817.5	643.6	558.4	535.7	1 071.8
Children's Bonus Bonds	KGVO	58.5	53.4	45.0	54.0	51.7	66.8	59.5	54.1	54.1	46.8
First Option Bonds	KIAR	34.3	..	..	..	–	..	..	..	..	..
Pensioners Guaranteed Income Bond	KJDW	590.7	687.2	603.5	662.9	274.2	323.9	142.7	216.4	371.3	0.3
Treasurer's account	KWNF	13.6	12.5	15.2	19.4	13.9	11.1	10.9	11.6	2.4	..
Individual Savings Account	ZAFC	257.8	265.9	397.8	405.6	335.4	276.4	261.3	1 015.1	1 394.2	835.0
Fixed Rate Savings Bonds	ZAFD	175.9	284.7	192.7	193.0	82.0	86.3	51.2	69.5	347.4	4 327.6
Guaranteed Equity Bonds	ECPU	..	..	27.2	274.8	227.9	317.1	81.4	62.1	56.0	99.9
Easy Access Savings Account	C3OM	..	..	..	..	126.9	903.5	608.6	513.2	933.4	3 763.5
Certificate of tax deposit	KQGL	121.4	76.5	77.6	59.6	145.2	114.8	110.6	100.2	163.7	1 301.7
Nationalised industries', etc temporary deposits	KQGM	40 343.3	56 106.6	62 150.0	55 395.1	47 958.6	25 022.0	22 039.1	35 224.0	51 365.0	60 200.9
Sterling Treasury bills (net receipt)	KQGO	..	..	..	..	–	..	..	..	..	..
ECU Treasury bills (net receipt)	KQGP	..	..	..	..	–	..	..	..	..	..
ECU Treasury notes (net receipt)	KDZZ	721.1	..	..	..	–	..	..	..	..	..
Ways and means (net receipt)	KQGQ	5 599.0	12 126.0	12 095.3	3 899.9	22 700.2	..	..	23 428.0	12 810.5	–
Other debt: payable in sterling :											
Interest free notes	KQGR	373.5	972.7	1 427.2	754.0	1 213.2	662.3	1 858.9	1 049.9	97.2	822.8
Other debt : payable in external currencies	KHCY	..	..	..	..	1 792.5	..	..	..	..	..
Total receipts	KHCZ	81 723	104 503	128 437	124 430	138 903	93 778	116 163	139 047	142 961	364 394
Repayment of debt											
Government securities: redemptions	KQGS	19 815.8	33 722.2	43 642.3	42 109.9	35 087.4	25 130.1	17 456.5	62 406.9	32 940.2	37 503.6
Statutory sinking funds	KQGT	2.0	2.0	1.9	1.9	1.8	1.8	0.4	..	..	..
Terminable annuities:											
National Debt Commissioners	KQGU	..	..	..	..	–	..	..	..	..	..
National savings securities:											
National savings certificates	KQGV	2 405.2	4 546.8	4 177.7	4 146.7	2 769.1	1 979.6	1 107.4	1 172.1	1 201.9	1 240.2
Capital bonds	KQGW	324.2	375.0	175.9	155.9	116.9	121.1	159.2	137.4	184.0	229.0
Income bonds	KQGX	1 686.3	857.0	933.8	1 144.2	977.1	879.5	724.6	719.2	712.8	2 145.1
Deposit bonds	KQGY	70.2	71.1	45.4	369.9	4.4	..	..	..	..	..
Yearly Plan	KQGZ	141.8	18.4	4.5	3.0	2.0	..	..	0.8	4.9	19.3
British savings bonds	KQHA	..	..	..	..	–	..	..	..	..	..
Premium savings bonds	KQHB	1 923.8	1 872.6	1 942.9	2 343.3	2 967.4	3 492.4	3 289.2	4 279.8	4 952.3	4 613.9
Residual Account	JT3G	..	..	..	..	..	..	..	..	..	14.9
Save As You Earn	KQHC	34.5	22.9	8.0	3.2	0.5	..	0.5	0.5	1.6	10.1
National savings stamps and gift tokens	KQHD	..	..	..	..	–	1.2	..	..	..	..
National Savings Bank Investments (repayments)	KQHE	1 886.3	1 654.1	1 415.8	1 350.1	1 342.7	1 554.0	1 153.3	1 172.4	976.8	1 058.2
Children's Bonus Bonds	KGVQ	69.3	95.0	114.5	92.6	79.8	84.5	95.8	105.7	108.5	106.1
First Option Bonds	KIAS	298.1	225.2	111.6	77.4	62.2	33.4	36.1	25.6	26.6	25.2
Pensioners Guaranteed Income Bond	KPOB	935.30	2 003.80	1 640.40	703.90	538.50	445.00	428.60	452.70	543.10	1 342.98
Treasurer's account	KWNG	16.4	13.9	16.5	16.9	14.2	16.2	18.3	11.7	47.1	18.6
Individual Savings Account	ZAFE	12.3	39.9	70.3	105.9	157.6	202.2	194.1	193.6	274.9	822.2
Fixed Rate Savings Bonds	ZAFF	2.8	62.1	110.1	133.6	153.1	92.1	105.0	77.2	104.2	246.8
Guaranteed Equity Bonds	JUWE	..	..	..	3.9	3.3	..	0.2	3.7	365.9	370.3
Easy Access Savings Account	C3ON	..	..	..	..	126.9	189.3	400.6	509.7	544.6	1 507.3
Certificates of tax deposit	KQHF	159.9	120.1	91.4	161.5	113.1	171.9	152.1	56.0	88.0	608.8
Tax reserve certificates	KQHG	..	..	..	..	..	..	..	..	..	..
Nationalised industries', etc temporary deposits	KQHH	41 089.4	56 004.0	63 127.9	55 695.6	47 757.7	25 949.5	21 943.1	35 686.5	48 265.0	55 847.8
Debt to the Bank of England	KPOC	..	..	..	..	–	..	..	..	..	..
Sterling Treasury bills (net repayment)	KQHJ	3 014.8	6 194.2	..	..	–	..	..	..	..	..
ECU Treasury bills (net repayment)	KJEG	2 492.9	..	..	..	–	..	..	..	..	..
ECU Treasury notes (net repayment)	KSPA	..	1 391.9	1 359.6	1 453.1	–	..	..	..	..	..
Ways and means (net repayment)	KQHK	..	..	..	..	..	9 760.2	36 207.3	..	..	3 161.7
Other debt: payable in sterling :											
Interest free notes	KQHL	246.4	458.2	1 723.3	1 393.3	990.5	300.4	222.3	586.4	474.4	1 092.9
Other	KQHM	..	..	..	..	..	..	..	..	..	..
Other debt : payable in external currencies	KQHN	98.1	1 835.6	2 838.1	1 960.3	47.0	46.5	98.9	52.4	–	..
Total payments	KQHO	76 726	111 586	123 552	113 426	93 313	70 451	83 794	107 650	91 817	111 985
Net borrowing	KQHP	4 997.30	..	4 884.70	11 004.40	45 590.10	23 327.30	32 369.30	31 397.00	51 143.80	252 409.34
Net repayment	KHDD	..	7 083.4	..	..	–	..	..	..	..	..

Note: the table excludes transactions in treasury bills issued for the Special Liquidity scheme

1 See chapter text.

Source: HM Treasury: 020 7270 4761

Government finance

18.8 Central government net cash requirement on own account (receipts and outlays on a cash basis)

£ million

| | Cash receipts | | | | | | | | Cash outlays | | | | |
| | HM Revenue and Customs | | | | | | | | | | | | |
	Total paid over [1]	Income tax [2]	Corpora-tion tax [2]	NICs [3]	V.A.T. [4]	Interest and dividends	Other receipts [5]	Total	Interest payments	Net acquisiti-on of company securities [6]	Net depart-mental outlays [7]	Total	Own account net cash requireme-nt
	1	2	3	4	5	6	7	8	9	10	11	12	13
	MIZX	RURC	ACCD	ABLP	EYOO	RUUL	RUUM	RUUN	RUUO	ABIF	RUUP	RUUQ	RUUX
2000	305 547	103 118	33 003	59 274	58 509	9 009	46 078	360 634	23 890	−251	297 933	321 572	−39 062
2001	316 517	111 874	33 520	62 973	60 282	8 611	24 643	349 771	23 132	−661	324 633	347 104	−2 667
2002	315 987	111 559	28 866	63 992	63 000	6 954	25 310	348 251	19 343	–	347 612	366 955	18 704
2003	325 138	113 712	28 489	69 360	67 525	7 335	25 329	357 802	20 348	−39	379 418	399 727	41 925
2004	347 514	121 493	31 160	77 026	71 907	6 855	25 137	379 506	21 027	–	400 631	421 658	42 152
2005	372 567	130 818	37 820	83 612	73 012	6 549	26 341	405 457	22 434	–	421 021	443 455	37 998
2006	401 362	140 616	47 108	87 156	76 103	6 640	28 115	436 117	25 834	−347	448 131	473 618	37 501
2007	422 465	149 968	43 912	96 656	80 301	8 251	30 083	460 799	25 537	−2 340	470 169	493 366	32 567
2008	428 380	157 500	46 487	98 504	80 709	9 354	30 556	468 290	26 033	19 714	544 720	590 467	122 177
2009	384 872	146 721	35 331	95 411	68 635	6 666	31 262	422 800	29 264	41 809	548 771	619 844	197 044
1999/00	291 280	96 032	34 322	56 354	56 395	8 637	22 660	322 577	24 320	−535	288 128	311 913	−10 664
2000/01	309 726	108 414	32 421	60 614	58 501	8 715	46 772	365 213	23 798	−81	304 245	327 962	−37 251
2001/02	314 959	111 028	32 041	63 168	61 026	7 843	25 001	347 803	22 126	−683	329 726	351 169	3 366
2002/03	317 174	111 102	29 268	64 553	63 451	7 425	24 725	349 324	19 687	−39	353 890	373 538	24 214
2003/04	331 133	116 194	28 077	72 457	69 075	7 172	25 348	363 653	21 251	–	385 119	406 370	42 717
2004/05	355 917	125 202	33 641	78 098	73 026	6 633	25 074	387 624	21 810	–	403 268	425 078	37 454
2005/06	382 067	133 519	41 829	85 522	72 856	6 393	27 022	415 482	23 121	−347	428 616	451 390	35 908
2006/07	406 337	147 134	44 308	87 274	77 360	6 754	27 359	440 450	26 279	–	451 062	477 341	36 891
2007/08	431 800	152 591	46 383	100 411	80 601	9 000	31 205	472 005	25 390	−2 340	478 576	501 626	29 621
2008/09	416 512	155 704	43 077	96 884	78 439	8 724	28 008	453 244	25 947	32 250	557 560	615 757	162 513
2007 Q3	107 134	37 488	12 465	24 165	19 301	1 986	9 934	119 054	6 486	–	114 418	120 904	1 850
Q4	101 691	31 137	12 957	22 764	21 327	2 504	7 070	111 265	6 473	–	124 364	130 837	19 572
2008 Q1	126 971	54 549	12 946	27 550	19 850	2 646	5 997	135 614	6 472	–	118 768	125 240	−10 374
Q2	97 153	34 333	8 509	23 517	20 087	2 252	8 154	107 559	6 449	–	131 441	137 890	30 331
Q3	108 990	39 286	12 742	24 801	21 235	2 266	9 143	120 399	6 566	−255	150 477	156 788	36 389
Q4	95 266	29 332	12 290	22 636	19 537	2 190	7 262	104 718	6 546	19 969	144 034	170 549	65 831
2009 Q1	115 103	52 753	9 536	25 930	17 580	2 016	3 449	120 568	6 386	12 536	131 608	150 530	29 962
Q2	85 700	31 145	6 338	22 729	16 104	1 892	9 631	97 223	8 516	−2 021	145 067	151 562	54 339
Q3	93 410	35 190	8 026	23 863	16 846	1 357	9 713	104 480	7 584	–	133 138	140 722	36 242
Q4	90 659	27 633	11 431	22 889	18 105	1 401	8 469	100 529	6 778	31 294	138 958	177 030	76 501

Relationships between columns 1+6+7=8; 9+10+11=12; 12-8=13

1 Comprises payments into the Consolidated Fund and all payovers of NICS excluding those for Northern Ireland.
2 Income tax includes capital gains tax and is net of any tax credits treated by HM Revenue and Customs as tax deductions.
3 UK receipts net of personal pension rebates; gross of Statutory Maternity Pay and Statutory Sick Pay.
4 Payments into Consolidated Fund.

5 Including some elements of expenditure not separately identified.
6 Mainly comprises privatisation proceeds.
7 Net of certain receipts, and excluding on-lending to local authorities and public corporations.

Sources: HM Revenue & Customs;
Office for National Statistics

18.9 HM Revenue and Customs taxes and duties

£ million

		Net receipts by HM Revenue and Customs						
	Total[1],[6]	Income tax and Capital gains tax[2],[3]	Corporation tax[4]	Inheritance tax[6]	Stamp duties	Petroleum revenue tax[5]	Payments into Consolidated Fund[6]	Advance corporation tax
	MDXD	RURC	ACCD	ACCH	ACCI	ACCJ	ACAB	ACCN
2005	183 481	130 818	37 820	3 134	9 910	1 799	170 130	−73
2006	206 851	140 616	47 108	3 507	13 074	2 546	192 715	−21
2007	213 705	149 968	43 912	3 804	14 634	1 387	200 127	–
2008	219 318	157 500	46 487	3 169	9 499	2 663	202 283	–
2009	192 540	146 721	35 331	2 337	7 104	1 047	171 509	–
2004/05	172 017	125 202	33 641	2 924	8 966	1 284	158 974	−33
2005/06	191 540	133 519	41 829	3 258	10 918	2 016	178 707	−84
2006/07	210 535	147 134	44 308	3 545	13 393	2 155	195 598	−4
2007/08	218 601	152 591	46 383	3 824	14 123	1 680	205 681	–
2008/09	212 187	155 704	43 077	2 837	8 002	2 567	193 539	–
2005 Q4	42 181	27 185	11 023	788	2 796	389	38 359	−52
2006 Q1	63 106	45 408	13 275	832	2 979	612	60 233	−17
Q2	42 814	30 604	7 882	874	3 089	365	39 406	−2
Q3	53 944	35 891	12 958	887	3 419	789	47 921	–
Q4	46 987	28 713	12 993	914	3 587	780	45 155	−2
2007 Q1	66 790	51 926	10 475	870	3 298	221	63 116	–
Q2	42 352	29 417	8 015	937	3 727	256	38 704	–
Q3	55 460	37 488	12 465	1 054	3 998	455	52 463	–
Q4	49 103	31 137	12 957	943	3 611	455	45 844	–
2008 Q1	71 686	54 549	12 946	890	2 787	514	68 670	–
Q2	46 490	34 333	8 509	808	2 573	267	41 394	–
Q3	56 375	39 286	12 742	787	2 240	1 320	51 626	–
Q4	44 767	29 332	12 290	684	1 899	562	40 593	–
2009 Q1	64 555	52 753	9 536	558	1 290	418	59 926	–
Q2	40 008	31 145	6 338	550	1 608	367	34 109	–
Q3	45 866	35 190	8 026	615	1 969	66	39 869	–
Q4	42 111	27 633	11 431	614	2 237	196	37 605	–

1 The total is not always equal to the sum of the individual taxes due to rounding.
2 Income tax and Capital gains tax combined.
3 Figures for income tax treat payments of the personal tax credits as negative tax to the extent that the credits are less than or equal to the tax liability of the family. Payments exceeding this liability are treated as public expenditure.
4 Including net advance corporation tax receipts shown separately in the final column.

5 Including net advance petroleum revenue tax.
6 Payments into the consolidated fund are not directly comparable to receipts Over the year payments into the consolidated fund will always be lower than total receipts because the public expenditure element of payments of tax being recorded in receipts. Because the public expenditure element of payments of tax credits (both personal and company) are deducted from the payments into the consolidated fund but have no impact on receipts. In addition, there is a timing difference between payments taking value and hence paid over to the consolidated fund and being recorded in receipts.

Sources: HM Revenue and Customs; National Statistics

18.10 British government and government guaranteed marketable securities[1]
Nominal values of official and market holdings by maturity[2],[3]

At 31 March each year

£ million

		1999	2000	2001	2002	2003	2004	2005	2006	2007	2008	2009
Total holdings	KQMO	291 788	290 629	285 915	278 808	292 777	321 051	354 884	411 770	442 857	478 779	713 224
Up to 5 years	KQMP	95 112	95 131	92 090	92 780	106 074	88 678	110 839	122 496	119 872	117 620	211 888
Over 5 and up to 15 years	KQMQ	124 603	116 910	120 101	106 044	101 465	131 665	123 729	151 841	167 525	168 623	210 685
Over 15 years (including undated)	KQMR	72 074	78 587	73 724	79 984	85 238	97 500	117 350	134 485	152 529	192 536	290 651
Official holdings:[3]												
Total	HHAW	6 394	6 204	8 210	7 558	10 650	9 118	7 433	25 409	23 305	25 754	133 080
Up to 5 years	HHAY	2 600	2 849	4 652	3 928	4 797	3 321	2 770	8 222	7 328	7 120	40 990
Over 5 and up to 15 years	HHAZ	2 989	2 567	3 009	2 844	4 115	4 015	3 063	9 620	9 511	10 329	39 808
Over 15 years (including undated)	HHBA	805	788	549	786	1 738	1 540	1 562	7 530	6 420	8 304	52 282
Market holdings:												
Total	HHBB	285 394	284 425	277 705	271 250	282 127	311 933	347 451	386 361	419 552	453 025	580 144
Up to 5 years	HHBD	92 512	92 282	87 438	88 852	101 277	85 357	108 070	114 274	112 545	110 500	170 898
Over 5 and up to 15 years	HHBE	121 614	114 343	117 092	103 200	97 350	127 650	120 666	142 221	158 014	158 294	170 877
Over 15 years (including undated)	HHBF	71 269	77 800	73 175	79 198	83 500	95 960	115 788	126 955	146 109	184 231	238 369

1 The government guaranteed securities of nationalised industries only. A relatively small amount of other government guaranteed securities is excluded.
2 Securities with optional redemption dates are classified according to the final redemption date. The nominal value of index-linked British Government Stock has been raised by the amount of accrued capital uplift.

3 Official holdings were changed following the introduction of the central bank sector in the UK national accounts. These holdings now principally include those of the Debt Management Office and other government departments. The Issue and Banking Departments of the Bank of England are classified within the central bank sector and are therefore part of market holdings.

Source: Office for National Statistics: 020 7014 2124

Government finance

18.11 Income tax: allowances and reliefs[1]
United Kingdom

£

		1999/00	2000/01	2001/02	2002/03	2003/04	2004/05	2005/06	2006/07	2007/08	2008/09	2009/10
Personal allowances												
Personal allowance	KDZP	4 335	4 385	4 535	4 615	4 615	4 745	4 895	5 035	5 225	6 035	6 475
Married couple's (both partners under 65)[2]	KDZR	1 970	..	..	..	..	..	..	..	..	..	..
Age allowance:												
Personal (aged 65-74)	KSOH	5 720	5 790	5 990	6 100	6 610	6 830	7 090	7 280	7 550	9 030	9 490
Personal (aged 75 or over)	KSOI	5 980	6 050	6 260	6 370	6 720	6 950	7 220	7 420	7 690	9 180	9 640
Married couple's (either partner between 65-74 but neither partner 75 or over)[2,3]	KEDI	5 125	5 185	5 365	5 465	5 565	5 725	5 905	6 065	6 285	6 535	..
Married couple's (either partner 75 or over)[2]	KEIY	5 195	5 255	5 435	5 535	5 635	5 795	5 975	6 135	6 365	6 625	6 965
Minimum married couple's allowance	C58D	1 970	2 000	2 070	2 110	2 150	2 210	2 280	2 350	2 440	2 540	2 670
Income limit[4]	KEOO	16 800	17 000	17 600	17 900	18 300	18 900	19 500	20 100	20 900	21 800	22 900
Additional personal allowance[2]	KEPG	1 970	..	..	..	..	..	..	..	..	..	..
Widow's bereavement allowance	KEPH	1 970	..	..	..	..	..	..	..	..	..	..
Blind person's allowance												
Single or married (one spouse blind)	KSOJ	1 380	1 400	1 450	1 480	1 510	1 560	1 610	1 660	1 730	1 800	1 890
Married (both spouses blind)	KSOK	2 760	2 800	2 900	2 960	3 020	3 120	3 220	3 320	3 460	3 600	3 780
Life Assurance Relief												
Percentage of gross premium	KFDR	12.5 or Nil	12.5 or Nil	12.5 or Nil	12.5 or Nil	12.5 or Nil	12.5 or Nil	12.5 or Nil	12.5 or Nil	12.5 or Nil	12.5 or Nil	12.5 or Nil

1 See chapter text.
2 The allowance was restricted to 20 per cent in 1994-95, 15 per cent from 1995-96 and 10 per cent from 1999-00.
3 In the 2009-10 tax year all Married Couples Allowance claimants in this category will become 75 at some point during the year and will therefore be entitled to the higher amount of allowance, for those aged 75 and over.

4 If the total income, less allowable deductions of a taxpayer aged 65 or over exceeds the limit, the age-related allowances are reduced by £1 for each £2 of income over the aged income level until the basic levels of the personal and married couple's allowances are reached.

Source: HM Revenue & Customs: 020 7147 3045

18.12 Rates of Income tax
United Kingdom

	2001/02		2002/03		2003/04		2004/05		2005/06	
	Bands of taxable income (£)[1]	Rate of tax - Percentages	Bands of taxable income (£)[1]	Rate of tax - Percentages	Bands of taxable income (£)[1]	Rate of tax - Percentages	Bands of taxable income (£)[1]	Rate of tax - Percentages	Bands of taxable income (£)[1]	Rate of tax - Percentages
Starting rate[2]	1 - 1 880	10	1 - 1 920	10	1 - 1 960	10	1 - 2 020	10	1 - 2 090	10
Basic rate[3]	1 881 - 29 400	22	1 921 - 29 900	22	1 961 - 30 500	22	2 021 - 31 400	22	2 091 - 32 400	22
Higher rate[4]	over 29 400	40	over 29 900	40	over 30 500	40	over 31 400	40	over 32 400	40

	2006/07		2007/08		2008/09		2009/10		20010/11	
	Bands of taxable income (£)[1]	Rate of tax - Percentages	Bands of taxable income (£)[1]	Rate of tax - Percentages	Bands of taxable income (£)[1]	Rate of tax - Percentages	Bands of taxable income (£)[1]	Rate of tax - Percentages	Bands of taxable income (£)[1]	Rate of tax - Percentages
Starting rate[2]	1 - 2 150	10	1 - 2 230	10	1 - 2 230	10[5]	-	-	-	
Basic rate[3]	2 151 - 33 300	22	2 231 - 34 600	22	2 321 - 34 800	20	1 - 37 400	20	1 - 37 400	20
Higher rate[4]	over 33 300	40	over 34 600	40	over 34 800	40	over 37 400	40	37 401 - 150 000	40
Additional rate									over 150 000	50

1 Taxable income is defined as gross income for income tax purposes less any allowances and reliefs available at the taxpayer's marginal rate.
2 The starting rate also applies to savings and dividends.
3 The basic rate of tax on dividends is 10% and savings income is 20%.
4 The higher rate of tax on dividends is 32.5%.
5 From 2008/09 there is a 10% starting rate for savings income only. If non-savings income is above this limit the 10% rate does not apply.

Source: HM Revenue & Customs: 020 7147 3045

18.13 Local Authorities: gross loan debt outstanding[1]
At 31 March each year

£ billion

		2005	2006	2007	2008	2009
United Kingdom						
Total debt	KQBR	52.9	59.7	62.3	66.2	67.2
Public Works Loan Board	KQBS	42.4	47.1	47.9	50.3	50.4
Northern Ireland Consolidated Fund	KQBT	0.3	..	..	..	..
Other debt	KQBU	10.5	..	..	..	..
England						
Total debt	C3OO	40.1	46.1	48.6	52.4	53.6
of which Public Works Loan Board	C3OP	32.2	36.6	37.6	40.2	40.6
Wales						
Total debt	C3OQ	3.7	3.8	3.8	4.0	3.8
of which Public Works Loan Board	C3OR	3.1	3.3	3.1	3.2	3.0
Scotland						
Total debt	KQBX	8.7	9.4	9.5	9.4	9.4
of which Public Works Loan Board	KQBY	*6.8*	*7.2*	*7.1*	*6.9*	*6.8*
Northern Ireland						
Total debt	KQBZ	0.3	0.3	0.3	0.4	0.4
of which						
Northern Ireland Consolidated Fund	KQBT	0.3	..	..	..	..

1 The sums shown exclude inter-authority loans.

Sources: Communities and Local Government: 020 7944 4176;
Public Works Loan Board: 020 7862 6610;
Department of Finance and Personnel for Northern Ireland: 028 9185 8132

18.14 Rateable Values[1]
England and Wales
At 1 April each year

		1999	2000	2001	2002	2003	2004	2005	2006	2007	2008	2009
Number of properties (Thousands)												
Commercial	KMIN	1 219	1 223	1 230	1 234	1 236	1 239	1 234	1 245	1 258	1 267	1 279
Shops and cafes	KMIO	484	478	476	473	469	466	462	459	457	456	455
Offices	KMIP	258	261	269	273	279	284	287	296	304	311	320
Other	KMIQ	477	484	485	487	488	490	485	490	497	500	504
On-licensed premises	KMIR	60	61	61	60	60	60	66	65	65	64	63
Entertainment and recreational:	KMIS	80	79	79	80	80	80	78	79	81	81	83
Cinemas	KMIT	1	1	1	1	1	1	1	1	1	1	1
Theatres and music-halls	KMIU	1	1	1	1	1	1	1	1	1	1	1
Other	KMIV	79	76	76	77	77	78	76	78	80	80	81
Public utility	KMIW	9	8	8	8	8	8	8	8	8	8	7
Educational and cultural	KMIX	41	41	42	42	42	43	45	45	45	45	45
Miscellaneous	KMIY	61	67	70	70	72	74	74	77	80	81	83
Industrial	KMIZ	250	250	251	250	250	250	252	251	252	249	246
Total	KMIH	1 720	1 729	1 740	1 745	1 749	1 754	1 756	1 771	1 788	1 796	1 806
Value of assessments (£ million)												
Commercial	KMHG	19 652	26 320	27 255	27 622	27 713	27 878	33 013	33 548	33 566	33 427	33 728
Shops and cafes	KMHH	5 840	6 801	6 972	6 953	6 863	6 845	8 257	8 311	8 289	8 251	8 321
Offices	KMHI	5 575	8 625	9 191	9 388	9 555	9 591	10 840	11 034	10 904	10 724	10 794
Other	KMHJ	8 237	10 894	11 092	11 281	11 295	11 441	13 916	14 203	14 373	14 452	14 613
On-licensed premises	KMHK	997	1 311	1 347	1 345	1 334	1 320	1 667	1 652	1 615	1 589	1 567
Entertainment and recreational	KMHL	1 045	1 310	1 369	1 430	1 416	1 362	1 467	1 483	1 481	1 478	1 466
Cinemas	KMHM	45	79	92	104	106	96	117	115	110	101	102
Theatres and music-halls	KMHN	20	24	25	26	26	26	34	35	35	35	36
Other	KMHO	980	1 207	1 252	1 300	1 284	1 240	1 316	1 333	1 337	1 342	1 328
Public utility	KMHP	3 361	3 828	3 411	3 460	3 444	3 410	3 680	3 668	3 668	3 656	3 471
Educational and cultural	KMHQ	1 672	1 829	1 872	1 902	1 895	1 904	2 359	2 411	2 407	2 397	2 417
Miscellaneous	KMHR	1 439	2 142	2 172	2 220	2 218	2 022	2 582	2 646	2 687	2 694	2 697
Industrial	KMHS	5 463	6 249	6 202	6 157	6 034	5 935	6 651	6 575	6 453	6 314	6 122
Total	KMHA	33 649	42 985	43 626	44 136	44 053	43 831	51 419	51 983	51 878	51 555	51 468

1 See chapter text.

Source: HM Revenue & Customs: 020 7147 2941

18.15 Revenue expenditure of local authorities

£ million

	2006/07 outturn	2007/08 outturn	2008/09 outturn	2009/10 budget
England				
Education[1]	37 942	40 135	42 148	42 991
Highways and Transport	5 316	5 636	5 710	6 332
Social care[2]	18 108	18 587	19 604	20 251
Housing (excluding HRA)[3]	14 963	15 844	16 985	17 130
Cultural, environmental and planning	9 658	10 139	10 489	10 533
of which:				
Cultural	3 129	3 188	3 297	3 274
Environmental	4 524	4 832	5 086	5 423
Planning and development	2 005	2 119	2 106	1 836
Police	11 542	11 704	11 548	12 218
Fire	2 193	2 233	2 104	2 311
Courts	62	70	73	71
Central services	3 430	3 541	3 776	3521
Other	128	360	639	202
Net current expenditure	103 341	108 249	113 076	115 559
Capital financing	2 993	3 004	2 971	3 595
Capital Expenditure charged to Revenue Account	1 103	1 095	1 670	1 750
Interest receipts	-1 481	-1 862	-1 926	-720
Pension Interest Costs and expected return on Pension assets	4 534	4 808	7 042	4 810
Other non-current expenditure[4]	3 350	3 448	3 654	3 711
Specific grants outside Aggregate External Finance (AEF)	-19 643	-20 761	-21 738	-21 011
Revenue expenditure	88 172	92 386	98 120	102 823
Specific and special grants inside AEF	-41 741	-44 486	-42 926	-44 038
Area Based Grant (ABG)	n/a	n/a	-3 051	-3 145
Net revenue expenditure	46 432	47 900	52 143	55 640
Appropriation to/from reserves (excluding pension reserves)	974	1 496	241	1 635
Appropriation to/from Pension Reserves	-6 025	-5 595	-6 423	-4 896
Other adjustments	16	2	2	10
Budget requirement	47 421	49 398	52 387	54 016
Police grant	-3 936	-4 028	-4 136	-4 253
Revenue support grant	-3 378	-3 105	-2 854	-4 501
Redistributed business rates	-17 506	-18 506	-20 506	-19 515
General Greater London Authority Grant	-38	-38	-48	-48
Other items	-111	-112	-85	-65
Council tax requirement	22 453	23 608	24 759	25 633
Scotland				
Net revenue expenditure on general fund	10 708	11 023	11 981	12 369

18.15 Revenue expenditure of local authorities
continued

£ million

	2006/07 outturn	2007/08 outturn	2008/09 outturn	2009/10 Budget
Wales[5]				
Education	2 213.0	2 325.6	2 427.5	2 483.5
Personal social services	1 253.6	1 302.9	1348.8	1 370.9
Housing[6]	716.7	759.4	878.2	841.3
Local environmental services[7]	353.9	356.4	393.0	410.0
Roads and transport	283.3	296.4	329.8	316.6
Libraries, culture, heritage, sport and recreation	259.9	267.4	285.8	270.3
Planning, economic development and community development	115.2	113.6	164.7	116.5
Council tax benefit and administration[8]	32.1	31.7	31.5	30.8
Debt financing costs: counties	278.0	289.0	320.5	318.9
Central administrative and other revenue expenditure: counties[9]	207.4	217.3	198.0	309.1
Total county and county borough council expenditure	5 713.1	5 959.8	6 377.8	6 467.8
Total police expenditure	601.4	623.3	642.6	675.3
Total fire expenditure	142.1	138.2	145.0	145.8
Total national park expenditure	15.8	17.8	18.0	16.1
Gross revenue expenditure	6 472.4	6 739.1	7 183.3	7 305.0
less specific and special government grants (except council tax benefit grant)	-1 529.7	-1 630.2	-1 809.0	-1 682.3
Net revenue expenditure	4 942.7	5 108.9	5 374.3	5 622.7
Putting to (+)/drawing from (-) reserves	24.6	97.0	14.0	-63.2
Budget requirement	4 967.3	5 205.9	5 388.4	5 559.6
Plus discretionary non-domestic rate relief	2.6	2.5	2.4	2.6
less revenue support grant	-2 951.8	-3 061.6	-3 104.6	-3 191.7
less police grant	-217.0	-225.0	-230.5	-236.3
less re-distributed non-domestic rates income	-730.0	-791.0	-868.0	-894.0
Council tax requirement	1 071.2	1 130.8	1 187.9	1 240.2
of which:				
Paid by council tax benefit grant from the Department for Work and Pensions	177.2	184.6	194.8	203.5
Paid directly by council tax payers	894.0	946.2	993.1	1 036.7

1 Includes mandatory student awards and inter-authority education recoupment.
2 Includes supported employment.
3 Includes mandatory rent allowances and rent rebates.
4 Includes:
(i) Gross expenditure on council tax benefit.
(ii) Expenditure on council tax reduction scheme.
(iii) Discretionary (non-domestic) rate relief.
(iv) Flood defence payments to the Environment Agency.
(v) Bad debt provision.
5 Service expenditure is shown excluding that financed by sales, fees and charges, but including that financed by specific and special government grants.
6 Includes housing benefit and private sector costs such as provision for the homeless. Includes rent rebates granted to HRA tenants which is 100% grant funded. Excludes council owned housing.

7 Includes cemeteries and crematoria, community safety, environmental health, consumer protection, waste collection/disposal and central services to the public such as birth registration and elections.
8 Excludes council tax benefit expednditure funded by the specific grant from the Department for Work and Pensions.
9 Includes agricultural services, coastal and flood defence and community councils. Also includes central administrative costs of corporate management, democratic representation and certain costs, such as those relating to back-year or additional pension contributions which should not be allocated to individual services, capital expenditure charged to the revenue account and is net of any interest expected to accrue on balances.

Sources: Communities and Local Government: 020 7944 4158;
Scottish Government, Statistical Support for Local Government: 0131 245 7034;
Welsh Assembly Government: 029 2082 5355

18.16 Financing of revenue expenditure
England and Wales
Years ending 31 March

£ million

		1999 /00	2000 /01	2001 /02	2002 /03	2003 /04	2004 /05	2005 /06	2006 /07	2007 /08	2008[1] /09	2009 /10
England[2]												
Revenue expenditure[3]												
Cash £m	KRTN	53 651	57 329	61 952	65 898	75 244	79 303	84 422	88 172	92 386	98 120	102 823
Government grants												
Cash £m	KRTO	26 421	27 809	31 469	32 634	41 777	45 258	45 838	49 093	51 656	53 015	55 985
Percentage of revenue expenditure	KRTP	49	49	50	50	56	57	54	56	56	54	54
Redistributed business rates[4]												
Cash £m	KRTQ	13 619	15 407	15 144	16 639	15 611	15 004	18 004	17 506	18 506	20 506	19 515
Percentage of revenue expenditure	KRTR	25	27	24	25	21	19	21	20	20	21	19
Council tax												
Cash £m	KRTS	13 278	14 200	15 246	16 648	18 946	20 299	21 315	22 453	23 608	24 759	25 633
Percentage of revenue expenditure	KRTT	25	25	25	25	25	26	25	25	26	25	25
Wales												
Gross revenue expenditure[5]	ZBXH	3 424	3 605	4 350	4 709	5 243	5 786	6 128	6 472	6 739	7 184	7 305
General government grants[6]	ZBXI	2 093	2 234	2 345	2 541	2 743	2 817	2 987	3 169	3 287	3 335	3 428
Specific government grants[7]	ZBXG	80	94	601	779	1 005	1 381	1 473	1 530	1 630	1 809	1 682
Share of redistributed business rates	ZBXJ	656	638	697	643	660	672	672	730	791	868	864
Council tax income[8]	ZBXK	596	670	716	776	861	924	1 012	1 071	1 131	1 188	1 240
Other[9]	ZBXL	−1	−31	−10	−30	−25	−8	−16	−27	−99	−16	61

1 Budget estimates.
2 Produced on a non-Financial Reporting Standard 17 (FRS17) basis.
3 The sum of government grants, business rates and local taxes does not normally equal revenue expenditure because of the use of reserves.
4 1993-94 to 2003-04 includes City of London Offset.
5 Gross revenue expenditure is total local authority expenditure on services, plus capital charges, but net of any income from sales, fees, and charges and other non-grant sources. It includes expenditure funded by specific grants. The figures have been adjusted to account for FRS17 pension costs.

6 Includes all unhypothecated grants, namely revenue support grant, police grant, council tax reduction scheme grant, transitional grant and the adjustment to reverse the transfer.
7 Comprises specific and supplementary grants, excluding police grant.
8 This includes community council precepts, and income covered by charge/council tax benefit grant, but excludes council tax reduction scheme.
9 This includes use of, or contributors to, local authority reserves and other minor adjustments.

Sources: Communities and Local Government: 020 7944 4158;
Welsh Assembly Government: 029 2082 5355

18.17 Capital expenditure and income
England

£ million

Financial year	Central government grants[1]	Other grants and contributions[2]	Use of usable capital receipts	BCA/SCE(R)Single Capital Pot	BCA/SCE(R)Separate Programme Element	Other borrowing and credit arrangements not supported by central government
	KRVM	I4V9	I4VA	I4VB	I4VC	I4VD
1999/00	1 161	571	1 599	1 051	1 250	..
2000/01	1 298	762	1 592	2 271	945	..
2001/02	2 027	757	1 975	1 173	1 378	..
2002/03	2 474	716	2 426	2 281	935	..
2003/04	2 642	869	1 988	2 583	1 326	..
2004/05	3 196	1 080	2 647	2 959	704	1 061
2005/06	3 909	1 377	2 812	2 932	947	2 251
2006/07	4 083	1 344	2 628	2 734	630	2 291
2007/08	7 007	2 019	2 665	2 296	630	3 186
2008/09	5 733	1 978	2 040	2 257	760	4 224

Financial year	Use of other resources [3]	Revenue financing of capital expenditure, of which:			Total resources used
		Housing revenue account	Major repairs reserve	General Fund	
	I4VE	I4VF	I4VG	I4VH	I4VI
1999/00	231	327	..	808	6 998
2000/01	304	218	..	896	8 288
2001/02	387	1 505	..	825	10 028
2002/03	375	175	1 465	825	11 672
2003/04	262	212	1 388	1 055	12 326
2004/05	..	187	1 440	1 130	14 404
2005/06	..	238	1 327	1 004	16 797
2006/07	..	240	1 337	1 185	16 472
2007/08	..	208	1 180	1 204	20 395
2008/09	..	228	1 224	1 789	20 233

1 2007-08 includes an exceptional item, £1.7 billion grant from DfT to GLA (TfL) for the £1.7 billion payment to Metronet.
2 Includes grants and contributions for private developers, Non-Departmental Public Bodies, National Lottery and European Structural Fund.

3 Use of monies set aside as provision for credit liabilities to finance capital expenditure (debt free authorities).
Source: Department for Communities and Local Government: 0303 444 2121

18.18 Local authority capital expenditure and receipts
England
Final outturn: Year ending 31 March

£ million

		2003 /04	2004 /05	2005 /06	2006 /07	2007 /08	2008 /09
Expenditure[1]							
Education	KRUD	2 780	3 087	3 492	3 442	3 711	4 542
Personal Social Services	KRUE	260	285	387	364	411	300
Transport[2]	KRUC	2 552	2 906	3 461	3 480	5 916	4 735
Housing[3]	KRUB	3 485	3 987	4 534	4 507	5 008	4 901
Arts and libraries	GEKZ	196	227	329	296	321	356
Agriculture and fisheries	GELA	72	66	93	96	85	82
Sport and recreation	KRUH	263	305	424	415	446	496
Other[4]	GELB	2 056	2 725	3 218	3 052	3 342	3 427
Fire and rescue	GELC	68	81	96	126	169	167
Police[5]	GELD	513	561	606	531	550	794
Magistrates courts	GELE	37	46	1	–	–	–
Total	KRUR	12 282	14 276	16 641	16 307	19 958	19 801
Receipts[6]							
Education	KRUT	221	210	217	261	272	102
Personal social services	KRUV	74	75	85	85	100	45
Transport	KRUU	92	101	87	130	301	41
Housing	KRUS	3 622	3 193	2 179	1 769	1 696	487
Arts and libraries	GELF	5	10	7	10	13	5
Agriculture and fisheries	GELG	53	45	63	65	69	39
Sport and recreation	KRUX	7	11	48	51	78	23
Other[4]	GELH	1 145	931	987	1 172	1 316	523
Fire and rescue	GELI	18	6	8	9	20	17
Police	GELJ	78	71	96	117	126	70
Magistrates court	GELK	6	8	1	–	..	1
Total[7]	KRVB	5 322	4 661	3 777	3 671	3 992	1 353

1 Includes aquisition of share and loan capital.
2 For 2007-08 Transport includes an exceptional item, the payment by the GLA (TfL) of £1.7 billion to Metronet.
3 For 2007-08 Housing includes an exceptional item, Liverpool's transfer of its housing stock to a registered social landlord which had the effect of increasing expenditure in 2007-08 by £500million.
4 Environmental services, consumer protection and employment services.
5 For 2008-09 Police includes a one-off acquisition of land and existing buildings by the Metropolitan Police.

6 Includes disposal of share and loan capital and disposal of other investments.
7 In 2008-09 capital receipts fell to £1.4 billion, a year on year decrease of 66%. This fall reflects the effect of the economic climate over that period on local authority sales of assets.

Source: Department for Communities and Local Government: 0303 444 2121

18.19 Local authorities capital expenditure and receipts
Wales
Final outturn: Year ending 31 March

£ million

		2004 /05	2005 /06	2006 /07	2007 /08	2008 /09	2009 /10
Expenditure							
Education	IY8Q	143.8	161.1	185.8	189.8	199.1	213.6
Social services	IY8R	16.8	20.5	18.7	18.5	28.4	25.4
Transport	IY8S	141.2	203.4	214.0	237.6	134.6	146.1
Housing	IY8T	242.3	257.5	267.0	247.1	224.0	217.1
Local environmental services	IY8U	272.8	298.3	354.9	409.7	325.1	263.8
Law, order and protective services	IY8V	43.4	41.5	36.5	43.1	71.6	61.7
Total expenditure	IY8W	860.3	982.3	1 077.0	1 145.9	982.8	927.7
Receipts							
Education	IY8X	10.2	4.6	6.1	12.2	14.7	3.6
Social services	IY8Y	1.3	0.2	3.7	1.5	..	..
Transport	IY8Z	1.2	4.5	0.8	0.4	10.2	9.3
Housing	IY92	147.7	88.2	75.1	54.9	38.5	7.3
Local environmental services	IY93	55.3	69.5	131.1	100.0	103.4	40.6
Law, order and protective services	IY94	1.2	1.4	1.1	4.2	16.0	2.7
Total receipts	IY95	216.8	168.5	218.0	173.2	185.6	66.6

Source: Welsh Assembly Government: 029 2082 5355

18.20 Expenditure of local authorities
Scotland

Years ending 31 March

£ thousand

		1999/00	2000/01	2001/02	2002/03	2003/04	2004/05	2005/06	2006/07	2007/08	2008/09
Out of revenue:[1] Total	KQTA	10 439 999	10 924 634	11 553 927	12 858 533	13 658 834	14 527 867	15 746 429	15 986 751	16 578 249	17 403 496
General Fund Services:	KQTB	7 429 626	7 884 168	8 428 217	9 290 268	10 139 679	10 964 598	12 021 453	12 143 056	12 653 585	13 255 975
Education	KQTC	2 855 945	3 037 780	3 283 827	3 533 853	3 872 786	4 180 675	4 406 876	4 596 832	4 747 148	4 869 127
Libraries, museums and galleries	KQTD	131 696	134 174	138 318	152 308	160 540	161 650	168 953	164 976	163 185	170 177
Social work	KQTE	1 519 191	1 632 843	1 793 732	2 173 752	2 400 652	2 621 134	2 808 040	2 994 486	3 192 214	3 408 851
Law, order and protective services	KQTF	1 006 000	1 047 034	1 088 791	1 130 693	1 226 067	1 306 085	1 501 854	1 469 644	1 506 432	1 631 037
Roads and Transport[2]	KQTG	527 018	564 738	506 326	601 454	611 721	635 329	673 167	625 341	633 828	678 922
Environmental services	KQTH	373 050	393 333	414 975	484 177	525 556	581 220	635 475	670 308	708 736	757 555
Planning	KQTI	198 285	194 771	223 414	265 315	282 572	299 182	351 617	366 803	372 445	437 261
Leisure and recreation	KQTJ	375 579	387 115	401 904	426 495	472 120	494 237	520 612	543 047	547 132	572 111
Other services	KQTL	435 155	465 612	572 136	515 661	585 425	681 288	948 167	702 554	782 035	730 934
Other general fund expenditure[3]	KQTM	7 707	26 768	4 794	6 560	2 240	3 798	6 692	9 065	430	–
Housing	KQTN	1 821 380	1 886 189	1 954 444	2 224 209	2 295 005	2 459 146	2 609 228	2 740 592	2 788 537	2 976 629
Trading services:	KQTO	87 321	80 355	61 899	74 062	92 782	106 445	103 461	102 336	100 104	110 042
Passenger transport	KQTR	336	162	343	427	441	282	353	355	315	397
Ferries	KQTS	9 709	10 005	9 650	11 493	11 768	13 759	14 308	18 483	21 907	23 872
Harbours, docks and piers	KQTT	15 923	13 604	10 912	12 222	13 405	12 407	11 995	8 495	8 312	276
Road bridges	KQTV	8 231	8 606	6 914	7 267	11 235	13 276	12 366	16 279	22 005	17 189
Slaughterhouses	KQTW	4	..	..	..	..	..	..	..	..	..
Markets	KQTX	14 106	23 844	16 657	17 995	14 824	15 353	17 447	16 793	18 461	20 250
Other trading services	KQTY	39 012	24 134	17 423	24 658	41 109	51 368	46 992	41 931	29 104	48 058
Loan charges:[4] Total	KQTZ	1 109 379	1 100 690	1 114 161	1 269 994	1 131 368	997 678	1 012 287	1 000 767	1 036 023	1 060 851
Allocated to :											
General Fund services	KMHV	701 515	708 822	739 351	738 870	772 852	772 648	792 404	782 002	806 806	854 918
Housing	KMHW	402 936	386 512	369 943	525 201	348 180	212 440	210 856	214 395	201 297	197 776
Trading services	KMHX	4 928	5 356	4 867	5 923	10 336	12 590	9 027	4 370	27 920	8 157
On capital works:[4] Total	KQUA	816 473	802 672	929 631	972 049	1 052 310	1 264 031	1 572 281	1 952 249	2 182 509	2 554 081
General Fund Services:	KQUB	557 119	538 843	610 485	662 869	767 122	1 006 150	1 160 818	1 462 620	1 652 425	1 850 660
Education	KQUC	136 508	127 781	143 268	157 439	172 227	199 387	310 054	402 865	464 827	479 258
Libraries, museums and galleries	KQUD	10 261	5 834	8 683	19 018	12 043	24 796	22 762	24 210	29 963	39 583
Social work	KQUE	22 097	21 539	31 359	30 116	31 966	33 450	37 877	50 327	65 449	63 233
Law, order and protective services	KQUF	37 132	35 761	39 901	53 268	65 477	65 154	51 146	60 287	68 680	101 062
Roads and Transport	KQUG	108 500	117 485	147 975	147 357	200 278	258 071	308 366	418 987	484 669	479 769
Environmental services	KQUH	14 936	17 944	16 396	17 957	20 567	40 773	55 020	43 104	101 325	121 267
Planning	KQUI	52 045	47 684	33 312	40 241	36 496	61 544	76 043	66 063	121 596	124 060
Leisure and recreation	KQUJ	52 365	44 516	39 240	50 558	71 486	74 116	83 681	98 275	136 029	167 505
Administrative buildings and equipment	KQUK	35 824	34 633	53 189	68 438	48 896	64 414	84 569	113 896	..	..
Other services	KQUL	87 451	85 666	97 162	78 477	107 686	184 445	131 300	184 606	179 887	274 923
Housing	KQUM	255 019	255 189	300 054	284 418	261 715	241 107	382 697	454 838	507 905	680 657
Trading Services:	KQUN	4 335	8 640	19 092	24 762	23 473	16 774	28 766	34 791	22 179	22 764
Ferries	KQUR	1 030	23	467	1	111	608	195	547	..	..
Harbours, docks and piers	KQUS	1 389	6 192	15 898	20 361	19 503	12 024	12 899	5 855	..	..
Airports	KQUT	..	607	663	1 031	609	572	663	798	..	..
Shipping, Airports, Transport piers & Ferry Terminals	J96X	..	..	..	..	..	..	..	..	18 654	14 018
Road bridges	KQUU	600	964	882	2 386	2 395	442	12 106	22 865	–	–
Slaughterhouses	KQUV	12	..	40	116	82	–	–	–	–	..
Other trading services	KMHY	1 304	854	1 142	867	773	3 128	2 903	4 726	3 525	8 746

1 Gross expenditure *less* inter-authority and inter-account transfers.
2 Including general fund support for transport (LA and NON-LA).
3 General fund contributions to Housing and Trading services (excluding transport), are also included in the expenditure figures for these services.
4 Expenditure out of loans, government grants and other capital receipts.

Source: Scottish Government, Statistical Support for Local Government: 0131 244 7033

18.21 Income of local authorities: classified according to source
Scotland

Years ending 31 March

£ thousand

		1998/99	1999/00	2000/01	2001/02	2002/03	2003/04	2004/05	2005/06	2006/07	2007/08	2008/09
Revenue account												
Non-Domestic Rates[1]	KQXA	1 437 646	1 440 522	1 662 691	1 553 926	1 718 104	1 804 423	1 895 941	1 897 073	1 883 769	1 859 727	1 962 800
Council tax	KPUC	1 146 366	1 193 693	1 273 316	1 363 399	1 459 212	1 532 071	1 614 808	1 720 305	1 811 577	1 889 913	1 908 972
Government grants												
General Revenue Funding[2]	KQXC	3 483 815	3 537 043	3 440 842	3 935 328	4 557 867	5 037 140	5 266 054	5 567 902	5 777 204	6 169 645	7 425 884
Council tax rebate grants	KPUD	274 940	275 789	279 459	285 131	293 606	307 733	344 899	354 067	359 159	354 030	351 165
Other grants and subsidies	KQXI	1 642 045	1 778 216	1 891 839	2 061 297	2 141 543	2 479 311	2 823 820	2 940 137	3 147 497	3 310 712	2 602 219
Sales	KQXJ	39 595	43 660	49 826	..	..	..	..	..	..	..	..
Fees and charges[3]	KQXK	1 668 223	1 682 385	1 776 455	1 789 428	1 954 337	1 785 672	1 845 161	1 951 315	2 039 217	2 125 114	2 253 653
Other income	KQXL	324 932	398 894	453 458	490 574	712 423	515 897	709 226	1 003 925	961 693	875 369	766 126
Capital account												
Sale of fixed assets	KQXM	335 037	303 582	149 504	165 016	207 388	222 844	355 069	366 302	451 353	513 913	229 805
Revenue contributions to capital	KQXP	204 982	213 564	210 912	147 760	239 778	212 533	219 593	247 693	199 749	173 668	196 836
Transfer from special funds	KMHZ	26 959	125 365	27 317	37 087	39 650	52 619	82 991	72 195	20 935	15 711	26 036
Other receipts[4]	KMGV	45 028	39 014	45 351	90 360	75 846	114 745	130 575	261 872	595 722	826 145	742 231

1 This is the Distributable Amount of Non-Domestic Rates.
2 Revenue Support Grant re-named General Revenue Funding from 2008-09.
3 From 2001-02 onwards, fees & charges incorporates sales.
4 Figures include public sector contributions from 2001-02 onwards.

Source: Scottish Government, Statistical Support for Local Government: 0131 244 7033

18.22 Income of local authorities from government grants[1]
Scotland

Year ending 31 March

£ thousand

		1999/00	2000/01	2001/02	2002/03	2003/04	2004/05	2005/06	2006/07	2007/08	2008/09
General fund services	KQYA	818 537	935 452	1 032 591	952 692	1 029 338	1 207 912	1 358 190	1 524 829	1 503 002	1 041 117
Education	KQYB	225 668	324 340	380 726	251 333	217 743	287 226	327 905	439 678	418 636	96 477
Libraries, museums and galleries	KQYC	507	634	1 137	5 359	1 517	763	818	1 394	1 523	1 869
Social work	KQYD	71 611	78 611	86 533	114 591	205 229	240 665	236 774	222 551	222 741	122 999
Law, order and protective services	KQYE	382 246	401 485	423 636	445 275	476 681	512 501	597 322	601 593	569 637	594 770
Roads and Transport[2]	KQYF	68 429	57 702	49 900	57 664	27 280	35 038	31 704	49 295	62 799	41 773
Environmental services	KQYG	71	301	2 272	5 407	18 120	39 971	45 338	55 173	59 112	7 219
Planning and Economic Development	KQYH	4 311	4 375	20 351	19 434	21 517	20 767	31 293	33 750	41 068	97 250
Leisure and recreation	KQYI	1 491	2 377	3 322	2 968	3 732	5 830	6 256	9 194	12 796	15 532
Other services	KQYK	64 203	65 627	64 714	50 661	57 619	65 151	80 780	112 201	114 690	63 228
Housing	KQYL	959 276	956 239	1 028 529	1 188 626	1 449 616	1 614 976	1 580 504	1 622 049	1 805 354	1 560 883
Trading services	KQYM	403	148	177	225	357	932	1 443	619	2 356	219
Grants not allocated to specific services[3]	KMGY	3 537 043	3 440 842	3 935 328	4 557 867	5 037 140	5 266 054	5 567 902	5 777 204	6 169 645	7 425 884
Total	KMGZ	5 315 259	5 332 681	5 996 625	6 699 410	7 516 451	8 089 874	8 508 039	8 924 701	9 480 357	10 028 103

1 Including grants for capital works.
2 Decrease in general fund services in 2008-09 is due to the rolling-up of ring-fenced grants into General Revenue Funding.
3 General revenue funding.

Source: Scottish Government, Statistical Support for Local Government: 0131 244 7033

18.23 Expenditure of local authorities
Northern Ireland

Years ending 31 March

£ thousand

		1997 /98	1998 /99	1999 /00	2000 /01	2001 /02	2002 /03	2003 /04	2004 /05	2005 /06	2006 /07	2007 /08
Libraries, museums and art galleries	KQVB	13 928	14 571	19 900	23 097	24 181	32 728	30 062	30 481	33 516	28 655	31 557
Environmental health services:												
Refuse collection and disposal	KQVC	56 246	56 360	62 226	65 289	73 336	90 148	94 715	102 633	113 768	121 879	136 181
Public baths	KQVD	2 585	2 634	1 750	1 724	1 423	..	..	..	..	..	..
Parks, recreation grounds, etc	KQVE	115 302	118 396	158 304	170 999	184 406	194 224	193 617	205 734	221 298	198 314	213 780
Other sanitary services	KQVF	39 682	42 923	44 214	45 552	48 784	52 075	55 349	59 906	66 294	68 641	74 624
Housing (grants and small dwellings												
acquisition)	KQVG	545	358	37	28	27	12	21	18	10	15	17
Trading services:												
Cemeteries	KQVI	5 626	5 887	5 973	6 151	6 538	7 208	7 980	8 455	8 520	7 752	8 726
Other trading services (including												
markets, fairs and harbours)	KQVJ	7 016	10 779	9 366	7 209	7 769	18 281	17 489	18 776	19 596	15 240	17 498
Miscellaneous	KQVK	63 375	161 790	86 649	89 881	98 244	79 645	114 971	105 031	128 304	141 717	160 606
Total expenditure	KQVA	304 305	413 698	388 419	409 930	444 708	474 321	490 619	531 034	591 306	582 213	642 991
Total loan charges	KQVL	34 823	26 413	..	..	..	..	..	..	..	..	..

Source: Department of the Environment for Northern Ireland: 028 9025 6086

External trade and investment

Chapter 19

External trade and investment

External trade

(Table 19.1 and 19.3 to 19.6)

The statistics in this section are on the basis of Balance of Payments (BoP). They are compiled from information provided to HM Revenue and Customs (HMRC) by importers and exporters on the basis of Overseas Trade Statistics (OTS) which values exports 'f.o.b.' (free on board) and imports 'c.i.f.' (including insurance and freight). In addition to deducting these freight costs and insurance premiums from the OTS figures, coverage adjustments are made to convert the OTS data to a BoP basis. Adjustments are also made to the level of all exports and European Union (EU) imports to take account of estimated under-recording. The adjustments are set out and described in the annual *United Kingdom Balance of Payments Pink Book* (Office for National Statistics (ONS)). These adjustments are made to conform to the definitions in the 5th edition of the *IMF Balance of Payments Manual*.

Aggregate estimates of trade in goods, seasonally adjusted and on a BoP basis, are published monthly in the ONS First Release UK Trade. More detailed figures are available from time series data on the ONS website (www.ons.gov.uk) and are also published in the Monthly Review of External Trade Statistics (Business Monitor MM24). Detailed figures for EU and non-EU trade on an OTS basis are published in *Overseas trade statistics: United Kingdom trade with the European Community and the world* (HMRC).

A fuller description of how trade statistics are compiled can be found in Statistics on *Trade in Goods* (Government Statistical Service Methodological Series) available at: www.statistics.gov.uk/STATBASE/Product.asp?vlnk=14943.

Overseas Trade Statistics

HMRC provide accurate and up to date information via the website: www.uktradeinfo.com

They also produce publications entitled 'Overseas Trade Statistics'.

Import penetration and export sales ratios

(Table 19.2)

The ratios were first introduced in the August 1977 edition of *Economic Trends* in an article entitled 'The Home and Export Performance of United Kingdom Industries'. The article described the conceptual and methodological problems involved in measuring such variables as import penetration.

The industries are grouped according to the 1992 Standard Industrial Classification. The four different ratios are defined as follows:

Ratio 1: percentage ratio of imports to home demand

Ratio 2: percentage ratio of imports to home demand plus exports

Ratio 3: percentage ratio of exports to total manufacturers' sales

Ratio 4: percentage ratio of exports to total manufacturers' sales plus imports

Home demand is defined as total manufacturers' sales plus imports minus exports. This is only an approximate estimate as different sources are used for the total manufacturers' sales and the import and export data. Total manufacturers' sales are determined by the Products of the European Community inquiry and import and export data are provided by HMRC.

Ratio 1 is commonly used to describe the import penetration of the home market. Allowance is made for the extent of a domestic industry's involvement in export markets by using Ratio 2; this reduces as exports increase.

Similarly, Ratio 3 is the measure normally used to relate exports to total sales by UK producers and Ratio 4 makes an allowance for the extent to which imports of the same product are coming into the UK.

International trade in services

(Tables 19.7 and 19.8)

These data relate to overseas trade in services and cover both production and non-production industries (excluding the public sector). In terms of the types of services traded these include royalties, various forms of consultancy, computing and telecommunications services, advertising and market research and other business services. A separate inquiry covers the film and television industries. The surveys cover receipts from the provision of services to residents of other countries (exports) and payments to residents of other countries for services rendered (imports).

Sources of data

The International Trade in Services (ITIS) surveys (which consist of a quarterly component addressed to the largest businesses and an annual component for the remainder) are based on a sample of companies derived from the Inter-departmental Business Register in addition to a reference list and from 2007 onwards a sample of approximately 5000 contributors from the Annual Business Inquiry (ABI). The companies are asked to show the amounts for their imports and exports against the geographical area to which they were paid or from which they were received, irrespective of where they were first earned.

The purpose of the ITIS survey is to record international transactions which impact on the UK's BoP. Exports and imports of goods are generally excluded, as they will have been counted in the estimate for Trade in Goods. However earnings from third country trade – that is, from arranging the sale of goods between two countries other than the UK and where the goods never physically enter the UK (known as merchanting) – are included. Earnings from commodity trading are also included. Together, these two comprise 'Trade Related Services'.

'Royalties' are a large part of the total trade in services collected in the ITIS survey. These cover transactions for items such as printed matter, sound recordings, performing rights, patents, licences, trademarks, designs, copyrights, manufacturing rights, the use of technical 'know-how' and technical assistance.

Balance of payments

(Tables 19.9 to 19.12)

Tables 19.9 to 19.12 are derived from *United Kingdom Balance of Payments: The Pink Book* 2009 edition. The following general notes to the tables provide brief definitions and explanations of the figures and terms used. Further notes are included in the *Pink Book*.

Summary of Balance of Payments

The BoP consists of the current account, the capital account, the financial account and the International Investment Position (IIP). The current account consists of trade in goods and services, income and current transfers. Income consists of investment income and compensation of employees. The capital account mainly consists of capital transfers and the financial account covers financial transactions. The IIP covers balance sheet levels of UK external assets and liabilities. Every credit entry in the balance of payments accounts should, in theory, be matched by a corresponding debit entry so that total current, capital and financial account credits should be equal to, and therefore offset by, total debits. In practice there is a discrepancy termed net errors and omissions.

The current account

Trade in goods

The goods account covers exports and imports of goods. Imports of motor cars from Japan, for example, are recorded as debits in the trade in goods account, whereas exports of vehicles manufactured in the UK are recorded as credits. Trade in goods forms a component of the expenditure measure of Gross Domestic Product (GDP).

Trade in services

The services account covers exports and imports of services, for example civil aviation. Passenger tickets for travel on UK aircraft sold abroad, for example, are recorded as credits in the services account, whereas the purchases of airline tickets from foreign airlines by UK passengers are recorded as debits. Trade in services, along with trade in goods, forms a component of the expenditure measure of GDP.

Income

The income account consists of compensation of employees and investment income and is dominated by the latter. Compensation of employees covers employment income from cross-border and seasonal workers which is less significant in the UK than in other countries. Investment income covers earnings (for example, profits, dividends and interest payments and receipts) arising from cross-border investment in financial assets and liabilities. For example, earnings on foreign bonds and shares held by financial institutions based in the UK are recorded as credits in the investment income account, whereas earnings on UK company securities held abroad are recorded as investment income debits. Investment income forms a component of Gross National Income (GNI) but not GDP.

Current transfers

Current transfers are composed of central government transfers (for example, taxes and payments to and receipts from, the EU) and other transfers (for example gifts in cash or kind received by private individuals from abroad or receipts from the EU where the UK government acts as an agent for the ultimate beneficiary of the transfer). Current transfers do not form a component either of GDP or of GNI. For example, payments to the UK farming industry under the EU Agricultural Guarantee Fund are recorded as credits in the current transfers account, while payments of EU agricultural levies by the UK farming industry are recorded as debits in the current transfers account.

External trade and investment

Capital account

Capital account transactions involve transfers of ownership of fixed assets, transfers of funds associated with acquisition or disposal of fixed assets and cancellation of liabilities by creditors without any counterparts being received in return. The main components are migrants transfers, EU transfers relating to fixed capital formation (regional development fund and agricultural guidance fund) and debt forgiveness. Funds brought into the UK by new immigrants would, for example, be recorded as credits in the capital account, while funds sent abroad by UK residents emigrating to other countries would be recorded as debits in the capital account. The size of capital account transactions are quite minor compared with the current and financial accounts.

Financial account

While investment income covers earnings arising from cross-border investments in financial assets and liabilities, the financial account of the balance of payments covers the flows of such investments. Earnings on foreign bonds and shares held by financial institutions based in the UK are, for example, recorded as credits in the investment income account, but the acquisition of such foreign securities by UK-based financial institutions are recorded as net debits in the financial account or portfolio investment abroad. Similarly, the acquisitions of UK company securities held by foreign residents are recorded in the financial account as net credits or portfolio investment in the UK.

International Investment Position

While the financial account covers the flows of foreign investments and financial assets and liabilities, the IIP records the levels of external assets and liabilities. While the acquisition of foreign securities by UK-based financial institutions are recorded in the financial account as net debits, the total holdings of foreign securities by UK-based financial institutions are recorded as levels of UK external assets. Similarly, the holdings of UK company securities held by foreign residents are recorded as levels of UK liabilities.

Foreign direct investment

(Tables 19.13 – 19.18)

Direct investment refers to investment that adds to, deducts from, or acquires a lasting interest in an enterprise operating in an economy other than that of the investor – the investor's purpose being to have an effective voice in the management of the enterprise. (For the purposes of the statistical inquiry, an effective voice is taken as equivalent to a holding of 10 per cent or more in the foreign enterprise.) Other investments in which the investor does not have an effective voice in the management of the enterprise are mainly portfolio investments and these are not covered here. Cross-border investment by public corporations or in property (which is regarded as direct investment in the national accounts) is not covered here, but is shown in the BoP. Similarly, foreign direct investment earnings data are shown net of tax in Tables 19.15 and 19.18 but are gross of tax in the BoP.

Direct investment is a financial concept and is not the same as capital expenditure on fixed assets. It covers only the money invested in a related concern by the parent company and the concern will then decide how to use the money. A related concern may also raise money locally without reference to the parent company.

The investment figures are published on a net basis; that is they consist of investments net of disinvestments by a company into its foreign subsidiaries, associate companies and branches.

Definitional changes from 1997

The new European System of Accounts (ESA(95)) definitions were introduced from the 1997 estimates. The changes were as follows:

i.   Previously, for the measurement of direct investment, an effective voice in the management of an enterprise was taken as the equivalent of a 20 per cent shareholding. This is now 10 per cent

ii. The Channel Islands and the Isle of Man have been excluded from the definition of the economic territory of the UK. Prior to 1987 these islands were considered to be part of the UK

iii. Interest received or paid was replaced by interest accrued in the figures on earnings from direct investment. There is deemed to be little or no impact arising from this definitional change on the estimates

New register sources available from 1998 have led to revisions of the figures from that year onwards. These sources gave an improved estimate of the population satisfying the criteria for foreign direct investment.

Definitional changes have been introduced from 1997 and the register changes from 1998. Data prior to these years have not been reworked in Tables 19.13 to 19.18. For clarity, the Offshore Islands are identified separately on the tables. Breaks in the series for the other definitional changes are not quantified but are relatively small. More detailed information on the effect of these changes appears in the business monitor MA4 – Foreign Direct Investment 2002, which was published in February 2003 and is available from the ONS website.

Sources of data

The figures in Tables 19.13 to 19.18 are based on annual inquiries into foreign direct investment for 2007. These were sample surveys which involved sending approximately 1,250 forms to UK businesses investing abroad, and 2,250 forms to UK businesses in which foreign parents and associates had invested. The tables also contain some revisions to 2006 as a result of new information coming to light in the course of the latest surveys. Further details from the latest annual surveys, including analyses by industry and by components of direct investment, are available in business monitor MA4. Initial figures were published on the ONS website in a First Release *Foreign Direct Investment 2008* in December 2009. Data for 2008 will be published in a First Release in December 2009, followed by the full business monitor MA4 in February 2009.

Country allocation

The analysis of inward investment is based on the country of ownership of the immediate parent company. Thus, inward investment in a UK company may be attributed to the country of the intervening overseas subsidiary, rather than the country of the ultimate parent. Similarly, the country analysis of outward investment is based on the country of ownership of the immediate subsidiary; for example, to the extent that overseas investment in the UK is channelled through holding companies in the Netherlands, the underlying flow of investment from this country is overstated and the inflow from originating countries is understated.

Further information

More detailed statistics on foreign direct investment are available on request from Richard Tonkin, Office for National Statistics, International Transactions Branch, Room 2.364, Government Buildings, Cardiff Road, Newport, South Wales, United Kingdom, NP10 8XG. Telephone: +44 (0)1633 456082, fax: +44 (0)1633 812855, email Richard.tonkin@ons.gov.uk.

19.1 Trade in goods[1]
United Kingdom
Balance of payments basis

£ million and indices (2005=100)

		1999	2000	2001	2002	2003	2004	2005	2006	2007	2008	2009
Value (£ million)												
Exports of goods	BOKG	166 166	187 936	189 093	186 524	188 320	190 874	211 608	243 633	220 858	251 643	227 670
Imports of goods	BOKH	195 217	220 912	230 305	234 229	236 927	251 774	280 197	319 945	310 612	345 024	309 460
Balance on trade in goods	BOKI	−29 051	−32 976	−41 212	−47 705	−48 607	−60 900	−68 589	−76 312	−89 754	−93 381	−81 790
Price index numbers												
Exports of goods	BQKR	94.1	95.2	94.1	94.0	95.8	95.8	100.0	102.5	103.4	118.0	121.0
Imports of goods	BQKS	97.0	100.2	99.4	96.8	96.2	95.7	100.0	103.5	104.6	118.4	121.9
Terms of trade[2]	BQKT	_97.0_	_95.0_	_94.7_	_97.1_	_99.6_	_100.1_	_100.0_	_99.0_	_98.9_	_99.7_	_99.3_
Volume index numbers												
Exports of goods	BQKU	80.1	89.9	91.8	90.7	90.5	91.9	100.0	111.5	100.4	100.8	89.0
Imports of goods	BQKV	71.2	77.9	82.0	85.8	87.4	93.5	100.0	110.4	107.2	105.2	91.8

1 See chapter text. Statistics of trade in goods on a balance of payments basis are obtained by making certain adjustments in respect of valuation and coverage to the statistics recorded in the _Overseas Trade Statistics._ These adjustments are described in detail in _The Pink Book 2009._
2 Export price index as a percentage of the import price index.

Source: Office for National Statistics: 01633 456294

19.2 Import penetration and export sales ratios for products of manufacturing industry[1,2]

United Kingdom: Standard Industrial Classification 1992

Ratios

			2005	2006	2007
Ratio 1 Imports/Home Demand		SIC Division			
Other mining and quarrying	BBAM	14	212	182	162
Food products and beverages	BBAN	15	26	27	28
Tobacco products	BBAO	16	17	15	15
Textiles	BAZJ	17	77	77	79
Wearing apparel: Dressing and dyeing of fur	BAZK	18	104	107	110
Tanning and dressing of leather: Luggage, handbags, saddlery, harness and footwear	BBAP	19	109	111	112
Wood products of wood and cork (except furniture) articles of straw and plaiting materials	BBAQ	20	35	33	36
Pulp, paper and paper products	BBAR	21	42	44	44
Publishing, printing and reproduction of recorded media	BBAS	22	6	6	7
Chemicals and chemical products	BAZL	24	91	95	97
Rubber and plastic products	BBAT	25	35	37	39
Other non metallic mineral products	BBAU	26	25	26	26
Basic metals	BBAV	27	90	88	98
Fabricated metal products (except machinery and equipment)	BBAW	28	24	27	27
Machinery and equipment not elsewhere classified	BBAX	29	67	72	74
Office machinery and computers	BBAY	30	150	232	151
Electrical machinery not elsewhere classified	BBAZ	31	68	74	76
Radio, television and communication equipment and apparatus	BBBA	32	184	−619	104
Medical, precision and optical instruments, watches and clocks	BBBB	33	85	96	86
Motor vehicles, trailers and semi-trailers	BBBC	34	70	71	74
Other transport equipment	BBBD	35	77	117	99
Furniture and manufacturing not elsewhere classified	BBBE	36	69	72	74
Total	BAZY		59	66	62
Ratio 2 Imports/Home Demand plus Exports					
Other mining and quarrying	BBBH	14	64	63	60
Food products and beverages	BBBI	15	23	24	25
Tobacco products	BBBJ	16	12	12	13
Textiles	BAZN	17	56	56	58
Wearing apparel: Dressing and dyeing of fur	BAZO	18	84	85	87
Tanning and dressing of leather: Luggage, handbags, saddlery, harness and footwear	BBBK	19	87	88	88
Wood products of wood and cork (except furniture) articles of straw and plaiting materials	BBBL	20	33	31	35
Pulp, paper and paper products	BBBM	21	36	38	38
Publishing, printing and reproduction of recorded media	BBBN	22	5	5	6
Chemicals and chemical products	BAZP	24	46	45	50
Rubber and plastic products	BBBO	25	28	29	31
Other non metallic mineral products	BBBP	26	22	22	23
Basic metals	BBBQ	27	49	53	54
Fabricated metal products (except machinery and equipment)	BBBR	28	21	22	23
Machinery and equipment not elsewhere classified	BBBS	29	42	43	44
Office machinery and computers	BBBT	30	77	84	88
Electrical machinery not elsewhere classified	BBBU	31	44	46	47
Radio, television and communication equipment and apparatus	BBBV	32	70	73	71
Medical, precision and optical instruments, watches and clocks	BBBW	33	47	50	48
Motor vehicles, trailers and semi-trailers	BBBX	34	48	49	51
Other transport equipment	BBBY	35	42	50	49
Furniture and manufacturing not elsewhere classified	BBBZ	36	53	55	56
Total	BBBF		41	43	44

19.2
continued

Import penetration and export sales ratios for products of manufacturing industry[1,2]

United Kingdom: Standard Industrial Classification 1992

Ratios

		SIC Division	2005	2006	2007
Ratio 3 Exports/Sales					
Other mining and quarrying	BBCM	14	195	178	158
Food products and beverages	BBCN	15	15	15	16
Tobacco products	BBCO	16	35	25	18
Textiles	BAZR	17	62	62	63
Wearing apparel: Dressing and dyeing of fur	BAZS	18	121	136	160
Tanning and dressing of leather: Luggage, handbags, saddlery, harness and footwear	BBCP	19	157	168	180
Wood products of wood and cork (except furniture) articles of straw and plaiting materials	BBCQ	20	6	6	6
Pulp, paper and paper products	BBCR	21	22	22	22
Publishing, printing and reproduction of recorded media	BBCS	22	9	8	9
Chemicals and chemical products	BAZT	24	92	96	97
Rubber and plastic products	BBCT	25	27	28	30
Other non metallic mineral products	BBCU	26	18	19	19
Basic metals	BBCV	27	89	85	97
Fabricated metal products (except machinery and equipment)	BBCW	28	18	20	19
Machinery and equipment not elsewhere classified	BBCX	29	65	71	72
Office machinery and computers	BBCY	30	209	398	350
Electrical machinery not elsewhere classified	BBDK	31	63	71	72
Radio, television and communication equipment and apparatus	BBDL	32	206	421	110
Medical, precision and optical instruments, watches and clocks	BBDM	33	84	96	85
Motor vehicles, trailers and semi-trailers	BBDN	34	60	61	63
Other transport equipment	BBDO	35	78	115	99
Furniture and manufacturing not elsewhere classified	BBDP	36	48	52	56
Total	BBCK		52	61	53
Ratio 4 Exports/Sales plus Imports					
Other mining and quarrying	BBDS	14	70	65	63
Food products and beverages	BBDT	15	12	12	12
Tobacco products	BBDU	16	31	22	15
Textiles	BAZV	17	28	27	27
Wearing apparel: Dressing and dyeing of fur	BAZW	18	20	20	21
Tanning and dressing of leather: Luggage, handbags, saddlery, harness and footwear	BBDV	19	21	21	22
Wood products of wood and cork (except furniture) articles of straw and plaiting materials	BBDW	20	4	4	4
Pulp, paper and paper products	BBDX	21	14	14	14
Publishing, printing and reproduction of recorded media	BBDY	22	8	8	9
Chemicals and chemical products	BAZX	24	50	52	49
Rubber and plastic products	BBDZ	25	19	20	21
Other non-metallic mineral products	BBEA	26	14	15	14
Basic metals	BBEB	27	45	40	44
Fabricated metal products (except machinery and equipment)	BBEC	28	14	16	14
Machinery and equipment not elsewhere classified	BBED	29	38	41	41
Office machinery and computers	BBEE	30	49	64	42
Electrical machinery not elsewhere classified	BBEF	31	35	38	38
Radio, television and communication equipment and apparatus	BBEG	32	62	112	32
Medical, precision and optical instruments, watches and clocks	BBEH	33	45	48	44
Motor vehicles, trailers and semi-trailers	BBEI	34	31	31	31
Other transport equipment	BBEJ	35	45	57	50
Furniture and manufacturing not elsewhere classified	BBEK	36	22	24	24
Total	BBDQ		30	35	30

1 See chapter text.
2 Division 13 (Mining of metal ores) has not been published since 1995. Division 23 (Coke, refined petroleum products and nuclear fuel) and SIC 24610 (Manufacture of explosives) are excluded from the analysis. SIC 27100 (Basic iron and steel and ferro-alloys) is not incorporated in PRODCOM and therefore also does not form part of the analysis.

Source: Office for National Statistics: 01633 456746

19.3 United Kingdom exports: by commodity[1,2]
Seasonally adjusted

£ million

		2000	2001	2002	2003	2004	2005	2006	2007	2008	2009
0. Food and live animals	BOGG	5 827	5 491	5 693	6 478	6 461	6 552	6 770	7 374	8 681	9 168
of which:											
01. Meat and meat preparations	BOGS	642	428	516	606	667	729	754	839	1 165	1 267
02. Dairy products and eggs	BQMS	660	614	625	760	780	718	712	807	885	835
04 & 08. Cereals and animal feeding stuffs	BQMT	1 604	1 383	1 444	1 681	1 553	1 554	1 587	1 791	2 283	2 344
05. Vegetables and fruit	BQMU	403	401	433	475	507	515	586	606	695	765
1. Beverages and tobacco	BQMZ	4 081	4 139	4 300	4 401	4 116	4 095	4 175	4 395	5 027	5 352
11. Beverages	BQNB	3 065	3 218	3 320	3 478	3 354	3 481	3 715	4 093	4 580	4 948
12. Tobacco	BQOW	1 016	921	980	923	762	614	460	302	447	404
2. Crude materials	BQOX	2 447	2 422	2 645	3 069	3 565	3 746	4 621	5 196	6 266	4 832
of which:											
24. Wood, lumber and cork	BQOY	72	70	81	106	117	131	146	144	126	84
25. Pulp and waste paper	BQOZ	78	81	106	180	244	283	338	417	481	357
26. Textile fibres	BQPA	496	440	472	492	520	516	542	499	543	576
28. Metal ores	BQPB	759	810	928	1 193	1 604	1 713	2 418	2 898	3 665	2 522
3. Fuels	BOPN	17 057	16 386	16 000	16 558	17 885	21 496	25 301	24 700	35 684	26 902
33. Petroleum and petroleum products	ELBL	15 584	14 815	14 321	14 608	16 200	19 794	23 173	22 756	32 145	24 529
32, 34 & 35. Coal, gas and electricity	BOQI	1 473	1 571	1 679	1 950	1 685	1 702	2 128	1 944	3 539	2 373
4. Animal and vegetable oils and fats	BQPI	156	149	210	266	205	235	271	327	360	386
5. Chemicals	ENDG	24 992	27 514	28 386	31 373	32 009	33 388	37 179	38 891	43 785	47 018
of which:											
51. Organic chemicals	BQPJ	5 718	6 090	5 698	6 070	6 040	6 702	8 009	7 601	8 389	9 107
52. Inorganic chemicals	BQPK	1 491	1 636	1 367	1 460	1 543	1 555	2 143	2 830	2 983	2 847
53. Colouring materials	CSCE	1 555	1 521	1 583	1 627	1 630	1 635	1 602	1 672	1 837	1 699
54. Medicinal products	BQPL	7 217	9 067	10 103	11 897	12 325	12 320	13 786	14 507	17 228	20 407
55. Toilet preparations	CSCF	2 597	2 714	2 823	3 122	3 105	3 219	3 443	3 689	3 945	4 144
57 & 58. Plastics	BQQA	3 366	3 416	3 526	3 703	3 847	4 298	4 445	4 612	4 859	4 403
6. Manufactures classified chiefly by material	BQQB	22 673	22 781	21 837	23 119	24 458	26 492	27 664	29 378	32 394	24 634
of which:											
63. Wood and cork manufactures	BQQC	255	261	270	322	291	255	273	272	243	222
64. Paper and paperboard manufactures	BQQD	2 096	2 081	2 019	2 097	1 996	2 043	2 014	2 124	2 335	2 271
65. Textile manufactures	BQQE	3 051	3 022	2 847	2 956	2 847	2 647	2 680	2 589	2 591	2 381
67. Iron and steel	BQQF	2 848	2 879	2 916	3 319	4 245	5 183	5 131	6 016	6 853	4 596
68. Non-ferrous metals	BQQG	3 171	3 033	2 552	2 567	3 228	3 862	4 827	5 778	6 866	3 987
69. Metal manufactures	BQQH	3 595	3 853	3 660	3 766	3 856	4 066	4 520	4 665	5 045	4 272
7. Machinery and transport equipment[3]	BQQI	87 812	87 240	84 395	79 650	78 376	89 379	110 393	82 713	89 189	79 595
71 - 716, 72, 73 & 74. Mechanical machinery	BQQK	22 140	24 244	22 704	24 231	23 808	25 795	28 244	28 969	32 273	29 353
716, 75, 76 & 77. Electrical machinery	BQQL	42 681	41 997	38 706	30 651	28 624	37 120	55 336	24 215	25 280	24 200
78. Road vehicles	BQQM	15 604	13 845	16 316	17 474	18 489	19 439	19 334	21 114	22 477	17 104
79. Other transport equipment	BQQN	7 387	7 154	6 669	7 294	7 455	7 025	7 479	8 415	9 159	8 938
8. Miscellaneous manufactures[3]	BQQO	21 206	21 948	21 985	22 543	22 917	25 105	25 973	26 695	28 468	27 779
of which:											
84. Clothing	CSCN	2 722	2 578	2 507	2 708	2 729	2 712	2 877	3 100	3 305	3 440
85. Footwear	CSCP	514	484	452	426	419	470	522	541	623	729
87 & 88. Scientific and photographic	BQQQ	7 333	7 775	7 212	7 281	7 040	7 245	7 344	7 063	8 062	8 318
9. Other commodities and transactions	BOQL	1 685	1 023	1 073	863	882	1 120	1 286	1 189	1 789	2 004
Total United Kingdom exports	BOKG	187 936	189 093	186 524	188 320	190 874	211 608	243 633	220 858	251 643	227 670

1 See chapter text. The numbers on the left hand side of the table refer to the code numbers of the *Standard International Trade Classification*, Revision 3, which was introduced in January 1988.
2 Balance of payments consistent basis.
3 Sections 7 and 8 are shown by broad economic category in table G2 of the *Monthly Review of External Trade Statistics*.

Source: Office for National Statistics: 01633 456294

19.4 United Kingdom imports: by commodity[1,2]
Seasonally adjusted

£ million

		2000	2001	2002	2003	2004	2005	2006	2007	2008	2009
0. Food and live animals	BQQR	13 310	14 269	14 874	16 452	17 211	18 593	19 814	21 324	25 287	26 346
of which:											
01. Meat and meat preparations	BQQS	2 366	2 689	2 793	3 267	3 441	3 619	3 800	3 992	4 618	4 877
02. Dairy products and eggs	BQQT	1 165	1 245	1 291	1 501	1 609	1 700	1 808	1 837	2 281	2 320
04 & 08. Cereals and animal feeding stuffs	BQQU	1 762	1 957	1 985	2 219	2 307	2 363	2 497	2 918	3 814	3 948
05. Vegetables and fruit	BQQV	3 894	4 101	4 374	4 766	4 919	5 447	5 783	6 204	7 054	7 060
1. Beverages and tobacco	BQQW	4 350	4 216	4 501	4 735	4 939	5 102	5 199	5 423	5 831	6 014
11. Beverages	EGAT	2 910	2 854	3 028	3 237	3 474	3 625	3 701	3 942	4 318	4 431
12. Tobacco	EMAI	1 440	1 362	1 473	1 498	1 465	1 477	1 498	1 481	1 513	1 583
2. Crude materials	ENVB	5 816	5 921	5 420	5 525	5 716	6 129	7 116	8 663	9 595	6 542
of which:											
24. Wood, lumber and cork	ENVC	1 193	1 168	1 236	1 366	1 337	1 358	1 453	1 805	1 410	1 164
25. Pulp and waste paper	EQAH	763	606	488	489	480	477	512	503	595	436
26. Textile fibres	EQAP	412	393	361	337	339	314	298	315	335	287
28. Metal ores	EHAA	1 811	1 997	1 448	1 430	1 647	1 999	2 672	3 790	4 658	2 262
3. Fuels	BQAT	10 016	10 795	10 279	12 311	17 547	25 921	30 888	31 928	48 578	35 199
33. Petroleum and petroleum products	ENXO	9 048	9 525	9 213	11 232	15 307	21 989	25 967	26 787	38 013	27 766
32, 34 & 35. Coal, gas and electricity	BPBI	968	1 270	1 066	1 079	2 240	3 932	4 921	5 141	10 565	7 433
4. Animal and vegetable oils and fats	EHAB	491	521	538	614	622	641	771	898	1 399	1 058
5. Chemicals	ENGA	20 633	22 745	23 987	26 139	27 929	29 208	31 727	34 645	37 928	38 992
of which:											
51. Organic chemicals	EHAC	5 374	5 529	5 673	6 102	6 802	7 183	7 692	8 620	8 460	8 318
52. Inorganic chemicals	EHAE	1 046	1 171	1 070	1 094	1 367	1 507	2 123	2 679	2 756	2 752
53. Colouring materials	CSCR	1 002	975	952	1 003	1 060	1 072	1 090	1 164	1 228	1 137
54. Medicinal products	EHAF	4 714	6 149	7 288	8 189	8 372	8 504	9 158	9 943	11 049	13 129
55. Toilet preparations	CSCS	2 005	2 261	2 499	2 745	2 881	3 035	3 336	3 448	3 915	4 165
57 & 58. Plastics	EHAG	4 144	4 096	4 063	4 403	4 749	5 038	5 409	5 699	6 219	5 590
6. Manufactures classified chiefly by material	EHAH	29 232	30 165	28 735	29 906	32 299	33 469	37 615	39 792	41 910	35 646
of which:											
63. Wood and cork manufactures	EHAI	1 245	1 340	1 436	1 449	1 585	1 505	1 575	1 733	1 731	1 477
64. Paper and paperboard manufactures	EHAJ	4 407	4 864	4 582	4 747	4 841	4 820	5 037	5 248	5 492	5 450
65. Textile manufactures	EHAK	4 365	4 303	4 149	4 089	4 124	3 844	4 018	4 084	4 073	3 816
67. Iron and steel	EHAL	2 731	3 051	3 047	3 237	4 199	4 402	4 981	5 958	6 575	3 832
68. Non-ferrous metals	EHAM	3 711	3 780	3 222	3 320	3 616	3 923	6 185	6 230	6 419	6 198
69. Metal manufactures	EHAN	4 065	4 324	4 501	4 765	4 977	5 355	5 852	6 563	6 985	5 942
7. Machinery and transport equipment[3]	EHAO	102 420	105 386	107 556	101 473	103 882	117 118	139 826	117 726	121 009	106 871
71 - 716, 72, 73 & 74. Mechanical machinery	EHAQ	17 867	18 618	18 901	18 951	19 725	21 848	22 613	25 776	28 916	24 179
716, 75, 76 & 77. Electrical machinery	EHAR	53 631	50 842	49 917	43 656	45 495	55 535	75 086	46 006	47 588	44 663
78. Road vehicles	EHAS	23 117	26 289	28 449	29 921	30 734	31 436	32 674	36 590	33 924	26 041
79. Other transport equipment	EHAT	7 805	9 637	10 289	8 945	7 928	8 299	9 453	9 354	10 581	11 988
8. Miscellaneous manufactures[3]	EHAU	32 798	35 023	36 889	38 168	39 822	42 175	44 919	47 939	50 921	50 063
of which:											
84. Clothing	CSDR	8 495	9 119	9 804	10 323	10 646	11 303	11 847	12 310	13 210	13 921
85. Footwear	CSDS	2 001	2 236	2 365	2 375	2 447	2 563	2 699	2 659	2 840	3 099
87 & 88. Scientific and photographic	EHAW	7 273	7 620	7 044	7 049	7 255	7 414	7 655	7 572	8 443	8 487
9. Other commodities and transactions	BQAW	1 846	1 264	1 450	1 604	1 807	1 841	2 070	2 274	2 566	2 729
Total United Kingdom imports	BOKH	220 912	230 305	234 229	236 927	251 774	280 197	319 945	310 612	345 024	309 460

1 See chapter text. The numbers on the left hand side of the table refer to the code numbers of the *Standard International Trade Classification,* Revision 3, which was introduced in January 1988.
2 Balance of payments consistent basis.
3 Sections 7 and 8 are shown by broad economic category in table G2 of the *Monthly Review of External Trade Statistics.*

Source: Office for National Statistics: 01633 456294

19.5 United Kingdom exports: by area[1,2]
Seasonally adjusted

£ million

		2000	2001	2002	2003	2004	2005	2006	2007	2008	2009
European Union:[3]	LGCK	112 459	114 406	114 737	111 286	111 650	121 486	152 357	127 813	141 428	124 509
EMU members:	QAKW	102 333	104 437	104 144	100 902	100 819	109 765	136 333	114 537	126 411	111 384
Austria	CHMY	1 146	1 224	1 265	1 264	1 095	1 332	1 699	1 376	1 468	1 283
Belgium & Luxembourg	CHNQ	10 322	9 893	10 552	11 374	10 510	11 394	15 082	12 122	13 579	11 058
Cyprus	BQGN	311	291	272	317	324	359	960	415	536	596
Finland	CHMZ	1 471	1 611	1 442	1 493	1 363	1 514	1 872	1 958	1 904	1 327
France	ENYL	18 577	19 249	18 757	18 885	18 562	19 931	28 693	18 103	18 117	17 162
Germany	ENYO	22 789	23 655	22 064	20 805	21 668	23 025	27 602	24 699	27 890	24 305
Greece	CHNT	1 267	1 156	1 234	1 286	1 408	1 367	1 469	1 350	1 661	1 626
Irish Republic	CHNS	12 372	13 835	15 422	12 224	14 134	16 294	17 480	17 801	19 069	15 915
Italy	CHNO	8 429	8 404	8 506	8 603	8 400	8 790	9 494	9 189	9 370	8 312
Malta	BQGY	206	215	228	260	259	240	319	362	449	393
Netherlands	CHNP	15 167	14 599	14 011	13 597	12 029	12 716	16 522	15 115	19 849	18 077
Portugal	CHNU	1 660	1 579	1 518	1 453	1 580	1 698	2 374	1 481	1 636	1 543
Slovakia	BQHB	157	203	201	237	224	259	272	382	457	377
Slovenia	BQHE	157	160	182	161	163	169	200	205	224	175
Spain	CHNV	8 302	8 363	8 490	8 943	9 100	10 677	12 295	9 979	10 202	9 233
Non-EMU members:[3]	BQIA	10 164	10 001	10 628	10 418	10 831	11 721	16 024	13 276	15 017	13 125
of which:											
Bulgaria	WYUF	85	122	134	154	155	220	237	202	253	200
Czech Rep	FKML	927	1 075	1 031	1 003	978	1 080	1 526	1 401	1 544	1 452
Denmark	CHNR	2 315	2 267	2 729	2 180	2 042	2 314	3 715	2 182	2 584	2 463
Estonia	AUEV	96	83	100	95	106	115	472	228	220	141
Hungary	QALC	613	612	750	856	934	834	855	863	1 008	852
Latvia	BQGQ	21 631	22 447	22 469	22 973	23 204	25 515	26 482	27 048	28 351	27 390
Lithuania	BQGU	131	137	149	189	142	167	238	311	282	174
Poland	ERDR	1 299	1 297	1 318	1 462	1 417	1 653	2 705	2 372	3 004	2 798
Romania	WMDB	381	341	432	509	609	647	637	668	755	689
Sweden	CHNA	4 211	3 951	3 873	3 823	4 356	4 588	5 246	4 904	5 198	4 247
Other Western Europe:	HCJD	7 223	6 786	6 334	6 629	7 031	9 730	9 221	9 232	10 757	9 628
of which:											
Iceland	EPLW	193	150	131	141	167	179	188	198	187	129
Norway	EPLX	2 018	1 813	1 696	1 886	1 939	2 211	2 125	2 697	2 850	2 806
Switzerland	EPLV	3 061	3 496	3 080	2 786	2 842	4 985	4 189	3 808	4 656	3 937
Turkey	EOBA	1 800	1 150	1 287	1 638	1 903	2 160	2 426	2 283	2 568	2 337
North America:	HBZQ	33 714	33 408	32 261	32 924	32 763	35 010	36 928	36 365	39 623	38 017
of which:											
Canada	EOBC	3 487	3 203	3 107	3 239	3 340	3 277	3 894	3 291	3 262	3 329
Mexico	EPJX	675	681	704	687	629	638	747	801	904	752
USA inc Puerto Rica	J9C5	29 549	29 519	28 452	28 997	28 794	31 095	32 287	32 274	35 436	33 868
Other OECD countries:	HCII	8 028	7 542	7 469	7 824	8 226	8 577	8 716	8 778	9 948	9 026
of which:											
Australia	EPMA	2 699	2 298	2 114	2 289	2 455	2 580	2 488	2 630	3 103	2 953
Japan	EOBD	3 672	3 673	3 583	3 710	3 863	3 900	4 109	3 866	3 908	3 562
New Zealand	EPMB	305	309	311	348	418	415	373	364	385	348
South Korea	ERDM	1 350	1 262	1 461	1 468	1 481	1 677	1 746	1 914	2 552	2 163
Oil exporting countries:	HDII	6 031	6 474	6 229	7 615	7 996	10 850	9 060	9 716	11 618	11 419
of which:											
Brunei	QALF	96	59	61	127	67	43	79	870	65	61
UAE inc Dubai	J8YH	1 568	1 617	1 600	2 044	2 689	5 440	3 550	2 700	3 833	3 624
Indonesia	FKMR	404	313	324	452	397	366	311	289	385	359
Kuwait	QATB	338	359	308	373	354	426	438	450	543	469
Nigeria	QATE	524	686	711	738	773	799	821	1 043	1 513	1 307
Saudi Arabia	ERDI	1 557	1 525	1 388	1 819	1 611	1 559	1 644	1 857	2 191	2 340
Rest of the World	HCHW	20 481	20 477	19 494	22 042	23 208	25 955	27 351	28 954	38 269	35 071
of which:											
Brazil	FKMO	775	808	880	825	789	836	918	1 108	1 694	1 786
China	ERDN	1 468	1 709	1 493	1 924	2 366	2 811	3 264	3 860	5 084	5 398
Egypt	QALL	498	452	463	458	667	543	577	686	944	1 001
Hong Kong	ERDG	2 673	2 683	2 411	2 481	2 630	3 087	2 864	2 726	3 676	3 736
India	ERDJ	2 058	1 772	1 755	2 284	2 234	2 798	2 693	2 968	4 135	2 948
Israel	ERDL	1 516	1 357	1 428	1 359	1 386	1 352	1 308	1 257	1 341	1 140
Malaysia	ERDK	907	1 029	877	1 028	991	1 088	877	975	1 135	1 046
Pakistan	FKMU	207	229	240	291	343	461	488	423	475	474
Philippines	FKMX	273	392	352	377	315	279	242	251	245	272
Russia	ERDQ	668	893	981	1 420	1 465	1 869	2 063	2 893	4 275	2 403
Singapore	ERDH	1 625	1 592	1 445	1 582	1 708	2 078	2 318	2 467	2 820	2 957
South Africa	EPME	1 413	1 534	1 597	1 766	1 874	2 073	2 184	2 244	2 658	2 252
Taiwan	ERDP	1 015	875	848	897	950	939	911	957	892	796
Thailand	ERDO	582	594	529	572	637	638	567	613	757	914

1 See chapter text.
2 Balance of payments consistent basis.
3 Includes Austria, Belgium, Bulgaria, Cyprus, Czech Republic, Denmark, Estonia, Finland, France, Germany, Greece, Hungary, Irish Republic, Italy, Latvia, Lithuania, Luxemburg, Malta, Netherlands, Poland, Portugal, Romania, Slovakia, Slovenia, Spain and Sweden.

Source: Office for National Statistics: 01633 456294

19.6 United Kingdom imports: by area[1,2]
Seasonally adjusted

£ million

		2000	2001	2002	2003	2004	2005	2006	2007	2008	2009
European Union:[3]	LGDC	117 644	126 973	136 931	137 404	142 523	158 163	183 749	169 799	180 896	161 555
EMU members	QAKX	106 290	114 901	123 927	123 483	127 065	139 911	158 092	149 719	157 883	140 278
Austria	CHNB	1 410	1 888	2 396	2 776	2 354	2 461	2 786	2 488	2 344	2 271
Belgium & Luxembourg	CHNY	10 927	12 159	13 201	13 205	13 846	15 155	18 183	15 820	17 325	15 761
Cyprus	BQGO	208	243	247	251	205	272	1 445	193	157	78
Finland	CHNC	2 765	2 965	2 791	2 663	2 336	2 431	3 118	2 619	2 784	2 497
France	ENYP	18 644	20 127	20 798	20 389	20 133	21 984	26 376	21 896	23 180	20 346
Germany	ENYS	28 462	30 192	32 442	33 667	35 381	39 169	42 660	44 565	44 647	39 603
Greece	CHOB	459	476	555	613	637	703	790	640	647	551
Irish Republic	CHOA	10 261	12 141	13 176	9 920	10 131	10 411	10 770	11 338	12 239	12 506
Italy	CHNW	9 514	9 860	10 675	11 481	12 184	12 673	12 775	13 316	14 148	12 102
Malta	BQGZ	126	144	168	185	184	177	161	179	138	108
Netherlands	CHNX	15 380	15 395	16 143	16 692	18 196	20 436	22 275	23 079	25 816	21 741
Portugal	CHOC	1 735	1 625	1 761	1 966	1 928	2 018	3 054	1 506	1 744	1 422
Slovakia	BQHC	136	177	211	259	261	370	815	1 273	1 627	1 566
Slovenia	BQHN	122	149	173	169	169	201	740	318	314	252
Spain	CHOD	6 141	7 360	9 190	9 247	9 120	11 450	12 144	10 489	10 773	9 493
Non-EMU members:[3]	BQIB	11 362	12 072	13 004	13 921	15 458	18 252	25 657	20 080	23 013	21 277
of which:											
Bulgaria	WYUT	85	101	116	124	150	169	208	239	207	176
Czech Rep	FKMM	802	1 097	1 250	1 412	1 291	1 883	2 987	2 983	3 577	3 399
Denmark	CHNZ	2 630	2 922	3 595	3 399	3 357	4 393	6 439	3 444	3 921	3 794
Estonia	BQGL	309	283	327	264	379	363	2 100	226	144	126
Hungary	QALD	683	710	846	1 120	1 579	1 860	2 348	2 377	2 524	2 159
Latvia	BQGR	406	439	485	525	693	725	833	605	376	303
Lithuania	BQGV	247	235	268	285	270	273	274	299	349	373
Poland	ERED	905	1 166	1 265	1 545	1 835	2 320	3 622	3 695	4 307	4 721
Romania	WMDC	336	448	522	679	786	803	861	938	806	783
Sweden	CHND	4 951	4 671	4 330	4 568	5 118	5 463	5 985	5 274	6 802	5 446
Other Western Europe:	HBTS	13 040	12 240	12 523	13 331	15 754	20 072	23 417	24 359	32 436	26 488
of which:											
Iceland	EPMW	365	281	289	296	355	346	402	415	458	481
Norway	EPMX	5 563	5 523	5 258	6 423	8 495	12 077	14 453	14 316	21 609	15 912
Switzerland	EPMV	5 485	4 544	4 595	3 759	3 447	3 884	4 372	4 746	5 256	5 231
Turkey	EOBU	1 450	1 669	2 164	2 619	3 250	3 510	3 946	4 632	4 874	4 581
North America:	HCRB	33 460	34 617	29 811	27 480	27 130	27 133	31 228	32 472	32 627	29 930
of which:											
Canada	EOBW	4 009	3 664	3 563	3 664	4 194	4 157	4 954	5 793	5 824	4 531
Mexico	EPJY	613	680	505	490	411	446	444	582	794	766
USA inc Puerto Rica	J9C6	28 838	30 270	25 742	23 326	22 525	22 530	25 830	26 095	26 009	24 613
Other OECD countries:	HDJQ	15 717	14 154	13 017	12 989	13 644	14 424	13 633	13 870	15 192	12 559
of which:											
Australia	EPNA	1 543	1 776	1 688	1 789	1 868	2 100	2 107	2 245	2 389	2 226
Japan	EOBX	10 214	9 080	8 079	8 085	8 109	8 669	7 857	7 885	8 546	6 660
New Zealand	EPNB	544	542	522	552	584	592	600	667	748	814
South Korea	ERDY	3 416	2 756	2 728	2 563	3 083	3 063	3 069	3 073	3 509	2 859
Oil exporting countries:	HCPC	4 258	3 969	3 780	3 923	4 866	6 017	6 992	6 387	7 995	7 637
of which:											
Brunei	QALG	95	35	33	51	63	25	70	57	27	47
UAE inc Dubai	J8YI	598	649	736	990	1 060	1 319	1 028	1 015	933	1 107
Indonesia	FKMS	1 081	1 128	1 006	875	918	839	958	925	1 184	1 196
Kuwait	QATC	314	296	271	313	396	367	741	696	1 090	731
Nigeria	QATF	89	65	90	83	106	152	206	271	911	632
Saudi Arabia	ERDU	977	933	677	715	1 158	1 714	1 232	821	673	596
Rest of the World	HCIF	36 793	38 352	38 167	41 800	47 857	54 388	60 926	63 725	75 878	71 291
of which:											
Brazil	FKMP	1 114	1 279	1 365	1 477	1 545	1 740	1 905	2 061	2 619	2 526
China	ERDZ	4 826	5 741	6 726	8 342	10 390	12 962	15 237	18 734	23 175	24 304
Egypt	QALM	411	406	416	432	495	349	662	538	640	679
Hong Kong	ERDS	5 917	5 754	5 561	5 500	5 761	6 602	7 338	6 939	8 081	7 663
India	ERDV	1 651	1 816	1 804	2 093	2 287	2 781	3 121	3 809	4 490	4 560
Israel	ERDX	1 025	939	880	861	920	1 002	965	1 045	1 155	1 082
Malaysia	ERDW	2 288	1 939	1 731	1 867	2 022	1 813	1 895	1 684	1 872	1 643
Pakistan	FKMV	363	421	472	519	554	487	511	512	630	692
Philippines	FKMY	1 155	1 155	944	713	655	712	742	717	629	394
Russia	EREC	1 496	2 047	1 950	2 454	3 506	5 010	5 740	5 248	6 928	4 609
Singapore	ERDT	2 395	2 067	1 959	2 672	3 379	3 828	3 756	4 247	4 007	3 542
South Africa	EPNE	2 553	2 841	2 685	2 949	3 272	3 937	3 904	3 060	4 739	3 801
Taiwan	EREB	3 561	2 784	2 385	2 198	2 341	2 226	2 339	2 418	2 598	2 241
Thailand	EREA	1 602	1 607	1 550	1 646	1 760	1 719	1 922	2 012	2 427	2 293

1 See chapter text.
2 Balance of payments consistent basis.
3 Includes Austria, Belguim, Bulgaria, Cyprus, Czech Republic, Denmark, Estonia, Finland, France, Germany, Greece, Hungary, Irish Republic, Italy, Latvia, Lithuania, Luxemburg, Malta, Netherlands, Poland, Portugal, Romania, Slovakia, Slovenia, Spain and Sweden.

Source: Office for National Statistics: 01633 456294

19.7 Services supplied (exports) and purchased (imports)[1,2]: 2007

£ million

	Exports	Imports	Net
Agricultural,Mining and On-site Processing services			
Agricultural	21	53	-33
Mining	85	16	68
Waste treatment and depollution	8	15	-8
Other on-slte processing services	347	86	261
Business and Professional services			
Accountancy,auditing, bookkeeping and tax consul	1 342	313	1 029
Advertising	1 972	1 534	437
Management consulting	1 185	424	761
Public relations services	211	60	151
Recruitment	388	141	247
Other Business Management	1 402	1 063	319
Legal Services	2 969	532	2 427
Market research and public opinion polling	426	268	158
Operational leasing services	375	462	-86
Procurement	216	234	-19
Property management	107	30	78
Research and development	5 271	2 235	3 006
Services between related enterprises	6 770	3 733	3 037
Other business and professional services	1 716	972	744
Communications services			
Postal and courier	396	669	-273
Telecommunications	2 740	2 501	239
Computer services			
Computer	4 695	2 366	2 329
Information services			
News agency services	596	36	561
Publishing services	344	91	253
Other information provision services	1 121	262	859
Construction Goods and Services			
Construction in the UK	133	369	-236
Construction outside the UK	863	436	428
Financial services			
Financial	10 371	3 257	7 114
Insurance Services			
Auxiliary services	1 546	96	1 450
Freight Insurance - Claims	1		1
Freigh Insurance - Premiums		13	-13
Life insurance and pension funding - Claims	1		1
Life insurance and pension funding - Premiums		5	-5
Reinsurance - Claims	13		13
Reinsurance - Premiums		34	-34
Other Direct insurance - Claims	37		37
Other Direct insurance - Premlums		161	-161
Merchanting and Other Trade related Services			
Merchanting	861		861
Other trade related services	1 630	438	1 192
Personal, Cultural and Recreational Services			
Audio-Visual and related services	162	70	92
Health services	6	7	-1
Training and educational services	37	14	23
Other personal, cultural and recreational services	361	105	256
Royalties and Licenses			
Use of Franchise and similar rights fees	1 571	1 751	-180
Other royalties and license fees	4 687	2 106	2 580
Purchases and sales of franchises and similar right	375	277	96
Purchases and sales of other royalties and licenses	407	516	-109
Technical services			
Architectural	272	12	260
Engineering	3 796	1 525	2 271
Surveying	107	28	79
Other technical services	1 086	510	576
Other Trade in Services			
Other Trade in services	2 581	1 281	1 299
World Total	**65 607**	**31 161**	**34 446**

1 Due to rounding, the sum of constituent items may not always equal the total shown.
2 Data excludes the following industries: Financial, Film and TV, Travel and
Transport, Public Sector (including Education). Note (-) Denotes nil or less
than £500,000. Note (..) Denotes disclosive data.

Source: Office for National Statistics: 01633 456644

19.8 International trade in services:[1,2] by country, 2007

£ million

	Receipts	Payments	Net
European Union			
Austria	598	147	451
Belgium	1 287	775	512
Bulgaria	85	43	42
Cyprus	155	101	54
Czech Republic	225	68	157
Denmark	570	191	379
Estonia	18	4	14
Finland	676	119	558
France	3 123	2 565	558
Germany	3 849	2 816	1 033
Greece	316	78	238
Hungary	212	116	96
Irish Republic	4 463	1 607	2 856
Italy	1 447	1 106	341
Latvia	22	8	14
Lithuania	18	23	-5
Luxembourg	1 053	228	826
Malta	30	15	15
Netherlands	4 121	1 191	2 930
Poland	226	252	-26
Portugal	267	143	124
Romania	112	24	87
Slovakia	52	18	34
Slovenia	..	..	11
Spain	1 198	636	563
Sweden	885	657	228
EU Institutions	..	..	3
Total European Union	**25029**	**12936**	**10293**
EFTA			
Iceland	63	5	58
Liechtenstein	52	29	23
Norway	1 027	310	717
Switzerland	3 553	1 120	2 433
Total EFTA	**4 695**	**1 464**	**3 231**
Other European countries			
Russia	682	284	398
Channel Islands	1 141	120	1 022
Isle of Man	118	13	106
Turkey	177	66	111
Rest of Europe	240	71	169
Europe Unallocated	2 185	1 120	1 065
Total Europe	**34 267**	**16 072**	**18 195**
Africa			
Nigeria	307	66	241
South Africa	517	180	337
Rest of Africa	987	283	705
Africa Unallocated	112	103	10
Total Africa	**1 924**	**632**	**1 292**
America			
Brazil	143	92	52
Canada	666	327	339
Mexico	127	37	90
USA	14 455	7 458	6 996
Rest of America	2 682	971	1 711
America Unallocated	420	134	286
Total America	**18 492**	**9 019**	**9 474**

19.8 International trade in services:[1,2] by country, 2007
continued

£ million

	Exports	Imports	Balances
Asia			
China	264	242	22
Hong Kong	383	460	-78
India	410	553	-142
Indonesia	72	18	54
Israel	200	147	53
Japan	1 201	999	202
Malaysia	151	40	111
Pakistan	55	17	38
Phillippines	34	38	-3
Saudi Arabia	1 592	542	1 050
Singapore	2 168	406	1 752
South Korea	300	117	184
Taiwan	120	126	-6
Thailand	108	49	59
Rest of Asia	2 099	856	1 244
Asia Unallocated	378	292	86
Total Asia	**9 536**	**4 900**	**4 636**
Australiasia and Oceania			
Australia	1 127	406	721
New Zealand	89	37	52
Rest of Australia and Oceania	36	9	27
Oceania Unallocated	10	2	8
Total Australasia and Oceania	**1 261**	**454**	**808**
Rest of World Unallocated	..	..	42
International organisations	..	..	..
World Total	**65 607**	**31 161**	**34 446**
Economic Zones			
OECD	46 626	23 591.4	23 024.7
NAFTA	14 506	7 819.41	6 686.38
Central and Eastern Europe	1 041	593.681	447.002
OPEC	3 297	1 066.27	2 230.64
ASEAN	2 576	558.78	2017.38
CIS	1 288	557.307	731.101
NICs1	2 971	1108.97	1861.99
Offshore Financial centres	6 548	1 985.79	4 472.29
ACP	1 627	604.934	1 021.97

1 Due to rounding, the sum of constituent items may not always equal the total shown.

2 Data excludes the following industries: Financial, Film and TV, Travel and Transport, Public Sector (including Education) and Law Society Members Note (..) Denotes disclosive data. Note (-) Denotes nil or less than £500,000.

Source: Office for National Statistics: 01633 456644

19.9 Summary of balance of payments,[1] 2008
United Kingdom

£ million

	Credits	Debits
1. Current account		
A. Goods and services	388 838	421 315
1. Goods	227 670	309 460
2. Services	161 168	111 855
2.1. Transportation	21 348	18 177
2.2. Travel	19 292	31 117
2.3. Communications	5 199	4 585
2.4. Construction	1 472	1 644
2.5. Insurance	8 501	1 079
2.6. Financial	43 159	12 077
2.7. Computer and information	7 423	3 628
2.8. Royalties and licence fees	8 213	6 122
2.9. Other business	42 120	28 548
2.10. Personal, cultural and recreational	2 323	1 085
2.11. Government	2 118	3 793
B. Income	175 571	146 915
1. Compensation of employees	916	1 604
2. Investment income	174 655	145 311
2.1 Direct investment	77 519	26 073
2.2 Portfolio investment	54 593	59 539
2.3 Other investment (including earnings on reserve assets)	42 543	59 699
C. Current transfers	16 998	31 612
1. General government	6 158	17 348
2. Other sectors	10 840	14 264
Total current account	**581 407**	**599 842**
2. Capital and financial accounts		
A. Capital account	5 854	2 225
1. Capital transfers	4 251	1 339
2. Acquisition/disposal of non-produced, non-financial assets	1 603	886
B. Financial account	–162 373	–172 598
1. Direct investment	29 320	11 852
Abroad		11 852
1.1. Equity capital		4 631
1.2. Reinvested earnings		28 655
1.3. Other capital[2]		–21 434
In United Kingdom	29 320	
1.1. Equity capital	23 323	
1.2. Reinvested earnings	13 411	
1.3. Other capital[3]	–7 414	
2. Portfolio investment	188 299	154 396
Assets		154 396
2.1. Equity securities		13 655
2.2. Debt securities		140 741
Liabilities	188 299	
2.1. Equity securities	44 245	
2.2. Debt securities	144 054	
3. Financial derivatives (net)		–14 450
4. Other investment	–379 992	–330 159
Assets		–330 159
4.1 Trade credits		–96
4.2 Loans		–116 466
4.3 Currency and deposits		–213 738
4.4 Other assets		141
Liabilities	–379 992	
4.1. Trade credits	–	
4.2. Loans	–61 434	
4.3. Currency and deposits	–318 462	
4.4. Other liabilities	–96	
5. Reserve assets		5 763
5.1. Monetary gold		–
5.2. Special drawing rights		8 522
5.3. Reserve position in the IMF		613
5.4. Foreign exchange		–3 282
Total capital and financial accounts	**–156 519**	**–170 373**
Total current, capital and financial accounts	**424 888**	**429 469**
Net errors and omissions	4 581	

1 See chapter text.
2 Other capital transaction on direct investment abroad represents claims on affiliated enterprises less liabilities to affiliated enterprises
3 Other capital transactions on direct investment in the United Kingdom represents liabilities to direct investors less claims on direct investors

Source: Office for National Statistics

19.10 Summary of balance of payments: balances (credits less debits)[1]
United Kingdom

£ million

			Current account									
	Trade in goods	Trade in services	Total goods and services	Compensati-on of employees	Investment income	Total income	Current transfers	Current balance	Current balance as % of GDP[2]	Capital account	Financial account	Net errors & omissions
	LQCT	KTMS	KTMY	KTMP	HMBM	HMBP	KTNF	HBOG	AA6H	FKMJ	HBNT	HHDH
1955	−315	42	−273	−27	149	122	43	−108	−0.6	−15	34	89
1956	50	26	76	−30	203	173	2	251	1.2	−13	−250	12
1957	−29	121	92	−32	223	191	−5	278	1.3	−13	−313	48
1958	34	119	153	−34	261	227	4	384	1.7	−10	−411	37
1959	−116	118	2	−37	233	196	–	198	0.8	−5	−68	−125
1960	−404	39	−365	−35	201	166	−6	−205	−0.8	−6	−7	218
1961	−144	51	−93	−35	223	188	−9	86	0.3	−12	23	−97
1962	−104	50	−54	−37	301	264	−14	196	0.7	−12	−195	11
1963	−123	4	−119	−38	364	326	−37	170	0.6	−16	−30	−124
1964	−551	−34	−585	−33	365	332	−74	−327	−1.0	−17	392	−48
1965	−263	−66	−329	−34	405	371	−75	−33	−0.1	−18	49	2
1966	−111	44	−67	−39	358	319	−91	161	0.4	−19	22	−164
1967	−601	157	−444	−39	354	315	−118	−247	−0.6	−25	179	93
1968	−708	341	−367	−48	303	255	−119	−231	−0.5	−26	688	−431
1969	−214	392	178	−47	468	421	−109	490	1.0	−23	−794	327
1970	−18	457	437	−56	527	471	−89	819	1.6	−22	−818	21
1971	205	617	822	−63	454	391	−90	1 123	2.0	−23	−1 330	230
1972	−736	722	−14	−52	350	298	−142	142	0.2	−35	477	−584
1973	−2 573	907	−1 666	−68	970	902	−336	−1 100	−1.5	−39	1 031	108
1974	−5 241	1 292	−3 949	−92	1 010	918	−302	−3 333	−4.0	−34	3 185	182
1975	−3 245	1 708	−1 537	−102	257	155	−313	−1 695	−1.6	−36	1 569	162
1976	−3 930	2 872	−1 058	−140	760	620	−534	−972	−0.8	−12	507	477
1977	−2 271	3 704	1 433	−152	−678	−830	−889	−286	−0.2	11	−3 286	3 561
1978	−1 534	4 215	2 681	−140	−300	−440	−1 420	821	0.5	−79	−2 655	1 913
1979	−3 326	4 573	1 247	−130	−342	−472	−1 777	−1 002	−0.5	−103	864	241
1980	1 329	4 414	5 743	−82	−2 268	−2 350	−1 653	1 740	0.8	−4	−2 157	421
1981	3 238	4 776	8 014	−66	−1 883	−1 949	−1 219	4 846	1.9	−79	−5 312	545
1982	1 879	4 261	6 140	−95	−2 336	−2 431	−1 476	2 233	0.8	6	−1 233	−1 006
1983	−1 618	5 406	3 788	−89	−1 050	−1 139	−1 391	1 258	0.4	75	−3 287	1 954
1984	−5 409	6 101	692	−94	−326	−420	−1 566	−1 294	−0.4	107	−7 130	8 317
1985	−3 416	8 499	5 083	−120	−2 609	−2 729	−2 924	−570	−0.2	185	−1 657	2 042
1986	−9 617	8 182	−1 435	−156	71	−85	−2 094	−3 614	−0.9	135	−122	3 601
1987	−11 698	8 604	−3 094	−174	−730	−904	−3 437	−7 435	−1.7	333	10 606	−3 504
1988	−21 553	6 388	−15 165	−64	−1 188	−1 252	−3 293	−19 710	−4.1	235	16 989	2 486
1989	−24 724	5 866	−18 858	−138	−2 309	−2 447	−4 228	−25 533	−4.9	270	13 614	11 649
1990	−18 707	6 643	−12 064	−110	−4 586	−4 696	−4 802	−21 562	−3.8	497	22 272	−1 207
1991	−10 223	6 312	−3 911	−63	−5 642	−5 705	−999	−10 615	−1.8	290	7 855	2 470
1992	−13 050	6 353	−6 697	−49	−1 037	−1 086	−5 228	−13 011	−2.1	421	16 311	−3 721
1993	−13 066	8 174	−4 892	35	−2 547	−2 512	−5 056	−12 460	−1.9	309	22 278	−10 127
1994	−11 126	8 161	−2 965	−170	1 521	1 351	−5 187	−6 801	−1.0	33	−3 240	10 008
1995	−12 023	11 165	−858	−296	−546	−842	−7 363	−9 063	−1.2	533	−1 717	10 247
1996	−13 722	14 312	590	93	−2 460	−2 367	−4 539	−6 316	−0.8	1 260	−940	5 996
1997	−12 342	16 801	4 459	83	241	324	−5 745	−962	−0.1	958	−7 294	7 298
1998	−21 813	15 003	−6 810	−10	11 813	11 803	−8 172	−3 179	−0.4	489	4 480	−1 790
1999	−29 051	15 562	−13 489	201	−1 244	−1 043	−7 322	−21 854	−2.4	747	29 505	−8 398
2000	−32 976	15 002	−17 974	150	1 812	1 962	−9 775	−25 787	−2.6	1 703	23 133	951
2001	−41 212	17 200	−24 012	66	9 359	9 425	−6 515	−21 102	−2.1	1 318	27 194	−7 410
2002	−47 705	19 632	−28 073	67	18 219	18 286	−8 870	−18 657	−1.7	932	24 204	−6 479
2003	−48 607	22 612	−25 995	59	17 464	17 523	−9 835	−18 307	−1.6	1 466	22 553	−5 712
2004	−60 900	28 414	−32 486	−494	18 339	17 845	−10 276	−24 917	−2.1	2 064	29 358	−6 505
2005	−68 589	25 742	−42 847	−610	22 465	21 855	−11 849	−32 841	−2.6	1 503	29 024	2 314
2006	−76 312	34 782	−41 530	−958	10 531	9 573	−11 885	−43 842	−3.3	975	38 225	4 642
2007	−89 754	44 807	−44 947	−734	21 509	20 775	−13 538	−37 710	−2.7	2 566	31 676	3 468
2008	−93 381	55 142	−38 239	−714	31 007	30 293	−14 029	−21 975	−1.5	3 241	15 182	3 552
2009	−81 790	49 313	−32 477	−688	29 344	28 656	−14 614	−18 435	−1.3	3 629	10 225	4 581

1 See chapter text.
2 Using series YBHA: GDP at current market prices.

Source: Office for National Statistics

19.11 Balance of payments:[1] current account
United Kingdom

£ million

		1999	2000	2001	2002	2003	2004	2005	2006	2007	2008	2009
Credits												
Exports of goods and services												
Exports of goods	LQAD	166 166	187 936	189 093	186 524	188 320	190 874	211 608	243 633	220 858	251 643	227 670
Exports of services	KTMQ	76 525	81 883	87 773	94 012	102 357	112 922	119 186	134 246	150 645	170 758	161 168
Total exports of goods and services	KTMW	242 691	269 819	276 866	280 536	290 677	303 796	330 794	377 879	371 503	422 401	388 838
Income												
Compensation of employees	KTMN	960	1 032	1 087	1 121	1 116	931	974	938	981	1 045	916
Investment income	HMBN	100 733	131 902	137 447	120 543	122 069	137 380	185 766	236 684	290 321	260 022	174 655
Total income	HMBQ	101 693	132 934	138 534	121 664	123 185	138 311	186 740	237 622	291 302	261 067	175 571
Current transfers												
General government	FJUM	3 542	2 465	4 991	3 663	3 968	4 177	4 294	4 383	4 315	5 621	6 158
Other sectors	FJUN	8 510	8 018	8 926	8 571	8 079	9 590	13 106	14 090	9 731	10 711	10 840
Total current transfers	KTND	12 052	10 483	13 917	12 234	12 047	13 767	17 400	18 473	14 046	16 332	16 998
Total	HBOE	356 436	413 236	429 317	414 434	425 909	455 874	534 934	633 974	676 851	699 800	581 407
Debits												
Imports of goods and services												
Imports of goods	LQBL	195 217	220 912	230 305	234 229	236 927	251 774	280 197	319 945	310 612	345 024	309 460
Imports of services	KTMR	60 963	66 881	70 573	74 380	79 745	84 508	93 444	99 464	105 838	115 616	111 855
Total imports of goods and services	KTMX	256 180	287 793	300 878	308 609	316 672	336 282	373 641	419 409	416 450	460 640	421 315
Income												
Compensation of employees	KTMO	759	882	1 021	1 054	1 057	1 425	1 584	1 896	1 715	1 759	1 604
Investment income	HMBO	101 977	130 090	128 088	102 324	104 605	119 041	163 301	226 153	268 812	229 015	145 311
Total income	HMBR	102 736	130 972	129 109	103 378	105 662	120 466	164 885	228 049	270 527	230 774	146 915
Current transfers												
General government	FJUO	7 271	7 778	7 340	9 085	10 657	12 225	13 637	13 881	14 087	14 714	17 348
Other sectors	FJUP	12 103	12 480	13 092	12 019	11 225	11 818	15 612	16 477	13 497	15 647	14 264
Total current transfers	KTNE	19 374	20 258	20 432	21 104	21 882	24 043	29 249	30 358	27 584	30 361	31 612
Total	HBOF	378 290	439 023	450 419	433 091	444 216	480 791	567 775	677 816	714 561	721 775	599 842
Balances												
Trade in goods and services												
Trade in goods	LQCT	−29 051	−32 976	−41 212	−47 705	−48 607	−60 900	−68 589	−76 312	−89 754	−93 381	−81 790
Trade in services	KTMS	15 562	15 002	17 200	19 632	22 612	28 414	25 742	34 782	44 807	55 142	49 313
Total trade in goods and services	KTMY	−13 489	−17 974	−24 012	−28 073	−25 995	−32 486	−42 847	−41 530	−44 947	−38 239	−32 477
Income												
Compensation of employees	KTMP	201	150	66	67	59	−494	−610	−958	−734	−714	−688
Investment income	HMBM	−1 244	1 812	9 359	18 219	17 464	18 339	22 465	10 531	21 509	31 007	29 344
Total income	HMBP	−1 043	1 962	9 425	18 286	17 523	17 845	21 855	9 573	20 775	30 293	28 656
Current transfers												
General government	FJUQ	−3 729	−5 313	−2 349	−5 422	−6 689	−8 048	−9 343	−9 498	−9 772	−9 093	−11 190
Other sectors	FJUR	−3 593	−4 462	−4 166	−3 448	−3 146	−2 228	−2 506	−2 387	−3 766	−4 936	−3 424
Total current transfers	KTNF	−7 322	−9 775	−6 515	−8 870	−9 835	−10 276	−11 849	−11 885	−13 538	−14 029	−14 614
Total (Current balance)	HBOG	−21 854	−25 787	−21 102	−18 657	−18 307	−24 917	−32 841	−43 842	−37 710	−21 975	−18 435

1 See chapter text.

Source: Office for National Statistics

19.12 Balance of payments:[1] summary of international investment position, financial account and investment income

United Kingdom £ billion

		1999	2000	2001	2002	2003	2004	2005	2006	2007	2008	2009
Investment abroad												
International investment position												
Direct investment	HBWD	438.3	618.8	616.9	637.2	691.1	678.1	705.9	741.7	913.9	1 050.3	1 019.9
Portfolio investment	HHZZ	838.3	906.1	937.4	844.0	935.8	1 092.1	1 360.9	1 531.1	1 693.8	1 664.3	1 878.1
Other investment	HLXV	1 097.3	1 379.7	1 521.9	1 545.2	1 813.7	2 118.0	2 714.8	2 916.6	3 750.2	4 216.6	3 576.3
Reserve assets	LTEB	22.2	28.8	25.6	25.5	23.8	23.2	24.7	22.9	26.7	36.3	40.1
Total	HBQA	2 396.1	2 933.4	3 101.9	3 051.9	3 464.5	3 911.4	4 806.3	5 212.3	6 384.6	6 967.5	6 514.5
Financial account transactions												
Direct investment	-HJYP	125.6	155.6	42.8	35.0	40.9	51.5	44.0	45.0	136.1	87.6	11.9
Portfolio investment	-HHZC	21.4	65.6	86.6	1.0	36.3	141.0	151.0	138.8	92.0	-123.5	154.4
Financial derivatives (net)	-ZPNN	-2.7	-1.6	-8.4	-1.0	5.4	7.9	-9.6	-7.4	19.0	35.5	-14.4
Other investment	-XBMM	41.5	241.7	170.7	70.4	260.4	325.2	501.3	395.9	747.3	-612.4	-330.2
Reserve assets	-LTCV	-0.6	3.9	-3.1	-0.5	-1.6	0.2	0.7	-0.4	1.2	-1.3	5.8
Total	-HBNR	185.2	465.2	288.5	105.0	341.4	525.8	687.3	571.9	995.7	-614.2	-172.6
Investment income												
Direct investment	HJYW	33.1	45.0	46.7	51.5	55.1	63.3	79.2	83.6	90.2	67.3	77.5
Portfolio investment	HLYX	25.9	33.0	34.9	32.5	32.5	36.7	45.4	55.1	66.1	67.5	54.6
Other investment	AIOP	40.6	52.9	54.9	35.8	33.6	36.7	60.5	97.3	133.3	124.4	41.8
Reserve assets	HHCB	1.2	1.0	1.0	0.8	0.8	0.7	0.7	0.6	0.6	0.8	0.8
Total	HMBN	100.7	131.9	137.4	120.5	122.1	137.4	185.8	236.7	290.3	260.0	174.7
Investment in the UK												
International investment position												
Direct investment	HBWI	250.2	310.4	363.5	340.6	355.5	383.3	494.2	578.3	630.2	672.3	694.7
Portfolio investment	HLXW	933.2	1 067.6	1 013.2	925.3	1 082.9	1 227.9	1 461.7	1 702.6	1 917.6	1 945.4	2 328.5
Other investment	HLYD	1 400.9	1 651.6	1 861.9	1 906.0	2 143.2	2 520.8	3 103.0	3 284.0	4 119.4	4 409.1	3 673.8
Total	HBQB	2 584.3	3 029.5	3 238.5	3 171.9	3 581.6	4 132.1	5 058.9	5 564.8	6 667.2	7 026.7	6 697.1
Financial account transactions												
Direct investment	HJYU	55.1	80.6	37.3	16.8	16.8	31.2	97.8	84.9	98.2	49.8	29.3
Portfolio investment	HHZF	106.3	172.2	40.8	49.7	105.6	97.3	129.0	153.9	203.3	185.8	188.3
Other investment	XBMN	53.3	235.6	237.6	62.6	241.5	426.6	489.5	371.3	725.9	-834.6	-380.0
Total	HBNS	214.7	488.3	315.7	129.2	364.0	555.2	716.3	610.1	1 027.4	-599.0	-162.4
Investment income												
Direct investment	HJYX	17.0	27.4	21.4	16.0	21.9	27.6	36.2	51.6	44.8	5.6	26.1
Portfolio investment	HLZC	32.2	32.4	36.1	33.3	32.9	38.7	47.6	57.6	66.5	74.1	59.5
Other investment	HLZN	52.7	70.2	70.5	53.0	49.8	52.7	79.6	117.0	157.5	149.4	59.7
Total	HMBO	102.0	130.1	128.1	102.3	104.6	119.0	163.3	226.2	268.8	229.0	145.3
Net investment												
International investment position												
Direct investment	HBWQ	188.1	308.4	253.5	296.6	335.6	294.7	211.7	163.4	283.8	378.1	325.2
Portfolio investment	CGNH	-94.9	-161.5	-75.7	-81.3	-147.0	-135.8	-100.8	-171.5	-223.8	-281.1	-450.4
Other investment	CGNG	-303.6	-271.9	-339.9	-360.8	-329.5	-402.9	-388.2	-367.3	-369.2	-192.5	-97.5
Reserve assets	LTEB	22.2	28.8	25.6	25.5	23.8	23.2	24.7	22.9	26.7	36.3	40.1
Net investment position	HBQC	-188.2	-96.2	-136.5	-120.0	-117.2	-220.7	-252.6	-352.6	-282.5	-59.2	-182.6
Financial account transactions												
Direct investment	HJYV	-70.5	-75.0	-5.5	-18.3	-24.1	-20.3	53.8	39.9	-38.0	-37.8	17.5
Portfolio investment	HHZD	84.9	106.6	-45.7	48.7	69.4	-43.7	-21.9	15.1	111.3	309.4	33.9
Financial derivatives	ZPNN	2.7	1.6	8.4	1.0	-5.4	-7.9	9.6	7.4	-19.0	-35.5	14.4
Other investment	HHYR	11.8	-6.1	66.9	-7.7	-18.9	101.4	-11.8	-24.6	-21.4	-222.2	-49.8
Reserve assets	LTCV	0.6	-3.9	3.1	0.5	1.6	-0.2	-0.7	0.4	-1.2	1.3	-5.8
Net transactions	HBNT	29.5	23.1	27.2	24.2	22.6	29.4	29.0	38.2	31.7	15.2	10.2
Investment income												
Direct investment	HJYE	16.1	17.6	25.3	35.5	33.2	35.7	43.0	32.0	45.4	61.8	51.4
Portfolio investment	HLZX	-6.4	0.5	-1.2	-0.8	-0.4	-2.0	-2.2	-2.4	-0.4	-6.6	-4.9
Other investment	CGNA	-12.2	-17.3	-15.7	-17.2	-16.1	-16.0	-19.0	-19.6	-24.1	-25.0	-17.9
Reserve assets	HHCB	1.2	1.0	1.0	0.8	0.8	0.7	0.7	0.6	0.6	0.8	0.8
Net earnings	HMBM	-1.2	1.8	9.4	18.2	17.5	18.3	22.5	10.5	21.5	31.0	29.3

1 See chapter text.

Source: Office for National Statistics

19.13 Net Foreign Direct Investment flows abroad analysed by area and main country[1,2]

£ million

		2004	2005	2006	2007	2008
Europe	GQBX	10 814	12 105	16 899	90 683	54 084
EU27	IY6N	11 917	13 337	4 038	69 836	49 557
Austria	CBJD	1 322	−301	−94	110	−185
Belgium	HIIL	−544	970	−4 356	1 037	1 533
Bulgaria	IY6O	−	11	−5	..	42
Cyprus	DG8D	18	69	98	365	509
Czech Republic	DG8O	23	24	−160	59	336
Denmark	CAUW	569	391	1 529	539	2 983
Estonia	DG8E	21	2	3	−3	−20
Finland	CBJE	−37	707	106	268	65
France	CAUX	793	3 138	1 175	4 536	5 006
Germany	CAUY	−366	−479	3 186	2 260	−578
Greece	CAUZ	−253	63	15	286	383
Hungary	DG8F	336	1 821	39	88	170
Irish Republic	CAVA	3 325	−1 181	5 161	3 995	−273
Italy	CAVB	667	191	−397	2 904	198
Latvia	DG8G	1	−1	4	65	142
Lithuania	DG8H	1	−4	1	−	..
Luxembourg	HIIM	−1 022	−1 213	−14 131	25 453	5 949
Malta	DG8I	178	142	891	−1 952	..
Netherlands	CAVC	4 805	4 821	1 350	22 176	9 568
Poland	DG8J	182	150	397	−500	−73
Portugal	CAVD	444	603	314	278	194
Romania	IY6P	11	101	40	117	227
Slovakia	DG8K	18	21	18	90	105
Slovenia	DG8L	−5	−5	14	9	11
Spain	CAVE	1 131	564	2 177	4 155	21 495
Sweden	CBJG	299	2 732	6 669	3 501	530
EFTA	CAVG	−6 667	547	6 926	3 620	2 447
of which						
Norway	CBJF	367	−831	3	1 060	1 625
Switzerland	CBJH	−7 007	1 330	6 948	2 653	878
Other European Countries	IY6Q	5 564	−1 779	5 935	17 227	2 079
of which						
Russia	GLAA	1 831	349	−13	1 334	3 938
UK offshore islands[3]	GLAC	3 528	−2 341	5 023	14 752	−3 074
The Americas	GQBZ	24 321	20 689	19 100	53 837	14 137
of which						
Bermuda	CBKZ	6 242	653	908	2 082	3 873
Brazil	CBLA	386	48	354	791	844
Canada	CAVK	1 143	3 372	8 130	15 468	−1 091
Chile	GQCA	675	790	25	110	−323
Colombia	GQCB	225	−687	315	126	160
Mexico	GLAD	1 386	168	334	128	366
Panama	GLAE	12	27	7	−18	−4
USA	CAVJ	9 732	15 041	−1 803	30 820	7 477
Asia	GQCI	7 689	5 399	7 992	7 734	8 617
Near and Middle East Countries	CBKF	486	398	1 219	2 044	3 037
of which						
Gulf Arabian countries[5]	GQCC	293	577	329	482	690
Other Asian Countries	GQCD	7 203	5 001	6 773	5 689	5 579
of which						
China	HIIN	539	598	374	1 138	1 036
Hong Kong	CAVN	5 303	1 547	1 674	1 503	1 029
India	GLAF	274	616	104	650	467
Indonesia	GLAG	−289	−116	196	−140	−71
Japan	CAVM	37	247	440	1 141	808
Malaysia	CBKN	428	244	241	216	365
Singapore	CBKQ	−161	−508	2 621	−1 265	−731
South Korea	GLAH	278	2 247	679	488	673
Thailand	GLAI	181	228	536	3	220
Australasia and Oceania	GQCE	1 026	423	3 132	2 149	8 015
of which						
Australia	CBJO	408	444	2 743	2 012	6 948
New Zealand	CBJP	258	−56	405	125	117
Africa	GQCF	5 863	5 843	−235	4 726	909
of which						
Kenya	GLAJ	47	73	62	97	75
Nigeria	CBJY	−44	−108	44	56	234
South Africa	CAVO	3 840	4 368	1 466	1 734	1 399
Zimbabwe	CBKD	91	18	8	4	−6
World Total	CDQD	49 713	44 458	46 887	159 129	85 762
OECD	GQCG	18 355	35 305	21 276	125 975	66 153
Central and Eastern Europe[4]	GQCH	36	158	76	−	55

1 Net foreign direct investment includes unremitted profits.
2 A minus sign indicates a net disinvestment abroad (ie a decrease in the amount due to the UK).
3 The UK Offshore Island consist of the Channel Islands & the Isle of Man, excluded from the definition of the economic territory of the UK from 1997.
4 From 2007 includes data for Bulgaria and Romania. Prior to 2003 also includes data for Czech Republic, Estonia, Hungary, Lithuania, Latvia, Poland, Slovakia and Slovenia.
5 Includes Abu Dhabi, Bahrain, Dubai, Iraq, Kuwait, Oman, Other Gulf States, Qatar, Saudi Arabia and Yemen.

Source: ONS Foreign Direct Investments Surveys: 01633 456082; Bank of England

19.14 Net Foreign Direct Investment international investment position abroad analysed by area and main country

£ million

		2004	2005	2006	2007	2008
Europe	GQCJ	382 104	387 324	402 593	527 997	582 034
EU27	IY6R	348 576	339 692	314 481	412 024	465 062
Austria	CDLZ	4 102	4 005	2 402	2 579	2 794
Belgium	HIIO	7 828	13 492	4 380	6 887	10 999
Bulgaria	IY6S	22	53	46	46	132
Cyprus	DG8Q	64	59	561	683	564
Czech Republic	DG8R	793	823	523	632	948
Denmark	CDLP	5 256	5 090	7 782	6 220	10 783
Estonia	DG8S	78	7	−1	7	25
Finland	CDMA	695	2 465	1 287	2 329	569
France	CDLQ	35 313	47 348	36 327	39 598	42 462
Germany	CDLR	12 164	20 753	17 602	19 766	23 897
Greece	CDLS	456	625	562	864	1 111
Hungary	DG8T	1 506	2 491	1 795	1 870	2 127
Irish Republic	CDLT	29 059	26 824	26 432	25 362	23 406
Italy	CDLU	11 322	10 872	7 924	12 786	10 613
Latvia	DG8U	25	22	27	..	95
Lithuania	DG8V	22	16	6	11	..
Luxembourg	HIIP	81 709	97 260	62 355	95 915	123 278
Malta	DG8W	1 528	−459	2 399	3 263	..
Netherlands	CDLV	131 143	64 511	92 783	138 769	124 449
Poland	DG8X	2 316	1 974	2 519	2 078	2 991
Portugal	CDLW	1 664	2 702	3 167	3 366	3 517
Romania	IY6T	260	356	247	402	675
Slovakia	DG8Y	103	93	136	184	388
Slovenia	DG8Z	54	3	53	..	51
Spain	CDLX	11 318	25 604	25 233	30 879	52 468
Sweden	CDMD	9 776	12 702	17 935	17 388	25 313
EFTA	CDLY	14 468	12 933	12 637	17 745	22 396
of which						
Norway	CDMC	4 934	4 498	2 116	2 370	4 115
Switzerland	CDME	9 104	7 979	10 239	15 124	18 057
Other European Countries	IY6U	19 060	34 700	75 475	98 228	94 576
of which						
Russia	GQAA	1 627	1 814	6 054	7 182	11 077
UK offshore islands[1]	GQAB	15 678	29 954	65 814	86 482	77 031
The Americas	GQCU	182 091	216 343	256 423	292 687	338 058
of which						
Bermuda	CDOA	7 561	10 604	13 889	13 839	23 386
Brazil	CDOB	3 922	3 220	2 824	3 717	6 601
Canada	CDML	8 922	12 812	19 188	28 980	29 878
Chile	GQCT	2 133	2 814	563	439	319
Colombia	GQCS	1 874	1 132	985	1 109	1 636
Mexico	GQAC	2 461	2 860	2 337	3 791	3 772
Panama	GQAD	132	166	..	..	168
USA	CDMM	140 321	164 405	180 629	202 117	239 038
Asia	GQCL	47 311	54 919	54 377	60 887	82 182
Near and Middle East Countries	CDNH	3 008	3 733	6 874	9 984	14 966
of which						
Gulf Arabian countries[3]	GQCM	2 062	3 013	4 756	6 320	9 131
Other Asian Countries	GQCR	44 303	51 187	47 503	50 903	67 215
of which						
China	HIIQ	1 882	2 685	2 228	2 719	4 222
Hong Kong	CDNN	19 165	20 432	22 256	25 517	32 417
India	GQAE	1 682	2 126	1 977	2 942	3 879
Indonesia	GQAF	1 178	1 168	982	825	1 049
Japan	CDMP	5 829	6 076	2 485	592	1 468
Malaysia	CDNQ	1 592	1 455	1 174	1 233	1 482
Singapore	CDNT	6 610	7 144	6 684	6 220	10 272
South Korea	GQAG	1 218	4 586	3 763	4 457	4 405
Thailand	GQAH	947	1 281	1 407	1 456	1 675
Australasia and Oceania	GQCN	16 888	16 694	12 665	16 173	18 051
of which						
Australia	CDMO	14 586	14 627	11 571	15 391	16 033
New Zealand	CDMQ	1 459	1 176	923	682	689
Africa	GQCQ	17 350	20 834	15 105	18 516	19 167
of which						
Kenya	GQAI	238	281	313	331	400
Nigeria	CDNA	950	924	1 011	744	1 094
South Africa	CDMR	10 964	13 733	8 255	9 533	8 295
Zimbabwe	CDNF	103	50	58	32	35
World Total	CDOO	645 744	696 113	741 163	916 261	1 039 491
OECD	GQCO	537 109	561 694	547 303	684 619	784 512
Central & Eastern Europe[2]	GQCP	534	640	515	65	270

1 The UK Offshore Islands consist of the Channel Islands & the Isle of Man, excluded from the definition of the economic territory of the UK from 1997.
2 Prior to 2007 includes data for Bulgaria and Romania. Prior to 2003 also includes data for Czech Republic, Estonia, Hungary, Lithuania, Latvia, Poland, Slovenia and Slovakia

3 Includes Abu Dhabi, Bahrain, Dubai, Iraq, Kuwait, Oman, Other Gulf States, Qatar, Saudi Arabia and Yemen.

Sources: ONS Foreign Direct Investment Surveys: 01633 456082; Bank of England

19.15 Net earnings from Foreign Direct Investment abroad analysed by area and main country[1,2]

£ million

		2004	2005	2006	2007	2008
Europe	GQCV	25 782	32 186	38 957	44 062	40 573
EU27	IY6V	20 708	23 904	28 337	34 284	34 405
Austria	CBLQ	296	301	186	247	170
Belgium	HIIR	653	818	875	1 312	1 550
Bulgaria	IY6W	–	9	3	–9	–5
Cyprus	DG94	22	37	171	366	318
Czech Republic	DG95	110	108	–64	72	–143
Denmark	CAWI	272	387	411	580	530
Estonia	DG96	3	..	11	5	6
Finland	CBLR	112	103	69	281	128
France	CAWJ	2 107	2 957	3 344	3 007	2 016
Germany	CAWK	2 328	2 685	2 189	2 890	2 728
Greece	CAWL	102	160	151	223	109
Hungary	DG97	202	295	83	96	72
Irish Republic	CAWM	2 461	2 835	2 525	3 049	1 615
Italy	CAWN	708	732	696	837	243
Latvia	DG98	–	..	5	4	–18
Lithuania	DG99	–	–	–	2	–1
Luxembourg	HIIS	2 191	4 006	7 626	8 030	13 208
Malta	DG9A	60	31	–185	–56	58
Netherlands	CAWO	6 651	5 344	7 251	9 725	9 044
Poland	DG9B	218	293	373	256	405
Portugal	CAWP	191	297	234	264	274
Romania	IY6X	19	26	43	76	108
Slovakia	DG9C	..	34	24	103	19
Slovenia	DG9D	..	17	5	11	14
Spain	CAWQ	694	1 023	918	1 021	985
Sweden	CBLT	1 271	1 395	1 395	1 896	974
EFTA	CAWS	2 382	3 334	3 759	4 987	5 016
of which						
Norway	CBLS	297	937	345	296	590
Switzerland	CBLU	2 084	2 396	3 411	4 377	4 125
Other European Countries	IY6Y	2 692	4 948	6 861	4 791	1 151
of which						
Russia	GQAJ	841	1 681	1 715	1 180	1 827
UK offshore islands[3]	GQAK	1 602	3 017	4 580	3 138	–1 109
The Americas	GQCX	21 113	26 585	26 461	28 527	11 718
of which						
Bermuda	CBNK	1 629	1 561	..	1 557	1 523
Brazil	CBNL	652	866	577	712	857
Canada	CAWW	1 340	1 895	1 769	1 653	–2 495
Chile	GQCY	820	1 164	771	777	674
Colombia	GQCZ	379	414	274	190	318
Mexico	GQAL	485	536	531	563	529
Panama	GQAM	44	50	23	42	..
USA	CAWV	14 332	18 244	17 112	19 110	7 397
Asia	GQDA	8 001	10 975	11 621	11 389	11 356
Near and Middle East Countries	CBMS	692	1 053	1 430	2 563	3 623
of which						
Gulf Arabian countries[5]	GQDB	549	688	717	983	1 685
Other Asian Countries	GQDC	7 309	9 922	10 191	8 826	7 733
of which						
China	HIIT	370	580	445	504	269
Hong Kong	CAYB	2 541	3 553	3 786	4 163	2 999
India	GQAN	427	626	715	798	662
Indonesia	GQAO	155	226	336	153	139
Japan	CAWY	440	482	388	145	351
Malaysia	CBNA	525	508	494	595	562
Singapore	CBND	1 651	2 510	2 285	478	785
South Korea	GQAP	340	683	532	519	637
Thailand	GQAQ	159	171	–121	23	–117
Australasia and Oceania	GQDD	3 623	3 157	3 065	3 716	3 795
of which						
Australia	CBMB	3 108	2 681	2 665	3 294	3 397
New Zealand	CBMC	279	359	388	379	327
Africa	GQDE	3 958	5 764	3 488	4 548	3 887
of which						
Kenya	GQAR	64	70	88	89	116
Nigeria	CBML	153	197	133	78	222
South Africa	CAWZ	2 706	3 768	1 620	2 236	1 220
Zimbabwe	CBMQ	87	16	10	6	–5
World Total	GLAB	62 476	78 667	83 591	92 242	71 329
OECD	GQDF	43 453	52 138	55 675	64 794	49 253
Central & Eastern Europe[4]	GQDG	74	76	62	–11	25

1 Net earnings equal profits of foreign branches plus UK companies' receipts of interest and their share of profits of foreign subsidiaries and associates. Earnings are after deduction of provisions for depreciation and foreign taxes on profits, dividends and interest.

2 A minus sign indicates net losses.

3 The UK Offshore Islands consists of the Channel Islands and the Isle of Man, excluded from the definition of the economic territory of the UK from 1997.

4 Prior to 2007 includes data for Bulgaria and Romania. Prior to 2003 also includes data for Czech Republic, Estonia, Hungary, Lithuania, Latvia, Poland, Slovenia and Slovakia.

5 Includes Abu Dhabi, Bahrain, Dubai, Iraq, Kuwait, Oman, Other Gulf States, Qatar, Saudi Arabia and Yemen.

Sources: ONS Foreign Direct Investments Survey: 01633 456082;
Bank of England

19.16 Net Foreign Direct Investment flows into the United Kingdom analysed by area and main country[1],[2]

£ million

		2004	2005	2006	2007	2008
Europe	GQDH	29 901	80 087	53 837	49 752	25 274
EU27	IY6Z	26 384	71 034	47 698	39 348	21 963
Austria	CBOB	−31	171	−61	183	67
Belgium	HIIU	1 542	23	670	317	−575
Bulgaria	IY72	..	..	..	1	..
Cyprus	DG9G	–	7	18	75	34
Czech Republic	DG9H	–	–	..	1	1
Denmark	CAYQ	−11	−1 246	13	−18	75
Estonia	DG9I	–	–	–	–	..
Finland	CBOC	32	238	44	21	−35
France	CAYR	1 703	9 643	2 356	−1 931	−3 503
Germany	CAYS	11 131	7 279	5 566	16 616	5 310
Greece	CAYT	13	14	17	17	11
Hungary	DG9J	..	1	3	1	–
Irish Republic	CAYU	936	723	816	829	727
Italy	CAYV	1 327	−42	282	288	−275
Latvia	DG9K	..	..	..	–	..
Lithuania	DG9L	..	–	–	–	..
Luxembourg	HIIV	−115	151	221	4 349	1 725
Malta	DG9M	–	1	2	6	18
Netherlands	CAYW	1 226	50 366	13 715	2 471	17 453
Poland	DG9N	–	1	50	−29	7
Portugal	CAYX	..	−6	9	123	−79
Romania	IY73	−34	..	..	4	1
Slovakia	DG9O	..	..	..	1	..
Slovenia	DG9P	..	..	..	3	1
Spain	CAYY	..	3 297	23 457	16 139	431
Sweden	CBOE	−14	393	508	−117	577
EFTA	CAZB	3 016	9 050	5 321	8 793	−2 384
of which						
Norway	CBOD	−798	927	171	423	240
Switzerland	CBOF	3 488	7 405	4 786	8 159	−1 371
Other European Countries	IY74	501	3	817	1 611	5 696
of which						
Russia	GQAS	..	..	..	332	1 769
UK offshore islands[3]	GQAT	476	−60	733	1 248	4 081
The Americas	GQDJ	−4 792	17 422	17 242	32 460	21 125
of which						
Brazil	HP5A	..	6	..	2	1
Canada	CAZF	683	1 632	3 509	799	7
USA	CAZE	−5 727	15 589	12 313	27 975	20 553
Asia	GQDK	4 081	−4 168	11 806	9 938	2 515
Near and Middle East Countries	GQAU	384	736	5 034	−979	−1 078
Other Asian Countries	GQAV	3 697	−4 904	6 772	10 919	3 593
of which						
China	HP5B	−26	13	12	16	−20
Hong Kong	GQAW	..	315	92	−1 919	737
India	HP5C	−15	138	265	151	2 578
Japan	CAZH	817	−5 575	3 726	5 816	−175
Singapore	GQAX	14	46	..	6 749	271
South Korea	GQAY	193	175	−85	5	210
Australasia and Oceania	GQDL	1 420	3 396	1 869	540	−222
of which						
Australia	CBOJ	1 412	3 396	1 479	588	−178
New Zealand	CBOK	8	–	54	−48	−26
Africa	GQAZ	−43	66	131	459	1 075
of which						
South Africa	CAZJ	−35	25	101	438	..
World Total	CBDH	30 566	96 803	84 885	93 148	49 766
OECD	GQBA	26 762	95 187	73 961	83 165	39 858
Central & Eastern Europe[4]	GQBB	−32	..	6	1	..

1 Net investment includes unremmited profits.
2 A minus sign indicates net disinvestment in the United Kingdom (ie, a decrease in the amount due to overseas countries).
3 The UK Offshore Islands consist of the Channel Islands & the Isle of Man, excluded from the definition of the economic territory of the UK from 1997.
4 Prior to 2007 includes data for Bulgaria and Romania. Prior to 2003 also includes data for Czech Republic, Estonia, Hungary, Lithuania, Latvia, Poland, Slovakia and Slovenia.

Sources: ONS Foreign Direct Investment Surveys: 01633 456082; Bank of England

19.17 Net Foreign Direct Investment international positions in the United Kingdom analysed by area and main country

£ million

		2004	2005	2006	2007	2008
Europe	GQDM	181 198	277 027	332 077	354 382	385 092
EU27	IY75	161 395	244 392	299 906	308 996	330 842
Austria	CDPF	366	561	848	1 030	1 096
Belgium	HIIW	4 338	4 481	5 609	4 545	4 159
Bulgaria	IY76	..	..	..	..	..
Cyprus	DG9S	78	100	162	437	496
Czech Republic	DG9T	6	3	..	8	18
Denmark	CDOV	2 359	1 404	4 344	5 530	8 970
Estonia	DG9U	–	–	–	..	..
Finland	CDPG	886	756	817	708	718
France	CDOW	41 100	56 309	59 998	54 303	49 965
Germany	CDOX	39 300	51 469	54 382	64 558	73 136
Greece	CDOY	100	103	121	174	238
Hungary	DG9V	12	9	12	12	20
Irish Republic	CDOZ	5 021	7 146	8 186	8 839	10 106
Italy	CDPA	6 708	6 122	4 482	4 901	4 089
Latvia	DG9W	–	..	..	..	..
Lithuania	DG9X	..	–	–	–	–
Luxembourg	HIIX	5 963	7 880	16 021	20 399	26 539
Malta	DG9Y	5	12	12	62	140
Netherlands	CDPB	47 579	95 579	119 843	110 903	135 764
Poland	DG9Z	7	21	96	75	76
Portugal	CDPC	113	111	122	222	302
Romania	IY77	..	..	..	..	..
Slovakia	DGA2	..	–	..	..	..
Slovenia	DGA3	..	..	..	9	14
Spain	CDPD	4 536	8 782	20 658	27 876	10 619
Sweden	CDPI	2 849	3 467	4 113	4 312	4 253
EFTA	CDPE	15 752	25 033	22 358	32 570	30 772
of which						
Norway	CDPH	242	1 085	969	1 522	1 406
Switzerland	CDPJ	14 685	21 624	19 033	28 936	27 828
Other European Countries	IY78	4 051	7 602	9 813	12 816	23 478
of which						
Russia	GQBC	..	..	..	179	970
UK offshore islands[1]	GQBD	3 500	7 059	9 111	11 963	21 646
The Americas	GQDU	140 090	174 037	200 709	202 062	230 359
of which						
Brazil	HP5D	..	77	134	21	9
Canada	CDPM	12 108	15 587	19 369	20 835	19 110
USA	CDPN	122 069	149 759	170 880	167 008	190 674
Asia	GQDO	24 800	24 101	39 436	53 166	47 620
Near and Middle East Countries	GQBE	2 765	2 970	10 160	6 449	4 493
Other Asian Countries	GQBF	22 035	21 131	29 275	46 717	43 127
of which						
China	HP5E	119	111	99	202	202
Hong Kong	GQBG	..	..	..	..	..
India	HP5F	164	518	798	1 376	3 439
Japan	CDPQ	12 300	10 513	14 766	25 479	29 156
Singapore	GQBH	925	1 034	4 046	12 197	1 549
South Korea	GQBI	635	638	798	779	883
Australasia and Oceania	GQDP	16 804	12 537	7 623	9 412	7 709
of which						
Australia	CDPP	16 631	12 313	7 093	8 974	7 439
New Zealand	CDPR	153	224	428	430	268
Africa	GQBJ	530	510	469	1 397	2 097
of which						
South Africa	CDPS	296	186	130	900	1 601
World Total	CDPZ	363 422	488 212	580 313	620 419	672 877
OECD	GQBK	340 870	458 185	535 218	564 201	608 395
Central & Eastern Europe[2]	GQBL	..	..	..	6	11

1 The UK Offshore Islands consist of the Channel Islands & Isle of Man, excluded from the definition of the economic territory of the UK from 1997.
2 Prior to 2007 includes data for Bulgaria and Romania. Prior to 2003 also includes data for Czech Republic, Estonia, Hungary, Lithuania, Latvia, Poland, Slovenia and Slovakia.

Sources: ONS Foreign Direct Investment Surveys 01633 456082; Bank of England

19.18 Net earnings from Foreign Direct Investment in the United Kingdom analysed by area and main country[1,2]

£ million

		2004	2005	2006	2007	2008
Europe	GQDQ	12 676	17 592	27 447	26 174	−18 433
EU27	IY79	11 330	15 278	22 919	24 144	−4 002
Austria	CBOR	61	60	207	211	−45
Belgium	HIIY	269	367	646	577	353
Bulgaria	IY7A	..	–	–	..	..
Cyprus	DGA6	20	24	44	66	57
Czech Republic	DGA7	–	–	..	1	1
Denmark	CBDL	311	326	204	−70	−458
Estonia	DGA8	–	–	..	..	..
Finland	CBOS	62	61	93	181	50
France	CBDM	3 842	5 121	5 329	3 489	425
Germany	CBDN	2 900	4 037	4 541	5 789	−74
Greece	CBDO	−4	49	70	104	212
Hungary	DGA9	–	1	3	1	–
Irish Republic	CBDP	471	724	1 012	1 202	−137
Italy	CBDQ	408	483	477	577	473
Latvia	DGB2	–	..	..	..	..
Lithuania	DGB3	..	1	1	–	–
Luxembourg	HIIZ	289	214	79	463	577
Malta	DGB4	–	–	3	7	28
Netherlands	CBDR	2 585	2 800	7 283	8 393	−7 081
Poland	DGB5	–	1	8	6	3
Portugal	CBDS	47	30	48	54	50
Romania	IY7B	..	..	..	–	..
Slovakia	DGB6	..	5	5	3	..
Slovenia	DGB7	..	..	..	..	..
Spain	CBDT	37	773	2 536	2 696	1 207
Sweden	CBOU	21	182	316	386	360
EFTA	CBDW	849	1 495	3 366	264	−16 342
of which						
Norway	CBOT	−20	82	169	194	249
Switzerland	CBOV	819	1 320	2 933	−286	−15 058
Other European Countries	IY7C	497	819	1 162	1 767	1 912
of which						
Russia	GQBM	..	..	..	7	−77
UK offshore islands[3]	GQBN	468	757	1 107	1 752	2 072
The Americas	GQDV	12 278	16 460	20 154	17 158	24 677
of which						
Brazil	HP5G	1	−4	−4	6	−6
Canada	CBEA	1 021	1 348	1 458	−250	−2 917
USA	CBDZ	10 981	14 156	16 828	15 060	26 144
Asia	GQDS	168	937	2 710	447	−1 307
Near and Middle East Countries	GQBO	188	354	564	237	216
Other Asian Countries	GQBP	−19	583	2 145	210	−1 524
of which						
China	HP5H	8	−63	−35	17	−38
Hong Kong	GQBQ	..	..	−597	..	−337
India	HP5I	−2	65	132	140	261
Japan	CBEC	608	1 089	1 956	−216	−1 994
Singapore	GQBS	32	85	259	609	166
South Korea	GQBT	23	72	104	125	134
Australasia and Oceania	GQDT	695	535	1 259	1 222	656
of which						
Australia	CBOZ	690	521	876	1 196	672
New Zealand	CBPA	5	13	46	25	−13
Africa	GQBU	59	65	80	137	166
of which						
South Africa	CBED	26	25	31	82	126
World Total	CBEV	25 876	35 588	51 650	45 138	5 756
OECD	GQBV	25 471	33 927	47 476	40 242	1 589
Central & Eastern Europe[4]	GQBW	1	..	..	..	..

1 Net earnings equal profits of United Kingdom branches plus overseas foreign investors' receipts of interest from, and their share of the profits of, United Kingdom subsidiaries and associates. Earnings are after deducting provisions for depreciation and UK tax.
2 A minus sign indicates net losses.
3 The UK Offshore Islands consist of the Channel Islands & the Isle of Man, excluded from the definition of the economic territory of the UK from 1997.
4 Prior to 2007 includes data for Bulgaria and Romania. Prior to 2003 also includes data for Czech Republic, Estonia, Hungary, Lithuania, Latvia, Poland, Slovenia and Slovakia.

Sources: ONS Foreign Direct Investment Surveys: 01633 456082; Bank of England

Research and development

Chapter 20

Research and development

Research and experimental development (R&D) is defined for statistical purposes as 'creative work undertaken on a systematic basis in order to increase the stock of knowledge, including knowledge of man, culture and society, and the use of this stock of knowledge to devise new applications'.

R&D is financed and carried out mainly by businesses, the Government, and institutions of higher education. A small amount is performed by non-profit-making bodies. Gross Expenditure on R&D (GERD) is an indicator of the total amount of R&D performed within the UK: it has been approximately 2 per cent of GDP in recent years. Detailed figures are reported each year in a Statistical Bulletin published in March. Table 20.1 shows the main components of GERD.

ONS conducts an annual survey of expenditure and employment on R&D performed by Government, and of Government funding of R&D. The survey collects data for the reference period along with future estimates. Until 1993 the detailed results were reported in the *Annual Review of Government Funded R&D*. From 1997 the results have appeared in the Science, Engineering and Technology (SET) Statistics published by the Department for Business, Innovation and Skills (BIS). Table 20.2 gives some broad totals for gross expenditure by Government (expenditure before deducting funds received by Government for R&D). Table 20.3 gives a breakdown of net expenditure (receipts are deducted).

ONS conducts an annual survey of R&D in business. Tables 20.4 and 20.5 give a summary of the main trends up to 2008. The latest set of results from the survey became available in a Statistical Bulletin dated 11 December 2009.

Revisions were made to the business data for the periods 2006 and 2007 and were published at the same time as the 2008 Business Enterprise R&D (BERD) Statistical Bulletin on 11 December 2009. The format of this report was used as it covers all aspects of the R&D data published by ONS.

Statistics on expenditure and employment on R&D in Higher Education Institutions (HEIs) are based on information collected by Higher Education Funding Councils and the Higher Education Statistics Agency (HESA). In 1994 a new methodology was introduced to estimate expenditure on R&D in HEIs. This is based on the allocation of various Funding Council Grants. Full details of the new methodology are contained in SET Statistics available on the BIS website at: www.dius.gov.uk/science/science_funding/set_stats

The most comprehensive international comparisons of resources devoted to R&D appear in Main Science and Technology Indicators published by the Organisation for Economic Co-operation and Development (OECD). The Statistical Office of the European Union and the United Nations also compile R&D statistics based on figures supplied by member states.

To make international comparisons more reliable the OECD have published a series of manuals giving guidance on how to measure various components of R&D inputs and outputs. The most important of these is the Frascati Manual, which defines R&D and recommends how resources for R&D should be measured. The UK follows the Frascati Manual as far as possible.

For information on available aggregated data on Research and Development please contact Mark Williams on 01633 456728 (email Mark.Williams@ons.gov.uk).

20.1 Cost of research and development: by sector[1]
United Kingdom

£ million and percentages

	2001		2002		2003		2004		2005		2006		2007		2008	
	£m	%	£m	%	£m	%	£m	%	£m	%	£m	%	£m	%	£m	%
Sector carrying out the work **Cash terms (£ million)**																
Government	1 160	6	1 053	5	1 243	6	1 240	6	1 238	6	1 252	5	1 256	5	1 305	5
Research councils	674	4	713	4	825	4	930	5	1 051	5	1 061	5	1 034	4	1 041	4
Business enterprise	12 239	66	12 484	65	12 505	63	12 662	63	13 734	62	14 144	62	15 631	63	15 896	62
Higher education	4 149	22	4 618	24	4 785	24	5 004	25	5 580	25	6 022	26	6 519	26	6 794	26
Private non-profit	325	2	374	2	369	2	406	2	502	2	513	2	557	2	604	2
Total	18 547	100	19 243	100	19 727	100	20 242	100	22 106	100	22 993	100	24 997	100	25 641	100
Sector providing the funds **Cash terms (£ million)**																
Government	2 299	12	2 215	11	2 650	13	2 778	14	2 584	12	2 531	11	2 978	12	2 896	11
Research councils	1 512	8	1 713	9	1 947	10	2 084	10	2 574	12	2 709	12	2 518	10	2 739	11
Higher education funding councils	1 474	8	1 626	8	1 665	8	1 804	9	1 928	9	2 085	9	2 234	9	2 227	9
Higher education	184	1	208	1	218	1	229	1	266	1	288	1	308	1	318	1
Business enterprise[2]	8 499	46	8 384	44	8 287	42	8 914	44	9 580	43	10 377	45	11 487	46	11 647	45
Private non-profit	889	5	962	5	931	5	961	5	1 022	5	1 076	5	1 153	5	1 264	5
Abroad	3 691	20	4 135	22	4 029	20	3 472	17	4 152	19	3 927	17	4 319	17	4 550	18
Total	18 547	100	19 243	100	19 727	100	20 242	100	22 106	100	22 993	100	24 997	100	25 641	100

1 See chapter text.
2 Including research associations and public corporations.

Source: Office for National Statistics: 01633 456763

20.2 Gross central government expenditure on research and development[1]
United Kingdom

£ million

	2003/04		2004/05		2005/06		2006/07		2007/08		2008/09	
	Intra-mural	Extra-mural[2]	Intra-mural	Extra-mural[2]	Intra-mural	Extra-mural[2]	Intra-mural	Extra-mural[2]	Intra-mural	Extra-mural[3]	Intra-mural	Extra-mural
Defence	380	2 364	357	2 283	365	2 223	361	1 851	279	1 941	262	1 812
Research councils	811	1 643	874	1 752	1 004	2 034	1 051	2 135	1 034	2 005	1 041	2 297
Higher education institutes	-	1 665	-	1 804	-	1 928	-	2 085	-	2 234	-	2 227
Other programmes	338	1 111	327	870	316	1 546	309	881	346	1 418	351	1 316
Total (excluding NHS)	1 529	6 783	1 558	6 709	1 685	7 731	1 721	6 952	1 659	7 598	1 654	7 652

1 See chapter text.
2 Extramural includes work performed overseas and excludes monies spent with other government departments.
3 From 2007/08 expenditure figure no longer includes VAT.

Source: Office for National Statistics: 01633 456763

20.3 Net central government expenditure on research and development:[1] by European Union objectives for research and development expenditure
United Kingdom

£ million

		1998 /99	1999 /00	2000 /01	2001 /02	2002 /03	2003 /04	2004 /05	2005 /06	2006 /07	2007 /08	2008 /09
Exploration and exploitation of the earth	KDVP	78.5	79.5	85.5	106.0	138.3	176.8	193.0	239.0	241.0	228.0	254.0
Infrastructure and general planning of land-use	KDVQ	103.5	104.4	102.4	100.3	101.0	118.7	88.0	70.0	89.0	117.0	125.0
Control of environmental pollution	KDVR	142.8	147.0	151.1	129.1	126.5	150.1	149.0	158.0	158.0	220.0	260.0
Protection and promotion of human health (ex NHS)	KDVS	450.1	519.5	530.6	571.6	597.8	1 163.7	1 227.3	1 258.0	1 394.0	811.0	897.0
Production, distribution and rational utilisation of energy	KDVT	28.0	29.0	31.9	36.8	40.3	28.4	35.0	21.0	43.0	56.0	69.0
Agricultural production and technology	KDVU	255.5	260.6	266.6	265.2	267.8	275.9	278.0	273.0	284.0	259.0	252.0
Industrial production and technology	KDVV	61.6	56.5	109.2	237.0	423.4	426.5	138.4	94.0	88.0	9.0	60.0
Social structures and relationships	KDVW	154.7	217.6	270.2	268.8	293.4	226.7	291.8	471.0	311.0	396.0	438.0
Exploration and exploitation of space	KDVX	142.50	142.70	146.30	139.80	155.50	168.60	168.90	192.00	153.00	177.00	205.00
Research financed from general university funds	KDVY	1 085.1	1 157.1	1 276.1	1 473.5	1 626.4	1 664.6	1 804.7	1 933.0	2 092.0	2 234.0	2 227.0
Non-oriented research	KDVZ	677.0	700.5	789.3	918.2	1 071.6	1 290.9	1 332.0	1 658.0	1 715.0	1 925.0	1 852.0
Other civil research[2]	KDWA	25.8	20.6	22.3	19.7	36.3	39.9	38.4	38.0	45.0	–	–
Defence	KDWB	2 144.2	2 275.9	2 245.1	2 063.0	2 739.7	2 682.2	2 582.7	2 528.0	2 132.0	2 150.0	2 003.0
Total (Excluding NHS)	KDWC	5 349.3	5 710.9	6 026.6	6 329.0	7 618.0	8 413.5	8 327.0	8 932.0	8 745.0	8 582.0	8 642.0

1 See chapter text.
2 Due to OECD changes to the NABS codes, from 2007 "Other Civil Research" no longer exists as a category.

Source: Office for National Statistics: 01633 456763

Research and development

20.4 Intramural expenditure on Business Enterprise research and development:[1] by industry

United Kingdom: At Current Prices and Constant 2008 Prices
£ million

		Total				Civil				Defence		
		2006	2007	2008		2006	2007	2008		2006	2007	2008
Current Prices												
Chemicals	KDWF	..	..	..	KDWP	4 201	4 608	4 946	KDWZ	..	..	..
Mechanical engineering	KDWG	997	1 170	909	KDWQ	464	681	492	KDXA	533	489	417
Electrical machinery	KJRT	1 273	1 292	1 320	KJTC	930	930	944	KJUL	343	362	376
Aerospace	KDWJ	1 832	2 070	1 714	KDWT	908	902	817	KDXD	924	1 168	897
Transport equipment	KDWK	..	..	..	KDWU	795	983	1 318	KDXE	..	..	..
Other manufacturing	KDWL	1 336	1 340	1 397	KDWV	1 266	1 240	1 282	KDXF	70	100	115
Manufacturing: Total	KDWE	10 555	11 584	11 736	KDWO	8 564	9 345	9 799	KDWY	1 991	2 239	1 937
Services	KDWM	3 404	3 834	3 928	KDWW	3 226	3 665	3 798	KDXG	178	169	130
Agriculture, hunting and forestry; fishing	HFRV	88	..	..	HFSA	88	..	..	MKFC	–	–	–
Extractive industries	HFRW	59	82	90	HFSB	59	82	90	MKFD	–	–	–
Electricity, gas and water supply	HFRX	21	35	33	HFSC	21	35	33	MKFE	–	–	–
Construction	HFRY	17	..	..	HFSE	17	..	..	MKFF	–	–	–
Other: Total	HFRU	185	212	232	HFRZ	185	212	232	MKFB	–	–	–
Total	KDWD	14 144	15 631	15 896	KDWN	11 975	13 222	13 829	KDWX	2 169	2 409	2 067
2008 Prices												
Chemicals	HFXA	..	..	..	HFXJ	4 428	4 721	4 946	HFYO	..	..	..
Mechanical engineering	HFXB	1 051	1 199	909	HFXK	489	698	492	HFYP	562	501	417
Electrical machinery	HFXC	1 342	1 324	1 320	HFYH	980	953	944	HFYQ	362	371	376
Aerospace	HFXD	1 931	2 121	1 714	HFYI	957	924	817	HFYR	974	1 197	897
Transport equipment	HFXE	..	..	..	HFYJ	838	1 007	1 318	HFYS	..	..	..
Other manufacturing	HFXF	1 409	1 372	1 397	HFYK	1 335	1 270	1 282	HFYT	74	102	115
Manufacturing: Total	HFWZ	11 127	11 868	11 736	HFXI	9 028	9 574	9 799	HFYN	2 099	2 294	1 937
Services	HFXG	3 589	3 928	3 928	HFYL	3 401	3 755	3 798	HFYU	188	173	130
Agriculture, hunting and forestry: fishing	HFSG	..	..	..	HFSL	..	..	..	MKFH	–	–	–
Extractive industries	HFSH	62	84	90	HFSM	62	84	90	MKFI	–	–	–
Electricity, gas and water supply	HFSI	22	36	33	HFSN	22	36	33	MKFJ	–	–	–
Construction	HFSJ	18	..	..	HFSO	18	..	..	MKFK	–	–	–
Other: Total	HFSF	195	217	232	HFSK	195	217	232	MKFG	–	–	–
Total	HFWY	14 909	16 014	15 896	HFXH	12 623	13 546	13 829	HFYM	2 286	2 468	2 067

1 See chapter text.

Source: Office for National Statistics: 01633 456763

20.5 Sources of funds for research and development within Business Enterprises[1]

United Kingdom

£ million and percentages

		Total				Civil				Defence		
		2006	2007	2008		2006	2007	2008		2006	2007	2008
Cash terms (£ million)												
Government funds	KDYM	1 060	1 064	1 046	KDYU	150	175	187	KDZC	910	889	859
Overseas funds	KDYN	3 262	3 630	3 739	KDYV	2 686	2 978	3 211	KDZD	576	652	527
Mainly own funds	KDYO	9 822	10 937	11 111	KDYW	9 139	10 069	10 430	KDZE	683	868	681
Total	KDYL	14 144	15 631	15 896	KDYT	11 975	13 222	13 829	KDZB	2 169	2 409	2 067
Percentages												
Government funds	KDYQ	7	7	7	KDYY	1	1	1	KDZG	42	37	42
Overseas funds	KDYR	23	23	24	KDYZ	22	23	23	KDZH	27	27	25
Mainly own funds	KDYS	69	70	70	KDZA	76	76	75	KDZI	31	36	33
Total	KDYP	100	100	100	KDYX	100	100	100	KDZF	100	100	100

1 See chapter text.

Source: Office for National Statistics: 01633 456763

Agriculture, fisheries and food

Chapter 21

Agriculture, fisheries and food

Output and input

(Tables 21.1 and 21.2)

For both tables, output is net of VAT collected on the sale of non-edible products. Figures for total output include subsidies on products, that is payments that have the purpose of influencing production, their prices or remuneration of the factors of production. Unspecified crops include turf, other minor crops and arable area payments for fodder maize. Eggs include the value of duck eggs and exports of eggs for hatching. Landlords' expenses are included within farm maintenance, miscellaneous expenditure and depreciation of buildings and works. Also included within 'Other farming costs' are livestock and crop costs, water costs, insurance premia, bank charges, professional fees, rates, and other farming costs.

Other subsidies

These are payments other than subsidies on products from which farmers can benefit as a consequence of engaging in agriculture. Include environment and countryside management schemes, organic farming schemes, support schemes for less favoured areas, Single Payment Scheme, animal disease compensation attributable to income, and other payments.

Compensation of employees and interest charges

Total compensation of employees excludes the value of work done by farm labour on own account, capital formation in buildings and work. 'Interest' relates to interest charges on loans for current farming purposes and buildings, less interest on money held on short-term deposit.

Rent

Rent paid (after deductions) is the rent paid on all tenanted land including 'conacre' land in Northern Ireland, less landlords' expenses and the benefit value of dwellings on that land. Rent received (after deductions) is the rent received by farming landowners from renting of land to other farmers, less landlords' expenses and the benefit value of dwellings on that land. Total net rent is the net rent flowing out of the agricultural sector paid to non-farming landowners, including that part of tenanted land in Northern Ireland.

Agricultural censuses and surveys

(Tables 21.3, 21.5 and 21.13)

The coverage for holdings includes all main and minor holdings for each country. Northern Ireland data are now based on all active farm business.

Estimated quantity of crops and grass harvested

(Table 21.4)

The estimated yield of sugar beet is obtained from production figures supplied by British Sugar plc in England and Wales. In Great Britain potato yields are estimated in consultation with the Potato Council Limited.

Forestry

(Table 21.6)

Statistics for state forestry are from Forestry Commission and Forest Service management information systems. For private forestry in Great Britain, statistics on new planting and restocking are based on records of grant aid and estimates of planting undertaken without grant aid, and softwood production is estimated from a survey of the largest timber harvesting companies. Hardwood production is estimated from deliveries of roundwood to primary wood processors and others, based on surveys of the UK timber industry, data provided by trade associations and estimates provided by the Expert Group on Timber and Trade Statistics.

Average weekly earnings and hours of agricultural and horticultural workers

(Tables 21.11 and 21.12)

Prior to 1998, data were collected from a monthly postal survey, which mainly covered male full-time workers. Between 1998 and 2002 the survey collected information on an annual basis via a telephone survey. The survey was reviewed in 2002 and it was concluded that the frequency of the survey should be increased to four times per year to enable the production of more representative annual estimates. The annual sample size has been retained and has been split between four quarterly telephone surveys.

From April 2009, publication of quarterly results ceased. Results are now published on an annual basis, for the 12 months ending in September. The annual data provides the more robust estimates of earnings and hours, however quarterly data collection continues in order to achieve a representative sample of workers across the year.

The survey covers seven main categories of workers, providing data which are used by the Agricultural Wages Board when considering wage claims and in considering the cost of labour in agriculture and horticulture.

Data on earnings represents the total earnings for workers aged 20 and over. Figures include all payments-in-kind, valued where applicable in accordance with the Agricultural Wages Order. Part-time workers are defined as those working less than 39 basic hours per week. Casual workers are those employed on a temporary basis.

Results can be found on the Department for Environment, Food and Rural Affairs (DEFRA) website at: www.defra.gov.uk

Fisheries

(Table 21.15)

Figures show the number of registered and licensed fishing vessels, based on information provided by the Registry of Shipping and Seamen and licence registers maintained by the Marine and Fisheries Agency for England and Wales, the Scottish Government and the Department of Agriculture and Rural Development in Northern Ireland.

Estimated average household food consumption – 'Family Food' Expenditure and Food Survey

(Table 21.16)

In 2008 the Expenditure and Food Survey (EFS) was renamed as the Living Costs and Food Survey (LCFS) when it became part of the Integrated Household Survey (IHS). The Expenditure and Food Survey started in April 2001, having been preceded by the National Food Survey (NFS) and the Family Expenditure Survey (FES). Both surveys were brought into one to provide value for money without compromising data quality. The EFS was effectively a continuation of the FES, extended to record quantities of purchases. This extension is now known as the Family Food Module of the LCFS. Estimates from the NFS prior to 2000 have been adjusted by aligning estimates for the year 2000 with corresponding estimates from the FES. From 2006 the survey moved onto a calendar year basis (from the previous financial year basis) in preparation for its integration to the Integrated Household Survey from January 2008.

The Living Costs and Food Survey is a voluntary sample survey of private households throughout the UK. The basic unit of the survey is the household, which is defined as a group of people living at the same address and sharing common catering arrangements. The survey is continuous, interviews being spread evenly over the year to ensure that seasonal effects are covered. Each household member over the age of seven keeps a diary of all their expenditure over a two-week period. A simplified version of the diary is used by those aged 7 to 15. The diaries record expenditure and quantities of purchases of food and drink rather than consumption of food and drink. Items of food and drink are defined as either household or eating out and are recorded in the form in which the item was purchased not how it was consumed. 'Household' covers all food that is brought into the household. 'Eating out' covers all food that never enters the household, for example restaurant meals, school meals and snacks eaten away from home.

In 2008 the Living Costs and Food Survey collected the diaries of 13,890 people within 5,845 households across the UK. The response rate for 2008 was 51 per cent in Great Britain and 54 per cent in Northern Ireland.

21.1 Production and income account at current prices[1]
United Kingdom

£ million

		1999	2000	2001	2002	2003	2004	2005	2006	2007	2008	2009[2]
Output[3]												
1.Total cereals:	C5X5	1 620.2	1 621.4	1 348.3	1 534.7	1 491.3	1 707.5	1 434.9	1 506.1	1 949.5	3 152.8	2 352.8
Wheat	KFKA	1 105.2	1 124.8	836.6	1 095.1	1 000.8	1 232.3	1 018.3	1 066.4	1 324.6	2 245.0	1 589.6
Rye	VQBG	1.8	22.0	5.6	1.2	1.4	1.6	1.3	1.4	2.3	1.9	1.8
Barley	KFKB	474.6	432.1	465.7	392.0	445.7	433.1	379.5	383.8	555.4	817.4	686.5
Oats and summer cereal mixtures	KFKC	37.9	41.7	39.8	45.5	42.5	39.7	34.8	53.6	66.2	87.1	72.9
Other cereals	VQBH	0.8	0.8	0.6	0.9	0.9	0.9	0.9	0.9	1.1	1.4	1.9
2.Total industrial crops	VQBI	783.3	699.4	773.8	859.8	812.3	798.5	814.1	731.6	769.0	1 164.5	1 108.1
Oilseeds	VQBJ	225.0	143.8	177.1	220.1	313.7	265.9	277.2	315.1	426.6	628.2	492.7
Oilseed rape	KFKG	194.8	139.0	171.5	217.4	303.8	256.7	261.2	307.2	422.3	617.8	475.4
Other oil seeds	KIBT	30.1	4.8	5.6	2.7	9.9	9.2	15.9	7.9	4.3	10.4	17.4
Sugar beet	KFKH	279.7	252.1	256.4	282.9	279.7	278.1	279.0	178.2	161.5	208.3	240.7
Other industrial crops	VQBK	278.7	303.4	340.3	356.8	218.9	254.4	257.9	238.3	180.9	328.0	374.6
Fibre plants	VQBL	2.3	1.3	1.7	1.0	1.8	1.2	0.9	0.9	0.4	1.0	0.2
Hops	KFKI	12.1	10.4	9.0	7.2	6.1	5.7	5.4	4.4	4.4	4.4	4.4
Others[4]	VQBM	264.2	291.7	329.6	348.5	211.1	247.5	251.7	233.0	176.0	322.6	370.0
3.Total forage plants	VQBO	75.9	80.9	103.4	90.3	103.7	93.3	94.9	85.9	106.3	109.9	127.7
4.Total vegetables and horticultural products	VQBP	1 667.5	1 561.1	1 612.6	1 591.1	1 672.6	1 621.5	1 690.0	1 748.1	1 848.0	1 903.2	1 932.5
5.Total potatoes (including seeds)	KFKO	769.4	477.1	701.4	505.0	548.3	695.2	531.1	638.4	684.4	767.2	644.3
6.Total fruit	KFKQ	256.9	232.2	238.8	251.2	310.3	315.8	388.1	382.8	467.4	544.5	570.6
7.Other crop products including seeds	VQBQ	42.0	37.7	37.5	25.5	31.6	31.0	52.0	47.9	43.2	44.6	45.8
8.Total crop output (Sum 1 to 7)	VQBR	5 215.2	4 709.7	4 815.8	4 857.6	4 970.0	5 262.7	5 004.9	5 140.8	5 867.7	7 686.6	6 781.8
9.Total livestock production	VQBS	4 326.7	4 358.0	4 277.9	4 573.0	4 813.5	4 813.9	4 908.4	5 093.8	5 230.7	6 576.4	7 140.1
Primarily for meat	KFLA	3 929.5	3 964.2	3 651.3	3 866.4	4 083.5	4 156.5	4 298.9	4 362.1	4 431.2	5 499.6	5 928.8
Cattle	KFKU	1 145.2	1 093.7	955.3	1 145.8	1 227.1	1 279.2	1 465.2	1 559.2	1 621.9	2 068.0	2 199.6
Pigs	KFKW	784.8	800.2	748.4	687.2	671.1	680.0	676.9	685.2	736.3	865.2	1 015.0
Sheep	VQBT	574.8	616.8	438.0	613.4	696.4	725.7	685.9	709.0	640.6	797.8	962.1
Poultry	KFXX	1 275.8	1 300.9	1 354.6	1 262.4	1 327.7	1 305.9	1 300.0	1 233.1	1 249.0	1 578.4	1 562.9
Other animals	KFKY	148.9	152.6	154.9	157.7	161.2	165.7	170.9	175.5	183.5	190.3	189.2
Gross fixed capital formation	KFLI	397.3	393.8	626.6	706.7	730.0	657.3	609.4	731.8	799.5	1 076.8	1 211.4
Cattle	KUJZ	206.9	192.9	371.3	392.2	447.7	337.4	360.9	447.3	492.9	784.5	813.1
Pigs	LUKB	6.9	5.6	5.3	7.4	7.0	7.6	6.2	8.0	5.3	6.4	9.1
Sheep	LUKA	56.7	63.9	122.5	177.5	145.8	176.4	111.5	146.0	152.6	123.7	200.6
Poultry	LUKC	126.8	131.4	127.5	129.5	129.5	135.9	130.8	130.5	148.7	162.2	188.5
10.Total livestock products	KFLF	2 963.1	2 711.4	3 088.2	2 834.3	3 030.7	3 037.7	3 009.5	2 918.1	3 285.9	4 018.6	3 692.9
Milk	KFLB	2 662.0	2 385.8	2 742.6	2 466.3	2 628.5	2 610.4	2 592.5	2 497.2	2 823.4	3 446.8	3 114.0
Eggs	KFLC	254.0	280.3	307.1	314.5	336.4	378.3	349.4	361.7	410.1	520.2	526.2
Raw wool	KFLD	21.4	22.7	17.2	19.1	20.8	20.1	19.5	11.5	11.6	10.4	9.9
Other animal products	KFLE	25.7	22.6	21.2	34.5	45.1	28.9	48.1	47.7	40.8	41.2	42.9
11.Total livestock output (9+10)	VQBV	7 289.8	7 069.4	7 366.0	7 407.4	7 844.2	7 851.5	7 917.8	8 012.0	8 516.7	10 595.0	10 833.1
12.Total other agricultural activities	LUOS	457 188	455 401	473 519	508 574	459 754	462 633	481 053	522 722	474 287	514 235	844
Agricultural services	LUKD	609.6	587.0	604.0	601.4	592.3	636.2	630.7	622.6	679.9	794.3	843.8
Leasing out quota	VQBW	116.5	51.2	28.1	42.8	40.2	82.0	8.6	0.9	0.4	0.4	0.2
13.Total inseparable non-agricultural activities	LUOT	273 476	370 184	367 736	450 749	480 252	573 382	712 489	810 993	889 723	1 136 074	809
14.Gross output at market prices (8+11+12+13)	LUOV	23 140	20 367	17 682	20 364	59 534	71 485	68 120	147 106	71 386	19 425	19 268
15.Total subsidies (less taxes) on product	LUOU	224 700	222 431	192 446	294 981	311 602	333 318	447 978	383 513	430 773	449 163	37
16.Output at basic prices (14+15)	KFLT	15 875.0	14 917.1	15 187.8	15 410.9	16 015.1	16 637.4	14 452.4	14 587.0	15 894.8	19 946.2	19 304.7
of which transactions within the agricultural industry												
Feed wheat	LUNQ	64.4	40.1	41.1	41.9	70.1	103.8	85.9	83.4	100.0	138.2	125.5
Feed barley	LUNR	147.9	137.8	148.9	144.6	149.2	148.6	136.1	142.0	177.9	207.7	157.3
Feed oats	LUNS	14.5	12.6	12.5	11.7	11.8	13.5	11.9	15.3	19.3	23.5	19.3
Seed potatoes	LUNT	29.0	6.9	13.8	12.0	4.1	9.2	12.5	15.9	8.5	12.6	10.6
Straw	LUNU	232.9	258.6	291.2	306.5	177.0	209.0	210.4	191.0	137.4	266.5	307.8
Contract work	LUNV	609.6	587.0	604.0	601.4	592.3	636.2	630.7	622.6	679.9	794.3	843.8
Leasing of quota	LUNW	116.5	51.2	28.1	42.8	40.2	82.0	8.6	0.9	0.4	0.4	0.2
Total capital formation in livestock	LUNX	397.3	393.8	626.6	706.7	730.0	657.3	609.4	731.8	799.5	1 076.8	1 211.4

21.1 Production and income account at current prices[1]
United Kingdom
continued

£ million

		1999	2000	2001	2002	2003	2004	2005	2006	2007	2008	2009[2]
Intermediate consumption												
17. Seeds	KFME	542.8	468.2	510.1	485.8	466.7	619.9	661.9	579.5	608.4	703.6	783.8
18. Energy	VQDO	621.9	697.9	683.4	647.0	600.0	669.1	778.8	831.2	897.0	1 165.7	1 023.0
Electricity	VQDQ	221.7	230.2	240.1	234.8	204.8	209.7	235.2	258.5	274.0	340.8	340.9
Fuels	VQDV	400.2	467.8	443.2	412.2	395.2	459.4	543.6	572.7	623.0	824.9	682.1
19. Fertilisers	KFMM	756.0	737.8	755.1	752.2	696.4	780.1	773.9	774.6	827.1	1 129.8	1 113.7
20. Pesticides	KFMN	621.0	579.4	526.2	531.2	501.1	576.1	547.2	517.6	570.7	689.9	674.4
21. Veterinary expenses	KCPC	270.0	255.8	241.2	250.1	253.4	279.1	280.3	284.5	302.4	337.4	342.3
22. Animal feed	KFMB	2 260.9	2 165.2	2 411.2	2 268.7	2 394.0	2 559.1	2 316.0	2 423.9	2 876.4	3 748.8	3 476.2
Compounds	LUNY	1 402.4	1 283.3	1 398.2	1 376.9	1 348.2	1 449.6	1 318.0	1 425.7	1 702.5	2 185.8	2 095.5
Straights	LUNZ	631.7	691.4	810.4	693.6	814.8	843.5	764.2	757.6	876.8	1 193.8	1 078.6
Feed purchased from other farms	LUOA	226.8	190.4	202.6	198.2	231.1	265.9	233.9	240.7	297.1	369.3	302.1
23. Total maintenance[5]	VQDW	1 013.4	939.0	980.6	957.0	967.9	1 012.1	994.6	1 014.3	1 077.2	1 141.0	1 231.7
Materials	KFMO	698.2	651.2	660.1	636.2	641.3	662.9	653.1	655.9	688.3	722.6	779.3
Buildings	KCPB	315.2	287.8	320.5	320.7	326.6	349.2	341.5	358.4	388.9	418.4	452.4
24. Agricultural services	LUOE	609.6	587.0	604.0	601.4	592.3	636.2	630.7	622.6	679.9	794.3	843.8
25. Other goods and services[5,6]	VQDX	2 265.6	2 083.4	2 031.9	2 061.5	2 122.3	2 361.9	2 345.1	2 318.5	2 379.4	2 578.0	2 647.9
26. Total intermediate consumption (Sum 17 to 25)	KCPM	8 961.0	8 513.8	8 743.7	8 554.8	8 594.2	9 493.7	9 328.4	9 366.8	10 218.4	12 288.6	12 136.8
27. Gross value added at market prices (14-26)	LUOG	4 700.4	4 391.7	4 694.3	4 914.2	5 444.8	4 976.1	4 912.1	5 135.4	5 617.0	7 600.1	7 130.8
28. Gross value added at basic prices (16-26)	JT3Z	6 914.0	6 403.3	6 444.0	6 856.0	7 420.9	7 143.7	5 124.0	5 220.2	5 676.5	7 657.6	7 167.8
29. Total consumption of Fixed Capital	KCPS	2 438.2	2 495.6	2 600.2	2 584.2	2 648.2	2 533.0	2 659.5	2 677.4	2 710.8	3 060.8	3 285.3
Equipment	KCPR	1 317.6	1 267.4	1 262.9	1 261.9	1 205.7	1 192.4	1 204.5	1 194.5	1 205.6	1 259.8	1 363.2
Buildings[5,7]	LUOH	701.3	691.2	686.4	689.5	692.3	673.9	675.7	685.3	696.4	707.5	725.2
Livestock	VQEA	419.3	537.0	650.8	632.9	750.1	666.7	779.3	797.6	808.7	1 093.5	1 196.9
Cattle	LUOI	208.2	281.1	348.4	353.2	441.2	363.6	489.6	499.4	503.3	745.5	755.6
Pigs	LUOK	7.7	8.0	6.1	7.8	7.7	8.6	7.3	7.3	6.1	6.8	8.3
Sheep	LUOJ	69.6	120.1	169.5	141.5	173.0	167.3	150.7	161.7	156.8	187.9	268.0
Poultry	LUOL	133.8	127.8	126.8	130.4	128.3	127.2	131.6	129.2	142.5	153.3	165.1
30. Net value added at market prices (27-29)	KCPT	2 262.2	1 896.1	2 094.2	2 329.9	2 796.6	2 443.1	2 252.6	2 458.0	2 906.2	4 539.3	3 845.5
31. Net value added at basic prices (28-29)	JT42	4 475.8	3 907.8	3 843.9	4 271.8	4 772.7	4 610.6	2 464.6	2 542.8	2 965.7	4 596.8	3 882.5
32. Compensation of employees[8]	LUOR	2 028.3	1 900.1	1 949.9	1 965.4	1 915.2	2 004.2	2 217.7	2 271.1	2 362.5	2 499.6	2 604.4
33. Other taxes on production	VQEB	−92.4	−92.2	−84.9	−80.6	−82.8	−95.7	−102.2	−98.9	−102.0	−105.6	−104.2
34. Other subsidies on production	VQEC	470.1	462.1	695.7	723.4	782.1	777.7	2 818.4	2 943.5	2 955.7	3 235.8	3 606.6
Animal disease compensation	LUOM	11.9	19.1	13.0	24.6	24.7	18.6	19.9	16.9	21.2	25.6	21.7
Set-aside	LUON	170.0	127.3	180.1	142.5	176.7	129.5	–	..	..	..	..
Agri-environment schemes[9]	ZBXC	128.5	140.3	164.1	196.1	222.6	257.0	287.6	376.1	460.0	490.3	496.8
Other including Single Payment Scheme[10]	VQED	159.6	175.4	338.5	360.2	358.1	372.6	2 510.9	2 550.5	2 474.4	2 719.9	3 088.1
35. Net value added at factor cost	LUOQ	4 853.5	4 277.7	4 454.7	4 914.6	5 472.0	5 292.6	5 180.8	5 387.4	5 819.4	7 727.0	7 384.8
36. Rent	KCPV	239.6	224.5	250.5	253.7	268.6	241.2	219.7	237.0	254.9	273.6	267.7
Paid[11]	ZBXE	322.0	303.3	328.5	339.6	364.7	346.5	304.7	325.6	352.3	368.8	367.1
Received[12]	ZBXF	−82.4	−78.8	−78.1	−85.9	−96.2	−105.2	−85.0	−88.6	−97.3	−95.2	−99.4
37. Interest[13]	KCPU	68.6	83.9	101.6	118.5	134.9	152.6	174.2	200.2	224.8	252.4	267.0
Total income from farming (35-32-36-37)	KCQB	1 997.6	1 540.9	1 711.7	2 235.3	2 854.9	2 550.1	2 210.7	2 343.7	2 568.2	4 361.7	4 069.1

1 See chapter text.
2 Provisional.
3 Output is net of VAT collected on the sale of non-edible products. Figures for total output include subsidies on products, but not other subsidies.
4 Includes straw and minor crops.
5 Landlords' expenses are included within 'Total maintenance', 'Other goods and services' and 'Total consumption of Fixed Capital of buildings'.
6 Includes livestock and crop costs, water costs, insurance premiums, bank charges, professional fees, rates and other farming costs.
7 A more empirically based methodology for calculating landlords' consumption of fixed capital was introduced in 2000. The new series has been linked with the old one using a smoothing procedure for the transition year of 1996.
8 Excludes the value of work done by farm labour on own account capital formation in buildings and works.

9 Includes environment and countryside management schemes and Organic Farming Schemes.
10 Includes Single Payment Scheme, support for less favoured areas and other payments received by farmers by virtue of engaging in agriculture.
11 Rent paid on all tenanted land (including 'conacre' land in Northern Ireland) less landlords' expenses, landlords' consumption of fixed capital and the benefit value of dwellings on that land.
12 Rent received by farming landowners from renting of land to other farmers less landlords' expenses. This series starts in 1996 following a revision to the methodology of calculating net rent.
13 Interest charges on loans for current farming purposes and buildings and works less interest on money held on short term deposit.

Source: Department for Environment, Food and Rural Affairs: 01904 455080

21.2 Output and input volume indices[1]
United Kingdom

Indices (2000=100)

		1999	2000	2001	2002	2003	2004	2005	2006	2007	2008	2009
Outputs												
1. Total cereals:	VQAN	92.5	100.0	80.4	97.4	91.6	93.5	89.5	88.6	81.5	102.6	93.7
Wheat	LUKH	88.9	100.0	70.1	96.0	86.5	93.2	89.7	88.7	79.6	103.0	87.0
Rye	VQAO	104.5	100.0	104.5	90.9	86.4	86.4	86.4	86.4	86.4	86.4	86.4
Barley	LUKI	102.4	100.0	105.3	97.2	101.4	91.8	87.5	83.7	81.5	97.2	107.2
Oats and summer cereal mixtures	LUKJ	84.1	100.0	96.9	118.0	116.8	97.5	83.1	114.4	111.7	122.7	118.4
Other cereals	VQAP	82.4	100.0	74.4	108.9	107.0	102.9	104.2	104.1	87.2	99.5	154.7
2. Total industrial crops:	VQAQ	117.6	100.0	93.3	105.6	109.3	105.7	103.4	96.2	87.1	103.3	104.2
Oil seeds	VQAR	167.0	100.0	100.3	124.0	153.1	139.8	167.2	161.5	178.9	183.8	176.3
Oilseed rape	VQAS	148.8	100.0	100.7	127.2	153.8	140.4	165.5	163.1	183.8	188.0	177.1
Other oil seeds	LUKN	708.3	100.0	89.0	39.0	130.4	120.2	195.9	116.5	46.0	69.4	131.7
Sugar beet	C5X4	116.6	100.0	91.8	105.3	101.0	99.6	95.7	81.5	74.2	84.2	91.7
Other industrial crops	VQAU	95.2	100.0	91.2	97.3	92.0	93.1	75.1	72.4	45.8	76.1	79.2
Fibre plants	VQAV	139.6	100.0	69.3	40.3	67.3	45.5	31.7	32.5	16.1	26.8	6.7
Hops	LUKP	112.4	100.0	94.3	94.5	72.4	72.4	61.9	51.1	51.1	51.1	51.1
Others[3]	VQAW	94.4	100.0	91.2	97.7	92.6	94.0	75.7	73.3	45.9	77.0	80.4
3. Total forage plants	VQAX	96.7	100.0	117.0	117.2	115.6	111.4	113.4	100.8	71.8	87.2	113.6
4. Total vegetables and horticultural Products:	VQAY	102.4	100.0	96.8	96.1	93.5	95.3	95.4	89.7	89.4	91.5	89.8
Fresh vegetables	LUKX	106.2	100.0	96.6	88.3	87.8	88.3	91.9	89.8	86.5	89.0	89.8
Plants and flowers	LUKZ	97.5	100.0	97.0	106.6	101.3	104.8	100.4	90.0	93.8	95.3	90.4
5. Total potatoes (including seeds)	LUKW	120.4	100.0	113.0	110.4	100.4	105.7	98.5	93.3	89.4	95.5	96.5
6. Total fruit	LUKY	108.2	100.0	105.8	99.8	109.7	130.0	148.5	149.7	176.5	182.8	193.2
7. Other crop products including seeds	VQAZ	101.8	100.0	101.2	69.0	83.0	84.6	123.6	111.5	100.7	106.5	92.9
8. Total crop output	VQBA	103.3	100.0	93.3	99.9	97.3	99.5	98.3	94.1	90.4	102.9	100.0
9. Total livestock production	VQBB	105.3	100.0	93.6	97.2	94.7	95.4	97.7	96.1	97.2	97.9	94.7
Mainly for meat processing	LULH	104.7	100.0	92.1	96.2	94.9	95.4	99.3	96.9	97.2	96.5	94.9
Cattle	LULC	103.1	100.0	88.6	102.7	105.9	104.5	118.9	114.0	116.7	114.7	113.8
Pigs	LULE	117.5	100.0	90.9	86.8	76.8	77.5	77.0	76.9	80.9	80.0	81.0
Sheep	LULD	104.1	100.0	71.8	81.8	83.3	88.6	89.9	89.7	89.3	86.8	83.3
Poultry	LULF	99.5	100.0	104.6	102.3	101.0	100.2	99.1	95.9	91.6	93.4	90.3
Other animals	LULG	100.0	100.0	99.7	99.8	99.3	99.1	99.6	99.0	99.3	99.1	99.1
Gross fixed capital formation	LULR	112.3	100.0	105.7	106.2	96.7	98.5	90.3	94.1	99.7	107.9	96.2
Cattle	LULN	112.7	100.0	115.8	110.6	109.2	101.8	97.6	98.6	101.1	120.4	97.6
Pigs	LULP	148.1	100.0	85.2	126.6	101.2	93.5	79.5	96.9	88.6	99.7	99.3
Sheep	LULO	147.5	100.0	155.6	173.6	119.4	148.3	116.3	138.4	153.3	106.7	113.6
Poultry	LULQ	96.7	100.0	67.8	68.9	68.9	72.3	69.6	69.4	79.1	86.3	100.3
10. Total livestock products	LULM	102.8	100.0	101.6	102.9	104.0	101.6	101.8	100.6	98.3	96.9	96.2
Milk	LULI	102.8	100.0	101.2	102.3	103.5	100.3	99.6	98.7	96.8	94.6	93.7
Eggs	LULJ	101.1	100.0	107.3	107.1	104.9	113.3	115.2	111.3	108.6	115.5	116.1
Raw wool	LULK	103.9	100.0	83.1	86.3	84.4	85.7	87.9	79.5	73.4	70.6	67.6
Other animal products	LULL	118.7	100.0	88.2	139.6	173.9	105.3	173.7	173.9	137.8	112.9	119.4
11. Total livestock output	VQBC	104.3	100.0	96.7	99.4	98.3	97.9	99.4	97.9	97.7	97.6	95.3
12. Total other agricultural activities	VQBD	116.2	100.0	98.9	100.7	98.7	109.8	96.2	92.0	98.4	112.7	117.3
Agricultural services	VQBE	105.9	100.0	102.9	102.5	100.9	106.3	103.3	100.0	107.0	122.6	127.6
Leasing out quota	VQBF	234.4	100.0	54.0	80.9	73.8	146.3	15.9	1.6	0.7	0.7	0.3
13. Total inseparable non-agricultural Activities	LULX	91.1	100.0	124.5	108.2	110.6	113.7	116.1	118.7	119.4	119.1	118.7

21.2
Output and input volume indices[1]
United Kingdom

continued

		1999	2000	2001	2002	2003	2004	2005	2006	2007	2008	2009[2]
14. Gross output at market prices	VQEG	104.0	100.0	96.6	100.0	98.4	99.6	99.5	97.1	95.9	101.2	98.9
15. Total subsidies (less taxes) on product	VQEE	108.2	100.0	86.0	98.8	99.6	99.6	108.5	99.9	94.5	89.3	98.3
16. Output at basic prices	LULY	104.6	100.0	95.2	99.8	98.5	99.5	100.1	97.6	96.4	101.7	99.5
of which transactions within the agricultural industry												
Feed wheat	LULZ	145.3	100.0	95.6	102.9	162.4	220.2	215.6	194.4	168.8	180.3	195.3
Feed barley	LUMA	100.5	100.0	107.5	114.1	107.2	96.7	99.8	97.6	86.1	80.5	84.3
Feed oats	LUMB	109.4	100.0	104.1	102.5	110.5	110.3	97.1	110.9	111.2	106.2	107.6
Seed potatoes	LUMC	141.1	100.0	109.9	109.7	43.5	65.8	131.2	138.2	53.1	76.5	75.1
Straw	LUMD	93.9	100.0	89.8	95.8	89.9	90.9	71.2	68.0	39.8	70.1	73.2
Contract work	LUME	105.9	100.0	102.9	102.5	100.9	106.3	103.3	100.0	107.0	122.6	127.6
Leasing of quota	LUMF	234.4	100.0	54.0	80.9	73.8	146.3	15.9	1.6	0.7	0.7	0.3
Total capital formation in livestock	LUMG	112.3	100.0	104.9	105.4	95.9	97.8	89.6	93.4	99.0	107.1	95.4
Intermediate Consumption												
17. Seeds	LUMO	111.9	100.0	99.2	84.7	82.1	75.9	92.6	100.0	112.7	108.0	106.8
Cereals	LUMM	102.0	92.1	90.8	88.5	77.8	81.4	..	..	..	..	..
Other	LUMN	99.2	98.6	103.5	101.1	100.4	99.0	..	..	..	..	..
18. Energy	VQEH	109.4	100.0	101.3	100.6	85.5	88.2	81.9	78.1	80.4	77.3	80.2
Electricity	VQEI	108.1	100.0	108.2	110.3	89.6	86.6	81.7	75.9	71.5	77.8	77.2
Fuels	VQEJ	110.1	100.0	97.8	95.8	83.5	88.9	81.9	79.0	84.6	77.2	81.7
19. Fertilisers	VQEK	114.2	100.0	87.4	91.2	78.2	79.8	71.4	67.6	63.7	62.0	60.1
20. Pesticides	LUMQ	101.4	100.0	93.9	95.8	90.5	99.3	92.3	86.4	93.8	111.1	109.2
21. Veterinary expenses	LUMW	104.3	100.0	95.6	100.0	97.6	104.4	105.6	100.2	105.3	123.4	124.5
22. Animal feed	LUML	102.9	100.0	104.4	101.9	105.8	107.7	105.6	105.4	103.8	105.4	105.3
Compounds	LUMH	108.8	100.0	102.9	102.3	102.2	103.3	99.5	104.4	107.6	106.9	105.0
Straights	LUMI	89.9	100.0	107.1	98.8	109.0	111.2	111.5	103.3	96.3	103.1	104.5
Feed purchased from other farms	LUMJ	110.7	100.0	104.7	111.0	119.9	125.2	125.7	120.5	106.5	104.6	110.8
23. Total maintenance[4]	VQEL	110.6	100.0	102.2	96.2	92.6	92.9	86.1	83.4	86.0	86.4	92.0
Materials	LUMU	109.5	100.0	98.5	91.0	86.3	85.4	78.7	75.2	77.7	77.6	81.6
Buildings	LUMT	113.1	100.0	110.5	108.1	107.1	110.2	103.4	102.9	105.6	107.0	116.9
24. Agricultural services	VQEM	105.9	100.0	102.9	102.5	100.9	106.3	103.3	100.0	107.0	122.6	127.6
25. Other goods and services[4,5]	VQEO	112.2	100.0	93.6	93.7	99.2	105.4	99.0	94.9	92.7	96.1	98.3
26. Total intermediate consumption	LUNE	108.1	100.0	98.4	96.7	95.6	98.5	95.0	92.7	93.5	96.1	97.3
27. Gross value added at market prices	LUNF	96.6	100.0	93.3	105.9	103.6	101.6	108.4	105.9	100.7	111.2	102.7
28. Total consumption of Fixed Capital	LUNN	101.3	100.0	96.3	92.1	91.6	91.1	91.7	88.6	87.3	92.7	88.7
Equipment	LUNI	102.3	100.0	97.7	96.1	94.7	94.0	92.4	90.3	89.8	91.2	93.6
Buildings[4,6]	LUNG	104.2	100.0	101.3	103.3	100.6	98.3	94.9	96.7	93.5	102.3	101.3
Livestock	VQES	94.3	100.0	88.1	74.6	77.0	78.2	85.0	77.2	76.2	83.8	72.5
Cattle	LUNJ	88.1	100.0	86.4	76.0	81.0	81.5	92.2	79.1	75.1	84.0	66.6
Pigs	LUNL	117.3	100.0	67.9	97.7	78.4	78.2	68.3	66.5	69.3	75.3	67.3
Sheep	LUNK	95.1	100.0	120.7	78.7	78.0	78.7	86.2	86.7	85.1	88.6	83.3
Poultry	LUNM	104.9	100.0	65.9	66.9	66.9	70.3	67.6	67.4	76.9	83.9	96.7
29. Net value added at market prices	LUNO	91.2	100.0	89.5	125.3	120.3	116.4	132.9	131.5	120.7	137.4	123.5

1 See chapter text.
2 Provisional.
3 Includes straw and minor crops.
4 Landlords' expenses are included within 'Total maintenance', 'Other goods and services' and 'Total consumption of Fixed Capital of buildings'.

5 Includes livestock and crop costs, water costs, insurance premiums, bank charges, professional fees, rates, and other farming costs.

Source: Department for Environment, Food and Rural Affairs: 01904 455080

21.3 Agriculture land-use
United Kingdom
Area at the June Survey[1]

Thousand hectares

		1999	2000	2001	2002	2003	2004	2005	2006	2007	2008	2009
Total agricultural area	BFAH	18 579	18 311	18 594	18 537	18 464	18 432	18 502	18 788	18 690	18 702	18 736
Total croppable land	JT3T	6 539.7	6 494.7	6 504.3	6 460.5	6 394.9	6 423.0	6 312.8	6 197.3	6 215.1	6 070.5	6 210.3
Crops	BFAA	4 709	4 665	4 493	4 604	4 475	4 589	4 437	4 415	4 439	4 740	4 694
Bare fallow[2]	BFAB	33	37	43	33	29	29	140	150	165	..	..
Uncropped arable land[3]	J8U3	604.7	603.8	843.4	644.3	718.1	588.7	698.8	663.0	599.2	194.3	254.5
Total tillage	KIJR	4 742	4 702	4 536	4 636	4 504	4 619	4 600	4 611	4 603	4 935	..
All grass under 5 years old	KFEM	1 226.5	1 225.6	1 205.1	1 242.6	1 200.5	1 245.8	1 193.3	1 137.1	1 176.0	1 141.0	1 261.8
Total arable land	KFEN	5 968	5 928	5 741	5 879	5 705	5 864	5 794	5 749	5 779	6 076	..
All grasses 5 years old and over	KFEO	5 448.9	5 363.1	5 584.0	5 518.6	5 683.4	5 620.2	5 711.1	5 967.3	5 964.9	6 035.6	6 081.2
Total permanent grass	JT3V	10 023.6	9 808.1	10 018.6	10 006.2	10 012.7	9 946.3	10 065.0	10 458.4	10 283.8	10 394.9	10 244.7
Total tillage and grass	KFEP	11 417	11 292	11 325	11 397	11 388	11 485	11 505	11 716	11 744	12 112	..
Sole right rough grazing	BFAD	4 575	4 445	4 435	4 488	4 329	4 326	4 354	4 491	4 313	4 359	4 164
Set aside	DMNF	572	567	800	612	689	559	535	513	440	..	..
All other land on agricultural holdings including woodland	BFAE	789	780	801	806	820	825	872	874	954	993	1 042
Woodland	JT3W	..	..	514.0	523.6	544.3	563.0	583.2	606.2	663.1	705.3	778.6
All other land	JT3X	..	..	287.4	282.2	276.3	262.2	288.8	267.5	291.4	288.5	263.8
Total land on agricultural holdings	BFAF	17 352	17 083	17 361	17 303	17 227	17 195	17 266	17 547	17 452	17 464	17 498
Common rough grazing (estimated)	BFAG	1 227	1 228	1 232	1 234	1 236	1 237	1 236	1 241	1 238	1 238	1 238
Crops	BFAA	4 709	4 665	4 493	4 604	4 475	4 589	4 437	4 415	4 439	4 740	4 694
Arable crops	JT3U	4 529.7	4 493.0	4 283.2	4 397.7	4 300.6	4 413.3	4 251.0	4 231.3	4 271.3	4 565.1	4 521.6
Cereals	BFAJ	3 141	3 348	3 014	3 245	3 057	3 130	2 919	2 864	2 885	3 274	3 134
Wheat	BFAK	1 847	2 086	1 635	1 996	1 837	1 990	1 867	1 836	1 830	2 080	1 814
Barley	BFAL	1 179	1 128	1 245	1 101	1 076	1 007	938	881	898	1 032	1 160
Oats	BFAM	92	109	112	126	121	108	90	121	129	135	131
Mixed corn	BFAN	2	2	3	4	4	..	..	..	..	..	..
Rye[4]	BFAO	8	7	5	5	4	6	..	..	..	..	..
Triticale	DMNH	13	16	14	14	15	15	13	13	16	..	..
Rye, mixed corn and triticale	J8U4	23	25	21	23	23	25	24	25	27	27	..
Other arable crops (excluding potatoes)	DMNI	1 211	979	1 141	1 024	1 098	1 136	1 211	1 245	1 245	1 152	..
Oilseed rape	BFAP	417	332	404	357	460	498	519	568	674	598	613
Sugar beet not for stock feeding[4]	BFAQ	183	173	177	169	162	154	148	130	125	120	116
Hops[5]	DMNJ	3	2	2	2	2	2	1	1	..	..	..
Peas for harvesting dry and field beans	DMNK	202	208	275	249	235	242	239	231	161	148	233
Linseed	DMNL	209	71	31	12	32	30	45	36	13	16	29
Maize	JT3Y	107.1	104.1	129.2	121.3	118.7	117.6	130.9	137.3	146.3	152.7	165.7
Other crops	DMNM	197	192	214	204	201	203	252	278	272	269	..
Potatoes	BFAR	178	166	165	158	145	148	137	140	140	144	147
Horticultural	BFAV	179	172	173	176	176	175	170	166	169	170	172
Vegetables grown in the open	DMNN	126	119	120	124	125	125	121	119	121	122	124
Orchard fruit[6]	BFBG	28	28	28	26	25	24	23	23	23	24	24
Soft fruit	DMNO	9	10	9	9	9	9	9	10	9	10	10
Ornamentals	DMNP	13	14	14	15	14	15	14	12	13	13	12
Glasshouse crops	DMNQ	2	2	2	2	2	2	2	2	2	2	2

1 Includes estimates for minor holdings for all countries. See chapter text.
2 The area of bare fallow has shown an increase of 378% in 2005. The rise in the bare fallow area in England is believed to be due to the way the farmers have described their land following the introduction of the Single Payment Scheme.
3 Includes all uncropped arable land i.e. bare fallow and arable land not in production managed under GAEC12 conditions.
4 Figures are for England and Wales only.
5 Figures are for England only from 2005. From 2007 are included in Other Crops.
6 Includes non-commercial orchards.

Source: Agricultural Departments: 01904 455333

21.4 Estimated quantity of crops and grass harvested[1]
United Kingdom

Thousand tonnes

		1999	2000	2001	2002	2003	2004	2005	2006	2007	2008	2009
Agricultural crops												
Wheat	BADO	14 867	16 704	11 580	15 973	14 282	15 468	14 863	14 735	13 221	17 227	14 379
Barley (Winter and Spring) .	BADP	6 581	6 492	6 660	6 128	6 360	5 799	5 495	5 239	5 079	6 144	6 769
Oats	BADQ	541	640	621	753	749	626	532	728	712	784	757
Sugar beet[2]	BADR	10 584	9 079	8 335	9 559	9 168	8 850	8 687	7 400	6 733	7 641	8 330
Potatoes	BADS	7 131	6 636	6 649	6 966	5 918	6 316	5 979	5 727	5 564	6 145	6 423
		1999	2000	2001	2002	2003	2004	2005	2006	2007	2008	2009
Horticultural crops												
Field vegetables												
Brussels sprouts	BADT	72.5	78.5	67.3	54.8	42.7	55.8	45.1	46.1	44.8	43.3	43.6
Cabbage (including savoys and spring greens)	BADU	308.9	295.2	273.2	295.4	255.2	245.6	290.9	262.7	254.8	216.3	231.0
Cauliflowers	BADV	191.7	172.4	156.1	107.4	116.5	126.3	168.3	133.2	123.7	122.1	108.5
Carrots	BADW	617.6	673.2	725.8	760.0	718.4	602.4	671.1	710.1	701.3	735.4	671.0
Turnips and swedes	BADX	117.5	123.3	132.1	141.8	103.9	96.5	97.0	103.1	105.7	106.2	116.5
Beetroot	BADY	69.5	63.4	67.1	68.6	56.3	58.8	53.1	51.0	57.3	56.8	55.2
Onions, dry bulb	BADZ	342.0	391.4	392.7	374.9	283.4	373.6	340.9	413.6	358.8	303.8	354.9
Peas, green for market (in pod weight)	BAEA	7.0	7.0	6.7	6.2	7.2	5.9	5.9	5.9	5.9	5.9	5.9
Peas, green for processing (shelled weight)	BAEB	152.0	143.1	184.5	161.0	169.3	167.6	131.1	129.0	124.4	97.8	166.9
Lettuce	BAEC	151.8	155.2	135.8	123.9	109.9	125.6	140.9	131.7	126.4	109.0	110.6
Protected crops												
Tomatoes	BAED	107.6	116.6	113.0	109.1	100.9	75.6	78.5	78.8	84.1	85.6	86.8
Cucumbers	BAEE	83.8	83.8	79.8	71.5	73.6	77.0	61.4	59.9	56.5	49.4	57.7
Lettuce	BAEF	20.6	19.9	18.7	20.9	16.0	16.6	10.4	8.1	8.2	7.8	6.8
Fruit												
Dessert apples	BFCD	97.8	133.9	101.3	104.4	84.0	69.0	92.2	118.0	129.3	106.2	121.1
Cooking apples	BFCE	85.9	112.4	107.5	107.4	95.3	74.9	78.2	100.1	111.5	136.9	105.9
Soft fruit	BFCF	60.1	65.9	65.6	64.6	67.1	79.9	86.0	105.4	107.7	124.1	150.6
Pears	BFBQ	26.3	22.7	26.6	38.5	34.2	29.6	22.7	23.4	28.4	20.6	23.5

1 See chapter text.
2 Figures are adjusted to constant 16% sugar content.

Source: Agricultural Departments: 01904 455332

21.5 Cattle, sheep, pigs and poultry on agricultural holdings[1]
United Kingdom
At June each year

Thousands

		1999	2000	2001	2002	2003	2004	2005	2006	2007	2008	2009
Total cattle and calves[2]	BFCG	11 423.4	11 134.6	10 602.1	10 345.3	10 508.2	10 588.1	10 770.2	10 578.8	10 303.9	10 107.0	10 025.5
of which:												
dairy cows	BFCH	2 440.3	2 335.8	2 251.2	2 227.2	2 191.0	2 128.8	1 997.7	1 978.8	1 954.0	1 908.9	1 856.9
beef cows	BFCI	1 924.3	1 842.2	1 708.3	1 657.0	1 697.6	1 736.0	1 750.9	1 737.1	1 698.2	1 670.2	1 625.6
heifers in calf	BFCJ	763	718	701	728	679	690	638	645	..	..	..
Total sheep and lambs	BFCM	44 656.2	42 264.1	36 716.5	35 834.3	35 811.6	35 817.5	35 416.0	34 722.5	33 945.8	33 131.0	32 038.1
of which:												
ewes and shearlings	CKUQ	21 457.8	20 448.6	17 921.2	17 630.1	17 579.5	17 630.4	16 935.3	16 636.9	16 063.6	15 616.2	14 912.0
lambs under one year old	BFCP	22 092.1	20 856.7	17 768.9	17 310.5	17 322.0	17 238.3	17 487.6	17 058.2	16 855.4	16 574.3	16 177.4
Total pigs	BFCQ	7 283.9	6 482.2	5 845.4	5 588.0	5 045.8	5 158.5	4 861.9	4 932.9	4 834.4	4 713.5	4 724.3
of which:												
sows in pig and other sows for breeding	CKUU	603.3	536.8	527.0	483.3	442.5	350.8	321.2	322.9	319.6	299.1	317.7
gilts in pig	CKUR	85.4	73.1	70.9	74.3	73.2	65.7	66.9	67.3	56.8	55.1	49.5
Total fowls	KPSV	165 156.9	169 772.7	179 879.7	168 996.5	178 799.5	181 759.2	173 908.7	173 080.5	167 666.9	166 199.8	159 288.1
of which:												
table fowls including broilers	CKUT	101 625.0	105 688.8	112 530.9	105 136.6	116 737.8	119 888.3	111 474.7	110 671.9	109 794.2	109 858.9	102 759.1
laying fowls[3]	CKUV	29 257.9	28 686.9	29 895.2	28 778.0	29 273.9	29 655.2	29 544.1	28 632.5	27 320.8	25 939.8	26 757.4
growing pullets	CKUW	9 582.7	9 461.1	9 366.6	9 783.7	8 285.8	8 155.8	10 928.3	9 624.7	8 936.3	9 313.3	8 356.0
fowls for breeding	JT3Q	9 401.2	10 667.0	12 082.8	11 307.0	10 987.6	10 125.2	8 561.5	9 272.9	11 461.5	9 068.3	9 608.9
turkeys, ducks, geese and all other poultry	JT3R	15 290.1	15 268.9	16 004.3	13 991.1	13 514.5	13 934.7	13 400.1	14 878.7	10 154.1	12 019.5	11 806.7

1 Includes estimates for minor holdings for all countries. See chapter text.
2 In 2007, cattle figures were sourced from the Cattle Tracing System (CTS) in England and Wales, the equivalent APHIS system in Northern Ireland and survey data in Scotland and are therefore not directly comparable with earlier years. To see comparable data for 2005-2007 please go to: http://statistics.defra.gov.uk/esg/statnot/june_uk.pdf
3 Excludes fowls laying eggs for hatching.

Sources: Department for Environment, Food and Rural Affairs;
Farming Statistics: 01904 455333

21.6 Forestry[1]
United Kingdom

		1980	1990	2000	2004	2005	2006	2007	2008	2009
Woodland area[2] - (Thousand hectares)										
United Kingdom	C5OF	2 175	2 400	2 793	2 816	2 825	2 829	2 837	2 841	2 841
England[3]	C5OG	948	958	1 103	1 114	1 119	1 121	1 124	1 127	1 128
Wales[3]	C5OI	241	248	289	286	286	285	285	285	284
Scotland[3]	C5OH	920	1 120	1 318	1 330	1 334	1 337	1 341	1 342	1 341
Northern Ireland	C5OJ	67	74	83	86	85	86	87	87	88
Forestry Commission/Forest Service[4]	C5OK	946	956	886	842	838	832	827	821	814
Other[5]	C5OL	1 230	1 443	1 907	1 974	1 987	1 997	2 010	2 020	2 027
Conifer	C5OM	1 372	1 576	1 663	1 651	1 647	1 642	1 640	1 635	1 628
Broadleaved[6]	C5ON	804	824	1 131	1 165	1 178	1 187	1 197	1 207	1 213

		1998 /99	1999 /00	2000 /01	2001 /02	2002 /03	2003 /04	2004 /05	2005 /06	2006 /07	2007 /08	2008 /09
New Planting[7] - (Thousand hectares)												
United Kingdom	C5OO	17.0	17.9	18.7	14.4	13.5	12.4	11.9	8.7	10.7	7.5	5.9
England	C5OP	5.1	5.9	5.9	5.4	5.9	4.6	5.3	3.7	3.2	2.6	2.1
Wales	C5OR	0.6	0.7	0.4	0.3	0.3	0.5	0.5	0.5	0.4	0.2	0.1
Scotland	C5OQ	10.5	10.4	11.7	8.0	6.7	6.8	5.7	4.0	6.6	4.2	3.4
Northern Ireland	C5OS	0.7	0.8	0.7	0.7	0.6	0.5	0.4	0.6	0.5	0.6	0.3
Forestry Commission/Forest Service	C5OT	0.2	0.3	0.3	0.8	0.9	0.2	0.1	0.3	0.2	0.2	0.9
Other[8]	C5OU	16.8	17.6	18.4	13.6	12.6	12.1	11.8	8.4	10.4	7.4	5.0
Conifer	C5OV	6.6	6.5	4.9	3.9	3.7	2.9	2.1	1.1	2.1	0.9	1.2
Broadleaved	C5OW	10.4	11.4	13.8	10.5	9.8	9.5	9.8	7.6	8.5	6.7	4.7
Restocking[7] - (Thousand hectares)												
United Kingdom	C5OX	14.1	15.2	15.3	13.9	14.5	14.9	16.1	15.9	19.0	18.9	15.9
England	C5OY	4.1	3.9	4.0	3.4	3.4	3.2	2.8	3.2	2.8	3.5	3.2
Wales	C5P2	3.0	2.6	2.2	1.9	1.9	1.8	1.8	2.8	3.0	2.3	2.2
Scotland	C5OZ	6.3	8.0	8.0	7.8	8.5	8.9	10.4	9.0	12.4	12.6	9.6
Northern Ireland	C5P3	0.7	0.6	1.1	0.9	0.7	1.1	1.0	0.9	0.8	0.5	0.8
Forestry Commission/Forest Service	C5P4	8.5	8.8	8.9	9.2	9.1	9.9	10.6	10.4	11.0	10.4	9.2
Other[8]	C5P5	5.6	6.4	6.4	4.7	5.3	5.0	5.5	5.5	8.0	8.5	6.7
Conifer	C5P6	11.3	11.9	12.3	11.5	12.0	12.1	13.0	12.5	15.3	14.8	12.1
Broadleaved	C5P7	2.8	3.3	3.0	2.4	2.5	2.8	3.0	3.4	3.6	4.1	3.8

		2000	2001	2002	2003	2004	2005	2006	2007	2008
Wood Production (volume - Thousand green tonnes[9])										
United Kingdom	C5P8	8 080	8 140	8 250	8 880	9 040	9 080	8 950	9 460	8 850
Softwood total	C5PA	7 430	7 500	7 630	8 320	8 520	8 490	8 510	9 020	8 420
Forestry Commission/Forest Service	C5PB	4 850	4 600	4 650	4 820	4 890	4 580	4 580	4 650	4 420
Non-Forestry Commission/Forest Service	C5PC	2 580	2 900	2 980	3 500	3 630	3 910	3 930	4 360	4 000
Hardwood[10]	C5PD	650	630	620	560	510	590	440	440	430

1 See chapter text.
2 Areas as at 31 March.
3 For England, Wales and Scotland, 1980 woodland area figures are the published results from the 1979-1982 Census of Woodlands and Trees and figures for 1990 are adjusted to reflect subsequent changes. From 1998 onwards they are based on results from the 1995-1999 National Inventory of Woodlands and Trees, adjusted to reflect subsequent changes.
4 The apparant fall in woodland cover in 2001 is due to the reclassification of Forestry Commission open land within the forest.
5 Includes private woodland and non-Forestry Commission / Forest Service public woodland.

6 Broadleaved includes coppice. For data based on 1979-82 Census, all scrub and other non-plantation woodland have been assumed to be broadleaved.
7 Figures shown are for the areas of new planting and restocking in the year to 31 March.
8 Includes grant aided planting on non-Forestry Commission/ Forest Service woodland and estimates for areas planted without the aid of grants.
9 Figures have been rounded to the nearest 10 thousand green tonnes.
10 Hardwood is timber from broadleaved species. Most hardwood production in the UK comes from non-FC/FS woodland; the figures are estimates based on reported deliveries to wood processing industries and others.

Source: Forest Service Agency;Forestry Commission: 0131 314 6171

21.7 Sales for food of agricultural produce and livestock
United Kingdom

			1999	2000	2001	2002	2003	2004	2005	2006	2007	2008	2009
Cereals:		Thousand											
Wheat[1]	KCQK	tonnes	5 668	5 617	5 672	5 628	5 611	5 600	5 642	5 625	5 702	..	..
Barley	KCQL	"	5 280	5 363	5 714	5 771	5 438	5 418	4 962	4 971	4 904	..	..
Oats[2]	KCQM	"	266	261	287	312	322	321	343	373	420	..	..
Potatoes[3]	KCQN	"	6 209	6 129	6 605	6 803	6 560	6 449	5 868	5 674	5 816	..	..
Milk:													
Utilised for liquid consumption	KCQO	Million litres	6 889	6 793	6 748	6 825	6 753	6 693	6 652	6 734	6 724	6 678	6 640
Utilised for manufacture	KCQP	"	6 973	6 532	6 752	6 883	7 140	6 724	6 490	6 266	6 085	5 840	5 705
Total available for domestic use[4]	KCQQ	"	14 234	13 730	13 940	14 100	14 290	13 765	13 478	13 325	13 146	12 816	12 852
		Million											
Hen eggs in shell	KCQR	dozens	738	712	753	747	730	773	772	743	720	754	747
Animals slaughtered:													
Cattle and calves:													
Cattle	KCQS	Thousands	2 217	2 275	2 072	2 184	2 188	2 290	2 302	2 593	2 616	2 588	2 575
Calves	KCQT	"	75	152	92	98	87	103	111	51	46	44	43
Total	KCQU	"	2 292	2 427	2 164	2 282	2 275	2 393	2 413	2 644	2 661	2 632	2 618
Sheep and lambs	KCQV	"	19 116	18 442	12 964	14 993	15 095	15 492	16 284	16 414	15 804	16 697	15 381
Pigs:													
Clean pigs	MBGD	"	14 350	12 370	10 446	10 260	9 133	9 150	8 971	8 900	9 274	9 192	9 297
Sows and boars	KCQZ	"	379	321	180	314	241	240	202	196	210	235	211
Total	KCRA	"	14 728	12 692	10 626	10 575	9 374	9 390	9 173	9 097	9 484	9 427	9 508
Poultry[5]	KCRB	Millions	863	844	867	862	882	881	903	886	874	862	866

Note: The figures for cereals and for animals slaughtered relate to periods of 52 weeks

1 Flour millers' receipts of home-grown wheat.
2 Oatmeal millers' receipts of home-grown oats.
3 Total sales for human consumption in the UK. Data for 2007 are provisional.

4 The totals of liquid consumption and milk used for manufacture may not add up to the total available for domestic use because of adjustments for dairy wastage, stock changes and other uses, such as farmhouse consumption, milk fed to stock and on farm waste.
5 Total fowls, ducks, geese and turkeys.

Source: Department for Environment, Food and Rural Affairs: 01904 455333

21.8 Estimates of producers of organic and in-conversion livestock[1]
United Kingdom

Thousand head

		2004	2005	2006	2007	2008
Cattle	IDR8	174.8	214.3	244.8	250.4	319.6
Sheep	IDR9	571.6	691.0	747.3	863.1	1 178.3
Pigs	IDS2	43.7	30.0	32.9	50.4	71.2
Poultry	IDS3	2 431.6	3 439.5	4 421.3	4 440.7	4 362.9
Goats	IDS4	0.5	0.5	0.6	0.5	0.4
Other Livestock	IDS5	1.2	1.5	4.3	3.4	4.4

Note: DEFRA have recalculated the basis on which these data are collected to make it clearer that they are an average for the year(see footnote 1).
1 Certification bodies record production data at various times of the year so figures should be treated with care as they will not represent an exact snapshot of organic livestock farming.

Sources: Department for Environment, Food and Rural Affairs;
Organic Statistics Team: 01904 455558

21.9 Producers of organic and in-conversion livestock, Organic producers, growers, processors and importers

United Kingdom

Number of producers or businesses

		2004	2005	2006	2007	2008
Producers of organic and in-conversion livestock						
North East	IDZ2	49	44	54	46	58
North West	IDZ3	122	87	102	104	95
Yorkshire and Humberside	IDZ4	82	54	82	82	85
East Midlands	IDZ5	135	110	125	121	127
West Midlands	IDZ6	196	162	196	174	190
Eastern	IDZ7	99	69	86	91	76
South West	IDZ8	761	553	724	706	705
South East (including London)	IDZ9	220	162	201	179	188
England	IE22	1 664	1 241	570	1 503	1 524
Wales	IE23	469	402	502	493	580
Scotland	IE24	385	293	296	285	282
Northern Ireland	IE25	119	110	140	167	176
United Kingdom	IE26	2 637	2 046	2 508	2 448	2 562

		2004	2005	2006	2007	2008
Producers and growers businesses						
North East	IE27	74	83	101	116	137
North West	IE28	169	176	168	173	211
Yorkshire and Humberside	IE29	134	149	138	155	190
East Midlands	IE2A	218	237	221	236	276
West Midlands	IE2B	325	337	335	351	408
Eastern	IE2C	258	259	253	267	315
South West	IE2D	1 020	1 123	1 152	1 282	1 631
South East (including London)	IE2E	409	463	417	423	556
England	IE2F	2 607	2 827	2 785	3 003	3 724
Wales	IE2G	623	667	688	710	857
Scotland	IE2H	689	653	595	686	671
Northern Ireland	IE2I	153	174	217	240	254
United Kingdom	IE2J	4 072	4 321	4 285	4 639	5 506
Processors and/or importers businesses[1]						
North East	IE2K	31	19	28	45	53
North West	IE2L	130	107	143	159	180
Yorkshire and Humberside	IE2M	126	121	141	164	191
East Midlands	IE2N	191	154	195	210	241
West Midlands	IE2O	139	114	143	169	188
Eastern	IE2P	249	209	255	289	298
South West	IE2Q	353	242	380	450	509
South East (including London)	IE2R	450	387	484	516	579
England	IE2S	1 669	1 353	1 769	2 002	2 239
Wales	IE2T	112	85	112	125	149
Scotland	IE2U	174	152	197	225	231
Northern Ireland	IE2V	35	36	50	52	56
United Kingdom	IE2W	1 990	1 626	2 128	2 404	2 675

Note: DEFRA have recalculated the basis on which these data are collected to make it clearer that they are an average for the year(see footnote 1).

1 Processors and importers include abattoirs, bakers, stores and wholesalers. The recorded location depends on the address registered with the Sector Bodies and so larger businesses may be recorded at their headquarters.

Sources: Department for Environment, Food and Rural Affairs; Organic Statistics Team:01904 455558

Agriculture, fisheries and food

21.10 Organic and in-conversion land and land use United Kingdom

Thousand hectares

		2004	2005	2006	2007	2008
Land, in-conversion						
North East	IDS6	4.6	6.6	6.9	4.8	9.8
North West	IDS7	2.5	3.2	1.8	3.3	3.8
Yorkshire and Humberside	IDS8	1.3	2.3	3.4	4.1	3.8
East Midlands	IDS9	1.2	2.4	2.1	3.1	3.7
West Midlands	IDT2	2.4	3.2	4.0	5.7	8.2
Eastern	IDT3	2.4	2.6	3.6	5.3	4.8
South West	IDT4	9.1	22.0	31.6	48.2	46.5
South East (including London)	IDT5	5.4	10.7	13.2	14.6	10.4
England	IDT6	28.8	53.2	66.5	89.0	91.1
Wales	IDT7	8.6	12.8	15.4	30.9	49.5
Scotland	IDT8	13.7	16.7	35.2	34.8	6.2
Northern Ireland	IDT9	1.6	3.2	4.0	3.2	2.3
United Kingdom	IDU2	52.7	86.0	121.1	157.9	149.1
Land, fully organic						
North East	IDU3	25.3	29.3	22.6	25.8	25.6
North West	IDU4	19.8	18.9	19.4	20.4	21.2
Yorkshire and Humberside	IDU5	8.6	9.0	9.0	9.6	10.9
East Midlands	IDU6	13.4	13.2	12.5	13.2	12.2
West Midlands	IDU7	26.8	27.0	26.3	28.2	29.7
Eastern	IDU8	10.3	11.8	10.8	12.7	13.2
South West	IDU9	90.5	94.0	93.4	106.3	123.9
South East (including London)	IDV2	34.9	35.2	35.8	42.5	47.2
England	IDV3	229.6	238.4	229.9	258.7	284.0
Wales	IDV4	55.6	58.0	63.5	65.1	75.1
Scotland	IDV5	331.6	231.2	200.1	193.1	225.1
Northern Ireland	IDV6	5.0	6.3	5.1	7.3	10.1
United Kingdom	IDV7	621.8	533.9	498.6	524.3	594.4

		2004	2005	2006	2007	2008
Land, in-conversion						
Cereals	IDV8	4.1	10.3	11.9	13.2	9.9
Other Crops	IDV9	2.7	3.5	3.4	3.5	2.5
Fruit and Nuts	IDW2	0.2	0.2	0.2	0.4	0.4
Vegetables (including potatoes)	IDW3	1.3	1.3	2.1	2.6	2.0
Herbs and ornamentals	IDW4	–	0.2	0.1	0.1	0.6
Temporary pasture	IDW5	10.4	15.9	22.9	34.2	31.0
Set aside	IDW6	2.3	1.3	1.4	1.1	..
Permanent pasture[1]	IDW7	27.2	47.5	72.1	93.6	96.0
Woodland	IDW8	0.6	3.5	4.2	5.6	2.7
Non cropping	IDW9	4.2	2.5	3.3	3.3	1.9
Other	IDX2	1.7	1.1	0.2	0.3	0.3
Unknown	IDX3	0.1	0.1	0.8	1.1	1.7
Total	IDX4	52.7	86.0	121.1	157.9	149.1
Land, fully organic						
Cereals	IDX5	35.1	37.4	35.5	38.4	47.3
Other Crops	IDX6	10.2	7.3	6.8	7.8	8.7
Fruit and Nuts	IDX7	1.5	1.5	1.6	1.6	1.5
Vegetables (including potatoes)	IDX8	12.7	12.4	13.5	14.3	17.7
Herbs and ornamentals	IDX9	0.2	0.6	0.6	0.5	4.9
Temporary pasture	IDY2	80.3	82.0	79.8	90.9	98.8
Set aside	IDY3	4.6	4.6	2.3	1.3	..
Permanent pasture[1]	IDY4	467.8	380.9	350.5	358.4	398.3
Woodland	IDY5	5.2	3.3	4.0	5.9	3.2
Non cropping	IDY6	5.9	4.7	5.4	4.7	4.4
Other	IDY7	2.4	3.2	0.4	0.4	1.0
Unknown	IDY8	0.4	0.4	0.6	1.4	8.6
Total	IDY9	621.8	533.9	498.6	524.3	594.4

Note: DEFRA have recalculated the basis on which these data are collected to make it clearer that they are a yearly average , not a snapshot.
1 Includes rough grazing.

Sources: Department for Environment, Food and Rural Affairs; Organic Statistics Team: 01904 455558

21.11 Average weekly and hourly earnings and hours of full-time male agricultural workers[1]

England and Wales: At September each year

		2004	2005	2006	2007	2008	2009
Average weekly earnings (£) 95% confidence interval	LQML	331.26 (+/-£12.46)	357.64 (+/-£13.62)	340.60 (+/-£22.05)	352.33 (+/-£13.62)	356.13 (+/-£18.97)	404.05 (+/-£19.93)
Average weekly hours worked 95% confidence interval	LQMM	46.2 (+/-1.2)	48.4 (+/-1.4)	46.1 (+/-2.4)	47.0 (+/-1.4)	46.6 (+/-2.3)	49.4 (+/-2.1)
Average earnings/hours (£) 95% confidence interval	LQMN	7.16 (+/-£0.17)	7.40 (+/-£0.17)	7.39 (+/-£0.21)	7.50 (+/-£0.16)	7.64 (+/-£0.16)	8.19 (+/-£0.17)
Number of workers in the sample		311	299	248	279	283	231

1 See chapter text.

Source: Department for Environment, Food and Rural Affairs: 01904 455332

21.12 Average weekly and hourly earnings and hours of agricultural workers[1] : by type, aged 20 and over

England and Wales: At September 2009

	Full-time		Part-time		Casual		
	Male	Female	Male	Female	Male	Female	Managers
Average weekly earnings (£) 95% confidence interval	404.05 (+/-£19.93)	329.78 (+/-£32.29)	158.52 (+/-£20.04)	148.10 (+/-£14.93)	227.08 (+/-£26.30)	160.47 (+/-£28.88)	571.75 (+/-£39.69)
Average weekly hours worked 95% confidence interval	49.4 (+/-2.1)	45.5 (+/-3.9)	20.8 (+/-2.6)	21.7 (+/-2.1)	33.0 (+/-3.4)	24.8 (+/-4.2)	..
Average earnings/hour (£) 95% confidence interval	8.19 (+/-£0.17)	7.25 (+/-£0.27)	7.61 (+/-£0.30)	6.82 (+/-£0.21)	6.88 (+/-£0.32)	6.46 (+/-£0.36)	..
Number of workers in the sample	231	103	102	105	119	63	158

1 See chapter text.

Source: Department for Environment, Food and Rural Affairs: 01904 455332

21.13 Workers employed in agriculture [1,2]: by type

United Kingdom

At June each year

Thousands

	Regular					Seasonal or casual			All			Salaried managers
	Total	Full - time		Part - time[6]		Total	Male	Female	Total	Male	Female	
		Male	Female	Male	Female							
	BANC	BAMY	BAMZ	BANA	BANB	BANF	BAND	BANE	BANI	BANG	BANH	KAYG
1995	157.4	90.4	13.0	30.0	24.1	83.7	56.5	27.2	241.2	176.8	64.3	7.7
1996	156.4	89.2	12.6	31.2	23.4	81.5	55.6	25.8	237.9	176.0	61.9	7.8
1997	154.4	87.5	12.6	31.2	23.1	80.9	55.3	25.5	235.2	174.0	61.2	7.8
1998[3,4]	155.6	88.0	13.1	29.7	24.7	79.5	55.6	23.8	235.0	172.8	62.2	12.1
1999	144.7	82.7	11.9	27.5	22.6	73.0	51.8	21.2	217.7	162.0	55.6	13.8
2000	128.9	73.4	10.3	24.6	20.6	64.4	45.9	18.5	193.3	143.9	49.4	11.1
2001[5]	120.8	69.0	10.9	22.0	18.9	63.2	44.6	18.6	184.0	135.6	48.5	13.4
	123.5	70.3	11.2	22.5	19.4	64.1	45.4	18.8	187.6	138.2	49.4	14.1
2002	116.3	64.7	11.5	21.7	18.4	64.2	46.2	18.0	180.6	132.6	47.9	13.4
2003	108.4	60.4	10.0	21.0	17.0	62.6	44.8	17.8	170.9	126.2	44.8	12.7
2004 Jun	108.8	58.1	9.8	23.5	17.4	68.3	49.6	18.6	177.0	131.2	45.8	15.2
2005 Jun	109.2	57.2	10.3	24.5	17.2	65.1	46.4	18.7	174.3	128.1	46.2	15.7
2006 Jun	105.4	53.6	10.4	24.3	17.1	64.0	44.4	19.6	169.4	122.3	47.1	14.6
2007 Jun	107.8	52.2	10.3	28.0	17.3	58.9	41.0	17.9	166.6	121.2	45.5	15.4
2008 Jun	111.1	54.7	11.3	27.9	17.2	61.7	43.2	18.6	172.8	125.8	47.1	15.1
2009 Jun	113.1	54.5	11.7	29.0	17.9	61.5	43.5	18.1	174.7	127.0	47.7	12.2

1 See chapter text. Includes estimates for minor holdings for all countries.
2 Figures exclude schoolchildren but include trainees employed under an official youth training scheme and paid at Agricultural Wages Board rates or above.
3 Results from 1998 onwards are not comparable with previous years, due to changes in the labour questions on the June Agricultural and Horticultural Census in England, Wales and Scotland.

4 From 1998, all farmers managing holdings for limited companies or other institutions in England and Wales were asked to classify themselves as salaried managers.
5 Due to an English register improvement only the top figure for 2001 is directly comparable with 2000, while the bottom figure for 2001 is only comparable with data from 2002.
6 Part time is defined as less than 39 hours per week in England and Wales, less than 38 hours per week in Scotland and less than 30 hours per week in Northern Ireland.

Sources: Department for Environment, Food and Rural Affairs;
Farming Statistics: 01904 455332

21.14 Summary of UK fishing industry
United Kingdom

£ million (unless otherwise stated)

		2000	2001	2002	2003	2004	2005	2006	2007	2008	2009
GDP for fishing[1]											
current pricegross value added at basic prices	QTUF	398	377	366	368	369	372	402	408	441	..
Output index (chain volume measures)2003 = 100	EWAC	112.0	110.4	111.2	100.0	107.2	93.5	91.3	94.5	93.8	
GDP for agriculture, forestry and fishing											
Current price gross value added at basic prices	QTOP	8 788	8 566	9 008	9 807	10 600	7 422	7 865	8 552	10 369	..
Output index (chain volume measures) 2003 = 100	GDQA	93.0	84.7	94.6	93.0	92.9	100.0	100.7	95.9	96.1	91.9
GDP at market prices											
Current price GDP at market prices	YBHA	976 533	1 021 828	1 075 564	1 139 746	1 202 956	1 254 058	1 325 795	1 398 882	1 448 391	1 395 872
Chain volume measures index 2003 = 100	YBEZ	88.4	90.6	92.5	95.1	97.9	100.0	102.9	105.5	106.1	100.8
Percentage contribution of GVA from fishing to GVA for agriculture, hunting, forestry & fishing											
Current prices		4.4%	4.5%	4.4%	4.1%	3.8%	3.5%	5.0%	5.1%	4.8%	4.3%
Current price gross value added for fishing[2] 2003=100	I3X3	106.0	100.0	100.0	100.0	100.0	101.0	109.0	111.0	120.0	..

		1999	2000	2001	2002	2003	2004	2005	2006	2007	2008
Fleet size at end of year[3]											
number of vessels	I3TC	8 039	7 818	7 721	7 578	7 096	7 022	6 716	6 752	6 763	6 573
Employment											
Number of fishermen	I3TD	16 896	15 649	14 958	14 205	13 122	13 453	12 831	12 934	12 662	12 761
Total landings by UK vessels[4]											
quantity ('000 tonnes)	I3TE	836.0	748.0	738.0	686.0	640.0	654.0	708.0	614.0	610.0	588.0
value	I3TF	588.0	550.0	574.0	546.0	528.0	513.0	513.0	610.0	645.0	629.0
Imports											
quantity ('000 tonnes)	I3TG	552.0	550.0	627.0	621.0	632.0	671.0	720.0	753.0	672.0	781.0
value[5]	I3TH	1 302.0	1 325.0	1 435.0	1 439.0	1 439.0	1 474.0	1 696.0	1 919.0	1 769.0	2 207.0
Exports											
quantity ('000 tonnes)	I3TI	351.0	365.0	391.0	389.0	480.0	478.0	461.0	416.0	431.0	416.0
value[5]	I3TJ	746.0	696.0	745.0	762.0	891.0	886.0	939.0	944.0	909.0	1 010.0

		1999	2000	2001	2002	2003	2004	2005	2006	2007	2008
Household consumption											
('000 tonnes)[6])	I3TK	447.0	443.0	483.0	479.0	485.0	487.0	494.0	525.0	539.0	527.0
Population ('000 persons)	I3TL	58 684	58 886	59 113	59 323	59 557	59 846	60 238	60 587	60 975	61 173
Consumer expenditure											
on fish	I3TM	2 063	2 172	2 298	2 405	2 397	2 447	2 661	2 987	3 516	3 685
on food	I3TN	57 040	63 958	59 804	67 959	68 227	70 743	72 400	74 430	77 196	79 583
Fish as a % of food[7]	I3TO	3.6	3.4	3.8	3.5	3.5	3.5	3.7	4.0	4.6	4.6
Landed Price index 1987 = 100	I3TP	144.0	149.0	156.0	153.0	157.0	166.0	182.0	204.0	214.0	223.0
Retail Price Index[8]	I3TQ	148.0	151.0	153.0	158.0	156.0	154.0	155.0	164.0	175.0	187.0

1 GDP for fish includes landings abroad.

2 Year on year comparisons may be affected by changes in the industrial classification of some contributors. For most businesses data are appropriate to a single activity heading; where information covers a mixture of activities, the business is classified according to the main activity.

3 The number of vessels includes those registered in the Channel Islands and the Isle of Man.

4 The quantity of landed fish is expressed in terms of liveweight. The figures relate to landings both into the UK and abroad.

5 Imports are valued at cost, including insurance and freight terms whereas exports are valued at free on board terms.

6 Data are derived from the National Food Survey prior to 2001, and from the Expenditure and Food Survey from 2001 onwards. Figures for 2001 onwards are based on financial year data.

7 Including non-alcoholic beverages.

8 The fish component of the RPI which includes canned and processed fish. The index is calculated on a monthly basis with January 1987 = 100.

Source: Fisheries Statistics Unit: 020 7270 8096

21.15

Fishing fleet[1]
United Kingdom
At 31 December each year

Numbers

		1999	2000	2001	2002	2003	2004	2005	2006	2007	2008	2009
By size												
10m and under	KSNF	5 409	5 273	5 227	5 287	5 113	5 092	4 833	4 896	4 521	4 520	4 435
10.01 - 12.19m	KSNG	577	547	536	514	486	465	449	445	446	439	430
12.20 - 17.00m	KSNH	468	467	442	409	405	393	387	384	378	379	372
17.01 - 18.29m	KSNI	154	131	143	129	121	115	112	111	110	106	102
18.30 - 24.38m	KSNJ	414	406	405	322	271	257	253	244	245	247	248
24.39 - 30.48m	KSNK	224	219	218	185	156	147	143	139	121	125	126
30.49 - 36.58m	KSNL	80	77	75	65	63	60	55	56	44	41	43
over 36.58m	KSNM	122	122	123	122	120	112	109	97	88	79	73
Total over 10m	KSNN	2 039	1 969	1 942	1 746	1 622	1 549	1 508	1 476	1 432	1 416	1 394
Total UK fleet[2]	KSNO	7 448	7 242	7 169	7 033	6 735	6 641	6 341	6 372	5 953	5 936	5 829
By segment												
Pelagic gears	KSNP	46	44	47	45	42	31	23	16	..	..	..
Beam trawl	KSNQ	114	111	116	113	162	102	96	93	..	..	..
Demersal, Seines and Nephrops	JZCI	1 235	1 208	1 158	969	853	852	812	785	..	..	..
Lines and Nets	KSNR	172	165	146	136	118	123	114	111	..	..	..
Shellfish: mobile	KSNS	243	211	229	228	191	166	155	151	..	..	..
Shellfish: fixed	KSNT	301	297	301	304	307	253	236	230	..	..	..
Distant water	KSNU	12	13	11	10	8	10	10	8	..	..	..
Under 10m	KSNV	5 916	5 769	5 713	5 773	5 587	5 395	4 276	4 131	..	..	..
Other: Mussel Dredgers	JZCJ	2	2	7	15	15	13	7	6	..	..	..
Total UK fleet[3]	I3TC	8 039	7 818	7 721	7 578	7 096	7 022	6 716	6 752	6 763	6 573	..

1 See chapter text.
2 Excluding Channel Islands and Isle of Man.
3 Including Channel Islands and Isle of Man.

Source: Fisheries Statistics Unit:020 72 728 096

Agriculture, fisheries and food

21.16 Estimated household food consumption[1]

Grammes per person per week

		Great Britain					United Kingdom							
		1997	1998	1999	2000		2001/02	2002/03	2003/04	2004/05	2005/06	2006	2007	2008
Liquid wholemilk[2] (ml)	KPQM	712	693	634	664	VQEW	599	555	585	484	460	477	420	410
Fully skimmed (ml)	KZBH	158	164	167	164	VQEX	160	166	154	158	159	163	173	158
Semi skimmed (ml)	KZBI	978	945	958	975	VQEZ	931	919	926	975	1 008	974	982	987
Other milk and cream (ml)	KZBJ	248	243	248	278	VQFA	333	350	358	366	385	395	397	392
Cheese	KPQO	109	104	104	110	VQFB	112	112	113	110	116	116	119	111
Butter	KPQP	38	39	37	39	VQFC	42	37	35	35	38	40	41	40
Margarine	KPQQ	26	26	20	21	VQFD	13	13	12	11	20	18	19	22
Low and reduced fat spreads	KZBK	77	69	71	68	VQFE	72	70	71	68	55	57	53	51
All other oils and fats (ml for oils)	KPQR	62	62	58	58	VQFF	70	70	68	68	70	69	68	72
Eggs (number)	KPQS	2	2	2	2	VQFG	2	2	2	2	2	2	2	2
Preserves and honey	KPQT	41	38	33	33	VQFH	35	34	33	34	35	34	33	34
Sugar	KPQU	128	119	107	105	VQFI	112	111	102	99	94	92	92	93
Beef and veal	KPQV	110	109	110	124	VQFJ	118	118	119	123	120	128	126	111
Mutton and lamb	KPQW	56	59	57	55	VQFK	51	51	49	50	53	54	55	45
Pork	KPQX	75	76	69	68	VQFL	61	61	56	56	52	55	54	55
Bacon and ham, uncooked	KPQY	72	76	68	71	VQFM	68	69	70	70	68	66	64	63
Bacon and ham, cooked (including canned)	KPQZ	41	40	39	41	VQFN	45	45	47	43	44	45	45	45
Poultry uncooked	JZCH	221	218	201	214	VQFO	206	199	200	197	212	207	208	207
Cooked poultry (not purchased in cans)	KYBP	33	33	35	39	VQFQ	44	45	48	49	48	48	43	44
Other cooked and canned meats	KPRB	52	49	48	51	VQFR	54	59	60	58	56	53	50	51
Offals	KPRC	7	5	5	5	VQFS	6	6	7	5	5	5	5	5
Sausages, uncooked	KPRD	63	60	58	60	VQFT	66	66	70	67	64	65	65	62
Other meat products	KPRE	209	216	221	239	VQFU	313	319	335	330	323	315	316	311
Fish, fresh and processed (including shellfish)	KPRF	70	70	70	67									
Canned fish	KPRG	31	29	31	32									
Fish and fish products, frozen	KPRH	46	46	42	44									
Fish, fresh chilled or frozen						VQAI	51	48	45	42	45	47	43	43
Other fish and fish products						VQAJ	105	106	111	115	122	123	122	118
Potatoes (excluding processed)	KPRI	745	715	673	707	VQFY	647	617	600	570	587	565	537	535
Fresh green vegetables	KPRJ	251	246	245	240	VQAK	229	231	228	225	235	221	224	203
Other fresh vegetables	KPRK	497	486	500	492	VQAL	502	505	505	536	567	566	566	557
Frozen potato products	KYBQ	106	111	113	120									
Other frozen vegetables	KPRL	94	88	87	80									
Potato products not frozen	JZCF	90	89	86	82									
Canned beans	KPRM	122	118	112	114									
Other canned vegetables (excl. potatoes)	KPRN	104	99	92	97									
Other processed vegetables (excl. potatoes)	LQZH	52	54	59	54									
All processed vegetables						VQAM	620	613	611	597	608	601	594	599
Apples	KPRO	179	181	169	180	VQGN	175	172	171	173	179	180	178	162
Bananas	KPRP	195	198	202	206	VQGO	203	208	211	217	225	226	230	219
Oranges	KPRQ	62	63	50	54	VQGP	55	62	64	57	59	55	59	49
All other fresh fruit	KPRR	276	274	290	304	VQGS	318	351	343	358	392	394	389	360
Canned fruit	KPRS	44	37	38	38	VQGT	40	39	40	38	36	39	35	32
Dried fruit, nuts and fruit and nut products	KPRT	35	34	30	35	VQGU	39	41	40	46	51	53	51	52
Fruit juices (ml)	KPRU	277	304	284	303	VQGX	327	333	322	280	350	366	340	325
Flour	KPRV	54	55	56	67	VQGY	55	61	52	55	60	54	54	63
Bread	KPRW	746	742	717	720	VQGZ	769	756	728	695	701	692	677	659
Buns, scones and teacakes	KPRX	43	41	40	43	VQHA	37	41	44	47	46	45	44	43
Cakes and pastries	KPRY	93	88	87	89	VQHB	139	122	120	117	122	120	115	111
Biscuits	KPRZ	138	137	132	141	VQHC	166	174	163	165	165	165	163	170
Breakfast cereals	KPSA	135	136	134	143	VQHE	133	132	134	131	135	135	130	130
Oatmeal and oat products	KPSB	16	11	13	15	VQHF	12	13	12	14	19	17	19	20
Other cereals and cereal products	JZCG	293	270	284	291	VQHG	345	366	360	354	378	378	387	375
Tea	KPSC	36	35	32	34	VQHK	34	34	31	31	33	30	30	30
Instant coffee	KPSD	11	12	11	11	VQHL	13	12	13	13	13	14	13	14
Canned soups	KPSE	70	71	67	71	VQHM	79	80	77	76	82	79	79	76
Pickles and sauces	KPSF	92	96	91	107	VQHN	121	123	121	120	125	128	129	130

1 See chapter text.
2 Including also school and welfare milk (pre-2001-02).

Sources: Living Costs and Food Survey;
Department for Environment Food and Rural Affairs/;
Office for National Statistics: 01904 455359

Production

Chapter 22

Production

Annual Business Inquiry

(Table 22.1)

The Annual Business Inquiry (ABI) estimates cover all UK businesses registered for Value Added Tax (VAT) and/or Pay As You Earn (PAYE) classified to the 2003 Standard Industrial Classification (SIC(2003)) headings listed in the tables. The ABI obtains details on these businesses from the Office for National Statistics (ONS) Inter-Departmental Business Register (IDBR).

As with all its statistical inquiries, ONS is concerned to minimise the form-filling burden of individual contributors and as such the ABI is a sample inquiry. The sample was designed as a stratified random sample of about 66,600 businesses; the inquiry population is stratified by SIC(2003) and employment using the information from the register.

The inquiry results are grossed up to the total population so that they relate to all active UK businesses on the IDBR for the sectors covered.

The results meet a wide range of needs for government, economic analysts and the business community at large. In official statistics the inquiry is an important source for the national accounts and input-output tables, and also provides weights for the indices of production and producer prices. Inquiry results also enable the UK to meet statistical requirements of the European Union.

Data from 1995 and 1996 were calculated on a different basis from those for 1997 and later years. In order to provide a link between the two data series, the 1995 and 1996 data were subsequently reworked to provide estimates on a consistent basis.

Revised ABI results down to SIC(2003) 4 digit class level for 1995–2007, giving both analysis and tabular detail, are available from the ONS website at: www.onsstatistics.gov.uk, with further extracts and bespoke analyses available on request. This service replaces existing publications.

Manufacturers' sales by industry

(Table 22.2)

This table shows the total manufacturers' sales for products classified to SIC(2003) and collected under the Products of the European Community Inquiry since its introduction in

1993. Some data are not available for confidentiality reasons or where data have not been published for a given period. Detailed product sales data together with exports and imports data are available in ONS's Product Sales and Trade quarterly and annual reports (PRQ and PRA series).

PRODCOM 2008 estimates are now aligned with the NACE Rev 2 (2007). Because many of the product descriptions for 2007 have been merged or split leading to the new PRODCOM List for 2008, PRODCOM 2008 estimates cannot be comprehensively compared with those of 2007 and previous years.

The PRODCOM 2007 estimates in table 22.2 of the Annual Abstract of Statistics will not be updated. PRODCOM estimates for 2008 and 2009 will be published in restructured tables in this publication in 2011.

PRODCOM 2008 estimates, in the revised structure, are currently available in Microsoft Excel format on the ONS website at: http://www.onsstatistics.gov.ukstatbase/Product.asp?vlnk=15281

Number of local units in manufacturing industries in 2003

(Table 22.3)

The table shows the number of local units (sites) in manufacturing by employment size band. The classification breakdown is at division level (two digit) as classified to SIC(2003) held on the Inter-Departmental Business Register (IDBR). This register became fully operational in 1995 and combines information on VAT traders and PAYE employers in a statistical register comprising 2.1 million enterprises (businesses) representing nearly 99 per cent of economic activity. *UK Business: Activity, Size and Location 2007* provides further details and contains detailed information regarding enterprises in the UK including size, classification, and local units in the UK including size, classification and location.

For further information on the IDBR see the ONS website at: www.statistics.gov.uk/idbr

Production of primary fuels

(Table 22.4)

This table shows indigenous production of primary fuels. It includes the extraction or capture of primary commodities and the generation or manufacture of secondary commodities. Production is always gross; that is, it includes the quantities used during the extraction or manufacturing process. Primary fuels are coal, natural gas (including colliery methane), oil, primary electricity (that is, electricity generated by hydro, nuclear wind and tide stations and also electricity imported from France through the interconnector) and renewables (includes solid renewables such as wood, straw and waste and gaseous renewables such as landfill gas and sewage gas). The figures are presented on a common basis expressed in million tonnes of oil equivalent. Estimates of the gross calorific values used for converting the statistics for the various fuels to these are given in the Digest of UK Energy Statistics available at: www.decc.gov.uk/en/content/cms/statistics/publications/dukes/dukes.aspx

Total inland energy consumption

(Table 22.5)

This table shows energy consumption by fuel and final energy consumption by fuel and class of consumer. Primary energy consumption covers consumption of all primary fuels (defined above) for energy purposes. This measure of energy consumption includes energy that is lost by converting primary fuels into secondary fuels (the energy lost burning coal to generate electricity or the energy used by refineries to separate crude oil into fractions) in addition to losses in distribution. The other common way of measuring energy consumption is to measure the energy content of the fuels supplied to consumers. This is called final energy consumption. It is net of fuel used by the energy industries, conversion, transmission and distribution losses. The figures are presented on a common basis, measured as energy supplied and expressed in million tonnes of oil equivalent. Estimates of the gross calorific values used for converting the statistics for the various fuels to these are given in the *Digest of UK Energy Statistics* available at: www.decc.gov.uk/en/content/cms/statistics/publications/dukes/dukes.aspx

So far as practicable the user categories have been grouped on the basis of the SIC(2003) although the methods used by each of the supply industries to identify end users are slightly different. Chapter 1 of the *Digest of UK Energy Statistics* gives more information on these figures.

Coal

(Table 22.6)

Since 1995, aggregate data on coal production have been obtained from the Coal Authority. In addition, main coal producers provide data in response to an annual Department of Energy and Climate Change (DECC) inquiry which covers production (deepmined and opencast), trade, stocks and disposals. HM Revenue & Customs (HMRC) also provides trade data for solid fuels. DECC collects information on the use of coal from the UK Iron and Steel Statistics Bureau and consumption of coal for electricity generation is covered by data provided by the electricity generators.

Gas

(Table 22.7)

Production figures, covering the production of gas from the UK Continental Shelf offshore and onshore gas fields and gas obtained during the production of oil, are obtained from returns made under the DECC's Petroleum Production Reporting System. Additional information is used on imports and exports of gas and details from the operators of gas terminals in the UK to complete the picture.

It is no longer possible to present information on fuels input into the gas industry and gas output and sales in the same format as in previous editions of this table. As such, users are directed to Chapter 4 of the 2002 edition of the *Digest of UK Energy Statistics*, where more detailed information on gas production and consumption in the UK is available.

DECC carry out an annual survey of gas suppliers to obtain details of gas sales to the various categories of consumer. Estimates are included for the suppliers with the smallest market share, since the DECC inquiry covers only the largest suppliers (that is, those known to supply more than 1,750 GWh per year).

Electricity

(Tables 22.8 to 22.10)

Tables 22.8 to 22.10 cover all generators and suppliers of electricity in the UK. The relationship between generation, supply, availability and consumption is as follows:

Electricity generated
less	electricity used on works
equals	electricity supplied (gross)
less	electricity used in pumping at pumped storage stations
equals	electricity supplied (net)
plus	imports (net of exports) of electricity
equals	electricity available
less	losses and statistical differences
equals	electricity consumed

In Table 22.8 'major power producers' are those generating companies corresponding to the old public sector supply system:

- AES Electric Ltd.
- Baglan Generation Ltd.
- Barking Power Ltd.
- British Energy plc

Production

- Centrica Energy
- Coolkeeragh ESB Ltd.
- Corby Power Ltd.
- Coryton Energy Company Ltd.
- Derwent Cogeneration Ltd.
- Drax Power Ltd.
- EDF Energy plc
- E.ON UK plc
- Energy Power Resources Ltd.
- Gaz De France
- GDF Suez Teesside Power Ltd
- Immingham CHP
- International Power plc
- Magnox Electric Ltd.
- Premier Power Ltd.
- RGS Energy Ltd.
- Rocksavage Power Company Ltd.
- RWE Npower plc
- Scottish Power plc
- Scottish and Southern Energy plc
- Seabank Power Ltd.
- SELCHP Ltd.
- Spalding Energy Company Ltd.
- Uskmouth Power Company Ltd.
- Western Power Generation Ltd.

Additionally, from 2007, the following major wind farm companies are included as 'major power producers':

- Airtricity
- Cumbria Wind Farms
- Fred Olsen
- H G Capital
- Renewable Energy Systems
- Vattenfall Wind

In Table 22.10 all fuels are converted to the common unit of million tonnes of oil equivalent, that is, the amounts of oil which would be needed to produce the output of electricity generated from those fuels.

More detailed statistics on energy are given in the *Digest of United Kingdom Energy Statistics 2009*. Readers may wish to note that the production and consumption of fuels are presented using commodity balances. A commodity balance shows the flows of an individual fuel through from production to final consumption, showing its use in transformation and energy industry own use.

Oil and oil products

(Tables 22.11 – 22.13)

Data on the production of crude oil, condensates and natural gases given in Table 22.11 are collected by DECC direct from the operators of production facilities and terminals situated on UK territory, either onshore or offshore, that is, on the UK Continental Shelf. Data are also collected from the companies on their trade in oil and oil products. These data are used in preference to the foreign trade as recorded by HMRC in *Overseas Trade Statistics*.

Data on the internal UK oil industry (that is, on the supply, refining and distribution of oil and oil products in the UK) are collected by the UK Petroleum Industry Association. These data, reported by individual refining companies and wholesalers and supplemented where necessary by data from other sources, provide the contents of Tables 22.12 and 22.13. The data are presented in terms of deliveries to the inland UK market. This is regarded as an acceptable proxy for actual consumption of products. The main shortcoming is that, while changes in stocks held by companies in central storage areas are taken into account, changes in the levels of stocks further down the retail ladder (such as stocks held on petrol station forecourts) are not. This is not thought to result in a significant degree of difference in the data.

Iron and steel

(Tables 22.14 – 22.16)

Iron and steel industry

The general definition of the UK iron and steel industry is based on groups 271 'ECSC iron and steel', 272 'Tubes', and 273 'Primary Transformation' of the UK SIC(92), except those parts of groups 272 and 273 which cover cast iron pipes, drawn wire, cold formed sections and Ferro alloys.

The definition excludes certain products which may be made by works within the industry, such as refined iron, finished steel castings, steel tyres, wheels, axles and rolled rings, open and closed die forgings, colliery arches and springs. Iron foundries and steel stockholders are also considered to be outside of the industry.

Statistics

The statistics for the UK iron and steel industry are compiled by the Iron and Steel Statistics Bureau (ISSB) Ltd from data collected from UK steel producing companies, with the exception of trade data which is based on HMRC data.

'Crude steel' is the total of usable ingots, usable continuously cast semi-finished products and liquid steel for castings.

'Production of finished products' is the total production at the mill of that product after deduction of any material which is immediately scrapped.

'Deliveries' are based on invoiced tonnages and will include deliveries made to steel stockholders and service centres by the UK steel industry.

For more detailed information on definitions etc please contact ISSB Ltd. on 020 7343 3900.

Minerals

(Table 22.19)

Table 22.19 gives, separately for Great Britain and Northern Ireland, the production of minerals extracted from the ground. The figures for chemicals and metals are estimated from the quality of the ore which is extracted. The data come from an annual census of the quarrying industry, which, for Great Britain, is conducted by ONS for Communities and Local Government and Business, Innovation and Skills (BIS) —formally known as Business, Enterprise and Regulatory Reform (BERR).

Building materials

(Table 22.20)

Table 22.20 gives the production and deliveries of a number of building materials which are closely associated with material extracted from the ground. The data come from surveys conducted by ONS on behalf of BIS.

Construction

(Tables 22.21 – 22.22)

Figures for the construction industry are based on SIC(2003).

The value of output represents the value of construction work done during the quarter in Great Britain and is derived from returns made by private contractors and public authorities with their own direct labour forces. The series (and the accompanying index of the volume of output) include estimates of the output of small firms and self-employed workers not recorded in the regular quarterly output inquiry.

The new orders statistics are collected from private contractors and analysed by the principal types of construction work involved. The series includes speculative work for eventual sale or lease undertaken on the initiative of the respondent where no formal contract or order is involved.

Engineering turnover and orders

(Tables 22.23 – 22.24)

The figures represent the output of UK-based manufacturers classified to Subsections DK and DL of the SIC(2003). They are derived from the monthly production inquiry (MPI) and include estimates for non-responders and for establishments which are not sampled.

New car registrations

(Table 22.25)

Mini –
Normally less than 1.0 CC
Bodystyle 'miniature'
Normally two-door
Length normally not exceeding 3050mm (10 feet)

Supermini –
Normally between 1.0–1.4 CC
Bodystyle bigger than mini
Length normally not exceeding 3745 mm (12.5 Feet)
Performance greater than mini

Lower Medium –
Normally between 1.3–2.0 CC
Length normally under 4470 mm (14.9 feet)

Executive –
Normally between 2.0–3.5 CC
Length normally under 4800 mm (16 feet)
Normally four-door

Luxury Saloon –
Normally upward from 3.5 CC
Most luxurious available

Specialist Sports –
Sports coupes
Sports saloons
Traditional sports

Dual Purpose –
4x4 off road

Production

Multi Purpose Vehicle –
4x2 or 4x4 estates with a seating capacity of up to eight
people

Drink and tobacco

(Tables 22.26 – 22.27)

Data for these tables are derived by HMRC from the
systems for collecting excise duties. Alcoholic drinks and
tobacco products become liable for duty when released for
consumption in the UK. Figures for releases include both
home-produced products and commercial imports. Production
figures are also available for potable spirits distilled and beer
brewed in the UK.

Alcoholic drink

(Table 22.26)

The figures for imported and other spirits released for home
consumption include gin and other UK produced spirits for
which a breakdown is not available.

Since June 1993 beer duty has been charged when the beer
leaves the brewery or other registered premises. Previously
duty was chargeable at an earlier stage (the worts stage) in
the brewing process and an allowance was made for wastage.
Figures for years prior to 1994 include adjustments to bring
them into line with current data. The change in June 1993
also led to the availability of data on the strength; a series in
hectolitres of pure alcohol is shown from 1994.

Made wine with alcoholic strength from 1.2 per cent to 5.5
per cent is termed 'coolers'. Included in 'coolers' are alcoholic
lemonade and similar products of appropriate strength. From
28 April 2002 duty on spirit-based 'coolers' (ready to drink
products) is charged at the same rate as spirits per litre of
alcohol. Made wine coolers include only wine based 'coolers'
from this period.

Tobacco products

(Table 22.27)

Releases of cigarettes and other tobacco products tend to be
higher in the period before a Budget. Products may then be
stocked, duty paid, before being sold.

22.1 Production and construction:[1] summary table
United Kingdom

Standard Industrial Classification 2003: Estimates for all firms

£ million

	Total turnover	Gross value added	Stocks and work in progress		Capital expenditure *less* disposals	Total employment costs
			At end of year	Change during year		
Standard Industrial Classification: Revised 2003						
Production and construction Sections C-F						
2003	678 072	228 976	67 044	1 845	25 663	118 540
2004	704 450	242 834	67 027	3 339	23 989	120 512
2005	743 738	255 974	70 536	4 038	27 292	123 310
2006	781 321	269 507	71 825	4 053	28 838	127 825
2007	828 697	285 824	76 835	4 996	32 152	132 620
Production industries (Revised definitions) Sections C-E						
2003	527 180	175 826	49 122	−401	22 448	91 317
2004	546 426	187 199	48 831	1 180	20 598	92 423
2005	577 426	192 666	50 261	1 807	23 890	93 364
2006	605 551	201 927	51 042	2 825	25 227	95 185
2007	632 513	211 167	52 941	2 834	27 649	96 433
Mining and quarrying Section C						
2003	32 329	18 173	814	−29	4 420	2 782
2004	34 159	17 890	798	30	3 992	2 755
2005	43 633	23 485	1 045	143	6 230	3 117
2006	48 386	24 832	1 028	107	5 897	3 353
2007	49 672	26 634	1 125	127	6 159	3 411
Mining and quarrying of energy producing materials Subsection CA						
2003	27 506	16 682	506	−47	4 116	1 957
2004	29 012	16 163	492	12	3 680	1 975
2005	37 270	21 686	716	89	5 944	2 258
2006	42 211	23 066	700	96	5 621	2 486
2007	44 850	24 996	860	119	5 820	2 681
Mining and quarrying except energy producing materials Subsection CB						
2003	4 823	1 491	308	18	304	825
2004	5 147	1 728	307	17	312	780
2005	6 363	1 799	329	55	286	860
2006	6 175	1 766	328	11	276	867
2007	4 822	1 638	265	7	338	729
Manufacturing (Revised definition) Section D						
2003	447 637	142 207	46 914	−371	12 677	84 597
2004	459 880	148 864	46 807	975	11 689	85 243
2005	472 235	146 913	47 805	1 488	11 322	85 432
2006	483 349	151 538	48 143	2 347	11 417	87 006
2007	504 469	157 864	50 035	2 761	12 002	87 724

22.1
continued

Production and construction:[1] summary table
United Kingdom
Standard Industrial Classification 2003: Estimates for all firms

£ million

	Total turnover	Gross value added	Stocks and work in progress		Capital expenditure *less* disposals	Total employment costs
			At end of year	Change during year		

Standard Industrial Classification: Revised 2003

Manufacture of food; beverages and tobacco
Subsection DA

2003	78 759	21 870	7 677	63	2 364	10 564
2004	81 985	22 516	7 846	177	1 966	10 632
2005	82 304	22 269	7 932	−40	2 115	11 098
2006	81 909	22 435	7 992	206	2 087	11 205
2007	81 954	22 995	8 406	657	2 409	11 156

Manufacture of textile and textile products
Subsection DB

2003	11 396	4 147	1 713	23	234	2 553
2004	10 840	3 825	1 639	7	117	2 333
2005	10 258	3 602	1 435	−10	118	2 283
2006	9 316	3 277	1 424	−18	119	1 996
2007	9 445	3 411	1 340	47	95	1 930

Manufacture of leather and leather products
Subsection DC

2003	974	375	145	−1	11	198
2004	920	326	138	−6	20	197
2005	771	301	112	4	–	167
2006	761	292	112	9	−1	190
2007	767	279	123	7	4	188

Manufacture of wood and wood products
Subsection DD

2003	7 134	2 669	713	49	211	1 444
2004	7 421	2 958	702	6	177	1 662
2005	7 488	2 952	699	44	189	1 560
2006	7 515	2 714	659	41	151	1 671
2007	8 484	3 224	786	121	235	1 850

Manufacture of pulp, paper and paper products; publishing and printing
Subsection DE

2003	44 767	18 684	2 637	78	1 338	11 056
2004	45 924	19 413	2 750	−30	1 251	11 063
2005	44 188	18 382	2 392	55	1 516	10 928
2006	43 404	18 386	2 250	95	1 156	11 149
2007	43 748	18 483	2 300	65	1 000	11 115

Manufacture of coke, refined petroleum products and nuclear fuel
Subsection DF

2003	25 348	2 213	1 269	−13	604	1 160
2004	27 881	2 651	1 362	97	484	1 131
2005	29 719	2 621	1 702	458	512	1 386
2006	30 965	2 825	1 715	5	291	1 186
2007	32 822	3 354	1 979	185	217	1 738

22.1
continued

Production and construction:[1] summary table
United Kingdom
Standard Industrial Classification 2003: Estimates for all firms

£ million

	Total turnover	Gross value added	Stocks and work in progress		Capital expenditure *less* disposals	Total employment costs
			At end of year	Change during year		

Standard Industrial Classification: Revised 2003

Manufacture of chemicals, chemical products and man-made fibres
Subsection DG

2003	49 779	15 700	6 190	−119	1 926	7 964
2004	51 375	17 240	5 941	−15	1 915	8 313
2005	60 460	18 070	6 407	−17	1 492	8 249
2006	62 129	19 047	6 706	512	1 798	8 213
2007	62 948	18 223	6 385	−179	2 337	8 318

Manufacture of rubber and plastic products
Subsection DH

2003	19 803	7 533	1 779	78	751	4 762
2004	20 790	7 799	1 878	116	579	4 960
2005	21 361	7 781	1 852	−25	475	4 841
2006	21 237	7 598	1 808	98	506	4 860
2007	21 639	7 789	1 909	123	463	4 767

Manufacture of other non-metallic mineral products
Subsection DI

2003	12 573	5 315	1 321	11	579	2 779
2004	13 715	5 846	1 434	87	525	3 041
2005	12 562	5 240	1 392	76	633	2 889
2006	13 476	5 503	1 453	59	649	2 952
2007	15 790	6 110	1 551	72	883	3 204

Manufacture of basic iron and of ferro-alloys
Subsection DJ

2003	38 125	14 623	3 744	216	1 121	9 584
2004	40 873	15 234	3 963	540	1 049	9 498
2005	43 300	15 417	4 339	302	879	9 787
2006	46 722	16 758	4 727	548	1 069	10 108
2007	50 346	17 717	5 186	400	1 080	10 134

Manufacture of machinery and equipment not elsewhere specified
Subsection DK

2003	32 078	11 785	4 913	134	644	7 914
2004	33 838	12 170	5 020	118	505	8 040
2005	34 591	12 251	5 021	95	500	8 057
2006	36 559	12 927	5 068	157	452	8 443
2007	39 004	13 302	5 069	114	568	8 304

Manufacture of electrical and optical equipment
Subsection DL

2003	46 638	15 302	5 228	−265	773	10 024
2004	41 545	15 206	5 210	160	703	9 389
2005	40 826	14 925	5 107	113	603	9 137
2006	40 922	15 729	4 860	99	677	9 228
2007	40 589	15 982	4 692	214	741	9 516

22.1

Production and construction:[1] summary table
United Kingdom
Standard Industrial Classification 2003: Estimates for all firms

£ million

	Total turnover	Gross value added	Stocks and work in progress		Capital expenditure *less* disposals	Total employment costs
			At end of year	Change during year		
Standard Industrial Classification: Revised 2003						
Manufacture of transport equipment Subsection DM						
2003	63 338	15 838	7 975	−688	1 659	10 963
2004	64 870	16 963	7 198	−429	1 913	11 274
2005	66 290	16 689	7 637	365	1 940	11 409
2006	69 054	17 542	7 652	403	2 007	12 035
2007	74 950	19 112	8 142	714	1 488	11 531
Manufacture not elsewhere classified Subsection DN						
2003	16 923	6 153	1 608	61	463	3 633
2004	17 902	6 718	1 724	147	486	3 710
2005	18 117	6 413	1 780	68	351	3 641
2006	19 381	6 504	1 718	134	455	3 769
2007	21 984	7 881	2 167	220	482	3 973
Electricity, gas and water supply Section E						
2003	47 214	15 446	1 393	−1	5 351	3 938
2004	52 386	20 445	1 227	175	4 917	4 425
2005	61 557	22 268	1 411	175	6 338	4 814
2006	73 817	25 558	1 871	371	7 912	4 826
2007	78 372	26 670	1 781	−53	9 488	5 298
Construction Section F						
2003	150 892	53 150	17 923	2 246	3 215	27 223
2004	158 025	55 636	18 195	2 159	3 391	28 088
2005	166 312	63 308	20 275	2 232	3 402	29 946
2006	175 770	67 579	20 783	1 228	3 611	32 640
2007	196 185	74 656	23 894	2 162	4 503	36 188

1 See chapter text.

Source: Office for National Statistics: 01633 456592

22.2 Manufacturers' sales: by industry[1]
United Kingdom
Standard Industrial Classification 2003

£ million

Industry		SIC (03)	2004	2005	2006	2007
Other mining and quarrying						
Quarrying of stone for construction	KSPF	14110	..	..	..	..
Quarrying of limestone, gypsum and chalk	KSPG	14120	..	..	..	..
Quarrying of slate	KSPH	14130	..	..	..	..
Operation of gravel and sand pits	KSPJ	14210	..	..	..	..
Mining of clays and kaolin	KSPK	14220	..	..	..	..
Mining of chemical and fertilizer minerals	KSPL	14300	..	..	..	..
Production of salt	KSPM	14400	..	..	..	..
Other mining and quarrying not elsewhere classified	KSPN	14500	46	52	42	37
Manufacture of food products and beverages						
Production and preserving of meat	KSPO	15110	3 927	4 166	4 319	4 320
Production and preserving of poultry meat	KSPP	15120	..	2 064	2 197	2 432
Bacon and ham production	KSPQ	15131	1 364	1 465	1 543	1 466
Other meat and poultry meat processing	KSPR	15139	3 993	4 174	3 976	4 189
Processing and preserving of fish and fish products	KSPS	15200	1 741	1 802	1 873	1 805
Processing and preserving of potatoes	KSPT	15310	1 233	..	1 286	1 336
Fruit and vegetable juice	KSPU	15320	567	586	712	775
Processing and preserving of fruit and vegetables not elsewhere classified	KSPV	15330	2 474	2 544	2 582	2 637
Crude oils and fats	KSPW	15410	399	446	372	397
Refined oils and fats	KSPX	15420	914	889	831	820
Margarine and similar edible fats	KSPY	15430	..	..	417	..
Operation of dairies	KTEH	15510	5 460	5 640	5 882	6 110
Ice cream	KSPZ	15520	..	467	432	438
Grain mill products	KSQA	15610	2 786	2 595	2 732	2 911
Starches and starch products	KSQB	15620	380	429	352	400
Prepared feeds for farm animals	KSPI	15710	2 419	2 151	2 365	2 685
Prepared pet foods	KSQC	15720	1 214	..	1 251	1 339
Bread; fresh pastry goods and cakes	KSQD	15810	4 407	4 186	4 367	4 596
Rusks and biscuits; preserved pastry goods and cakes	KSQE	15820	..	3 211	3 089	..
Sugar	KSQF	15830	1 133	1 077	1 056	1 045
Cocoa; chocolate and sugar confectionery	KSQG	15840	3 384	3 175	3 623	3 609
Macaroni, noodles, couscous and similar farinaceous products	KSQH	15850	..	..	468	..
Processing of tea and coffee	KSQI	15860	1 420	1 502	1 636	..
Condiments and seasonings	KSQJ	15870	1 129	1 129	1 235	1 217
Homogenised food preparations and dietetic foods	KSQK	15880	..	42	47	35
Manufacture of other food products not elsewhere classified	KSQL	15890	2 200	2 300	2 401	2 519
Distilled potable alcoholic beverages	KSQM	15910	2 216	..	..	..
Production of ethyl alcohol from fermented materials	KSQN	15920	..	..	..	..
Wines	KSQO	15930	52	..	..	..
Cider and other fruit wines	KSQP	15940	..	458	453	..
Other non-distilled fermented beverages	KSQQ	15950	–	–	–	..
Beer	KSQR	15960	4 072	3 805	3 896	3 578
Malt	KSQS	15970	255	239	242	..
Mineral waters and soft drinks	KSQT	15980	..	3 021	3 241	3 273
Manufacture of tobacco products						
Tobacco products	KSQU	16000	1 838	1 718	1 875	1 626
Manufacture of textiles						
Preparation and spinning of textile fibres	KSQV	17100	486	433	398	386
Textile weaving	KSQW	17200	690	626	593	578
Finishing of textiles	KSQX	17300	472	490	476	468
Soft furnishings	KSQY	17401	576	564	635	646
Canvas goods, sacks etc	KSQZ	17402	101	80	100	..
Household textiles	KSRA	17403	654	643	645	686
Carpets and rugs	KSRB	17510	690	711	770	773
Cordage, rope, twine and netting	KSRC	17520	76	84	76	85

22.2

Manufacturers' sales: by industry[1]
United Kingdom
Standard Industrial Classification 2003

£ million

Industry	SIC (03)	2004	2005	2006	2007
Manufacture of textiles continued					
Nonwovens and articles made from nonwovens, except apparel	KSRD	17530	149	150	160	169
Lace	KSRE	17541	16	19	16	..
Narrow fabrics	KSRF	17542	145	133	124	110
Other textiles not elsewhere classified	KSRG	17549	435	468	453	382
Knitted and crocheted fabrics	KSRH	17600	197	..	..	..
Knitted and crocheted hosiery	KSRI	17710	230	..	..	..
Knitted and crocheted pullovers, cardigans and similar	KSRJ	17720	219	193	176	155
Manufacture of wearing apparel; dressing and dyeing of fur					
Leather clothes	KSRK	18100	7	5	2	4
Workwear	KSRL	18210	263	225	220	198
Men's outerwear	KSRM	18221	249	182	158	167
Other women's outerwear	KSRN	18222	792	632	622	541
Men's underwear	KSRO	18231	171	..	102	63
Women's underwear	KSRP	18232	392	350	368	..
Hats	KSRQ	18241	35	..	31	28
Other wearing apparel and accessories	KSRR	18249	315	280	276	265
Dressing/dyeing of fur; articles of fur	KSRS	18300	4	4	3	3
Tanning and dressing of leather; manufacture of luggage, handbags, saddlery, harness and footwear					
Tanning and dressing of leather	KSRT	19100	..	..	..	200
Luggage, handbags and the like, saddlery and harness	KSRU	19200	140	128	127	132
Footwear	KSRV	19300	250	227	212	217
Manufacture of wood and of products of wood and cork, except furniture; manufacture of articles of straw and plaiting materials					
Sawmilling and planing of wood, impregnation of wood	KSRW	20100	752	786	834	994
Veneer sheets	KSRX	20200	801	790	838	874
Builders' carpentry and joinery	KSRY	20300	3 209	3 500	3 683	3 950
Wooden containers	KSRZ	20400	413	438	453	513
Other products of wood	KSSA	20510	380	408	373	437
Articles of cork, straw and plaiting materials	KSSB	20520	6	5	5	6
Manufacture of pulp, paper and paper products					
Paper and paperboard	KSSC	21120	2 775	2 787	2 798	2 759
Corrugated paper and paperboard, sacks and bags	KSSD	21211	551	513	543	603
Cartons, boxes, cases and other containers	KSSE	21219	3 100	2 899	2 881	3 050
Household and sanitary goods and toilet requisites	KSSF	21220	2 071	..	1 628	1 661
Paper stationery	KSSG	21230	580	581	555	..
Wallpaper	KSSH	21240	184	..	102	..
Manufacture of printed labels	EQ2T	21251	481	461	463	492
Manufacture of unprinted labels	EQ2U	21252	49	..	..	..
Manufacture of other articles of paper and paperboard not elsewhere classified	EQ2V	21259	292	228	203	380
Publishing, printing and reproduction of recorded media					
Publishing of books	KSSJ	22110	3 247	3 118	3 201	3 458
Publishing of newspapers	KSSK	22120	4 320	4 135	4 241	4 120
Publishing of journals and periodicals	KSSL	22130	7 303	7 632	7 544	7 304
Publishing of sound recordings	KSSM	22140	..	296	266	296
Other publishing	KSSN	22150	549	576	588	598
Printing of newspapers	KSSO	22210	235	..	..	193
Printing not elsewhere classified	KSSP	22220	9 148	8 859	8 576	8 993
Bookbinding and finishing	KSSQ	22230	414	422	365	353
Composition and plate-making	KSSR	22240	346	..	344	350
Other activities related to printing	KSSS	22250	819	712	652	687
Reproduction of sound recording	KSST	22310	209	242	128	65
Reproduction of video recording	KSSU	22320	272	197	123	..
Reproduction of computer media	KSSV	22330	..	26	..	6
Manufacture of chemicals and chemical products					
Industrial gases	KSSW	24110	528	525	565	599
Dyes and pigments	KSSX	24120	936	1 019	1 044	1 047
Other inorganic basic chemicals	KSSY	24130	1 090	1 165	1 169	1 211
Other organic basic chemicals	KSSZ	24140	5 825	5 740	7 169	7 101
Fertilizers and nitrogen compounds	KSTA	24150	786	863	846	945

22.2
continued

Manufacturers' sales: by industry[1]
United Kingdom
Standard Industrial Classification 2003

£ million

Industry	SIC (03)	2004	2005	2006	2007
Manufacture of chemicals and chemical products continued					
Plastics in primary forms	KSTB	24160	3 740	3 783	3 577	3 549
Synthetic rubber in primary forms	KSTC	24170	..	..	..	464
Pesticides and other agro-chemical products	KSTD	24200	470	433	424	393
Paints, varnishes and similar coatings, printing ink and mastic	KSTE	24300	2 776	2 673	2 706	2 822
Basic pharmaceutical products	KSTF	24410	734	895	1 057	797
Pharmaceutical preparations	KSTG	24420	8 761	9 568	9 731	10 960
Soap and detergents, cleaning and polishing preparations	KSTH	24510	1 805	1 661	1 646	1 753
Perfumes and toilet preparations	KSTI	24520	2 171	1 769	1 848	1 888
Explosives	KSTJ	24610	110	120	..	..
Glues and gelatines	KSTK	24620	400	438	460	382
Essential oils	KSTL	24630	..	504	564	..
Photographic chemical material	KSTM	24640	250	260	247	218
Prepared unrecorded media	KSTN	24650	..	..	31	27
Other chemical products not elsewhere classified	KSTO	24660	1 992	1 969	2 079	2 085
Man-made fibres	KSTP	24700	587	482	616	577
Manufacture of rubber and plastic products					
Rubber tyres and tubes	KSTQ	25110	569	..	551	..
Retreading and rebuilding of rubber tyres	KSTR	25120	99	..	..	..
Other rubber products	KSTS	25130	1 549	1 529	1 554	1 624
Plastic plates, sheets, tubes and profiles	KSTT	25210	3 755	4 202	4 348	4 389
Plastic packing goods	KSTU	25220	..	..	..	..
Builders' ware of plastic	KSTV	25230	4 478	4 393	4 344	4 230
Other plastic products	KSTW	25240	3 414	3 259	3 386	3 647
Manufacture of other non-metallic mineral products					
Flat glass	KSTX	26110	..	..	..	..
Shaping and processing of flat glass	KSTY	26120	1 026	1 044	1 050	1 084
Hollow glass	KSTZ	26130	638	632	560	525
Glass fibres	KSUA	26140	322	357	358	381
Manufacturing and processing of other glass including technical glassware	KSUB	26150	253	177	131	117
Ceramic household and ornamental articles	KSUC	26210	..	..	..	268
Ceramic sanitary fixtures	KSUD	26220	..	180	179	..
Ceramic insulators and insulating fittings	KSUE	26230	..	22	25	31
Other technical ceramic products	KSUF	26240	21	20	21	22
Other ceramic products	KSUG	26250	..	..	..	..
Refractory ceramic products	KSUH	26260	335	331	334	332
Ceramic tiles and flags	KSUI	26300	97	98	91	92
Bricks, tiles and construction products in baked clay	KSUJ	26400	656	650	652	614
Cement	KSUK	26510	763	..	860	963
Lime	KSUL	26520	..	78	..	..
Plaster	KSUM	26530	125	131	158	152
Concrete products for construction purposes	KSUN	26610	2 278	2 209	2 183	2 234
Plaster products for construction purposes	KSUO	26620	392	427	..	..
Ready mixed concrete	KSUP	26630	1 017	898	1 257	1 502
Mortars	KSUQ	26640	143	147	..	..
Fibre cement	KSUR	26650	85	96	..	101
Other articles of concrete, plaster and cement	KSUS	26660	116	100	87	81
Cutting, shaping and finishing of stone	KSUT	26700	386	..	435	453
Abrasive products	KSUU	26810	167	180	171	143
Other non-metallic mineral products not elsewhere classified	KSUV	26820	718	759	793	..
Manufacture of basic metals					
Cast iron tubes	KSUW	27210	164	178	211	199
Steel tubes	KSUX	27220	1 053	1 254	1 498	1 690
Cold drawing	KSUY	27310	141	146	133	142

22.2
continued

Manufacturers' sales: by industry[1]
United Kingdom
Standard Industrial Classification 2003

£ million

Industry	SIC (03)	2004	2005	2006	2007
Manufacture of basic metals continued					
Cold rolling of narrow strip	KSUZ	27320	124	116	120	140
Cold forming or folding	KSVA	27330	..	..	..	..
Wire drawing	KSVB	27340	..	235	..	259
Precious metals production	KSVD	27410	247	280	302	322
Aluminium production	KSVE	27420	1 781	1 781	2 343	2 339
Lead, zinc and tin production	KSVF	27430	..	305	454	522
Copper production	KSVG	27440	786	685	..	652
Other non-ferrous metal production	KSVH	27450	638	755	981	1 306
Casting of iron	KSVI	27510	433	438	396	371
Casting of steel	KSVJ	27520	109	135	139	149
Casting of light metals	KSVK	27530	323	303	337	396
Casting of other non-ferrous metals	KSVL	27540	262	226	215	205
Manufacture of fabricated metal products, except machinery and equipment					
Metal structures and parts of structures	KSVM	28110	5 386	5 917	6 189	7 328
Builders' carpentry and joinery of metal	KSVN	28120	1 009	1 202	1 163	1 259
Tanks, reservoirs and containers of metal	KSVO	28210	294	313	373	421
Central heating radiators and boilers	KSVP	28220	652	805	..	..
Steam generators, except central heating hot water boilers	KSVQ	28300	..	..	..	..
Forging, pressing, stamping and roll forming of metal	KSVR	28400	1 965	2 056	2 057	2 135
Treatment and coating of metals	KSVS	28510	1 163	1 274	1 345	1 335
General mechanical engineering	KSVT	28520	2 798	2 933	3 429	3 732
Cutlery	KSVU	28610	25	21	24	23
Tools	KSVV	28620	805	755	735	757
Locks and hinges	KSVW	28630	597	566	547	567
Steel drums and similar containers	KSVX	28710	122	138	127	118
Light metal packaging	KSVY	28720	1 079	1 093	1 176	1 194
Wire products	KSVZ	28730	500	534	630	665
Fasteners, screw machine products, chain and spring	KSWA	28740	623	618	581	606
Other fabricated metal products not elsewhere classified	KSWB	28750	1 662	1 618	1 689	1 714
Manufacture of machinery and equipment not elsewhere classified					
Engines and turbines, except aircraft, vehicles and cycle engines	KSWC	29110	2 307	2 446	2 614	2 773
Pumps	KSWD	29121	1 157	1 220	1 233	1 412
Compressors	KSWE	29122	1 177	1 086	1 240	1 333
Taps and valves	KSWF	29130	1 164	1 237	1 269	1 423
Bearings, gears, gearing and driving elements	KSWG	29140	863	936	976	1 021
Furnaces and furnace burners	KSWH	29210	269	258	253	277
Lifting and handling equipment	KSWI	29220	2 948	3 101	3 165	3 261
Non-domestic cooling and ventilation equipment	KSWJ	29230	2 827	2 794	2 943	3 275
Other general purpose machinery not elsewhere classified	KSWK	29240	2 003	2 192	2 347	2 474
Agricultural tractors	KSWL	29310	739	658	698	748
Other agricultural and forestry machinery	KSWM	29320	510	497	547	565
Manufacture of portable hand held power tools	EQ2W	29410	146	148	..	..
Manufacture of other metal working machine tools	EQ2X	29420	529	544	553	622
Manufacture of other machine tools n.e.c.	EQ2Y	29430	271	252	300	296
Machinery for metallurgy	KSWO	29510	71	81	77	87
Machinery for mining	KSWP	29521	540	824	..	818
Earth-moving equipment	KSWQ	29522	..	1 287	1 429	1 854
Equipment for concrete crushing and screening and roadworks	KSWR	29523	..	..	..	940
Machinery for food, beverage and tobacco processing	KSWS	29530	683	644	647	774
Machinery for textile, apparel and leather production	KSWT	29540	106	94	93	91
Machinery for paper and paperboard production	KSWU	29550	200	160	..	135
Other special purpose machinery not elsewhere classified	KSWV	29560	1 721	1 614	1 584	1 707
Weapons and ammunition	KSWW	29600	2 094	107	94	73

22.2
continued

Manufacturers' sales: by industry[1]
United Kingdom
Standard Industrial Classification 2003

£ million

Industry	SIC (03)	2004	2005	2006	2007
Manufacture of machinery and equipment not elsewhere classified continued					
Electric domestic appliances	KSYR 29710	2 047	1 706	1 724	1 741
Non-electric domestic appliances	KSWX 29720	487	445	468	478
Manufacture of office machinery and computers					
Office machinery	KSWY 30010	367	446	412	313
Computers and other information processing equipment	KSWZ 30020	4 042	3 635	2 224	1 546
Manufacture of electrical machinery and apparatus not elsewhere classified					
Electric motors, generators and transformers	KSXA 31100	2 142	2 318	2 642	2 756
Electricity, distribution and control apparatus	KSXB 31200	2 410	2 398	2 426	2 682
Insulated wire and cable	KSXC 31300	989	928	1 103	1 093
Accumulators, primary cells and batteries	KSXD 31400	318	267	207	260
Lighting equipment and electric lamps	KSXE 31500	1 090	1 104	1 049	1 100
Electrical equipment for engines and vehicles not elsewhere classified	KSXF 31610	924	871	799	850
Other electrical equipment not elsewhere classified	KSXG 31620	1 670	1 773	1 887	1 865
Manufacture of radio, television and communication equipment and apparatus					
Electronic valves and tubes and other electronic components	KSXH 32100	2 995	2 710	2 450	2 304
Telegraph and telephone apparatus and equipment	KSXI 32201	941	883	1 005	828
Radio and electronic capital goods	KSXJ 32202	1 707	1 755	..	1 730
Television and radio receivers, sound or video recording etc	KSXK 32300	2 502	2 017	2 143	2 092
Manufacture of medical, precision and optical instruments, watches and clocks					
Medical and surgical equipment and orthopaedic appliances	KSXL 33100	2 262	2 510	2 599	2 771
Instruments and appliances for measuring, checking, testing etc	KSXM 33200	4 841	4 956	5 131	5 731
Industrial process control equipment	KSXN 33300	709	820	835	1 028
Optical instruments and photographic equipment	KSXO 33400	958	949	952	1 005
Watches and clocks	KSXP 33500	52	53	42	39
Manufacture of motor vehicles, trailers and semi-trailers					
Motor vehicles	KSXQ 34100	22 485	23 914	22 645	25 543
Bodies (coachwork) for motor vehicles (excluding caravans)	KSXR 34201	..	702	722	714
Trailers and semi-trailers	KSXS 34202	1 118	1 186	1 039	1 131
Caravans	KSXT 34203	593	..	..	..
Parts and accessories for motor vehicles and their engines	KSXU 34300	9 678	9 531	9 324	9 428
Manufacture of other transport equipment					
Building and repairing of ships	KSXV 35110	1 552	465	492	480
Building and repairing of pleasure and sporting boats	KSXW 35120	640	768	813	873
Railway and tramway locomotives and rolling stock	KSXX 35200	2 103	..	1 317	..
Aircraft and spacecraft	KSXY 35300	11 904	9 552	9 709	10 667
Motorcycles	KSXZ 35410	..	..	..	..
Bicycles	KSYA 35420	54	49	45	25
Invalid carriages	KSYB 35430	..	..	106	109
Other transport equipment not elsewhere classified.	KSYC 35500	83	..	..	..
Manufacture of furniture; manufacturing not elsewhere classified					
Chairs and seats	KSYD 36110	2 871	2 885	2 801	2 849
Other office and shop furniture	KSYE 36120	1 046	1 099	1 108	1 220
Other kitchen furniture	KSYF 36130	970	940	1 047	1 158
Other furniture	KSYG 36140	1 884	1 775	1 875	2 091
Mattresses	KSYH 36150	591	542	546	523
Striking of coins and medals	KSYI 36210	..	..	..	..
Jewellery and related articles not elsewhere classified	KSYJ 36220	385	338	444	434
Musical instruments	KSYK 36300	43	42	31	32
Sports goods	KSYL 36400	336	326	293	311
Games and toys	KSYM 36500	354	354	322	352
Imitation jewellery	KSYN 36610	25	31	35	37
Brooms and brushes	KSYO 36620	130	..	110	127
Miscellaneous stationers' goods	KSYP 36631	..	174	177	159
Other manufacturing not elsewhere classified	KSYQ 36639	390	423	419	447

1 See chapter text. PRODCOM data is published on the ONS website in the PRA and PRQ series of reports.

Source: Office for National Statistics: 01633 456746

22.3 Number of local units in manufacturing industries, March 2008[1]
United Kingdom
Standard Industrial Classification 2003 Division by Employment Sizeband

Numbers

	Employment size								
	0 - 4	5 - 9	10 - 19	20 - 49	50 - 99	100 - 249	250 - 499	500+	Total
Division									
15/16 Food products; beverages and tobacco	3 895	2 070	1 360	1 090	550	500	240	175	9 880
17 Textiles and textile products	2 860	830	545	420	195	105	20	5	4 980
18 Wearing apparel; dressing and dyeing of fur	2 455	690	380	235	80	25	5	0	3 870
19 Leather and leather products	430	140	80	65	25	15	0	0	755
20 Wood and wood products	5 485	1 480	965	545	160	70	15	0	8 720
21 Pulp, paper and paper products	940	275	255	320	165	160	35	5	2 155
22 Publishing, printing and reproduction of recorded media	20 065	3 895	2 330	1 490	550	325	95	50	28 800
23 Coke, refined petroleum products and nuclear fuel	160	50	25	20	20	15	15	10	315
24 Chemicals, chemical products and man-made fibres	1 885	580	495	530	335	245	110	55	4 235
25 Rubber and plastic products	3 015	1 330	1 180	1 020	500	330	70	15	7 460
26 Other non-metallic mineral products	3 515	1 020	670	565	265	180	40	10	6 265
27 Basic metals	800	270	230	250	145	100	30	15	1 840
28 Fabricated metal products, except machinery and equipment	17 420	4 940	3 480	2 475	850	335	60	15	29 575
29 Machinery and equipment not elsewhere classified	7 085	2 205	1 755	1 420	535	365	105	55	13 525
30 Office machinery and computers	775	140	75	75	30	25	10	10	1 140
31 Electrical machinery and apparatus not elsewhere classified	2 880	735	640	595	245	180	50	20	5 345
32 Radio, television and communication equipment and apparatus	1 695	365	250	270	105	90	35	15	2 825
33 Medical, precision and optical instruments, watches and clocks	2 935	880	710	580	255	140	55	15	5 570
34 Motor vehicles, trailers and semi-trailers	1 775	505	360	350	190	160	75	60	3 475
35 Other transport equipment	1 750	390	285	195	120	110	50	55	2 955
36/37 Manufacturing not elsewhere classified	12 750	3 170	1 640	985	315	180	45	15	19 100
Total manufacturing (15/37)	94 570	25 960	17 710	13 495	5 635	3 655	1 160	600	162 785

1 The data in this table is taken from the NS publication,
UK Business: Activity, Size and Location 2008.
The count of units refers to local units, i.e. individual sites, rather than whole businesses. All counts have been rounded to avoid disclosure.

Source: Office for National Statistics: 01633 812293

22.4 Production of primary fuels[1]
United Kingdom

Million tonnes of oil equivalent

		1998	1999	2000	2001	2002	2003	2004	2005	2006	2007	2008
Coal	HFZQ	25.8	23.2	19.6	20.0	18.8	17.6	15.6	12.7	11.4	10.7	11.4
Petroleum[2]	HGCY	145.3	150.2	138.3	127.8	127.0	116.2	104.5	92.9	84.0	83.9	78.6
Natural Gas[3]	HGDB	90.2	99.1	108.4	105.9	103.6	102.9	96.4	88.2	80.0	72.1	69.7
Primary electricity[4]	HGDN	24.0	22.9	20.2	21.2	20.6	20.4	18.7	19.0	17.9	14.9	13.0
Renewable energy[5]	HGDO	2.1	2.2	2.3	2.5	2.8	3.0	3.1	3.7	4.0	4.4	4.4
Total Production	HGDP	287.2	297.7	288.7	277.4	272.9	260.2	238.4	216.5	197.2	186.0	176.9

1 See chapter text.
2 Includes crude oil, natural gas liquids and feedstocks.
3 Includes colliery methane.

4 Nuclear, natural flow hydro-electricity and generation at wind stations.
5 Includes solar and geothermal heat, solid renewable sources (wood, waste, etc), and gaseous renewable sources (landfill gas, sewage gas).

Source: Department of Energy and Climate Change: 0300 068 5060

22.5 Total inland energy consumption
United Kingdom

Heat supplied basis

Million tonnes of oil equivalent

		1998	1999	2000	2001	2002	2003	2004	2005	2006	2007	2008
Inland energy consumption of primary fuels and equivalents[1]	KLWA	230.8	230.7	233.7	236.3	229.9	232.0	233.5	234.7	232.6	226.6	224.4
Coal[2]	KLWB	40.9	36.7	38.6	41.0	37.7	40.5	39.0	39.8	43.5	40.9	37.9
Petroleum[3]	KLWC	76.0	75.2	75.9	75.4	74.0	73.5	75.3	77.3	77.1	75.6	74.4
Primary electricity	KLWD	25.0	24.2	21.4	22.1	21.3	20.6	19.4	19.8	18.5	15.4	13.9
Natural gas	KLWE	86.9	92.5	95.6	95.4	94.2	94.5	96.6	93.9	89.2	90.1	93.0
Renewables and waste	GYUY	2.1	2.2	2.3	2.5	2.8	3.1	3.5	4.1	4.4	4.7	5.3
less Energy used by fuel producers and losses in conversion and distribution	KLWF	74.7	74.1	74.5	75.4	73.2	73.8	73.6	74.4	74.2	71.2	69.3
Total consumption by final users[1]	KLWG	155.9	156.5	159.2	160.9	156.5	158.0	159.8	160.2	158.3	155.3	154.9
Final energy consumption by type of fuel												
Coal (direct use)	KLWH	3.7	3.5	2.7	2.7	2.2	2.1	2.0	1.7	1.6	1.7	1.8
Coke and breeze	KLWI	0.9	0.9	0.8	0.8	0.7	0.7	0.6	0.6	0.5	0.5	0.5
Other solid fuel[4]	KLWJ	0.7	0.6	0.4	0.5	0.5	0.3	0.3	0.4	0.4	0.4	0.4
Coke oven gas	KLWK	0.4	0.2	0.2	0.2	0.1	0.1	0.1	0.1	0.1	0.1	0.1
Natural gas (direct use)	KLWL	55.9	55.1	57.1	57.8	55.2	56.7	57.1	55.3	52.9	50.6	51.7
Electricity	KLWM	27.1	27.8	28.3	28.6	28.7	28.9	29.1	29.8	29.6	29.4	29.4
Petroleum (direct use)[5]	KLWN	66.1	65.1	66.3	67.1	66.1	66.8	68.6	70.4	71.0	70.3	68.1
Renewables[6]	GYVA	0.9	0.7	0.7	0.7	0.7	0.7	0.7	0.7	0.9	1.2	1.8
Heat	JT3J	..	2.5	2.5	2.3	2.1	1.8	1.3	1.3	1.2	1.1	1.1
Final energy consumption by class of consumer												
Agriculture	KLWP	1.4	1.3	1.2	1.3	1.2	1.0	0.9	1.0	0.9	0.9	0.9
Iron and steel industry	KLWQ	4.0	3.8	2.2	2.3	2.0	1.9	1.9	1.8	1.9	1.7	1.5
Other industries	KLWR	30.5	30.5	33.1	33.2	32.0	32.4	31.3	31.9	31.0	29.9	29.1
Railways[7]	KLWS	1.3	1.4	1.4	1.4	1.4	1.4	1.4	1.5	1.5	1.4	1.5
Road transport	KLWT	41.0	41.4	41.1	41.1	41.9	41.8	42.2	42.4	42.7	43.2	42.2
Water transport	KLWU	1.2	1.1	1.0	0.8	0.7	1.2	1.2	1.4	1.8	1.6	1.8
Air transport	KLWV	10.2	11.0	12.0	11.8	11.7	11.9	12.9	13.9	14.0	13.9	13.4
Domestic	KLWW	46.1	46.1	46.9	48.2	47.0	47.7	48.6	47.2	45.8	44.2	45.6
Public administration	KLWX	8.1	8.2	8.1	8.0	7.0	6.7	7.2	7.2	7.1	6.7	6.9
Commercial and other services	KLWY	12.0	11.8	12.2	12.8	11.6	12.0	12.2	12.1	11.8	11.8	12.0

1 Includes heat sold from 1999.
2 Includes net trade and stock change in other solid fuels.
3 Refinery throughput of crude oil, *plus* net foreign trade and stock change in petroleum products. Petroleum products not used as fuels (chemical feedstock, industrial and white spirits, lubricants, bitumen and wax) are excluded.

4 Includes briquettes, ovoids, Phurnacite, Coalite, etc., and wood, waste etc., used for heat generation.
5 Includes manufactured liquid fuels from 1994.
6 Predominantly used for renewable heat: includes liquid biofuels from 2006, consumption of renewable electricity is included under 'Electricity'.
7 Includes fuel used at transport premises.

Source: Department of Energy and Climate Change: 0300 068 5060

Production

22.6 Coal: supply and demand[1]
United Kingdom

Million tonnes

		1997	1998	1999	2000	2001	2002	2003	2004	2005	2006	2007	2008
Supply													
Production of deep-mined coal	KLXA	30.3	25.7	20.9	17.2	17.3	16.4	15.6	12.5	9.6	9.4	7.7	8.1
Production of opencast coal	KLXB	16.7	14.3	15.3	13.4	14.2	13.1	12.1	12.0	10.4	8.6	8.9	9.5
Total	KLXC	47.0	40.0	36.2	30.6	31.5	29.5	27.8	24.5	20.0	18.1	16.5	17.6
Recovered slurry, fines, etc	KLXD	1.5	1.1	0.9	0.6	0.4	0.4	0.5	0.6	0.5	0.4	0.5	0.4
Imports	KLXE	19.8	21.2	20.3	23.4	35.5	28.7	31.9	36.2	44.0	50.5	43.4	43.9
Total	KLXF	68.3	62.4	57.4	54.6	67.5	58.7	60.2	61.3	64.5	69.0	60.4	61.9
Change in stocks at collieries and opencast sites	KSOL	0.7	−0.2	0.6	−3.5	−0.1	0.9	−0.9	−0.4	−0.1	−0.3	−0.1	0.1
Total supply	KLXI	67.6	62.7	56.8	58.2	67.5	57.8	61.0	61.7	64.6	68.7	60.3	62.0
Home consumption													
Total home consumption	KLXW	63.1	63.2	55.7	59.9	63.9	58.6	63.0	60.5	61.9	67.5	62.9	58.2
Overseas shipments and bunkers	KLXX	1.1	1.0	0.8	0.7	0.5	0.5	0.5	0.6	0.5	0.4	0.5	0.6
Total consumption and shipments	KLXY	64.2	64.1	56.5	60.6	64.4	59.1	63.6	61.1	62.4	67.9	63.4	58.8
Change in distributed stocks[2]	KLXZ	3.0	−1.1	0.6	−2.3	3.5	−1.4	−2.4	0.5	1.9	1.9	−2.9	4.1
Balance[3]	KLYA	0.4	−0.3	−0.3	−0.1	−0.4	0.1	−0.2	0.1	0.3	−1.1	−0.2	−0.9
Stocks at end of year													
Distributed[2]	KLYB	15.3	14.2	14.8	12.4	15.9	14.5	12.1	12.6	14.5	16.4	13.5	17.6
At collieries and opencast sites	KSOM	4.8	4.6	5.2	1.6	1.6	2.5	1.6	1.2	1.1	0.8	0.7	0.8
Total stocks	KLYE	20.1	18.8	19.9	14.1	17.5	17.0	13.7	13.8	15.6	17.2	14.2	18.4

1 See chapter text. Figures relate to periods of 52 weeks. For 1998, figures relate to 52 weeks estimate for period ended 26 December 1998.
2 Excludes distributed stocks held in merchant yards etc., mainly for the domestic market, and stocks held by the industrial sector.
3 This is the balance between supply and consumption, shipments and changes in known distributed stocks.

Source: Department of Energy and Climate Change: 0300 068 5044

22.7 Fuel input and gas output: gas consumption[1,2]
United Kingdom

Giga-watt hours

		2000	2001	2002	2003	2004	2005	2006	2007	2008
Analysis of gas consumption										
Transformation sector	I77I	349 454	336 525	351 856	344 410	362 668	351 448	331 528	374 646	397 246
Electricity generation	I77G	324 563	312 939	329 847	324 580	340 824	328 960	309 505	352 737	374 084
Heat generation[3]	I77H	24 891	23 586	22 009	19 830	21 844	22 488	22 023	21 909	23 161
Energy industry use total	I77N	77 941	91 451	91 260	88 907	88 468	86 273	79 240	73 260	69 196
Oil and gas extraction	I77J	65 555	78 457	79 364	76 837	77 753	74 187	70 138	65 305	62 231
Petroleum refineries	KIKN	3 641	4 189	3 350	2 773	3 076	4 274	2 542	2 441	1 887
Coal extraction and coke manufacture	I77K	241	220	196	188	150	114	112	91	95
Blast furnaces	I77L	712	375	222	539	728	941	611	719	718
Other	I77M	7 792	8 210	8 128	8 570	6 761	6 757	5 837	4 703	4 265
Final consumption total	I77F	678 142	683 753	653 151	669 457	673 860	652 570	622 671	598 161	610 561
Iron and steel industry	KIKR	8 953	8 502	8 791	10 327	9 715	8 469	8 406	7 311	6 818
Other industries	KIKS	174 488	171 341	156 375	155 890	144 238	142 923	137 328	127 949	125 683
Domestic	KIKT	369 909	379 426	376 372	386 486	396 411	384 009	365 850	352 943	363 315
Public administration	KIKU	44 552	46 232	42 998	44 362	51 934	50 319	48 816	44 486	47 288
Commercial	I77D	36 216	37 098	36 224	39 537	37 595	35 097	34 277	35 943	37 958
Agriculture	KIKV	1 522	2 329	2 346	2 324	2 355	2 261	2 013	1 999	2 161
Miscellaneous	KIKW	28 166	27 452	19 265	20 510	21 591	19 814	18 068	17 302	18 066
Non energy use	I77E	14 336	11 373	10 780	10 021	10 021	9 678	7 913	10 228	9 273
Total gas consumption	I77O	1 105 537	1 111 729	1 096 267	1 102 774	1 124 996	1 090 291	1 033 439	1 046 067	1 077 003

1 See chapter text. The breakdown of consumption by industrial users is made according to the 2003 Standard Industrial Classification.
2 Natural gas plus colliery methane.
3 Heat generation data are not available before 1999. For earlier years gas used to generate heat for sale is allocated to final consumption by the sector producing the heat.

Source: Department of Energy and Climate Change: 0300 068 5042

22.8 Electricity: generation, supply and consumption[1]
United Kingdom

Gigawatt-hours

		1998	1999	2000	2001	2002	2003	2004	2005	2006	2007	2008
Electricity generated												
Major power producers: total	KLUA	333 764	336 608	341 783	353 066	353 994	362 600	358 313	362 156	361 232	361 410	355 284
Conventional thermal and other[2]	AWLC	134 009	118 762	131 062	132 744	126 694	146 382	139 105	140 405	156 813	144 596	127 763
Combined cycle gas turbine stations	KJCS	93 832	114 620	117 935	123 846	132 016	121 076	131 182	130 689	118 495	139 826	158 734
Nuclear stations	KLUC	99 486	95 133	85 063	90 093	87 848	88 686	79 999	81 618	75 451	63 028	52 486
Hydro-electric stations:												
Natural flow	KLUE	4 237	4 431	4 331	3 215	3 927	2 568	3 908	3 826	3 693	4 144	4 224
Pumped storage	KLUF	1 624	2 902	2 694	2 422	2 652	2 734	2 649	2 873	3 853	3 859	4 089
Renewables other than hydro	KLUG	576	761	698	738	856	1 154	1 471	2 744	2 928	5 957	7 988
Other generators: total	KLUH	28 938	31 543	35 285	31 721	33 252	35 609	35 616	36 148	36 060	35 634	34 365
Conventional thermal and other[2]	AWLD	19 091	19 419	19 094	16 621	15 788	17 244	14 419	13 407	12 354	13 865	12 951
Combined cycle gas turbine stations	KJCT	5 428	7 141	10 859	8 979	10 577	10 879	11 852	11 792	11 561	11 516	11 009
Hydro-electric stations (natural flow)	KLUK	881	905	755	840	860	660	936	1 096	900	946	944
Renewables other than hydro	KILA	3 538	4 078	4 577	5 283	6 028	6 825	8 408	9 853	11 246	9 308	9 461
All generating companies: total	KLUL	362 702	368 151	377 068	384 787	387 246	398 209	393 929	398 304	397 292	397 044	389 649
Conventional thermal and other[2]	AWYH	153 100	138 181	150 156	149 365	142 482	163 626	153 524	153 812	169 167	158 461	140 714
Combined cycle gas turbine stations	KJCU	99 260	121 761	128 794	132 825	142 593	131 955	143 034	142 481	130 056	151 342	169 743
Nuclear stations	KLUN	99 486	95 133	85 063	90 093	87 848	88 686	79 999	81 618	75 451	63 028	52 486
Hydro-electric stations:												
Natural flow	KLUP	5 118	5 336	5 086	4 055	4 787	3 228	4 844	4 922	4 593	5 090	5 168
Pumped storage	KLUQ	1 624	2 902	2 694	2 422	2 652	2 734	2 649	2 873	3 853	3 859	4 089
Renewables other than hydro	KLUR	4 114	4 839	5 275	6 021	6 884	7 979	9 879	12 597	14 174	15 265	17 449
Electricity used on works: Total	KLUS	17 408	16 706	16 304	17 394	17 126	18 136	17 032	17 817	18 504	17 699	16 317
Major generating companies	KLUT	16 140	15 461	14 952	16 066	15 746	16 747	15 582	16 209	17 031	16 099	14 671
Other generators	KLUU	1 268	1 245	1 352	1 328	1 380	1 389	1 451	1 608	1 472	1 600	1 646
Electricity supplied (gross)												
Major power producers: total	KLUV	317 624	321 147	326 831	336 999	338 248	345 854	342 732	345 947	344 201	345 311	340 613
Conventional thermal and other[2]	AWYI	127 788	112 919	124 828	126 434	120 495	139 137	132 240	133 513	148 520	136 825	120 707
Combined cycle gas turbine stations	KJCV	93 005	112 768	116 110	121 344	129 384	118 546	128 983	128 179	116 398	137 561	156 225
Nuclear stations	KLUX	90 590	87 672	78 334	82 985	81 090	81 911	73 682	75 173	69 237	57 249	47 673
Hydro-electric stations:												
Natural flow	KLUZ	4 225	4 409	4 316	3 203	3 914	2 559	3 901	3 821	3 680	4 114	4 209
Pumped storage	KLVA	1 569	2 804	2 603	2 340	2 562	2 641	2 559	2 776	3 722	3 846	4 075
Renewables other than hydro	KLVB	447	574	640	692	802	1 059	1 367	2 486	2 643	5 717	7 724
Other generators: total	KLVC	27 670	30 298	33 933	30 393	31 873	34 220	34 165	34 539	34 588	34 034	32 719
Conventional thermal and other[2]	AWYJ	18 250	18 643	18 499	15 996	15 211	16 711	13 986	13 026	12 007	13 471	12 573
Combined cycle gas turbine stations	KJCW	5 157	6 785	10 318	8 531	10 049	10 336	11 260	11 204	10 984	10 941	10 460
Hydro-electric stations (natural flow)	KLVF	869	894	743	829	849	653	919	930	885	930	927
Renewables other than hydro	KIKZ	3 393	3 977	4 374	5 037	5 764	6 519	7 999	9 380	10 712	8 693	8 759
All generating companies: total	KLVG	345 294	351 445	360 764	367 392	370 121	380 074	376 897	380 486	378 789	379 345	373 332
Conventional thermal and other[2]	AWYK	146 038	131 562	143 327	142 430	135 706	157 136	146 226	146 539	160 527	150 296	133 280
Combined cycle gas turbine stations	KJCX	98 162	119 553	126 428	129 875	139 433	128 882	140 243	139 383	127 382	148 502	166 685
Nuclear stations	KLVI	90 590	87 672	78 334	82 985	81 090	81 911	73 682	75 173	69 237	57 249	47 673
Hydro-electric stations:												
Natural flow	KLVK	5 094	5 303	5 059	4 032	4 763	3 212	4 820	4 751	4 565	5 044	5 136
Pumped storage	KLVL	1 569	2 804	2 603	2 340	2 562	2 641	2 559	2 776	3 722	3 846	4 075
Renewables other than hydro	KLVM	3 840	4 551	5 014	5 729	6 566	7 578	9 366	11 866	13 355	14 410	16 483
Electricity used in pumping												
Major power producers	KLVN	2 594	3 774	3 499	3 210	3 463	3 546	3 497	3 707	4 918	5 071	5 371
Electricity supplied (net): Total	KLVO	342 700	347 671	357 266	364 182	366 657	376 528	373 399	376 780	373 871	374 274	367 961
Major power producers	KLVP	315 030	317 373	323 332	333 789	334 785	342 308	339 235	342 240	339 283	340 240	335 242
Other generators	KLVQ	27 670	30 298	33 933	30 393	31 873	34 220	34 165	34 539	34 588	34 034	32 719
Net imports	KGEZ	12 468	14 244	14 174	10 399	8 414	2 160	7 490	8 321	7 517	5 215	11 022
Electricity available	KGIZ	355 168	361 915	371 440	374 581	375 072	378 687	380 889	385 100	381 387	379 488	378 983
Losses in transmission etc	KGKW	29 818	29 862	31 146	32 077	30 963	32 070	33 175	30 101	28 456	27 453	28 478
Electricity consumption: Total	KGKX	325 350	332 053	340 294	342 504	344 109	346 617	347 714	354 999	352 931	352 035	350 505
Fuel industries	KGKY	8 406	8 037	9 703	8 625	10 060	9 752	8 142	7 850	7 997	10 064	8 377
Final users: total	KGKZ	316 944	324 016	330 593	333 879	334 049	336 865	339 571	347 150	344 934	341 972	342 128
Industrial sector	KGLZ	108 443	112 250	115 286	112 495	113 296	114 006	116 466	121 199	118 555	117 614	114 124
Domestic sector	KGMZ	109 410	110 308	111 842	115 337	114 534	115 761	115 526	116 811	116 449	115 051	117 841
Other sectors	KGNZ	99 091	101 457	103 465	106 047	106 219	107 098	107 579	109 140	109 930	109 307	110 163

1 See chapter text.
2 Includes electricity supplied by gas turbines and oil engines and plants producing electricity from renewable resources other than hydro.

Source: Department of Energy and Climate Change: 0300 0685050

Production

22.9 Electricity: plant capacity and demand
United Kingdom
At end of December

Megawatts

		2000	2001	2002	2003	2004	2005	2006	2007	2008
Major power producers:[1]										
Total declared net capability	GUFY	72 193	73 382	70 369	71 471	73 293	73 941	74 996	76 052	76 450
Conventional steam stations	GUFZ	34 835	34 835	30 687	31 867	31 982	32 292	33 608	33 734	32 426
Combined cycle gas turbine stations	GUGA	19 349	20 517	21 800	22 037	23 783	24 263	24 859	24 854	26 494
Nuclear stations[2]	GUGB	12 486	12 486	12 240	11 852	11 852	11 852	10 969	10 979	10 979
Gas turbines and oil engines	GUGC	1 291	1 291	1 433	1 537	1 495	1 356	1 444	1 445	1 258
Hydro-electric stations:										
Natural flow	GUGD	1 327	1 348	1 304	1 273	1 276	1 273	1 294	1 293	1 412
Pumped storage	GUGE	2 788	2 788	2 788	2 788	2 788	2 788	2 726	2 744	2 744
Renewables other than hydro	GUGF	117	117	117	117	117	117	96	1 002	1 136
Other generators:										
Total capacity of own generating plant[3]	GUGG	6 258	6 296	6 336	6 793	6 829	7 422	7 389	6 912	7 092
Conventional steam stations[4]	GUGH	3 544	3 464	3 325	3 480	3 275	3 269	3 059	3 033	2 975
Combined cycle gas turbine stations	GUGI	1 709	1 777	1 854	1 927	1 968	2 182	2 106	2 076	2 069
Hydro-electric stations (natural flow)	GUGJ	158	160	162	129	132	120	123	127	127
Renewables other than hydro	GUGK	847	895	995	1 257	1 454	1 852	2 101	1 675	1 921
All generating companies: Total capacity[3]	GUGL	78 451	79 678	76 705	78 264	80 122	81 363	82 385	82 964	83 542
Conventional steam stations[4]	GUGM	38 379	38 299	34 012	35 347	35 257	35 561	36 667	36 767	35 401
Combined cycle gas turbine stations	GUGN	21 058	22 294	23 654	23 964	25 751	26 445	26 965	26 930	28 563
Nuclear stations	GUGO	12 486	12 486	12 240	11 852	11 852	11 852	10 969	10 979	10 979
Gas turbines and oil engines	GUGP	1 291	1 291	1 433	1 537	1 495	1 356	1 444	1 445	1 258
Hydro-electric stations:										
Natural flow	GUGQ	1 485	1 508	1 466	1 402	1 408	1 393	1 417	1 420	1 539
Pumped storage	GUGR	2 788	2 788	2 788	2 788	2 788	2 788	2 726	2 744	2 744
Renewables other than hydro	GUGS	964	1 012	1 112	1 374	1 571	1 969	2 197	2 677	3 057
Major power producers:[1]										
Simultaneous maximum load met[5]	GUGT	58 452	58 589	61 717	60 501	61 013	61 697	59 071	61 527	60 289
System load factor[6] **(percentages)**	GUGU	67.0	69.0	65.0	67.0	67.0	66.0	69.0	66.0	67.0

1 See chapter text.
2 Nuclear generators are now included under "major power producers" only.
3 Capacity figures for other generators are as at end-December of the previous year.

4 For other generators, conventional steam stations cover all types of stations not separately listed.
5 Maximum load in year to end of March.
6 The average hourly quantity of electricity available during the year ending March expressed as a percentage of the maximum demand.

Source: Department of Energy and Climate Change : 0300 0685050

22.10 Electricity: fuel used in generation
United Kingdom
At end of December[1]

Million tonnes of oil equivalent

		1997	1998	1999	2000	2001	2002	2003	2004	2005	2006	2007	2008
Major power producers:[1] **total all fuels**	KGPS	71.50	74.90	73.60	74.40	77.38	75.79	77.53	76.82	78.19	78.75	75.96	74.13
Coal	FTAJ	27.71	28.72	24.51	27.77	30.57	28.62	31.57	30.37	31.65	35.00	31.93	28.94
Oil[2]	FTAK	1.38	0.85	0.82	0.77	0.82	0.69	0.70	0.60	0.90	1.00	0.80	1.20
Gas	KGPT	19.3	20.3	24.2	24.4	23.8	25.0	24.5	26.2	25.4	23.9	27.5	29.6
Nuclear[3]	FTAL	22.99	23.44	22.22	19.64	20.77	20.10	20.04	18.16	18.37	17.13	14.04	11.91
Hydro (natural flow)	FTAM	0.28	0.36	0.38	0.37	0.28	0.34	0.22	0.34	0.33	0.32	0.36	0.37
Other fuels used by UK companies	KGPU	0.200	0.200	0.200	0.200	0.300	0.300	0.400	0.500	0.800	0.700	0.932	1.211
Net imports	KGPV	1.4	1.1	1.2	1.2	0.9	0.7	0.2	0.6	0.7	0.6	0.4	0.9
Other generators: total all fuels	KGPW	6.7	7.1	7.3	8.0	7.6	8.0	8.7	8.4	8.9	8.7	8.6	8.4
Transport undertakings													
Gas	KGPX	0.200	0.200	0.200	0.200	0.200	0.200	0.008	0.002	0.003	0.002	0.002	0.002
Undertakings in industrial sector													
Coal	KGPY	1.2	1.2	1.0	0.9	1.0	1.0	1.0	0.9	0.9	0.9	0.9	1.0
Oil	KGPZ	0.8	0.7	0.7	0.8	0.6	0.6	0.5	0.5	0.5	0.5	0.5	0.6
Gas	KGQM	2.2	2.5	2.7	3.3	2.9	3.2	3.4	3.1	2.8	2.6	2.8	2.8
Hydro (natural flow)	KGQO	0.1	0.1	0.1	0.1	0.1	0.1	0.1	0.1	0.1	0.1	0.1	0.1
Other fuels	KGQP	2.186	2.420	2.640	2.770	2.740	2.968	3.660	3.781	4.619	4.599	4.217	3.909
All generating companies: total fuels	KGQQ	78.20	82.00	80.90	82.40	84.90	83.80	86.20	85.20	87.10	87.50	84.50	82.50
Coal	KGQR	28.3	29.9	25.5	28.7	31.6	29.6	32.5	31.3	32.6	35.9	32.9	29.9
Oil	KGQS	2.0	1.5	1.5	1.5	1.4	1.3	1.2	1.1	1.4	1.5	1.3	1.8
Gas	KGQT	21.7	23.0	27.1	27.9	26.9	28.4	27.9	29.3	28.2	26.5	30.3	32.4
Nuclear[3]	KGQU	22.0	23.4	22.2	19.6	20.8	20.1	20.0	18.2	18.4	17.1	14.0	11.9
Hydro (natural flow)	KGQV	0.4	0.4	0.5	0.4	0.3	0.4	0.3	0.4	0.4	0.4	0.4	0.4
Other fuels used by UK companies[4]	KGQW	2.351	2.597	2.863	3.007	2.993	3.242	4.041	4.321	5.437	5.331	5.149	5.119
Net imports	KGQX	1.4	1.1	1.2	1.2	0.9	0.7	0.2	0.6	0.6	0.6	0.4	0.9

1 See chapter text.
2 Includes oil used in gas turbine and diesel plant for lighting up coal fired boilers and Orimulsion.

3 Nuclear generators are now included under "major power producers" only.
4 Main fuels included are coke oven gas, blast furnace gas, waste products from chemical processes and sludge gas.

Source: Department of Energy and Climate Change: 0300 0685050

22.11

Indigenous petroleum production, refinery receipts, imports and exports of oil[1]

Thousand tonnes

		1997	1998	1999	2000	2001	2002	2003	2004	2005	2006	2007	2008
Total indigenous petroleum production[2]	KMBA	128 234	132 633	137 099	126 245	116 678	115 944	106 073	95 374	84 721	76 578	76 575	71 665
Crude petroleum:[3]													
Refinery receipts total	KMBB	97 023	93 797	88 286	88 014	83 343	84 784	84 585	89 821	86 135	83 213	81 117	80 725
Foreign trade[4]													
Imports	KMBF	49 994	47 958	44 869	54 387	53 551	56 968	54 177	62 516	58 886	59 443	57 357	60 074
Exports	AXRB	79 400	84 610	91 797	92 918	86 930	87 144	74 898	64 504	54 098	50 195	50 999	48 410
Net imports	AXRC	−29 406	−36 652	−46 928	−38 531	−33 378	−30 176	−20 720	−1 988	4 787	9 249	6 358	11 664
Petroleum products													
Foreign trade													
Imports[4]	BHMI	8 705	11 327	12 650	14 212	17 234	14 900	16 472	18 545	22 512	26 828	25 093	23 916
Exports[4]	AXRD	26 755	24 375	21 730	20 677	19 088	23 444	23 323	30 495	29 722	29 009	30 017	28 811
Net imports[4]	AXRE	−18 049	−12 957	−7 834	−6 464	−1 854	−8 544	−6 851	−11 950	−7 211	−2 181	−4 924	−4 895
International marine bunkers	BHMK	2 961	3 080	2 329	2 079	2 274	1 913	1 764	2 085	2 055	2 348	2 371	2 594

1 See chapter text. The term 'indigenous' is used in this table to cover oil produced on the UK Continental Shelf. This includes small amounts produced onshore.
2 Crude oil *plus* condensates and petroleum gases derived at onshore treatment plants.

3 Includes process (partly refined) oils.
4 Foreign trade as recorded by the petroleum industry and may differ from figures published in *Overseas Trade Statistics*.

Source: Department of Energy and Climate Change : 0300 068 5038

22.12

Throughput of crude and process oils and output of refined products from refineries[1]

United Kingdom

Thousand tonnes

		1998	1999	2000	2001	2002	2003	2004	2005	2006	2007	2008
Throughput of crude and process oils	KMAU	93 797	88 285	88 014	83 343	84 784	84 585	89 821	86 135	83 213	81 117	80 725
less: Refinery fuel:	KMAA	6 177	5 538	5 252	5 059	5 677	5 456	5 417	5 602	4 639	4 639	4 531
Losses	KMAB	1 004	1 550	1 632	1 233	788	56	−7	371	374	−153	290
Total output of refined products	KMAC	86 616	81 197	81 130	77 051	78 319	79 073	84 411	80 162	78 200	76 788	75 903
Gases:												
Butane and propane	KMAE	1 961	1 975	1 917	1 764	2 139	2 281	2 150	2 184	2 105	2 259	2 248
Other petroleum	KMAF	394	361	288	272	537	715	520	427	661	517	469
Naphtha and other feedstock	KMAG	2 316	2 430	3 082	3 428	3 153	3 503	3 168	3 019	2 734	2 561	1 863
Aviation spirit	KMAH	–	16	30	101	28	26	31	32	26	–	..
Motor spirit	KMAJ	27 166	25 230	23 445	21 455	22 944	22 627	24 589	22 620	21 443	21 313	20 319
Industrial and white spirit	KMAK	135	129	122	121	121	104	100	136	107	70	55
Kerosene:												
Aviation turbine fuel	KMAL	7 876	7 249	6 484	5 910	5 365	5 277	5 615	5 167	6 261	6 176	6 549
Burning oil	KMAM	3 442	3 553	3 078	3 088	3 506	3 521	3 613	3 325	3 374	2 968	3 092
Gas/diesel oil	KMAN	27 542	25 755	28 229	26 748	28 343	27 380	28 647	28 486	26 037	26 452	26 971
Fuel oil	KMAO	11 125	10 446	10 296	10 179	8 507	9 495	11 308	10 155	11 279	10 433	10 496
Lubricating oil	KMAP	1 125	907	702	656	509	576	1 136	936	617	547	514
Bitumen	KMAQ	2 172	1 644	1 438	1 707	1 918	1 925	2 196	1 912	1 749	1 628	1 485
Petroleum wax	KMAR	59	261	437	416	430	460	94	98	16	12	8
Petroleum coke	KMAS	678	648	657	513	441	612	633	660	606	676	662
Other products	KMAT	625	593	927	692	378	569	607	1 005	1 189	1 175	1 174

1 See chapter text. Crude and process oils comprise all feedstocks, other than distillation benzines, for treatment at refinery plants. Refinery production does not cover further treatment of finished products for special grades such as in distillation plant for the preparation of industrial spirits.

Source: Department of Energy and Climate Change: 0300 068 5038

Production

22.13 Deliveries of petroleum products for inland consumption[1]
United Kingdom

Thousand tonnes

		1998	1999	2000	2001	2002	2003	2004	2005	2006	2007	2008
Total (including refinery fuel)	KMCA	78 438	77 974	77 196	76 413	76 233	77 154	79 059	80 735	79 749	77 716	75 951
Total (excluding refinery fuel)	KMCB	72 261	72 436	71 944	71 354	70 556	71 697	73 642	75 133	75 110	73 234	71 420
Butane and propane	ECAQ	2 368	2 249	2 070	2 097	2 553	3 019	3 114	3 314	3 127	2 853	3 294
Other Petroleum Gases (includes Ethane)	ECAR	1 752	2 041	1 886	2 077	2 181	2 114	1 918	2 021	1 920	1 815	1 801
Naphtha	ECAS	2 882	3 100	2 344	1 592	1 592	2 332	2 029	1 916	2 278	1 947	848
Aviation spirit	KMCI	36	45	52	59	50	46	49	52	46	33	30
Motor spirit:												
Retail deliveries:												
Leaded Premium / Lead Replacement Petrol[2]	KMCK	4 595	2 629	1 462	838	401	183	74	25	19	..	..
Super Premium Unleaded[2]	KMCL	409	480	403	420	706	861	810	924	719	814	1 032
Premium Unleaded	KMCM	16 432	19 480	19 008	19 100	19 167	18 291	17 795	16 954	16 704	15 991	15 035
Total Retail Deliveries	ECAT	21 436	21 409	20 873	20 358	20 274	19 335	18 679	17 903	17 442	16 806	16 067
Commercial consumers:												
Leaded Premium / Lead Replacement Petrol[2]	KMCO	91	61	44	34	19	19	14	1	2	..	..
Super Premium Unleaded[2]	KMCP	4	6	6	9	17	22	26	16	63	25	41
Premium Unleaded	KMCQ	318	311	480	538	499	542	765	811	637	764	570
Total Commercial Consumers	ECAU	413	378	530	581	535	583	805	828	702	789	611
Total Motor spirit	BHOD	21 848	21 787	21 403	20 940	20 808	19 919	19 484	18 732	18 144	17 594	16 678
Industrial and white spirits	KMCS	179	174	170	151	157	147	281	284	156	167	145
Kerosene:												
Aviation turbine fuel	BHOE	9 241	9 939	10 806	10 614	10 519	10 764	11 637	12 497	12 641	12 574	12 142
Burning oil	KMCT	3 575	3 633	3 839	4 236	3 578	3 569	3 950	3 869	4 017	3 631	3 694
Gas/diesel oil:												
Derv fuel:												
Retail Deliveries	ECAV	6 602	7 137	7 181	7 846	8 153	9 057	9 517	10 679	11 453	12 344	12 870
Commercial Consumers	ECAW	8 541	8 371	8 451	8 213	8 774	8 655	8 997	8 757	8 693	8 718	7 743
Total Derv fuel	BHOI	15 143	15 508	15 632	16 059	16 926	17 712	18 514	19 436	20 146	21 065	20 613
Other gas/diesel oil (includes Mdf)	ECAX	7 908	7 454	7 576	6 960	6 099	6 326	6 017	6 797	6 565	6 109	5 967
Fuel oil	BHOK	2 935	2 414	2 120	2 579	1 723	1 540	2 064	1 965	2 151	2 209	2 439
Lubricating oils	BHOL	1 967	1 928	1 975	1 935	2 002	1 959	1 991	1 906	1 610	1 563	1 741
Bitumen	BHOM	813	790	801	846	829	868	914	750	713	672	510
Petroleum wax	KMCU	18	37	32	33	51	57	50	72	48	39	46
Petroleum coke	KMCV	887	660	776	702	893	880	1 145	1 042	925	544	928
Miscellaneous products	KMCW	537	388	463	475	596	449	476	484	628	419	544

1 See chapter text.
2 With effect from 2007, deliveries of Lead Replacement Petrol are now included with Super Premium Unleaded.

Source: Department of Energy and Climate Change: 0300 068 5038

22.14 Iron and steel:[1] summary of steel supplies, deliveries and stocks
United Kingdom

		2000	2001	2002	2003	2004	2005	2006	2007	2008
Supply, disposal and consumption - (Finished product weight - Thousand tonnes)										
UK producers' home deliveries	KLTA	7 255	6 762	6 506	6 227	7 083	6 279	6 757	6 519	6 198
Imports excluding steelworks receipts	KLTB	6 387	6 978	6 793	6 893	7 272	6 297	7 403	7 848	6 913
Total deliveries to home market (a)	KLTC	13 642	13 740	13 299	13 120	14 355	12 576	14 160	14 367	13 111
Total exports (producers, consumers, merchants)	KLTD	7 446	6 512	6 320	7 007	7 455	8 408	7 862	9 131	8 657
Exports by UK producers	KLTE	7 163	6 182	5 594	6 202	6 275	6 594	6 852	7 645	7 398
Derived consumers' and merchants' exports (b)	KLTF	283	330	708	806	1 179	1 814	1 010	1 486	1 259
Net home disposals (a)-(b)	KLTG	13 359	13 410	12 591	12 314	13 176	10 762	13 150	12 881	11 852
Estimated home consumption	KLTI	13 359	13 410	12 591	12 114	13 176	10 762	13 150	12 881	11 852
Stocks - (Finished product weight - Thousand tonnes)										
Producers										
- ingots & semis	KLTJ	727	705	690	706	765	869	790	725	688
- finished steel	KLTK	1 039	981	932	917	901	947	876	862	607
Estimated home consumption - (Crude steel equivalent - Million tonnes)										
Crude steel production[2]	KLTN	15.15	13.54	11.53	13.13	13.77	13.23	13.90	14.39	13.52
Producers' stock change	KLTO	..	..	..	..	..	0.18	–	–0.08	–0.30
Re-usable material	KLTP	..	..	..	..	..	..	–	..	..
Total supply from home sources	KLTQ	15.48	13.68	11.61	13.13	13.77	13.20	13.90	14.47	13.82
Total imports[3]	KLTR	8.43	9.11	9.86	9.32	10.31	9.82	10.30	10.38	8.92
Total exports[3]	KLTS	8.61	7.53	7.39	8.65	9.15	8.93	10.40	10.28	9.73
Net home disposals	KLTT	15.30	15.26	14.08	14.20	14.99	13.09	14.70	14.57	13.01
Estimated home consumption	KLTV	15.30	15.26	14.08	14.20	14.99	13.09	14.70	14.57	13.01

1 See chapter text. The figures relate to periods of 52 weeks.
2 Includes liquid steel for castings only up to 2003.

3 Based on HM Customs Statistics, reflecting total trade rather than producers' trade.

Source: Iron and Steel Statistics Bureau: 020 8686 9050 ext 126

Production

22.15

Iron and steel:[1] **iron ore, manganese ore, pig iron and iron and steel scrap**
United Kingdom

Thousand tonnes

		1998	1999	2000	2001	2002	2003	2004	2005	2006	2007	2008
Iron ore[2]	KLOF	19 532	18 754	16 991	15 113	13 185	15 766	16 013	15 991	16 539	16 607	15 338
Manganese ore[2]	KLOG	22	14	36	4	4	..	6	3	6	3	4
Pig iron (and blast furnace ferro-alloys)												
Average number of furnaces in blast during period	KLOH	9	9	8	7	5	6	6	6	7	7	6
Production Steelmaking iron	KLOI	12 746	12 139	10 890	9 870	8 561	10 228	10 180	10 189	10 696	10 960	10 137
In blast furnaces: total	KLOL	12 746	12 139	10 890	9 870	8 561	10 228	10 180	10 189	10 696	10 960	10 137
In steel works	KLOM	12 746	12 139	10 890	9 870	8 561	10 228	10 180	10 189	10 696	10 960	10 137
Consumption of pig iron: total	KLOO	12 746	12 139	10 890	9 870	8 561	10 228	10 180	10 189	10 696	10 960	10 137
Iron and steel scrap												
Steelworks and steel foundries Circulating scrap	KLOQ	2 380	2 488	2 287	2 019	1 882	1 926	1 787	1 737	1 669	1 658	1 589
Purchased receipts	KLOR	4 045	3 433	3 327	3 001	2 271	2 617	3 371	2 779	3 171	3 425	3 429
Consumption	KLOS	6 408	5 884	5 675	5 006	4 216	4 469	5 123	4 531	4 811	5 144	4 888
Stocks (end of period)	KLOT	253	290	229	224	161	234	242	228	257	196	326

1 See chapter text. The figures relate to periods of 52 weeks.
2 Consumption.

Source: Iron and Steel Statistics Bureau: 020 8686 9050 ext 126

22.16 Iron and steel:[1] furnaces and production of steel
United Kingdom

Number and thousand tonnes

		1998	1999	2000	2001	2002	2003	2004	2005	2006	2007	2008
Steel furnaces (numbers[2])	KLPA	190	181	181	181	173	..	..	..	..	..	..
Oxygen converters	KLPC	11	11	11	11	8	..	..	..	..	..	..
Electric	KLPD	179	170	170	170	165	..	..	..	..	..	..
Production of crude steel	KLPF	17 315	16 284	15 155	13 543	11 667	13 268	13 766	13 239	13 905	14 392	13 521
by process												
Oxygen converters	KLPH	13 426	12 634	11 551	10 271	8 956	10 630	10 667	10 550	11 203	11 362	10 478
Electric	KLPI	3 889	3 650	3 604	3 272	2 711	2 639	3 099	2 685	2 702	3 030	3 043
by cast method												
Cast to ingot	KLPK	784	534	539	369	339	354	383	281	206	201	224
Continuously cast	KLPL	16 346	15 637	14 470	13 024	11 182	12 766	13 383	12 958	13 698	14 191	13 296
Steel for castings	KLPM	185	127	146	150	146	148	..	..	..	..	..
by quality												
Non alloy steel	KLPN	16 145	15 263	14 004	12 482	10 657	12 294	12 809	12 376	..	13 613	12 695
Stainless and other alloy steel	KLPO	1 170	1 035	1 151	1 061	1 010	974	957	863	760	779	826
Production of finished steel products (All quantities)[3]												
Rods and bars for reinforcement (in coil and lengths)	KLPP	1 133	893	812	755	487	294	769	730	902	1 113	1 109
Wire rods and other rods and bars in coil	KLPQ	1 492	1 407	1 408	1 389	1 394	1 316	1 392	1 035	962	869	803
Hot rolled bars in lengths	KLPR	1 791	1 542	1 545	1 449	1 267	1 107	1 179	1 142	1 249	1 350	1 252
Bright steel bars[4]	KLPS	336	311	337	296	271	273	277	233	226	239	226
Light sections other than rails	KLPT	318	264	183	201	188	116	136	130	149	162	157
Heavy sections	KGQZ	2 346	2 303	1 915	1 931	1 873	1 774	1 694	1 414	1 527	1 436	1 425
Hot rolled plates, sheets and strip in coil and lengths	KLPW	8 454	7 893	7 293	5 841	5 756	6 145	6 437	5 823	6 010	5 639	4 969
Cold rolled plates and sheets in coil and lengths	KLPX	4 288	3 914	3 612	2 944	2 951	2 958	3 001	2 769	2 726	2 520	2 315
Cold rolled strip[4]	KLPZ	259	233	218	201	179	186	156	131	98	81	73
Tinplate	KLQW	772	736	753	602	562	493	507	471	421	443	462
Other coated sheet	KLQX	2 610	2 475	2 471	1 773	1 786	1 811	1 713	1 644	1 773	1 661	1 472
Tubes and pipes[4]	KLQY	1 276	1 100	1 061	1 096	940	1 066	1 076	932	993	991	882
Forged bars[4]	KLQZ	3	2	1	1	1	..	..	..	..	..	..

1 See chapter text. The figures relate to periods of 52 weeks.
2 Includes steel furnaces at steel foundries, only up to 2003.
3 Includes material for conversion into other products listed in the table.
4 Based on producers' deliveries.

Source: Iron and Steel Statistics Bureau: 020 8686 9050 ext 126

22.17 Non-ferrous metals
United Kingdom

Thousand tonnes

		1996	1997	1998	1999	2000	2001	2002	2003	2004	2005	2006
Copper												
Production of refined copper:												
Primary	KLAA	13.0	9.1	6.4	1.7	–	–	–	–	–	–	–
Secondary	KLAB	43.6	51.3	47.4	49.0	–	–	–	–	–	–	–
Home consumption:												
Refined	KLAC	396.0	408.3	374.1	305.3	322.7	285.9	260.7	242.2	243.4	165.4	172.1
Scrap (metal content)	KLAD	81.0	69.0	64.6	112.5	132.4	127.0	120.0	120.0	120.0	120.0	120.0
Stocks (end of period)[1,2]	KLAE	6.6	12.8	7.5	7.3	10.4	7.3	7.3	7.3	7.3	7.3	7.3
Analysis of home consumption												
(refined and scrap):[3,4] total	KLAF	477.3	477.4	438.7	417.8	455.1	412.9	380.7	362.2	363.4	285.4	292.1
Wire[5]	KLAG	309.4	312.5	287.2	276.1	310.2	151.8	–	–	–	–	–
Rods, bars and sections	KLAH	58.3	58.3	53.6	46.9	43.6	21.6	–	–	–	–	–
Sheet, strip and plate	KLAI	34.0	36.5	30.5	27.7	32.3	16.9	–	–	–	–	–
Tubes	KLAJ	75.6	70.1	67.4	67.1	69.4	22.4	–	–	–	–	–
Zinc												
Slab zinc:												
Production	KLAL	96.9	107.7	99.6	132.8	99.6	99.6	99.6	16.6	–	–	–
Home consumption	KLAM	195.7	194.8	187.9	198.9	206.5	197.1	202.4	176.2	150.1	161.7	161.7
Stocks (end of period)	KLAN	10.5	10.1	10.6	10.9	10.9	9.5	9.2	8.9	8.9	8.9	8.9
Other zinc (metal content):												
Consumption	KLAO	41.3	41.5	37.3	41.6	46.3	48.2	51.8	52.3	55.4	–	–
Analysis of home consumption												
(slab and scrap): total	KLAP	237.1	236.5	221.6	232.1	237.9	226.6	230.4	229.1	234.3	–	–
Brass	KLAQ	39.1	41.6	36.6	33.6	34.4	32.2	30.0	30.0	31.2	–	–
Galvanized products	KLAR	110.3	108.4	103.8	116.6	120.9	111.8	117.3	115.5	118.4	–	–
Zinc sheet and strip	KLAS	3.0	3.3	3.3	3.3	3.3	3.3	3.4	3.3	3.3	–	–
Zinc alloy die castings	KLAT	46.5	46.5	46.5	46.5	46.5	46.5	46.5	46.5	46.5	–	–
Zinc oxide	KLAU	20.7	20.6	20.4	21.1	21.8	21.8	22.2	22.8	23.9	–	–
Other products	KLAV	17.5	16.1	11.0	11.0	11.0	11.0	11.0	11.0	11.0	–	–
Refined lead												
Production[6,7]	KLAW	351.4	384.1	349.7	351.0	328.0	366.3	374.6	364.6	245.9	304.4	318.7
Home consumption[7,8]												
Refined lead	KLAX	272.8	270.4	275.5	283.3	294.0	298.3	305.7	314.7	330.4	281.7	300.0
Scrap and remelted lead[7]	KLAY	43.4	39.1	38.4	32.2	39.5	40.6	40.7	34.1	40.8	–	–
Stocks (end of period)[9]												
Lead bullion	KLAZ	32.9	15.5	20.9	17.1	10.0	17.2	17.2	24.0	23.0	23.0	23.0
Refined soft lead at consumers	KLBA	28.8	29.1	27.4	25.7	25.8	26.1	25.6	25.3	25.9	25.9	25.9
In LME Warehouses (UK)	KLBB	3.0	2.4	0.1	0.1	0.1	0.1	0.1	0.1	0.1	0.1	–
Analysis of home consumption												
(refined and scrap): total	KLBC	316.2	309.5	313.9	315.5	334.8	338.9	347.1	348.9	371.2	281.6	300.0
Cables	KLBD	9.8	9.7	9.7	9.6	9.6	9.6	9.7	9.7	9.7	–	–
Batteries (excluding oxides)	KLBE	52.3	54.7	51.6	47.4	50.5	48.2	48.2	51.9	54.1	–	–
Oxides and compounds:												
Batteries	KLBF	54.9	56.1	54.4	53.1	55.9	54.7	54.7	55.9	59.0	–	–
Other uses	KLBG	56.1	54.5	56.4	57.0	56.8	53.8	53.8	60.6	64.5	–	–
Sheets and pipes	KLBH	94.1	91.1	96.1	94.9	102.3	102.3	107.9	109.7	111.4	–	–
Solder	KLBJ	7.4	7.4	7.4	7.4	7.4	7.4	7.4	7.2	7.4	–	–
Alloys	KLBK	12.1	9.4	9.4	11.9	16.5	24.3	26.8	25.9	33.4	–	–
Other uses	KLBL	29.5	26.6	28.9	34.1	35.8	38.6	38.6	28.0	31.7	–	–

22.17 Non-ferrous metals
United Kingdom
continued

		1996	1997	1998	1999	2000	2001	2002	2003	2004	2005	2006
Tin												
Tin ore (metal content):												
Production	KLBM	2.1	2.3	0.4	–	–	–	–	–	–	–	–
Tin metal:[10]												
Production[11]	KLBO	–	–	–	–	–	–	–	–	–	–	–
Home consumption[11]	VQIX	10.5	10.4	10.6	9.6	10.0	10.3	6.9	7.1	5.3	3.2	4.1
Exports and re-exports[12]	KLBQ	0.6	0.3	3.4	0.1	0.1	0.4	0.3	0.3	0.6	1.7	11.8
Stocks (end of period):												
Consumers	KLBR	1.0	1.0	1.0	1.0	1.0	1.0	1.0	1.0	1.0	1.0	1.0
Analysis of home consumption (excluding scrap): total	KLBT	10.5	10.4	17.5	16.5	17.0	18.8	18.8	1.9	18.4	–	–
Tinplate	KLBU	3.6	2.8	2.6	3.0	3.0	3.0	1.9	1.9	3.0	–	–
Alloys	KLBV	3.5	3.4	12.1	11.2	11.6	2.6	1.9	1.9	2.6	–	–
Solder	KLBW	1.1	1.1	1.1	0.6	0.8	1.5	1.9	1.9	1.5	–	–
Other uses	KLBX	0.4	0.4	0.4	0.4	0.4	0.4	1.9	1.9	0.4	–	–
Aluminium												
Ingot production												
Primary	KLBY	240.0	247.7	258.4	269.7	305.1	340.8	344.3	342.7	359.6	368.5	360.3
Secondary[13]	KLCA	260.0	242.7	274.8	285.3	241.3	248.6	205.4	205.4	205.4	204.2	204.2
Wrought remelt production[14]	C6EW	500.0	490.4	533.2	555.0	546.4	589.4	549.7	548.1	565.0	572.7	654.5
Wrought and cast despatches												
Bar, section and tube[15]	C6EX	149.6	160.8	168.0	181.7	184.7	177.1	168.3	158.7	157.0	–	–
Plate, sheet, strip and circles	C6EY	327.9	350.4	352.5	349.7	419.1	384.8	312.2	274.3	267.3	–	–
Castings	KLCH	156.0	152.4	148.0	137.3	134.9	138.2	159.4	127.5	139.7	103.0	158.6
Exports												
Primary ingot	C6EZ	53.1	219.6	68.7	233.6	347.7	263.3	250.4	271.2	335.9	379.1	350.2
Secondary ingot	KLCC	152.2	153.3	156.6	143.1	84.2	59.9	35.7	26.9	30.8	–	–
Extruded products	C6F2	45.8	56.8	59.7	47.5	25.5	20.7	15.3	14.2	15.8	–	–
Rolled products	C6F3	155.5	157.7	160.1	166.6	222.9	198.3	208.8	193.9	192.2	–	–
Refined nickel												
Production (including ferro-nickel)	KLCM	38.6	36.1	39.1	39.5	38.0	33.8	33.8	26.8	38.6	37.6	36.8

1 Unwrought copper (electrolytic, fire refined and blister).
2 Reported stocks of refined copper held by consumers and those held in London Metal Exchange (LME) warehouses in the United Kingdom.
3 2001 figures only cover the period January to June.
4 Copper content.
5 Consumption for high-conductivity copper and cadmium copper wire represented by consumption of wire rods, production of which for export is also included.
6 Lead reclaimed from secondary and scrap material and lead refined from bullion and domestic ores.

7 Figures for production and consumption of refined lead include antimonial lead, and for scrap and remelted lead, exclude secondary antimonial lead.
8 Including toll transactions involving fabrication.
9 Excluding goverment stocks.
10 Including production from imported scrap and residues refined on toll.
11 Primary and secondary metal.
12 Including re-exports on toll transactions.
13 Predominantly from old scrap.
14 Predominantly using recycled scrap from fabrication.
15 Excluding forging bars.

Sources: World Bureau of Metal Statistics: 01920 461274;
Aluminium Federation: 0121 456 1103

Production

22.18 Fertilisers
Years ending 30 June

Thousand tonnes

		1999	2000	2001	2002	2003	2004	2005	2006	2007	2008	2009
Nutrient Content												
Nitrogen (N):												
Straight	KGRM	819	819	714	751	664	662	691	631	656	744	733
Compounds	KGRN	465	449	448	446	467	463	370	372	352	292	180
Phosphate (P_2O_5)	KGRO	347	317	279	283	282	278	259	235	224	215	129
Potash (K_2O)	KGRP	451	409	369	391	375	375	352	325	317	325	208
Compounds - total product	KGRQ	3 013	2 851	2 471	2 511	2 558	2 550	2 221	2 134	2 039	1 827	1 116

Source: Agricultural Industries Confederation: 01733 385230

22.19 Minerals: production[1]
United Kingdom

Thousand tonnes

		1998	1999	2000	2001	2002	2003	2004	2005	2006	2007	2008
Great Britain												
Limestone	KLEA	85 382	82 714	80 810	83 492	88 013	84 445	86 846	81 830	82 598	83 482	74 324
Sandstone	KLEB	13 545	11 870	12 056	11 897	11 788	11 665	11 929	11 609	11 827	11 978	9 558
Igneous rock	KLEC	39 838	45 294	44 633	45 053	44 544	45 305	46 193	45 992	47 867	50 684	47 009
Clay/shale	KLED	12 230	11 355	10 838	10 426	10 306	10 680	11 164	10 898	10 432	10 104	8 459
Industrial sand	KLEE	4 662	4 092	4 095	3 848	3 833	4 073	5 011	4 146	5 174	4 909	4 777
Chalk	KLEF	9 934	9 667	9 213	8 205	8 587	8 066	7 997	7 105	7 376	7 565	5 874
Fireclay	KLEG	577	545	595	459	491	528	402	395	228	338	180
Barium sulphate	KLEH	64	59	54	70	56	..	..	62	44	54	46
Calcium fluoride	KLEI	52	46	21	46	22	..	..	44	133	..	..
Lead	KLEK	1	1	..	1	..	..	..	1	4	..	..
Iron ore: crude	KLEN	2	1	1	1	1	–	..	–	–	..	..
Iron ore: iron content	KLEO	1	1	1	..	..	–	..	–	–	..	..
Calcspar	KLEP	15	..	..	12	..	–	..	–	..	..	..
China clay	KILC	2 866	2 841	2 779	2 804	2 467	2 378	2 148	1 908	..	1 821	1 321
Chert and flint	KLER	..	6	..	2	2	..	2	2	..	1	1
Fuller's earth	KLES	111	83	103	..	33	19	11	..	–	..	..
Salt[2]	I8AV	..	..	..	..	..	..	..	5 770	5 224	5 320	5 287
Dolomite	KLEY	15 632	13 698	13 069	14 314	12 946	..	..	11 514	12 100	7 622	5 510
Gypsum	KLEZ	..	..	..	..	..	..	1 686	..	..	..	..
Slate[3]	KLFA	425	361	479	551	742	832	901	928	865	1 428	1 058
Soapstone and talc	KLFB	5	6	5	5	6	6	4	6	4	3	2
Sand and gravel (land-won)	KLFC	73 016	74 785	74 877	74 599	69 889	68 090	73 061	69 368	66 268	66 724	59 506
Sand and gravel (marine dredged)	KLFD	12 952	13 424	14 356	13 611	12 832	12 131	12 996	13 024	13 974	13 777	12 621
Northern Ireland												
Sand and gravel	KLFG	5 300	5 517	5 073	6 194	5 512	4 894	5 084	5 803	5 150	8 086	7 134
Basalt and igneous rock (other than granite)	KLFH	6 107	7 861	9 480	6 448	6 681	6 051	6 844	7 112	6 087	8 225	6 481
Limestone	KLFI	3 892	4 219	3 538	4 746	4 514	4 887	5 634	5 588	6 385	5 904	3 739
Sandstone[4]	KLFJ	6 584	3 615	2 844	8 070	6 574	6 594	6 915	7 076	6 211	4 828	2 697
Others[5]	KLFN	473	1 579	3 098	753	242	1 055	1 266	2 090	1 698	2 468	2 931

1 See chapter text.
2 Includes rock salt, salt from brine and salt in brine.
3 Roofing and vertically hanging slates, includes 'true' slate and stone slates produced from thinly bedded sandstones and limestones. Also includes 'true' and stone slates sold as sawn slabs for decorative cladding.
4 Prior to 1993 the 'Sandstone' heading was called 'Grit and conglomerate'. The new heading is all encompassing and was confirmed as correct with the Geological Survey in Northern Ireland.
5 Rock salt, Chalk, Dolomite, Fireclay and Granite.

Source: Office for National Statistics: 01633 812082

22.20 Building materials and components[1]
Great Britain

	Building bricks (millions)		Concrete blocks (000 sq m)		Concrete roofing tiles (000 sq m of roof covered)		Slate[2] (tonnes)		Cement[3] (000 tonnes)		RMX[4] (000 cu m)	Sand and gravel (000 tonnes)
	Production	Deliveries	Production	Deliveries	Production	Deliveries	Production	Deliveries	Production	Deliveries	Deliveries	Deliveries
	BLDA	QXIH	BLDM	QXII	BLDN	QXIJ	BLDQ	QXIK	QXIM	QXIL	BLDP	BLDS
2000	239	241	7 518	7 377	2 230	2 087	7 155	7 495	1 038	988	1 920	7 322
2001	230	235	7 327	7 376	2 069	2 036	7 760	7 852	924	888	1 917	8 121
2002	229	235	7 623	7 612	2 085	2 033	7 913	7 972	924	897	1 883	7 126
2003	231	245	7 973	8 032	1 786	1 783	6 591	6 543	935	923	1 857	6 896
2004	239	236	8 021	7 905	1 728	1 617	..	..	950	923	1 905	6 779
2005	229	214	7 500	7 463	2 143	2 041	..	..	935	917	1 869	6 708
2006	209	200	7 292	7 251	1 978	2 010	..	..	956	935	1 919	6 491
2007	206	201	7 496	7 395	1 963	1 984	..	..	991	970	1 962	6 293
2008	161	150	5 645	5 595	1 674	1 660	..	..	839	828	1 671	6 221
2009	101	116	4 200	4 220	1 173	1 301	..	5 626	..	..	1 172	4 896
2007 Q3	208	213	7 749	7 728	1 710	2 180	..	..	1 043	1 004	2 068	6 628
Q4	195	179	7 386	6 824	2 009	1 971	..	..	964	929	1 895	6 054
2008 Q1	193	167	7 044	6 285	1 903	1 807	..	..	870	850	1 731	6 051
Q2	195	180	6 744	6 571	1 938	1 893	..	..	934	939	1 924	6 758
Q3	158	141	4 965	5 436	1 552	1 659	..	..	840	832	1 634	6 447
Q4	97	111	3 829	4 086	1 301	1 283	..	..	713	691	1 394	5 628
2009 Q1	96	96	4 031	3 883	1 221	1 094	..	5 242	587	594	1 194	4 877
Q2	125	128	4 488	4 397	1 018	1 312	5 418	6 011	668	657	1 212	5 120
Q3	107	128	4 257	4 641	1 193	1 482	5 271	5 655	666	666	1 209	4 959
Q4	77	111	4 022	3 958	1 260	1 316	5 540	5 597	..	..	1 074	4 627
2008 Jan	159	144	7 212	5 593	..	..	..	..	746	776	..	..
Feb	196	171	6 955	6 665	..	..	..	..	916	941	..	..
Mar	225	185	6 965	6 597	..	..	..	..	947	834	..	..
Apr	198	192	7 213	7 000	..	..	..	..	939	1 001	..	..
May	187	173	6 385	6 396	..	..	..	..	928	914	..	..
Jun	200	173	6 633	6 318	..	..	..	..	936	901	..	..
Jul	167	144	5 687	6 016	..	..	..	..	921	924	..	..
Aug	134	133	4 410	5 014	..	..	..	..	810	744	..	..
Sep	174	146	4 796	5 279	..	..	..	..	789	828	..	..
Oct	136	125	4 616	5 178	..	..	..	..	835	854	..	..
Nov	100	109	4 035	4 057	..	..	..	..	757	702	..	..
Dec	55	99	2 836	3 024	..	..	..	..	547	518	..	..
2009 Jan	62	81	3 750	3 561	..	..	..	..	516	505	..	..
Feb	95	81	3 802	3 540	..	..	..	..	545	570	..	..
Mar	132	127	4 543	4 548	..	..	..	..	701	707	..	..
Apr	114	121	4 580	4 447	..	..	..	..	618	637	..	..
May	122	126	4 158	4 144	..	..	..	..	711	629	..	..
Jun	140	137	4 725	4 600	..	..	..	..	675	704	..	..
Jul	106	141	4 740	4 863	..	..	..	..	705	697	..	..
Aug	84	107	3 417	4 264	..	..	..	..	637	606	..	..
Sep	131	137	4 614	4 797	..	..	..	..	656	696	..	..
Oct	120	137	4 740	4 818	..	..	..	..	758	696	..	..
Nov	71	111	4 372	4 072	..	..	..	..	667	605	..	..
Dec	41	83	2 954	2 984	..	..	..	..	..	..	..	..

1 See chapter text.
2 Excluding slate residue used as fill.
3 United Kingdom; Great Britain from January 2002.
4 United Kingdom; RMX stands for ready mixed concrete.

Sources: Department for Business, Innovation and Skills; (formerly BERR) : 020 7215 1555

22.21 Volume of construction output by all agencies[1] by type of work at constant 2005 prices (seasonally adjusted)

Standard Industrial Classification 2003. Great Britain.

£ millions

	New work							Repair and maintenance						All work (seasonally adjusted volume index numbers)
	New housing for			Other new work for				Housing		Other work for				
				Public sector	Private sector		Total new work					Total repair and maintenance	Total all work	
					Private sector									
	Public sector	Private sector	Infrastructure	Public sector	Industrial	Commercial		Public	Private	Public sector	Private sector			
	BLAC	BLAD	BAXF	BLAE	BLAF	BLAG	BLAB	BLBK	BLBL	BLAJ	BLAK	BLAH	FGAY	SFZX
2006	3 281	18 714	6 008	9 679	4 767	19 695	62 145	8 352	14 858	8 276	14 733	46 219	108 364	101.3
2007	3 778	18 410	6 189	9 205	4 785	22 178	64 544	7 987	15 054	7 398	15 968	46 407	110 952	103.7
2008[3]	3 483	14 853	7 120	10 646	3 861	22 529	62 492	8 170	15 507	8 106	15 440	47 224	109 716	102.5
2006 Q4	758	4 748	1 427	2 375	1 276	5 256	15 839	2 018	3 674	1 876	3 952	11 521	27 360	102.3
2007 Q1	991	4 612	1 389	2 292	1 242	5 213	15 738	2 188	3 668	1 915	3 933	11 704	27 442	102.6
Q2	1 012	4 674	1 532	2 257	1 227	5 450	16 152	1 967	3 849	1 822	3 891	11 528	27 680	103.5
Q3	932	4 696	1 655	2 311	1 161	5 708	16 464	1 891	3 583	1 844	4 026	11 344	27 808	103.9
Q4	843	4 428	1 613	2 346	1 154	5 807	16 190	1 941	3 955	1 817	4 119	11 832	28 022	104.7
2008 Q1	892	4 266	1 786	2 498	1 120	5 929	16 493	2 010	3 749	2 000	4 059	11 818	28 311	105.8
Q2	865	3 855	1 840	2 607	964	5 685	15 817	2 128	3 981	2 033	4 063	12 206	28 023	104.8
Q3	884	3 536	1 828	2 734	934	5 702	15 617	2 095	3 723	2 119	3 791	11 729	27 346	102.2
Q4[3]	842	3 196	1 666	2 807	842	5 212	14 565	1 937	4 055	1 954	3 526	11 471	26 036	97.3
2009 Q1[3]	773	2 885	1 886	2 976	683	4 629	13 833	1 916	3 389	1 871	3 316	10 491	24 324	90.9
Q2[3]	795	2 782	2 028	3 350	628	4 568	14 151	1 936	3 389	1 783	3 201	10 310	24 461	91.4
Q3[2]	909	2 455	1 960	3 592	604	4 078	13 597	2 118	3 586	2 244	3 409	11 357	24 954	93.3

1 Estimates of unrecorded output by small firms and self-employed workers, and output by the public sector's direct labour department are included.
2 Provisional.
3 Revised

Sources: Office for National Statistics;
Tel : 020 7215 1953

Note: Responsibility for these statistics transferred from BERR (formerly DTI) to the ONS on 1st March 2008.

22.22 Value of new orders obtained by contractors for new work[1] at current prices

Great Britain

£ millions

	New housing[2]			Other new work					
	Public and housing association	Private	Total	Infrastructure	Other public	Private industrial	Private commercial	Total	New work total
	BLBC	BLBD	FGAU	BAWT	BAWU	BAWV	BAWW	BLBE	FHAA
2006	2 653	13 468	16 121	4 319	6 162	3 634	17 528	31 643	47 764
2007	2 964	13 109	16 073	5 633	7 324	3 306	18 288	34 551	50 624
2008	2 501	7 670	10 171	6 361	9 400	2 456	13 235	31 452	41 623
2007 Q1	1 056	3 473	4 529	1 677	1 651	876	4 189	8 393	12 922
Q2	707	3 547	4 254	1 533	1 912	851	5 386	9 680	13 934
Q3	568	3 150	3 718	1 225	1 992	756	4 588	8 562	12 279
Q4	634	2 939	3 572	1 198	1 770	824	4 125	7 916	11 489
2008 Q1	797	2 658	3 455	1 780	2 283	711	3 982	8 756	12 211
Q2	669	2 268	2 937	1 895	2 211	526	3 510	8 141	11 078
Q3	582	1 502	2 084	1 389	2 681	669	3 360	8 099	10 183
Q4	452	1 243	1 694	1 297	2 225	551	2 383	6 456	8 150
2009 Q1	623	1 191	1 814	1 909	1 710	299	1 789	5 707	7 521
Q2	523	1 406	1 929	2 516	2 502	398	1 860	7 276	9 205
Q3	743	1 228	1 971	2 365	2 676	338	1 575	6 954	8 925
Q4[4]	615	1 543	2 158	1 656	2 050	403	1 683	5 792	7 950
2009 Jun	176	405	580	469	716	166	694	2 044	2 625
Jul	388	429	817	872	1 139	99	544	2 653	3 470
Aug	195	344	539	857	721	106	498	2 181	2 720
Sep	161	454	615	637	816	133	533	2 120	2 735
Oct[4]	233	521	755	443	682	131	629	1 885	2 640
Nov[4]	140	654	793	381	768	148	593	1 889	2 682
Dec[3]	242	368	610	833	600	123	461	2 017	2 627

1 Including the value of speculative building when work starts on site.
2 Excluding orders for home improvement work.
3 Provisional.
4 Revised

Sources: Office for National Statistics;
Tel : 020 7215 1953

Note: Responsibility for these statistics transferred from BERR (formerly DTI) to the ONS on 1st March 2008.

22.23 Total engineering: total turnover of UK based manufacturers[1]
Values at current prices

£ millions

	Total			Home			Export		
	Orders on Hand	New Orders	Turnover	Orders on Hand	New Orders	Turnover	Orders on Hand	New Orders	Turnover
	HP62	HP65	HP5X	HP64	HP67	HP5Z	HP63	HP66	HP5Y
2004	27 256.9	79 680.2	79 961.2	19 980.7	48 174.6	48 555.3	7 276.2	31 505.3	31 405.7
2005	28 502.9	79 077.7	77 831.5	20 436.9	48 276.8	47 820.8	8 066.0	30 801.0	30 011.0
2006	29 131.0	81 089.5	80 461.3	19 729.9	47 417.5	48 124.5	9 401.1	33 672.2	32 336.9
2007	32 770.9	87 991.6	84 351.6	22 981.2	53 546.9	50 295.7	9 789.7	34 444.5	34 055.8
2008	33 126.4	87 203.1	86 847.6	22 583.8	50 824.9	51 222.3	10 542.6	36 378.1	35 625.4
2007 Q3	32 497.1	23 464.0	21 023.3	22 199.4	14 414.8	12 607.4	10 297.7	9 049.2	8 415.9
Q4	32 770.9	21 964.2	21 690.3	22 981.2	13 747.6	12 965.8	9 789.7	8 216.6	8 724.5
2008 Q1	34 144.2	22 824.4	21 451.1	23 108.1	13 134.8	13 007.7	11 036.1	9 689.7	8 443.3
Q2	34 828.8	22 771.9	22 087.3	23 143.8	12 957.2	12 921.5	11 685.0	9 814.7	9 165.8
Q3	35 191.8	21 770.3	21 407.3	24 047.3	13 533.7	12 630.3	11 144.5	8 236.5	8 777.0
Q4	33 126.4	19 836.5	21 901.9	22 583.8	11 199.2	12 662.8	10 542.6	8 637.2	9 239.3
2009 Q1	31 384.0	16 937.9	18 680.3	21 360.4	9 654.7	10 878.0	10 023.6	7 283.3	7 802.3
Q2	31 292.0	17 964.3	18 056.4	21 222.7	10 546.5	10 684.2	10 069.3	7 417.8	7 372.2
Q3	31 610.6	18 238.1	17 919.4	21 385.9	10 900.1	10 736.8	10 224.7	7 338.0	7 182.6
2008 Mar	34 144.2	7 653.0	7 537.1	23 108.1	4 189.8	4 584.7	11 036.1	3 463.3	2 952.4
Apr	34 348.7	7 557.7	7 353.2	22 897.2	4 126.6	4 337.5	11 451.5	3 431.1	3 015.7
May	34 713.4	7 488.5	7 123.9	23 191.3	4 511.1	4 217.1	11 522.0	2 977.4	2 906.8
Jun	34 828.8	7 725.7	7 610.2	23 143.8	4 319.5	4 366.9	11 685.0	3 406.2	3 243.3
Jul	34 436.1	6 881.5	7 274.3	23 223.0	4 381.1	4 302.0	11 213.1	2 500.4	2 972.3
Aug	34 062.8	6 152.4	6 525.7	22 774.6	3 442.3	3 890.7	11 288.2	2 710.0	2 634.9
Sep	35 191.8	8 736.4	7 607.3	24 047.3	5 710.3	4 437.6	11 144.5	3 026.1	3 169.8
Oct	33 912.4	6 408.3	7 687.7	22 889.4	3 269.5	4 427.4	11 022.9	3 138.7	3 260.4
Nov	32 928.6	6 106.8	7 090.6	22 375.9	3 618.5	4 132.1	10 552.6	2 488.3	2 958.6
Dec	33 126.4	7 321.4	7 123.6	22 583.8	4 311.2	4 103.3	10 542.6	3 010.2	3 020.3
2009 Jan	32 346.9	4 971.7	5 751.2	21 867.7	2 637.9	3 354.0	10 479.2	2 333.8	2 397.2
Feb	31 892.4	5 444.0	5 898.5	21 496.6	3 005.2	3 376.2	10 395.8	2 438.9	2 522.3
Mar	31 384.0	6 522.2	7 030.6	21 360.4	4 011.6	4 147.8	10 023.6	2 510.6	2 882.8
Apr	30 954.3	5 488.9	5 918.6	21 303.3	3 329.9	3 387.0	9 651.1	2 159.0	2 531.6
May	31 333.0	6 031.2	5 652.6	21 269.7	3 395.7	3 429.3	10 063.3	2 635.5	2 223.3
Jun	31 292.0	6 444.2	6 485.2	21 222.7	3 820.9	3 867.9	10 069.3	2 623.3	2 617.3
Jul	31 773.7	6 414.7	5 932.9	21 543.5	3 947.2	3 626.4	10 230.2	2 467.4	2 306.5
Aug	31 837.2	5 546.0	5 482.5	21 559.6	3 302.5	3 286.4	10 277.6	2 243.5	2 196.1
Sep	31 610.6	6 277.4	6 504.0	21 385.9	3 650.4	3 824.0	10 224.7	2 627.1	2 680.0
Oct	31 675.5	6 608.2	6 543.4	21 634.8	3 959.8	3 711.0	10 040.8	2 648.5	2 832.4
Nov	31 212.6	5 853.3	6 316.2	21 425.9	3 456.7	3 665.6	9 786.7	2 396.5	2 650.6

1 New methodology was introduced from January 2008 affecting all historic estimates. See details in February ELMR in-brief page 3 found at: http://nswebcopy/elmr/02_08/downloads/ELMR_Feb08.pdf published on 11 February.

Source: Office for National Statistics

Production

22.24 Manufacture of machinery and equipment not elsewhere classified[1]
Values at current prices

£ million

	Total			Home			Export		
	Orders on Hand	New Orders	Turnover	Orders on Hand	New Orders	Turnover	Orders on Hand	New Orders	Turnover
	HP6B	HP6E	HP68	HP6D	HP6G	HP6A	HP6C	HP6F	HP69
2004	13 669.4	33 228.0	33 524.0	10 192.8	20 242.2	20 652.8	3 476.6	12 985.8	12 871.3
2005	13 484.9	35 353.8	35 538.4	9 515.9	20 975.7	21 652.4	3 969.0	14 378.6	13 885.9
2006	14 095.2	38 110.7	37 500.3	9 260.9	22 047.4	22 302.1	4 834.3	16 063.6	15 198.2
2007	14 937.5	42 063.0	41 220.9	10 060.3	25 493.3	24 694.2	4 877.2	16 569.8	16 526.8
2008	16 271.8	45 888.6	44 554.6	11 155.7	26 646.6	25 551.3	5 116.1	19 242.2	19 003.3
2004 Q3	14 652.4	7 827.9	8 275.1	10 745.3	4 878.9	5 064.8	3 907.1	2 949.0	3 210.5
Q4	13 669.4	8 087.7	9 070.7	10 192.8	5 153.3	5 705.7	3 476.6	2 934.5	3 365.1
2005 Q1	14 361.2	9 200.2	8 508.3	10 349.8	5 455.7	5 298.6	4 011.4	3 744.6	3 209.7
Q2	14 482.6	8 972.7	8 851.2	10 367.1	5 404.6	5 387.3	4 115.5	3 568.1	3 463.9
Q3	13 961.1	8 343.8	8 865.5	9 998.9	5 030.8	5 398.9	3 962.1	3 313.3	3 466.6
Q4	13 484.9	8 837.1	9 313.4	9 515.9	5 084.6	5 567.6	3 969.0	3 752.6	3 745.7
2006 Q1	13 854.0	9 176.5	8 807.3	9 374.6	5 032.7	5 173.9	4 479.5	4 143.9	3 633.4
Q2	14 196.0	9 558.4	9 216.5	9 607.2	5 698.3	5 465.7	4 588.8	3 860.3	3 750.9
Q3	14 239.9	9 555.5	9 511.5	9 571.9	5 727.1	5 762.2	4 668.0	3 828.4	3 749.3
Q4	14 095.2	9 820.3	9 965.0	9 260.9	5 589.3	5 900.3	4 834.3	4 231.0	4 064.6
2007 Q1	13 794.4	9 494.2	9 795.0	9 239.4	5 960.9	5 982.6	4 555.1	3 533.3	3 812.4
Q2	14 234.4	10 482.7	10 042.7	9 465.3	6 179.3	5 953.3	4 769.1	4 303.5	4 089.5
Q3	15 237.0	11 484.1	10 481.6	10 127.8	6 959.2	6 296.8	5 109.1	4 524.9	4 184.8
Q4	14 937.5	10 602.0	10 901.6	10 060.3	6 393.9	6 461.5	4 877.2	4 208.1	4 440.1
2008 Q1	16 077.7	12 198.5	11 058.3	10 328.5	6 717.1	6 448.8	5 749.2	5 481.6	4 609.5
Q2	16 557.9	11 944.9	11 464.7	10 760.9	6 840.3	6 408.0	5 797.1	5 104.6	5 056.8
Q3	17 872.9	12 325.3	11 010.5	12 485.1	8 068.9	6 344.8	5 387.7	4 256.4	4 665.7
Q4	16 271.8	9 419.9	11 021.1	11 155.7	5 020.3	6 349.7	5 116.1	4 399.6	4 671.3
2009 Q1	15 213.2	7 828.5	8 887.0	10 511.8	4 757.8	5 401.7	4 701.3	3 070.8	3 485.5
Q2	15 082.6	8 278.5	8 409.1	10 166.9	4 834.3	5 179.1	4 915.7	3 444.2	3 229.9
Q3	15 197.4	8 374.0	8 259.2	10 035.5	4 951.2	5 082.8	5 161.9	3 422.7	3 176.4
2007 Nov	15 212.6	3 835.0	3 816.2	10 100.2	2 122.5	2 242.5	5 112.4	1 712.5	1 573.7
Dec	14 937.5	3 102.6	3 377.8	10 060.3	2 014.4	2 054.4	4 877.2	1 088.2	1 323.4
2008 Jan	16 003.0	4 523.4	3 457.9	10 598.5	2 563.4	2 025.2	5 404.6	1 960.1	1 432.7
Feb	15 910.0	3 638.3	3 731.3	10 428.4	2 030.8	2 200.8	5 481.6	1 607.6	1 530.5
Mar	16 077.7	4 036.8	3 869.1	10 328.5	2 122.9	2 222.8	5 749.2	1 913.9	1 646.3
Apr	16 143.9	3 913.6	3 847.5	10 253.8	2 108.0	2 182.7	5 890.0	1 805.6	1 664.8
May	16 533.5	4 077.9	3 688.2	10 681.0	2 513.0	2 085.8	5 852.5	1 564.9	1 602.4
Jun	16 557.9	3 953.4	3 929.0	10 760.9	2 219.3	2 139.5	5 797.1	1 734.1	1 789.6
Jul	16 552.5	3 825.7	3 831.2	10 958.0	2 371.6	2 174.5	5 594.4	1 454.1	1 656.7
Aug	16 789.0	3 497.5	3 261.0	11 147.8	2 091.8	1 902.1	5 641.2	1 405.7	1 358.9
Sep	17 872.9	5 002.1	3 918.3	12 485.1	3 605.5	2 268.2	5 387.7	1 396.6	1 650.1
Oct	17 019.6	3 119.4	3 972.7	11 680.8	1 480.6	2 284.9	5 338.8	1 638.8	1 687.8
Nov	16 277.3	2 807.3	3 549.6	11 282.5	1 654.3	2 052.6	4 994.8	1 153.0	1 497.0
Dec	16 271.8	3 493.2	3 498.8	11 155.7	1 885.4	2 012.2	5 116.1	1 607.8	1 486.5
2009 Jan	15 841.7	2 297.6	2 727.6	10 963.2	1 490.0	1 682.5	4 878.5	807.6	1 045.2
Feb	15 498.8	2 489.3	2 832.2	10 576.1	1 285.0	1 672.2	4 922.7	1 204.3	1 160.1
Mar	15 213.2	3 041.6	3 327.2	10 511.8	1 982.8	2 047.0	4 701.3	1 058.9	1 280.2
Apr	14 785.3	2 339.8	2 767.7	10 243.3	1 409.4	1 677.9	4 542.0	930.4	1 089.8
May	15 455.1	3 319.1	2 649.3	10 392.7	1 834.3	1 684.9	5 062.4	1 484.8	964.4
Jun	15 082.6	2 619.6	2 992.1	10 166.9	1 590.6	1 816.3	4 915.7	1 029.0	1 175.7
Jul	15 391.0	3 096.2	2 787.8	10 367.5	1 966.5	1 765.9	5 023.5	1 129.7	1 021.8
Aug	15 494.4	2 674.7	2 571.2	10 289.0	1 504.2	1 582.8	5 205.4	1 170.4	988.5
Sep	15 197.4	2 603.1	2 900.2	10 035.5	1 480.5	1 734.1	5 161.9	1 122.6	1 166.1
Oct	15 055.9	2 948.2	3 089.7	10 011.0	1 707.5	1 732.0	5 044.9	1 240.7	1 357.7
Nov	14 811.3	2 651.0	2 895.6	9 881.6	1 566.9	1 696.3	4 929.7	1 084.1	1 199.3

1 Note: New methodology was introduced from January 2008 affecting all historic estimates. See details in February ELMR in-brief page 3 found at: http://nswebcopy/elmr/02_08/downloads/ELMR_Feb08.pdf published on 11 February.

Source: Office for National Statistics

22.25 New Car Registrations
Segment totals

		1999	2000	2001	2002	2003	2004	2005	2006	2007	2008	2009
Mini	JW9C	39 635	52 203	47 899	40 370	38 940	36 171	27 195	23 297	21 512	28 094	68 098
Supermini	JW9D	593 745	688 686	773 995	831 264	873 690	839 604	732 756	753 872	770 601	726 006	742 153
Lower Medium	JW9F	703 611	661 502	741 817	771 319	719 164	729 690	761 328	694 428	722 012	605 817	530 849
Upper Medium	JW9G	513 218	476 860	507 736	505 026	480 220	459 061	427 278	393 999	386 414	340 796	283 552
Executive	JW9H	115 509	104 583	109 433	114 382	118 579	109 667	111 112	100 339	104 468	98 572	90 114
Luxury Saloon	JW9I	12 375	11 406	11 053	10 193	13 500	13 620	11 678	13 227	13 120	9 977	6 547
Specialist Sports	JW9J	68 845	67 208	65 358	60 108	65 178	73 940	64 681	65 047	65 731	50 256	46 467
4x4/SUV	JW9K	98 926	99 212	121 556	137 582	159 144	179 439	187 392	175 805	176 290	136 525	132 472
Multi-Purpose	JW9L	51 750	59 987	79 922	93 387	110 635	126 077	116 297	124 850	143 859	135 752	94 747
Total	JW9M	2 197 615	2 221 647	2 458 769	2 563 631	2 579 050	2 567 269	2 439 717	2 344 864	2 404 007	2 131 795	1 994 999

1 See chapter text.

Source: www.smmt.co.uk

Production

22.26 Alcoholic drink[1]
United Kingdom

			1999	2000	2001	2002	2003	2004	2005	2006	2007	2008	2009[4]
Spirits[2]		Thousand hectolitres of alcohol											
Production	KMEA	"	4 705	4 210	4 368	4 508	4 553	4 081	4 365	4 485	5 498	6 072	4 261
Released for home consumption													
Home produced whisky	KMEE	"	323	314	321	321	318	319	301	283	286	289	258
Spirit-based Ready-to-drink[3]	SNET	"	..	..	..	105	124	114	84	65	52	42	31
Imported and other	KMEG	"	596	615	647	689	744	792	822	767	832	816	802
Total	KMEH	"	919	929	968	1 115	1 187	1 226	1 206	1 114	1 170	1 147	1 091
Beer		Thousand hectolitres											
Production	BFNK	"	57 854	55 279	56 802	56 672	58 014	57 461	56 255	53 768	51 341	49 611	45 141
Released for home consumption	BAYL	"	58 917	57 007	58 234	59 384	60 301	59 194	57 572	55 751	53 465	51 498	46 722
Production	JYXJ	Thousand hectolitres of pure alcohol	2 364	2 299	2 358	2 352	2 414	2 433	2 338	2 250	2 160	2 062	1 891
Released for home consumption	JYXK	"	2 428	2 382	2 429	2 473	2 515	2 499	2 398	2 335	2 247	2 145	1 953
Wine of fresh grapes													
Released for home consumption		Thousand hectolitres											
Fortified	KMEM	"	316	289	287	325	296	298	306	302	305	324	219
Still table	KMEN	"	8 391	8 864	9 534	10 319	10 647	11 768	12 117	11 655	12 559	12 402	11 729
Sparkling	KMEO	"	576	543	515	578	640	676	721	715	838	757	731
Total	KMEP	"	9 284	9 696	10 336	11 222	11 584	12 742	13 143	12 672	13 702	13 483	12 680
Made-wine													
Released for home consumption													
Still	JTI9	"	413	428	360	366	338	351	334	316	343	374	390
Sparkling	JTJ2	"	3	3	4	2	1	1	–	1	5	7	2
Coolers[3]	KJDD	"	1 802	2 800	3 712	1 606	423	508	597	528	720	611	597
Total made wine	JTJ3	"	2 218	3 232	4 075	1 974	762	859	931	844	1 068	993	989
Cider and perry													
Released for home consumption	KMER	"	6 022	6 006	5 911	5 939	5 876	6 139	6 377	7 523	8 046	8 412	9 404

1 See chapter text.
2 Potable spirits distilled.
3 Made wine with alcoholic strength 1.2% to 5.5%. Includes alcoholic lemon-ade of appropriate strength and similar products. From 28 April 2002, duty on spirit-based "coolers" is charged at the same rate as spirits per litre of alcohol. Coolers for calendar year 2002 includes only wine based "coolers".
4 Provisional

Sources: HM Revenue & Customs UK Trade Information website:;
http://www.uktradeinfo.com/index.cfm?task=bulletins

22.27 Tobacco products: released for home consumption[1]
United Kingdom

	Million			Thousand kilogrammes			
	Cigarettes			Other tobacco products			Total tobacco products other than cigarettes
	Home-produced	Imported	Total	Cigars	Hand-rolling	Other[2]	
	LUQN	LUQO	LUQP	LUQQ	LUQR	LUQS	LUQT
2005	45 922	4 322	50 244	758	3 189	499	4 445
2006	44 392	4 570	48 962	689	3 454	439	4 581
2007	41 955	3 794	45 749	602	3 644	398	4 643
2008	42 053	3 680	45 733	546	4 154	381	5 081
2009[3]	43 989	3 586	47 575	534	5 076	397	6 007
2009 Apr	6 902	665	7 567	107	801	51	959
May	1 056	7	1 063	18	149	18	185
Jun	2 757	239	2 996	39	316	30	385
Jul	3 701	320	4 021	34	440	32	506
Aug	3 495	296	3 791	43	410	30	483
Sep	4 114	291	4 405	44	473	35	552
Oct	3 479	283	3 761	42	368	33	443
Nov[3]	3 339	283	3 622	50	427	37	515
Dec[3]	4 771	395	5 166	45	546	42	633

1 See chapter text.
2 Other includes other smoking and chewing tobacco.
3 Provisional.

Sources: HM Revenue and Customs Statistical Bulletins at;
http://www.uktradeinfo.com/index.cfm?task=bulletins

Banking, insurance

Chapter 23

Banking, insurance

Other banks balance sheet

(Table 23.3)

The table includes the business of all monthly and quarterly reporting banks in the UK.

The Channel Islands and Isle of Man are not treated as part of the UK for statistical purposes. Banking institutions in the Channel Islands and Isle of Man no longer have the option of being within the UK banking sector and their business, along with the business of offshore island branches of UK mainland banks, is excluded from the figures within this table. Additionally, the business of the UK banking sector with offshore island residents and entities are classified as 'non-residents'.

The table also contains details of business with building societies.

The aggregate balance sheet of the banking sector is reported on an accrual basis (accrued amounts that are payable and receivable are shown under liabilities and assets respectively). Additionally, acceptances are shown under both liabilities and assets.

The balance sheet of the Banking Department of the Bank of England is excluded from this table, and other banks business with the Issue Department is classified as 'UK banks'.

Data for 1999 reflect the acquisition of Birmingham Midshires Building Society by Halifax during that year.

Data for the end of 2000 reflect the entry of Bradford and Bingley plc to the banking sector during the year. Data for the end of 2000 also reflect the new reporting during the year of agency business as a result of collateral management via repurchase agreements (repos) and reverse repos.

Bank lending to, and bank deposits from, UK residents

(Tables 23.4 and 23.5)

These are series statistics based on the Standard Industrial Classification (SIC) 1992 (which was revised slightly in 2003).

Table 23.4. Until the third quarter of 2007, the analysis of lending covered loans, advances (including under reverse repos), finance leasing, acceptances and facilities (all in Sterling and other currencies) provided by reporting banks to their UK resident non-bank non-building society customers, as well as bank holdings of sterling and euro commercial paper issued by these resident customers. Following a review of statistical data collected, acceptances and holdings of sterling and euro commercial paper are no longer collected at the industry level detail with effect from fourth quarter 2007 data. Total lending therefore reflects loans and advances (including under reverse repos) only, from fourth quarter 2007 data.

Table 23.5 includes borrowing under sale and repo. Adjustments for transit items are not included.

Figures for both tables are supplied by monthly reporting banks and grossed to cover quarterly reporters. Following the transition of building societies' statistical reporting from the Financial Services Authority to the Bank of England on 1st January 2008, both tables will include data reported by building societies from the first quarter of 2008 onwards. They exclude lending to building societies and to residents of the Channel Islands and Isle of Man.

Building societies

(Table 23.13)

Building society figures are sourced from societies' annual returns and for each year relate to accounting years ending on dates between 1 February and 31 January of the following year. Figures are society-only as opposed to group consolidated.

Consumer credit

(Table 23.14)

Figures for net lending refer to changes in amounts outstanding adjusted to remove distortions caused by

revaluations of debt outstanding, such as write-offs. Class 3 loans are advanced under the terms of the Building Societies Act 1986.

A high proportion of credit advanced in certain types of agreement, notably on credit cards, is repaid within a month. This reflects use of such agreements as a method of payment rather than a way of obtaining credit. As from December 2006 the Bank of England has ceased to update the separate data on consumer credit provided by other specialist lenders, retailers and insurance companies previously contained in these tables. These categories have been merged into 'other consumer credit lenders'.

23.1 Bank of England Balance Sheet
Liabilities and assets outstanding at end of period

£ million

Consolidated statement

	Liabilities							Assets									
	Notes in circulation	Reserve balances	Standing facility deposits	Short term open market operations	Foreign currency public securities issued	Cash ratio deposits	Other liabilities	Standing facility assets	Short term open market operations	Of which 1 week sterling reverse repo	of which fine-tuning sterling reverse repo	of which other maturity within maintenance period reverse repos	Longer term sterling reverse repo	Ways and Means advances to HMG	Bonds and other securities acqured via market transactions	Other assets	Total assets/liabil
	B55A	B56A	B57A	B58A	B59A	B62A	B63A	B65A	B66A	B67A	B68A	BL59	B69A	B72A	B73A	B74A	B75A
2009	51 077	147 356	–	–	3 731	2 599	35 669	–				–	25 541	370	13 174	201 347	240 431
2009 Feb	44 494	33 700	–	–	2 893	2 427	40 951	–	–	–	–	–	126 261	9 392	11 873	20 878	168 404
Mar	45 465	50 892	–	–	4 365	2 427	46 411	–	–	–	–	–	126 827	4 142	14 014	28 376	173 360
Apr	47 022	68 723	–	–	4 089	2 427	40 949	–	–	–	–	–	129 716	370	13 602	55 232	198 920
May	45 921	102 669	–	–	3 932	2 427	38 983	–	–	–	–	–	120 779	370	13 305	86 668	221 122
Jun	46 029	129 525	–	–	3 754	2 547	32 493	–	–	–	–	–	100 648	370	13 183	108 517	222 718
Jul	46 509	153 035	–	–	3 732	2 547	31 873	–	11 560	11 560	–	–	79 651	370	13 028	133 086	237 695
Aug	46 556	137 850	–	–	3 716	2 547	29 843	–	–	–	–	–	58 174	370	13 165	148 802	220 511
Sep	46 736	139 814	–	–	3 712	2 547	33 180	–	–	–	–	–	47 883	370	13 375	164 361	225 989
Oct	46 998	146 633	–	–	3 681	2 547	30 108	–	–	–	–	–	33 560	370	13 472	182 564	229 966
Nov	47 234	150 483	–	–	3 661	2 545	31 298	–	–	–	–	–	29 522	370	13 551	191 778	235 221
Dec	51 077	147 356	–	–	3 731	2 599	35 669	–	–	–	–	–	25 541	370	13 174	201 347	240 431
2010 Jan	49 496	156 592	–	–	3 753	2 574	33 069	–	–	–	–	–	24 797	370	12 601	207 716	245 484

Issue Department

	Liabilities		Assets							
	Notes in circulation	Notes in Banking Departemnt	Short term open market operations	Of which 1 week sterling reverse repo	of which fine-tuning sterling reverse repo	Longer term sterling reverse repo	Ways and Means advances to HMG	Bonds and other securities acqured via market transactions	Other assets	Total assets/liabilities
	AEFA	AEFB	BL29	BL32	BL33	BL34	B54A	BL35	BL36	BL37
2009	51 077		–	–	–	20 395	370	5 439	24 874	51 077
2009 Mar	45 465		–	–	–	9 799	4 142	5 435	26 088	45 465
Apr	47 022		–	–	–	9 719	370	5 433	31 501	47 022
May	45 921		–	–	–	9 719	370	5 433	30 400	45 921
Jun	46 029		–	–	–	9 769	370	5 417	30 474	46 029
Jul	46 509		11 560	11 560	–	9 770	370	5 417	19 392	46 509
Aug	46 556		–	–	–	13 405	370	5 417	27 364	46 556
Sep	46 736		–	–	–	18 517	370	5 493	22 356	46 736
Oct	46 998		–	–	–	23 740	370	5 493	17 394	46 998
Nov	47 234		–	–	–	22 799	370	5 493	18 571	47 234
Dec	51 077		–	–	–	20 395	370	5 439	24 874	51 077
2010 Jan	49 496		–	–	–	19 712	370	5 439	23 975	49 496
Feb	49 486		–	..	..	..	..	..	..	..

Banking Department

	Liabilities						Assets								
	Reserve balances	Standing facility deposits	Short term open market operations	Foreign currency public securities issued	Cash ratio deposits	Other liabilities	Standing facility assets	Short term open market operations	Of which 1 week sterling reverse repo	of which fine-tuning sterling reverse repo	Longer term sterling reverse repo	Bonds and other securities acqured via market transactions	Bank of England notes	Other assets	Total assets/liabilitie
	BL38	BL39	BL42	BL43	BL44	BL45	BL47	BL48	BL49	BL52	B3J2	BL53	BL54	BL55	BL56
2009	147 356	–	–	3 731	2 599	60 542	–	–	–	–	5 146	7 735	–	201 347	214 228
2009 Feb	33 700	–	–	2 893	2 427	61 311	–	–	–	–	116 463	6 929	–	20 878	144 270
Mar	50 892	–	–	4 365	2 427	72 499	–	–	–	–	117 028	8 579	–	28 376	153 983
Apr	68 723	–	–	4 089	2 427	72 450	–	–	–	–	119 997	8 169	–	55 232	183 399
May	102 669	–	–	3 932	2 427	69 383	–	–	–	–	111 060	7 872	–	86 668	205 600
Jun	129 525	–	–	3 754	2 547	62 966	–	–	–	–	90 879	7 766	–	108 517	207 162
Jul	153 035	–	–	3 732	2 547	51 265	–	–	–	–	69 881	7 611	–	133 086	210 578
Aug	137 850	–	–	3 716	2 547	57 207	–	–	–	–	44 769	7 748	–	148 802	201 319
Sep	139 814	–	–	3 712	2 547	55 536	–	–	–	–	29 366	7 882	–	164 361	201 609
Oct	146 633	–	–	3 681	2 547	47 503	–	–	–	–	9 820	7 979	–	182 564	200 363
Nov	150 483	–	–	3 661	2 545	49 869	–	–	–	–	6 723	8 058	–	191 778	206 559
Dec	147 356	–	–	3 731	2 599	60 542	–	–	–	–	5 146	7 735	–	201 347	214 228
2010 Jan	156 592	–	–	3 753	2 574	57 044	–	–	–	–	5 085	7 163	–	207 716	219 964

Source: Bank of England

23.2

Value of inter-bank clearings
United Kingdom

£ billion

		2004	2005	2006	2007	2008	2009
Bulk paper clearings							
Cheque and Credit Clearing Company							
Cheques[1]	KCYY	1 111	1 062	1 076	1 157	1 076	870
Euro Debits	JT8O	..	..	..	..	3	3
Credits	KCYZ	63	57	56	58	52	42
Inter-bank Cheque and Credit	JT8P	1 174	1 119	1 132	1 215	1 130	915
High-value clearings							
Faster Payments Scheme[3]	JT8N	..	..	..	..	33	106
CHAPS Sterling	KCZB	52 348	52 672	59 437	69 352	73 626	64 617
Electronic clearing (BACS)							
Standing Orders/Direct Credits[2]	JT8J	2 133	2 353	2 584	2 812	3 006	2 970
Direct Debits	JT8L	750	797	845	884	935	886
Euro Direct Credits	JT8M	..	..	..	..	5	5
Total Bacs	KCZC	2 883	3 150	3 429	3 696	3 946	3 861
Total all Inter-Bank Clearings	JT8Q	56 405	56 941	63 998	74 263	88 127	69 500

1 Figures for 2004 - 2007 include Euro Debits.
2 Figures for 2004 - 2007 include Euro Direct Credits.
3 The UK Faster Payments Services was launched on 27th May 2008.

Source: APACS - The UK payments association: 020 7711 6223

23.3 Monetary Financial Institutions (Excluding Central Bank) Balance sheet , Liabilities and Assets

Amount outstanding at end of period

£ million

	Sterling liabilities										Sterling liabilities	
	Sterling liabilities: (UK) Sight deposits				Sterling liabilities: (UK) Time deposit							
	MFIs	UK Public sector	Other UK residents	Non-reside-nts	MFIs	UK Public sector	Other UK residents	Of which cash ISAs	Of which SAYE	Non-reside-nts	Notes outstanding and cash loaded cards	Acceptances granted
	B3GL	B3MM	B3NM	B3OM	B3HL	B3PM	B3QM	B3SM	B3RM	B3TM	B3LM	B3XM
2010 Jan	121 490	22 182	891 466	135 562	321 044	14 858	1 042 519	164 928	896	351 674	5 961	1 185
Feb	119 953	20 093	893 892	128 942	321 601	13 796	1 042 524	164 754	910	350 760	5 777	1 104
Changes												
	B4GA	B4CF	B4BH	B4DD	B4HA	B4DF	B4CH	B4DH	B4FH	B4ED	B4IJ	B4BK
2010 Jan	−7 806	2 323	−5 156	3 024	15 567	−780	−4 587	−323	14	−9 776	−38	20
Feb	−1 537	−2 639	2 977	−6 575	561	−1 061	33	−174	15	−607	−184	−81

	Sterling liabilities (continued)										
	Sterling liabilities: (UK) under sale and repurchase agreements				Sterling liabilities						
	MFIs	UK Public sector	Other UK residents	Non-residen-ts	CDs and other short term paper issued	Total sterling deposits	Sterling items in suspense and transmission	Net derivatives	Accrued amounts payable	Sterling capital and other internal funds	Total sterling liabilities
	B3IL	B3UM	B3VM	B3WM	B3YM	B3ZM	B3GN	B3HN	B3IN	B3JN	B3KN
2010 Jan	182 486	8 568	140 472	28 956	208 943	3 471 404	67 489	2 416	31 612	486 329	4 065 211
Feb	178 712	6 601	137 658	27 757	206 118	3 449 510	69 144	19 512	33 087	491 164	4 068 194
Changes											
	B4IA	B4EF	B4EH	B4FD	B4EJ	B4FJ	B4AK	B4GJ	B4CJ	B4DJ	B4JJ
2010 Jan	11 159	2 166	7 740	8 248	3 581	25 723	22 820	7 229	−1 087	62 965	117 612
Feb	−3 775	−1 968	−2 814	−1 199	−3 065	−21 750	1 656	17 096	1 475	−9 390	−11 097

	Foreign currency liabilities(including euro)							
	Foreign currency liabilities: (UK) Sight and time deposits				Foreign currency liabilities: (UK) Sale and repurchase agreements			
	MFIs	UK Public sector	Other UK residents	Non-residents	MFIs	UK Public sector	Other UK residents	Non-residents
	B3JL	B3LN	B3MN	B3NN	B3KL	B3PN	B3QN	B3RN
2010 Jan	242 647	732	246 760	1 981 093	121 467	845	88 953	455 611
Feb	248 570	666	265 733	2 133 743	134 175	2 325	98 540	501 841
Changes								
	B4GB	B4FG	B4FI	B4GE	B4HB	B4GG	B4GI	B4HE
2010 Jan	−14 918	8	−2 960	−73 107	1 139	−2 379	4 627	85 899
Feb	−4 046	−94	7 555	65 230	7 722	1 407	5 911	25 112

23.3
continued

Monetary Financial Institutions (Excluding Central Bank) Balance sheet , Liabilities and Assets

Amount outstanding at end of period

£ million

	Acceptances granted	CDs and other short term paper issued	Total foreign currency deposits	Items in suspense and transmission	Net derivatives	Accrued amounts payable	Capital and other internal funds	Total foreign currency liabilities	Total liabilities
	B3KQ	B3SN	B3TN	B3UN	B3VN	B3WN	B3XN	B3YN	B3ZN
2010 Jan	1 049	770 717	3 909 874	225 284	−52 004	26 523	135 873	4 245 550	8 310 762
Feb	1 200	798 510	4 185 303	232 634	−76 526	26 568	136 379	4 504 357	8 572 551
Changes									
	B4HM	B4CM	B4DM	B4GM	B4EM	B4AM	B4BM	B4FM	B4JM
2010 Jan	−26	14 096	12 379	124 670	3 423	−3 623	2 954	139 804	257 415
Feb	101	−10 388	98 510	3 036	−26 317	−386	5 121	79 964	68 866

Sterling Assets

	Sterling assets:with UK central bank		Market loans UK				Advances(UK)			
	Cash ratio deposits	Other	MFIs	MFIs CDs	MFIs commercial paper	Non-residents	UK Public sector	Other UK residents	Non-residents	Notes and coin
	B3VO	B3WO	B3NL	B3OL	B3PL	B3XO	B3NP	B3OP	B3PP	B3UO
2010 Jan	2 575	155 508	438 411	24 211	1 400	210 599	10 535	2 072 823	84 046	9 785
Feb	2 575	151 608	437 129	24 332	1 583	205 353	10 675	2 070 599	86 859	10 199
Changes										
	B3YR	B3ZR	B4DC	B4JB	B4BC	B4BD	B4JE	B4JG	B4HC	B4II
2010 Jan	−25	10 947	7 403	1 056	−20	17 953	361	−2 346	−738	−2 629
Feb	−	−3 900	−1 282	122	183	−5 114	141	−311	2 993	414

Sterling assets (continued)

	Sterling assets: (UK) Acceptances granted				Bills (UK)				Claims under sale and repurchase agreements (UK)			
	MFIs	UK Public sector	Other UK residents	Non-residents	Treasury bills	MFIs bills	Other UK residents	Non-residents	MFIs	UK Public sector	Other UK residents	Non-residents
	B3QL	B3YO	B3ZO	B3GP	B3HP	B3RL	B3IP	B3JP	B3SL	B3KP	B3LP	B3MP
2010 Jan	1	−	902	282	22 967	40	186	1 604	167 638	512	124 066	32 617
Feb	1	−	838	265	16 066	40	189	1 444	163 782	20	117 996	33 809
Changes												
	B4EC	B4FF	B3TR	B4GD	B4BA	B4IB	B4HG	B4IC	B4FA	B4BF	B4AH	B4CD
2010 Jan	−	−	46	−25	148	−39	7	..	10 650	−1 556	−1 691	5 949
Feb	−	−	−64	−17	−6 901	−	3	..	−3 856	−492	−6 071	1 192

Source: Bank of England

Banking, insurance

23.3 Monetary Financial Institutions (Excluding Central Bank) Balance sheet , Liabilities and Assets
continued

Amount outstanding at end of period

£ million

Sterling assets (continued)

	Investments					Items in suspense and collection	Accrued amount receivable	Other assets	Total sterling assets
	British government securities	Other UK Public sector	MFIs	Other UK residents	Non-residents				
	B3QP	B3RP	B3TL	B3SP	B3TP	B3UP	B3VP	B3WP	B3XP
2010 Jan	38 720	396	103 330	382 116	45 706	77 848	33 323	17 888	4 060 043
Feb	43 298	407	102 216	374 341	46 763	78 481	32 460	21 103	4 034 441
Changes									
	B4CA	B4IE	B4CC	B4IG	B4JC	B4BJ	B4HI	B4JI	B4AJ
2010 Jan	3 016	−15	23 091	8 206	−1 563	21 123	1 157	−471	100 200
Feb	4 940	11	−1 009	−12 087	−835	632	−862	−240	−32 570

Foreign currency assets (including euro)

	Market loans and advances					Claims under sale and repurchase agreements				Acceptances granted	Bills
	MFIs	MFIs CDs etc.	UK public sector	Other UK residents	Non-residents	MFIs	UK public sector	Other UK residents	Non-residents		
	B3UL	B3VL	B3YP	B3ZP	B3GQ	B3WL	B3HQ	B3IQ	B3JQ	B4IP	B3LQ
2010 Jan	249 536	6 061	85	305 316	1 891 384	130 716	1 261	148 429	454 557	1 049	54 101
Feb	257 029	5 650	88	317 384	2 056 245	139 352	524	157 623	517 703	1 200	56 403
Changes											
	B4EB	B4AF	B4DG	B4DI	B4EE	B4FB	B4EG	B4EI	B4FE	B4HP	B4GL
2010 Jan	−12 736	−1 065	13	5 618	−37 731	5 808	237	16 153	32 005	−26	−2 129
Feb	−2 742	−621	−1	−1 633	81 999	3 348	−775	3 293	42 155	101	−268

Foreign currency assets (including euro)(continued)

	Investments					Items in suspense & collection	Accrued amounts receivable	Other assets	Total foreign currency assets	Total assets	Holdings of own sterling acceptances	Holdings of own FC acceptances
	British govt securities	Other public sector	MFIs	Other UK residents	Non-residents							
	B3MQ	B3NQ	B3XL	B3OQ	B3PQ	B3QQ	B3RQ	B3SQ	B3TQ	B3UQ	B3IM	B3JM
2010 Jan	7	–	36 501	82 478	575 805	242 043	32 019	39 371	4 250 718	8 310 762	275	407
Feb	14	2	35 365	85 334	598 839	232 513	34 479	42 364	4 538 110	8 572 551	264	468
Changes												
	B4EA	B4CG	B4AG	B4CI	B4DE	B4JL	B4FL	B4HL	B4IL	B4IM	B3VR	B3XR
2010 Jan	7	–	−3 699	−946	18 245	142 592	−4 145	−994	157 208	257 408	–	16
Feb	6	2	−2 448	−465	−3 759	−18 908	1 037	1 100	101 422	68 852	−11	39

See Supplementary Information Also see footnotes in Bank of England Monetary and Financial Statistics Table B1.4

Source: Bank of England

23.4 Industrial analysis of bank lending to UK residents[1]
Not seasonally adjusted

£ million

	UK residents		Agriculture, hunting and forestry	Fishing	Mining & quarrying	Manufacturing			
	Total	of which sterling				Total	Food, beverages & tobacco	Textiles & leather	Pulp, paper, publishing & printing

Amounts outstanding (sterling & other currencies)

Loans & advances (including under repo & sterling commercial paper)

	TBOA	TBOB	TBOC	TBOD	TBOE	TBOF	TBOG	TBOH	TBOI
2006	1 793 840	1 460 380	9 620	413	4 205	47 476	11 434	1 512	6 405
2007	..	..	..	..	..	—	..	..	..

Acceptances

	TBQA	TBQB	TBQC	TBQD	TBQE	TBQF	TBQG	TBQH	TBQI
2006	1 190	956	—	—	1	104	5	28	1
2007	..	..	..	..	..	—	..	..	..

Total

	TBSA		TBSC	TBSD	TBSE	TBSF	TBSG	TBSH	TBSI
2008	2 630 295		10 714	356	17 457	65 033	19 428	1 588	7 735
2009	2 514 259		11 149	347	7 060	48 789	11 168	1 469	8 302

of which in sterling

	TBUA		TBUC	TBUD	TBUE	TBUF	TBUG	TBUH	TBUI
2008	2 078 569		10 139	347	2 205	32 684	9 359	953	4 354
2009	2 073 612		10 673	338	1 922	28 730	7 300	955	4 164

Facilities granted

	TCAA		TCAC	TCAD	TCAE	TCAF	TCAG	TCAH	TCAI
2008	3 087 455		13 925	453	28 557	108 737	28 914	2 374	12 548
2009	2 975 139		14 302	405	23 383	94 754	21 504	2 216	13 536

of which in sterling

	TCCA		TCCC	TCCD	TCCE	TCCF	TCCG	TCCH	TCCI
2008	2 362 723		13 317	444	3 180	49 345	12 918	1 427	6 388
2009	2 334 244		..	393	2 918	45 401	10 557	1 382	6 123

Manufacturing					Electricity, gas and water supply			
Chemicals, man-made fibres, rubber & plastics	Non-metallic mineral products & metals	Machinery, equipment & transport equipment	Electrical, medical & optical equipment	Other manufacturing	Electricity, gas & heated water	Cold water purification & supply	Construction

Amounts outstanding (sterling & other currencies)

Loans & advances (including under repo & sterling commercial paper)

	TBOJ	TBOK	TBOL	TBOM	TBON	TBOO	TBOP	TBOQ
2006	5 681	6 122	6 678	3 741	5 903	7 075	4 235	20 671
2007	..	..	..	..	..	—	..	..

Acceptances

	TBQJ	TBQK	TBQL	TBQM	TBQN	TBQO	TBQP	TBQQ
2006	4	10	8	14	33	—	—	15
2007	..	..	..	..	..	..	..	..

Total

	TBSJ	TBSK	TBSL	TBSM	TBSN	TBSO	TBSP	TBSQ
2008	..	8 035	10 604	..	6 158	9 766	3 964	31 706
2009	..	6 756	7 697	..	4 852	8 021	3 518	26 333

of which in sterling

	TBUJ	TBUK	TBUL	TBUM	TBUN	TBUO	TBUP	TBUQ
2008	3 191	3 703	4 968	2 128	4 027	7 606	3 933	30 629
2009	2 662	4 017	4 141	1 926	3 565	5 922	3 485	25 611

Facilities granted

	TCAJ	TCAK	TCAL	TCAM	TCAN	TCAO	TCAP	TCAQ
2008	..	12 608	17 976	8 811	11 438	18 313	7 802	43 141
2009	..	11 366	15 422	7 296	7 788	15 805	7 233	39 160

of which in sterling

	TCCJ	TCCK	TCCL	TCCM	TCCN	TCCO	TCCP	TCCQ
2008	4 715	5 998	8 771	3 419	5 709	11 698	6 975	40 340
2009	4 792	6 293	7 885	3 025	5 344	9 651	6 413	36 495

23.4 Industrial analysis of bank lending to UK residents[1]
Not seasonally adjusted
continued

£ million

	Wholesale and retail trade					Real estate, renting, computer and other business activities		
Total	Sale & repair of motor vehicles & fuel	Other wholesale trade	Other retail trade & repair	Hotels and restaurants	Transport, storage & communication	Total	Development, buying, selling, renting of real estate	Renting of machinery & equipment

Amounts outstanding (sterling & other currencies)

Loans & advances (including under repo & sterling commercial paper)

	TBOR	TBOS	TBOT	TBOU	TBOV	TBOW	TBOX	TBOY	TBPA
2005	40 548	9 293	13 312	17 943	25 064	20 836	177 152	137 281	6 661
2006	42 368	10 167	14 401	17 800	25 707	26 361	209 942	162 332	6 881

Acceptances

	TBQR	TBQS	TBQT	TBQU	TBQV	TBQW	TBQX	TBQY	TBRA
2005	151	7	120	25	–	–	721	714	–
2006	160	4	99	58	1	1	812	800	–

Total

	TBSR	TBSS	TBST	TBSU	TBSV	TBSW	TBSX	TBSY	TBTA
2008	56 778	9 929	23 726	23 124	32 260	32 454	310 911	250 265	9 931
2009	47 438	11 260	15 639	20 539	..	29 600	300 783	249 284	7 766

of which in sterling

	TBUR	TBUS	TBUT	TBUU	TBUV	TBUW	TBUX	TBUY	TBVA
2008	42 861	9 292	12 905	20 664	31 101	23 257	290 342	242 033	8 094
2009	40 314	10 881	10 313	19 119	31 742	21 805	285 896	242 599	6 596

Facilities granted

	TCAR	TCAS	TCAT	TCAU	TCAV	TCAW	TCAX	TCAY	TCBA
2008	84 998	12 741	33 528	38 730	37 840	51 623	373 289	292 979	11 608
2009	73 645	14 217	25 525	33 903	38 110	46 966	359 753	288 737	9 776

of which in sterling

	TCCR	TCCS	TCCT	TCCU	TCCV	TCCW	TCCX	TCCY	TCDA
2008	61 914	11 488	18 283	32 143	34 908	32 810	340 935	279 854	9 136
2009	56 681	13 066	15 402	28 213	35 707	30 663	332 399	276 677	7 811

	Real estate, renting, computer and other business activities					Recreational, personal & community service activities		Financial intermediation (excl. insurance & pension funds)	
Computer & related activities	Legal, accountancy, consultancy & other business activities	Public administration & defence	Education	Health & social work	Recreational, cultural & sporting activities	Personal & community services activities	Total	Financial leasing corporations	

Amounts outstanding (sterling & other currencies)

Loans & advances (including under repo & sterling commercial paper)

	TBPB	TBPC	TBPD	TBPE	TBPF	TBPH	TBPG	TBPI	TBPJ
2006	4 431	36 299	17 227	7 498	15 854	12 255	5 594	491 121	41 068
2007	..	..	..	..	..	..	..	–	..

Acceptances

	TBRB	TBRC	TBRD	TBRE	TBRF	TBRH	TBRG	TBRI	TBRJ
2006	–	12	–	–	–	–	5	90	–
2007	..	..	..	..	..	..	..	–	..

Total

	TBTB	TBTC	TBTD	TBTE	TBTF	TBTH	TBTG	TBTI	TBTJ
2008	5 405	46 103	31 792	10 544	21 475	14 473	6 801	832 114	46 520
2009	4 767	..	13 270	11 522	22 084	13 630	6 686	700 908	39 408

of which in sterling

	TBVB	TBVC	TBVD	TBVE	TBVF	TBVH	TBVG	TBVI	TBVJ
2008	2 814	37 401	31 282	10 357	20 987	12 951	6 010	489 665	35 863
2009	3 137	33 564	12 140	11 371	21 684	12 409	6 100	415 759	28 855

Facilities granted

	TCBB	TCBC	TCBD	TCBE	TCBF	TCBH	TCBG	TCBI	TCBJ
2008	7 648	61 054	35 091	13 882	24 490	19 697	8 966	918 210	50 171
2009	6 896	54 345	16 182	14 913	25 324	17 886	8 784	796 179	42 778

of which in sterling

	TCDB	TCDC	TCDD	TCDE	TCDF	TCDH	TCDG	TCDI	TCDJ
2008	3 862	48 083	33 733	13 441	23 620	16 188	7 686	515 363	39 213
2009	4 192	43 719	14 892	14 663	24 618	15 201	7 757	437 238	31 604

23.4 Industrial analysis of bank lending to UK residents[1]
continued — Not seasonally adjusted

£ million

Financial intermediation (excl. insurance & pension funds)

	Non-bank credit grantors, excl. credit unions	Credit unions	Factoring corporations	Mortgage & housing credit corporations	Investment & unit trusts excl. money market mutual funds	Money market mutual funds	Bank holding companies	Securities dealers (f)	Other financial intermediaries
Amounts outstanding (sterling & other currencies)									
Loans & advances (including under repo & sterling commercial paper)									
	TBPK	TBPL	TBPM	TBPN	TBPO	TBPP	TBPQ	TBPR	TBPS
2005	17 833	28	4 633	62 869	20 394	1 377	19 707	165 421	93 916
2006	21 496	60	5 593	84 959	20 131	674	17 969	183 551	115 620
Acceptances									
	TBRK	TBRL	TBRM	TBRN	TBRO	TBRP	TBRQ	TBRR	TBRS
2005	15	5	–	–	–	–	–	–	27
2006	15	5	–	–	–	–	–	–	69
Total									
	TBTK	TBTL	TBTM	TBTN	TBTO	TBTP	TBTQ	TBTR	TBTS
2008	25 159	83	7 072	193 203	11 584	394	53 455	199 874	294 771
2009	24 438	67	6 514	83 584	8 836	121	37 790	188 606	311 544
of which in sterling									
	TBVK	TBVL	TBVM	TBVN	TBVO	TBVP	TBVQ	TBVR	TBVS
2008	21 910	82	5 742	163 752	6 701	29	38 478	33 073	184 036
2009	21 977	66	5 797	81 133	5 152	29	33 072	33 834	205 844
Facilities granted									
	TCBK	TCBL	TCBM	TCBN	TCBO	TCBP	TCBQ	TCBR	TCBS
2008	27 131	95	7 367	198 340	43 856	481	56 078	206 022	328 669
2009	26 402	76	6 982	88 134	47 897	159	44 707	199 054	339 991
of which in sterling									
	TCDK	TCDL	TCDM	TCDN	TCDO	TCDP	TCDQ	TCDR	TCDS
2008	23 269	94	5 965	167 258	12 820	29	39 368	33 582	193 764
2009	23 444	75	6 054	85 168	8 746	29	33 942	34 484	213 691

	Activities auxiliary to financial intermediation			Individuals & individual trusts		
	Insurance companies & pension funds	Fund management activities	Other	Total	Lending secured on dwellings inc. bridging finance	Other loans & advances
Amounts outstanding (sterling & other currencies)						
Loans & advances (including under repo & sterling commercial paper)						
	TBPT	TBPU	TBPV	TBPW	TBPX	TBPY
2008	..	..	..	897 468	756 624	140 844
2009	..	..	..	1 008 611	876 113	132 497
Acceptances						
	TBRT	TBRU	TBRV			
2006	1	–	–			
2007	..	–	..			
Total						
	TBTT	TBTU	TBTV	TBTW	TBTX	TBTY
2008	30 682	34 605	178 901	897 468	756 624	140 844
2009	22 445	43 538	155 966	1 008 611	876 113	132 497
of which in sterling						
	TBVT	TBVU	TBVV	TBVW	TBVX	TBVY
2008	25 679	14 089	97 580	894 864	..	139 287
2009	18 928	10 506	101 712	1 006 567	..	131 205
Facilities granted						
	TCBT	TCBU	TCBV	TCBW	TCBX	TCBY
2008	57 298	44 463	182 114	1 014 567	813 460	201 107
2009	55 549	53 140	159 861	1 113 807	924 223	189 584
of which in sterling						
	TCDT	TCDU	TCDV	TCDW	TCDX	TCDY
2008	30 798	15 184	99 292	1 011 551	812 385	199 166
2009	23 539	11 314	103 082	1 111 460	923 471	187 990

1 See chapter text.

Source: Bank of England: 020 7601 3236

23.5 Industrial analysis of bank deposits from UK residents[1]

£ million

	Total from UK residents	Agriculture, hunting and forestry	Fishing	Mining & quarrying	Manufacturing			
					Total	Food, beverages & tobacco	Textiles & leather	Pulp, paper, publishing & printing

Amounts outstanding (sterling & other currencies)

Deposit liabilities (including under repos)

	TDAA	TDAB	TDAC	TDAD	TDAE	TDAF	TDAG	TDAH
2008	2 249 663	5 265	175	10 586	38 884	3 595	1 121	3 738
2009	2 314 921	5 076	202	7 483	44 808	3 207	1 283	4 192

of which in sterling

	TDCA	TDCB	TDCC	TDCD	TDCE	TDCF	TDCG	TDCH
2008	1 848 495	5 024	162	2 868	28 101	2 370	850	3 030
2009	1 968 754	4 815	193	2 185	31 545	2 593	1 026	3 505

	Manufacturing					Electricity, gas and water supply		
	Chemicals, man-made fibres, rubber & plastics	Non-metallic mineral products & metals	Machinery, equipment & transport equipment	Electrical, medical & optical equipment	Other manufacturing	Electricity, gas & heated water	Cold water purification & supply	Construction

Amounts outstanding (sterling & other currencies)

Deposit liabilities (including under repos)

	TDAI	TDAJ	TDAK	TDAL	TDAM	TDAN	TDAO	TDAP
2008	6 314	4 559	9 349	6 131	4 077	5 447	3 030	18 236
2009	8 280	5 442	11 735	6 373	4 295	5 104	2 966	18 671

of which in sterling

	TDCI	TDCJ	TDCK	TDCL	TDCM	TDCN	TDCO	TDCP
2008	4 188	3 782	6 542	3 830	3 511	4 380	2 999	17 725
2009	3 659	4 310	8 914	4 143	3 394	3 769	2 913	18 263

	Wholesale and retail trade				Hotels and restaurants	Transport, storage & communication	Real estate, renting, computer and other business activities		
	Total	Sale & repair of motor vehicles & fuel	Other wholesale trade	Other retail trade & repair			Total	Development, buying, selling, renting of real estate	Renting of machinery & equipment

Amounts outstanding (sterling & other currencies)

Deposit liabilities (including under repos)

	TDAQ	TDAR	TDAS	TDAT	TDAU	TDAV	TDAW	TDAX	TDAY
2008	30 494	4 063	13 462	12 969	4 380	19 347	121 623	33 600	1 750
2009	32 867	4 192	14 282	14 393	4 652	17 788	128 596	35 714	1 912

of which in sterling

	TDCQ	TDCR	TDCS	TDCT	TDCU	TDCV	TDCW	TDCX	TDCY
2008	25 856	3 561	10 288	12 006	4 198	15 075	109 549	32 623	1 564
2009	28 259	3 864	10 952	13 443	4 578	14 088	111 148	34 944	1 608

23.5 Industrial analysis of bank deposits from UK residents[1]
continued

£ million

	Real estate, renting, computer and other business activities					Recreational, personal & community service activities		Financial intermediation (excl. insurance & pension funds)	
	Computer & related activities	Legal, accountancy, consultancy & other business activities	Public administration & defence	Education	Health & social work	Recreational, cultural & sporting activities	Personal & community services activities	Total	Financial leasing corporations

Amounts outstanding (sterling & other currencies)

Deposit liabilities (including under repos)

	TDAZ	TDBA	TDBB	TDBC	TDBD	TDBF	TDBE	TDBG	TDBH
2008	9 547	76 727	54 071	10 285	14 525	16 353	15 918	647 181	7 356
2009	9 862	81 107	57 099	11 199	15 287	17 562	16 488	703 175	4 979

of which in sterling

	TDCZ	TDDA	TDDB	TDDC	TDDD	TDDF	TDDE	TDDG	TDDH
2008	7 856	67 506	50 794	9 914	13 154	15 234	15 358	422 201	6 304
2009	8 332	66 264	53 445	10 731	14 443	16 332	15 699	511 014	3 994

Financial intermediation (excl. insurance & pension funds)

	Non-bank credit grantors, excl. credit unions	Credit unions	Factoring corporations	Mortgage & housing credit corporations	Investment & unit trusts excl. money market mutual funds	Money market mutual funds	Bank holding companies	Securities dealers	Other financial intermediaries

Amounts outstanding (sterling & other currencies)

Deposit liabilities (including under repos)

	TDBI	TDBJ	TDBK	TDBL	TDBM	TDBN	TDBO	TDBP	TDBQ
2008	6 248	443	829	108 501	37 969	376	65 164	143 714	276 582
2009	8 606	514	841	115 982	34 200	498	67 516	131 651	338 387

of which in sterling

	TDDI	TDDJ	TDDK	TDDL	TDDM	TDDN	TDDO	TDDP	TDDQ
2008	3 900	443	678	106 490	23 260	233	45 368	36 246	199 278
2009	6 864	514	756	114 225	25 659	303	48 376	40 126	270 198

Insurance companies & pension funds	Activities auxiliary to financial intermediation		Individuals & individual trusts
	Placed by fund managers	Other	

Amounts outstanding (sterling & other currencies)

Deposit liabilities (including under repos)

	TDBR	TDBS	TDBT	TDBU
2008	65 978	111 869	154 853	901 162
2009	57 738	88 046	157 179	922 934

of which in sterling

	TDDR	TDDS	TDDT	TDDU
2008	55 637	52 161	101 373	896 732
2009	48 984	42 945	114 721	918 685

1 See chapter text.

Source: Bank of England: 020 7601 3236

Banking, insurance

23.6 Public sector net cash requirement and other counterparts to changes in money stock during the year

Not seasonally adjusted

£ million

		1999	2000	2001	2002	2003	2004	2005	2006	2007	2008	2009
Public sector net cash requirement (surplus)	ABEN	−3 205	−36 864	−2 019	18 010	37 160	41 915	41 278	33 916	31 089	125 369	205 186
Sales of public sector debt to M4 private sector	IDH8	−1 448	13 639	7 716	−9 258	−32 438	−32 007	−11 257	−20 082	−16 293	..	..
M4 lending[1]	AVBS	78 029	111 202	82 574	107 553	127 820	156 084	158 087	218 445	238 491	270 535	136 626
External and foreign currency finance of the public sector	VQDC	6 199	3 616	3 875	2 486	−13 441	−2 395	−30 708	−33 554	−38 366	−36 146	−21 179
Other external and foreign currency flows[2]	AVBW	−44 902	7 178	−21 631	−25 132	−27 124	4 288	33 643	−874	−37 241	148 653	−159 956
Net non-deposit liabilities (increase)	AVBX	−2 943	−31 050	−10 791	−25 130	−20 377	−67 401	−39 903	−29 964	−4 451	−172 812	−49 636
Money stock (M4)	AUZI	33 329	67 198	58 994	68 834	73 271	100 014	150 869	167 024	188 522	258 700	134 380

1 Bank and building society lending, plus holdings of commercial bills by the Issue Department of the Bank of England.
2 Including sterling lending to non-residents sector.

Source: Bank of England: 020 7601 5468

23.7 Money stock and liquidity

£ million

		1999	2000	2001	2002	2003	2004	2005	2006	2007	2008	2009
Amounts outstanding at end-year												
Notes and coin in circulation with the M4 private sector[1]	VQKT	26 269	28 174	30 450	31 889	34 010	36 410	38 508	40 539	43 001	46 173	47 952
UK private sector sterling non-interest bearing sight deposits[2]	AUYA	42 130	45 867	50 548	45 594	51 274	50 845	55 208	54 800	62 051	72 664	124 126
Money stock (M2)[3]	VQXV	558 334	597 523	649 980	703 920	777 347	845 654	922 687	996 645	1 071 416	1 123 753	1 184 765
Money stock M4	AUYM	816 601	884 873	942 594	1 008 750	1 081 299	1 179 192	1 328 321	1 498 936	1 674 847	1 937 137	2 048 927
Changes during the year[4]												
Notes and coin in circulation with the M4 private sector[1]	VQLU	2 582	1 957	2 284	1 493	2 189	2 461	2 156	2 053	2 536	3 136	4 185
UK private sector sterling non-interest bearing sight deposits[2]	AUZA	5 354	3 533	4 914	−6 761	5 321	−227	5 699	−409	9 292	587	35 522
Money stock (M2)[3]	AUZE	41 992	39 123	52 813	53 698	72 255	68 901	78 428	72 764	65 042	48 558	..
Money stock M4	AUZI	33 329	67 198	58 994	68 834	73 271	100 014	150 869	167 024	188 522	258 700	134 380

1 The estimates of levels of coin in circulation include allowance for wastage, hoarding, etc.
2 Non-interest bearing deposits are confined to those with institutions included in the United Kingdom banks sector (See Table 23.3).
3 M2 comprises the UK non-monetary financial institutions and non-public sector, i.e. M4 private sector's holdings of notes and coin together with its sterling denominated retail deposits with UK monetary financial institutions.
4 As far as possible the changes exclude the effect of changes in the number of contributors to the series, and also of the introduction of new statistical returns. Changes are not seasonally adjusted.

Source: Bank of England: 020 7601 5468

23.8 Selected retail banks' base rate[1]
Operative between dates shown

Percentage rates

Date of change	New rate	Date of change	New rate	Date of change	New rate
1986 Jan 9	12.50	Oct 5	15.00		
Mar 19	11.50			1999 Jan 7	6.00
Apr 8	11.00-11.50	1990 Oct 8	14.00	Feb 4	5.50
Apr 9	11.00			Apr 8	5.25
Apr 21	10.50	1991 Feb 13	13.50	Jun 10	5.00
May 23	10.00-10.50	Feb 27	13.00	Sep 8	5.00-5.25
May 27	10.00	Mar 22	12.50	Sep 10	5.25
Oct 14	10.00-11.00	Apr 12	12.00	Nov 4	5.50
Oct 15	11.00	May 24	11.50		
		Jul 12	11.00	2000 Jan 13	5.75
1987 Mar 10	10.50	Sep 4	10.50	Feb 10	6.00
Mar 18	10.00-10.50				
Mar 19	10.00	1992 May 5	10.00	2001 Feb 8	5.75
Apr 28	9.50-10.00	Sep 16[2]	12.00	Apr 5	5.50
Apr 29	9.50	Sep 17[2]	10.00-12.00	May 10	5.25
May 11	9.00	Sep 18	10.00	Aug 2	5.00
Aug 6	9.00-10.00	Sep 22	9.00	Sep 18	4.75
Aug 7	10.00	Oct 16	8.00-9.00	Oct 4	4.50
Oct 23	9.50-10.00	Oct 19	8.00	Nov 8	4.00
Oct 29	9.50	Nov 13	7.00		
Nov 4	9.00-9.50			2003 Feb 6	3.75
Nov 5	9.00	1993 Jan 26	6.00	Jul 10	3.50
Dec 4	8.50	Nov 23	5.50	Nov 6	3.75
1988 Feb 2	9.00	1994 Feb 8	5.25	2004 Feb 5	4.00
Mar 17	8.50-9.00	Sep 12	5.75	May 6	4.25
Mar 18	8.50	Dec 7	6.25	Jun 10	4.50
Apr 11	8.00			Aug 5	4.75
May 17	7.50-8.00	1995 Feb 2[2]	6.25-6.75		
May 18	7.50	Feb 3	6.75	2005 Aug 4	4.50
Jun 2	7.50-8.00	Dec 13	6.50		
Jun 3	8.00			2006 Aug 3	4.75
Jun 6	8.00-8.50	1996 Jan 18	6.25	Nov 9	5.00
Jun 7	8.50	Mar 8	6.00		
Jun 22	8.50-9.00	Jun 6	5.75	2007 Jan 11	5.25
Jun 23	9.00	Oct 30	5.75-6.00	May 10	5.50
Jun 28	9.00-9.50	Oct 31	6.00	Jul 5	5.75
Jun 29	9.50			Dec 6	5.50
Jul 4	9.50-10.00	1997 May 6	6.25		
Jul 5	10.00	Jun 6	6.25-6.50	2008 Feb 7	5.25
Jul 18	10.00-10.50	Jun 9	6.50	Apr 10	5.00
Jul 19	10.50	Jul 10	6.75	Oct 8	4.50
Aug 8	10.50-11.00	Aug 7	7.00	Nov 6	3.00
Aug 9	11.00	Nov 6	7.25	Dec 4	2.00
Aug 25	11.00-12.00				
Aug 26	12.00	1998 Jun 4	7.50	2009 Jan 8	1.50
Nov 25	13.00	Oct 8	7.25	Feb 5	1.00
		Nov 5	6.75	Mar 5	0.50
1989 May 24	14.00	Dec 10	6.25		

1 Data obtained from Barclays Bank, Lloyds/TSB Bank, HSBC Bank and
National Westminster Bank whose rates are used to compile this series.
2 Where all the rates did not change on the same day a spread is shown.

Source: Bank of England: 020 7601 4444

23.9 Average three month sterling money market rates[1]

Percentage rates

	1998	1999	2000	2001	2002	2003	2004	2005	2006	2007	2008	2009
Treasury bills:[2] KDMM												
January	6.80	5.28	5.72	5.49	3.83	3.80	3.92	4.66	4.39	5.30	5.12	0.90
February	6.88	5.04	5.83	5.46	3.87	3.50	4.01	4.69	4.38	5.34	5.02	0.72
March	6.95	4.92	5.86	5.23	3.97	3.47	4.13	4.77	4.40	5.33	4.88	0.60
April	7.00	4.90	5.92	5.12	3.97	3.45	4.20	4.70	4.42	5.43	4.83	0.63
May	7.01	4.93	5.95	4.98	3.95	3.44	4.40	4.66	4.50	5.55	4.95	0.53
June	7.29	4.76	5.85	4.99	3.98	3.47	4.61	4.62	4.54	5.67	5.11	0.50
July	7.22	4.76	5.83	5.01	3.84	3.31	4.67	4.46	4.53	5.77	5.08	0.44
August	7.19	4.85	5.81	4.72	3.77	3.40	4.71	4.41	4.75	5.79	4.95	0.40
September	6.94	5.12	5.78	4.43	3.79	3.52	4.69	4.40	4.84	5.69	4.74	0.38
October	6.54	5.23	5.75	4.16	3.75	3.65	4.68	4.40	4.94	5.61	3.68	0.43
November	6.31	5.20	5.68	3.78	3.80	3.81	4.66	4.42	5.01	5.50	1.99	0.47
December	5.72	5.46	5.62	3.83	3.84	3.83	4.68	4.43	5.08	5.30	1.29	0.36
Eligible bill: KDMY[3]												
January	7.28	5.63	5.90	5.64	3.91	3.87	3.94	4.75	..	..	..	..
February	7.24	5.28	6.01	5.56	3.92	3.65	4.06	4.78	..	..	..	..
March	7.25	5.11	5.98	5.37	3.99	3.54	4.19	4.88	..	..	..	..
April	7.24	5.02	6.05	5.21	4.04	3.52	4.28	4.84	..	..	..	..
May	7.20	5.08	6.09	5.06	4.01	3.52	4.42	4.80	..	..	..	..
June	7.42	4.94	6.03	5.08	4.04	3.45	4.68	4.76	..	..	..	..
July	7.49	4.89	5.97	5.07	3.94	3.39	4.75	4.57	..	..	..	..
August	7.40	4.94	5.97	4.82	3.86	3.42	4.85	4.51	..	..	..	..
September	7.20	5.16	5.95	4.57	3.86	3.59	4.83	..	..	..	..	..
October	6.91	5.42	5.92	4.26	3.82	3.69	4.79	..	..	..	..	..
November	6.52	5.43	5.88	3.85	3.84	3.88	4.78	..	..	..	..	..
December	6.05	5.59	5.78	3.88	3.71	3.90	4.77	..	..	..	..	..
Interbank rate: AMIJ												
January	7.48	5.80	6.06	5.76	3.98	3.91	3.99	4.80	4.54	5.45	5.61	2.28
February	7.46	5.43	6.15	5.69	3.98	3.69	4.10	4.82	4.52	5.52	5.61	2.08
March	7.48	5.30	6.15	5.47	4.06	3.58	4.23	4.92	4.53	5.50	5.86	1.83
April	7.44	5.23	6.21	5.33	4.11	3.58	4.33	4.88	4.57	5.61	5.90	1.48
May	7.41	5.25	6.23	5.17	4.08	3.57	4.46	4.83	4.65	5.72	5.79	1.30
June	7.63	5.12	6.14	5.19	4.11	3.57	4.73	4.78	4.69	5.83	5.90	1.21
July	7.71	5.07	6.11	5.19	3.99	3.42	4.79	4.59	4.68	5.98	5.80	1.03
August	7.66	5.18	6.14	4.93	3.92	3.45	4.89	4.53	4.90	6.34	5.76	0.80
September	7.38	5.32	6.12	4.65	3.93	3.63	4.87	4.54	4.98	6.58	5.87	0.62
October	7.14	5.94	6.08	4.36	3.90	3.73	4.83	4.53	5.09	6.21	6.18	0.56
November	6.89	5.78	6.00	3.93	3.91	3.91	4.82	4.56	5.18	6.36	4.40	0.60
December	6.38	5.97	5.89	3.99	3.95	3.95	4.81	4.59	5.25	6.35	3.21	0.61
Certificate of deposits: KOSA												
January	7.44	5.74	6.02	5.73	3.96	3.90	3.98	4.80	4.54	5.45	5.61	2.29
February	7.42	5.38	6.10	5.66	3.96	3.68	4.09	4.82	4.52	5.51	5.60	2.06
March	7.43	5.26	6.09	5.44	4.04	3.57	4.22	4.91	4.53	5.52	5.85	1.79
April	7.40	5.19	6.17	5.30	4.08	3.57	4.32	4.86	4.57	5.69	5.89	1.43
May	7.37	5.22	6.19	5.15	4.06	3.56	4.45	4.82	4.65	5.84	5.79	1.27
June	7.59	5.09	6.10	5.16	4.09	3.56	4.72	4.78	4.69	5.94	5.89	1.14
July	7.66	5.03	6.08	5.17	3.97	3.41	4.79	4.60	4.68	6.11	5.80	0.92
August	7.61	5.14	6.09	4.90	3.90	3.44	4.89	4.53	4.89	6.35	5.75	0.69
September	7.34	5.28	6.08	4.62	3.91	3.62	4.87	4.54	4.98	6.54	5.86	0.51
October	7.09	5.86	6.05	4.33	3.88	3.72	4.83	4.52	5.09	6.21	6.16	0.50
November	6.82	5.72	5.98	3.91	3.89	3.90	4.81	4.56	5.18	6.34	4.40	0.58
December	6.32	5.89	5.85	3.96	3.93	3.94	4.80	4.58	5.24	6.35	3.21	0.58
Local authority deposits: KDPX[4]												
January	7.43	5.76	6.03	5.73	3.85	3.87	3.91	..	..	..	..	..
February	7.40	5.38	6.09	5.62	3.88	3.61	4.08	..	..	..	..	..
March	7.40	5.27	6.08	5.39	4.01	3.55	4.12	..	..	..	..	..
April	7.38	5.17	6.12	5.26	4.05	3.54	4.31	..	..	..	..	..
May	7.34	5.19	6.14	5.13	4.06	3.54	4.45	..	..	..	..	..
June	7.56	5.07	6.09	5.10	4.05	3.57	4.75	..	..	..	..	..
July	7.64	5.01	6.04	5.12	3.95	3.39	4.82	..	..	..	..	..
August	7.55	5.11	6.06	4.86	3.87	3.43	4.92	..	..	..	..	..
September	7.35	5.19	6.05	4.58	3.88	3.61	4.90	..	..	..	..	..
October	7.08	5.83	6.03	4.29	3.86	3.71	4.85	..	..	..	..	..
November	6.85	5.64	5.96	3.82	3.87	3.90	4.84	..	..	..	..	..
December	6.35	5.88	5.80	3.87	3.93	3.92	4.82	..	..	..	..	..

1 A full definition of these series is given in Section 7 of the ONS Financial Statistics Explanatory Handbook.
2 Average rate of discount at weekly (Friday) tender.
3 This series discontinued at end of August 2005.
4 This series discontinued at end of December 2004.

Source: Bank of England: 020 7601 4444

23.10 Average foreign exchange rates[1]

	1998	1999	2000	2001	2002	2003	2004	2005	2006	2007	2008	2009
Sterling exchange rate index (1990 = 100)[2] AGBG												
January	104.7	99.6	108.5	104.4	106.9	104.0	102.4	102.1	102.7	..	..	..
February	104.7	100.8	108.4	104.1	107.4	102.4	104.8	103.3	102.8	..	..	..
March	106.8	102.8	108.4	105.0	106.5	100.6	105.0	103.2	102.1	..	..	..
April	107.1	103.4	110.1	105.8	107.1	99.8	105.2	104.4	101.9	..	..	..
May	103.4	104.2	108.5	106.6	105.3	97.9	104.6	103.6	104.1	..	..	..
June	105.4	104.7	104.6	106.8	103.6	99.6	105.8	104.9		..	..	..
July	105.3	103.5	105.6	107.2	105.3	99.4	105.9	102.1		..	..	..
August	104.6	103.3	107.4	105.1	105.4	99.0	105.2	102.8		..	..	..
September	103.3	104.7	106.2	106.1	106.5	99.2	103.3	103.9		..	..	..
October	100.7	105.4	109.2	105.8	106.7	99.8	102.2	103.1		..	..	..
November	100.6	105.7	107.3	106.1	105.9	100.4	101.7	103.2		..	..	..
December	100.4	106.7	106.4	106.5	105.5	100.3	103.2	103.3		..	..	..
Effective Sterling exchange rate index (Jan 2005 = 100) BK67												
January	100.4	96.3	102.9	98.5	100.6	99.9	100.2	100.0	99.1	105.4	96.5	76.7
February	100.1	97.1	102.5	98.1	100.8	98.5	102.5	101.0	98.9	104.9	96.0	78.6
March	101.8	98.8	102.3	98.8	100.1	96.8	102.2	101.1	98.4	103.4	94.5	76.6
April	102.1	98.8	103.7	99.4	100.9	96.1	102.2	102.0	98.4	104.1	92.7	78.6
May	98.9	99.6	101.7	99.8	99.5	94.9	101.8	101.0	101.2	103.8	92.7	80.2
June	100.9	99.6	98.7	99.6	98.2	96.6	103.1	101.8	100.9	104.4	92.8	83.7
July	100.8	98.4	99.4	100.2	100.4	96.1	103.2	98.8	100.9	105.1	92.9	83.2
August	100.3	98.7	100.6	98.8	100.3	95.5	102.4	99.7	102.9	104.4	91.4	83.4
September	99.6	99.8	99.1	99.9	101.4	95.8	100.7	100.7	102.9	103.2	89.6	80.9
October	97.4	100.7	101.7	99.7	101.7	96.9	99.8	99.7	103.1	102.7	89.1	79.1
November	97.2	100.6	100.1	99.8	101.1	97.5	99.7	99.4	103.4	101.7	83.2	80.7
December	97.2	101.3	99.8	100.4	100.8	97.9	101.3	99.5	104.4	99.8	77.9	80.1
Sterling/US Dollar AUSS												
January	1.6	1.7	1.6	1.5	1.4	1.6	1.8	1.9	1.8	2.0	2.0	1.4
February	1.6	1.6	1.6	1.5	1.4	1.6	1.9	1.9	1.7	2.0	2.0	1.4
March	1.7	1.6	1.6	1.4	1.4	1.6	1.8	1.9	1.7	1.9	2.0	1.4
April	1.7	1.6	1.6	1.4	1.4	1.6	1.8	1.9	1.8	2.0	2.0	1.5
May	1.6	1.6	1.5	1.4	1.5	1.6	1.8	1.9	1.9	2.0	2.0	1.5
June	1.7	1.6	1.5	1.4	1.5	1.7	1.8	1.8	1.8	2.0	2.0	1.6
July	1.6	1.6	1.5	1.4	1.6	1.6	1.8	1.8	1.8	2.0	2.0	1.6
August	1.6	1.6	1.5	1.4	1.5	1.6	1.8	1.8	1.9	2.0	1.9	1.7
September	1.7	1.6	1.4	1.5	1.6	1.6	1.8	1.8	1.9	2.0	1.8	1.6
October	1.7	1.7	1.5	1.5	1.6	1.7	1.8	1.8	1.9	2.0	1.7	1.6
November	1.7	1.6	1.4	1.4	1.6	1.7	1.9	1.7	1.9	2.1	1.5	1.7
December	1.7	1.6	1.5	1.4	1.6	1.8	1.9	1.7	2.0	2.0	1.5	1.6
Sterling/Euro THAP												
January	1.5	1.4	1.6	1.6	1.6	1.5	1.4	1.4	1.5	1.5	1.3	1.1
February	1.5	1.5	1.6	1.6	1.6	1.5	1.5	1.4	1.5	1.5	1.3	1.1
March	1.6	1.5	1.6	1.6	1.6	1.5	1.5	1.4	1.5	1.5	1.3	1.1
April	1.5	1.5	1.7	1.6	1.6	1.5	1.5	1.5	1.4	1.5	1.3	1.1
May	1.5	1.5	1.7	1.6	1.6	1.4	1.5	1.5	1.5	1.5	1.3	1.1
June	1.5	1.5	1.6	1.6	1.6	1.4	1.5	1.5	1.5	1.5	1.3	1.2
July	1.5	1.5	1.6	1.6	1.6	1.4	1.5	1.5	1.5	1.5	1.3	1.2
August	1.5	1.5	1.6	1.6	1.6	1.4	1.5	1.5	1.5	1.5	1.3	1.2
September	1.5	1.5	1.6	1.6	1.6	1.4	1.5	1.5	1.5	1.5	1.3	1.1
October	1.4	1.5	1.7	1.6	1.6	1.4	1.4	1.5	1.5	1.5	1.3	1.1
November	1.4	1.6	1.7	1.6	1.6	1.4	1.4	1.5	1.5	1.4	1.2	1.1
December	1.4	1.6	1.6	1.6	1.6	1.4	1.4	1.5	1.5	1.4	1.1	1.1

1 Working day average. A full definition of these series is given in Section 7 of the ONS Explanatory Handbook.
2 Series discontinued from 31 May 2006.

Source: Bank of England: 020 7601 4444

23.11 Average zero coupon yields[1]

Percentage rates

	1998	1999	2000	2001	2002	2003	2004	2005	2006	2007	2008	2009
Nominal Five Year Yield ZBRG												
January	6.18	4.30	6.28	5.07	4.90	4.15	4.61	4.43	4.11	5.06	4.31	2.79
February	6.10	4.46	6.13	5.04	4.94	3.85	4.63	4.53	4.17	5.08	4.33	2.66
March	6.09	4.69	5.89	4.86	5.22	3.93	4.56	4.73	4.33	5.00	4.04	2.41
April	5.93	4.66	5.80	4.96	5.21	4.09	4.80	4.54	4.48	5.20	4.27	2.59
May	5.95	4.95	5.82	5.14	5.22	3.85	5.01	4.31	4.67	5.32	4.64	2.69
June	6.04	5.28	5.61	5.25	5.05	3.72	5.15	4.17	4.69	5.59	5.17	2.91
July	6.12	5.49	5.58	5.26	4.88	3.98	5.07	4.16	4.69	5.55	4.93	3.08
August	5.80	5.75	5.65	5.03	4.54	4.36	4.96	4.23	4.74	5.25	4.56	2.91
September	5.32	6.00	5.65	4.90	4.31	4.46	4.83	4.12	4.67	5.02	4.37	2.74
October	4.94	6.25	5.46	4.74	4.36	4.73	4.65	4.26	4.76	4.95	4.12	2.64
November	4.92	5.86	5.33	4.55	4.38	4.91	4.58	4.29	4.73	4.64	3.53	2.79
December	4.51	5.90	5.14	4.88	4.34	4.71	4.43	4.21	4.80	4.57	3.02	2.81
Nominal Ten Year Yield ZBRH												
January	5.96	4.24	5.62	4.75	4.85	4.39	4.76	4.50	4.02	4.76	4.46	3.77
February	5.91	4.39	5.44	4.90	4.90	4.22	4.78	4.54	4.10	4.79	4.61	3.80
March	5.85	4.60	5.18	4.64	5.18	4.34	4.67	4.74	4.26	4.72	4.45	3.33
April	5.69	4.53	5.14	4.90	5.19	4.48	4.92	4.58	4.46	4.94	4.64	3.49
May	5.73	4.83	5.23	5.05	5.22	4.23	5.06	4.38	4.58	5.03	4.84	3.73
June	5.60	5.07	5.05	5.11	5.05	4.13	5.13	4.25	4.60	5.31	5.14	3.82
July	5.65	5.24	5.09	5.10	4.95	4.43	5.04	4.28	4.59	5.29	4.99	3.91
August	5.41	5.25	5.18	4.88	4.68	4.59	4.95	4.29	4.58	5.05	4.69	3.81
September	5.03	5.51	5.25	4.91	4.47	4.68	4.86	4.17	4.47	4.91	4.54	3.76
October	4.93	5.68	5.09	4.77	4.60	4.88	4.72	4.31	4.53	4.88	4.60	3.67
November	4.83	5.11	4.98	4.58	4.62	5.03	4.65	4.26	4.45	4.67	4.33	3.87
December	4.44	5.19	4.80	4.83	4.55	4.87	4.49	4.17	4.53	4.65	3.68	4.02
Nominal Twenty Year Yield ZBRI												
January	5.94	4.36	4.45	4.33	4.72	4.45	4.70	4.43	3.84	4.33	4.40	4.48
February	5.88	4.44	4.38	4.42	4.73	4.39	4.73	4.44	3.90	4.38	4.57	4.56
March	5.78	4.60	4.25	4.44	4.99	4.56	4.63	4.66	4.05	4.36	4.53	4.23
April	5.61	4.53	4.35	4.74	5.02	4.68	4.81	4.53	4.26	4.56	4.70	4.50
May	5.67	4.75	4.40	4.85	5.08	4.49	4.91	4.37	4.31	4.63	4.78	4.63
June	5.42	4.77	4.37	4.98	4.94	4.46	4.89	4.27	4.36	4.86	4.88	4.72
July	5.45	4.67	4.38	4.89	4.82	4.71	4.82	4.31	4.34	4.81	4.83	4.67
August	5.30	4.53	4.49	4.69	4.58	4.69	4.70	4.31	4.29	4.62	4.68	4.37
September	4.91	4.62	4.63	4.88	4.39	4.75	4.65	4.19	4.17	4.59	4.64	4.20
October	4.87	4.56	4.61	4.75	4.55	4.82	4.59	4.28	4.18	4.60	4.78	4.20
November	4.73	4.07	4.39	4.47	4.60	4.88	4.50	4.18	4.11	4.49	4.83	4.37
December	4.47	4.20	4.30	4.64	4.57	4.76	4.40	4.06	4.19	4.50	4.29	4.48
Real Ten Year Yield ZBRJ												
January	3.10	2.00	2.10	2.22	2.52	2.00	1.94	1.75	1.29	1.78	1.30	1.53
February	3.06	1.91	2.17	2.27	2.50	1.74	1.96	1.77	1.32	1.80	1.33	1.25
March	3.00	1.85	2.05	2.33	2.53	1.79	1.81	1.87	1.41	1.70	1.02	1.19
April	2.91	1.70	2.08	2.56	2.43	1.96	1.93	1.76	1.54	1.91	1.20	1.08
May	2.92	1.91	2.14	2.58	2.43	1.81	2.05	1.70	1.63	2.05	1.36	1.09
June	2.85	1.89	2.12	2.54	2.33	1.67	2.10	1.65	1.68	2.21	1.36	1.08
July	2.77	1.90	2.14	2.56	2.42	1.85	2.07	1.65	1.65	2.19	1.29	1.23
August	2.65	2.19	2.25	2.42	2.33	1.95	2.03	1.61	1.55	1.97	1.17	1.16
September	2.59	2.31	2.28	2.51	2.20	2.05	1.97	1.51	1.49	1.79	1.25	1.06
October	2.67	2.26	2.33	2.53	2.36	2.15	1.89	1.57	1.57	1.75	2.06	0.70
November	2.40	2.05	2.34	2.39	2.33	2.21	1.88	1.54	1.47	1.48	2.58	0.77
December	2.11	1.98	2.23	2.58	2.24	2.03	1.76	1.47	1.56	1.50	2.19	0.80
Real Twenty Year Yield ZBRK												
January	3.06	2.07	2.01	1.88	2.26	2.07	1.96	1.59	0.97	1.23	0.92	1.05
February	3.05	1.99	1.95	1.88	2.30	1.98	1.90	1.59	0.99	1.25	1.03	1.19
March	2.98	1.93	1.78	1.99	2.32	2.07	1.77	1.72	1.10	1.19	0.88	1.19
April	2.85	1.81	1.84	2.25	2.25	2.12	1.85	1.64	1.28	1.36	1.02	1.14
May	2.83	1.99	1.91	2.32	2.25	2.03	1.88	1.57	1.33	1.46	1.00	1.05
June	2.63	1.97	1.87	2.27	2.17	1.97	1.88	1.53	1.39	1.54	0.84	1.01
July	2.58	2.00	1.90	2.24	2.24	2.16	1.87	1.54	1.31	1.52	0.83	1.00
August	2.53	2.14	1.96	2.16	2.15	2.14	1.82	1.49	1.21	1.31	0.67	0.87
September	2.49	2.26	1.96	2.31	2.06	2.18	1.80	1.40	1.12	1.24	0.80	0.89
October	2.59	2.22	1.99	2.32	2.22	2.22	1.76	1.40	1.13	1.25	1.33	0.74
November	2.36	1.92	1.94	2.12	2.25	2.21	1.71	1.29	1.03	1.09	1.37	0.71
December	2.14	1.87	1.87	2.24	2.21	2.08	1.60	1.20	1.11	1.08	1.24	0.77

1 Working day average. Calculated using the Variable Roughness Penalty (VRP) model.

Source: Bank of England: 020 7601 4444

23.12 Average rates on representative British Government Stocks[1]

Percentage rates

	1998	1999	2000	2001	2002	2003	2004	2005	2006	2007	2008	2009
5 Year Conventional Rate[2] KORP												
January	6.33	4.25	6.36	5.17	4.94	4.15	4.59	4.43	4.27	..	..	..
February	6.24	4.41	6.23	5.13	4.96	3.88	4.46	4.61	4.31	..	..	..
March	6.26	4.65	6.01	4.94	5.23	3.93	4.44	4.77	4.41	..	..	..
April	6.11	4.66	5.95	4.97	5.26	4.08	4.66	4.58	4.44	..	..	..
May	6.14	4.93	5.97	5.15	5.48	3.83	4.89	4.36	4.44	..	..	..
June	6.31	5.27	5.78	5.32	5.10	3.68	5.08	4.24	4.66	..	..	..
July	6.14	5.49	5.75	5.34	4.92	3.72	4.98	4.11	4.62	..	..	..
August	5.84	5.80	5.81	5.09	4.57	4.30	4.88	4.22	4.84	..	..	..
September	5.34	6.04	5.81	4.94	4.25	4.42	4.76	4.18	4.91	..	..	..
October	4.88	6.24	5.66	4.78	4.38	4.70	4.57	4.23	5.00	..	..	..
November	4.86	5.89	5.50	4.59	4.40	4.88	4.52	4.31	4.39	..	..	..
December	4.45	5.91	5.27	4.88	4.34	4.68	4.42	4.27	–	..	..	..
10 year Conventional Rate KORQ												
January	6.07	4.16	5.75	4.86	4.84	4.37	4.78	4.51	4.19	5.21	4.33	1.65
February	6.02	4.32	5.56	4.88	4.91	4.25	4.75	4.60	4.25	5.25	4.28	1.53
March	5.97	4.54	5.29	4.75	5.15	4.51	4.65	4.79	4.39	5.15	4.00	1.33
April	5.81	4.48	5.25	4.95	5.23	4.64	4.91	4.60	4.47	5.34	4.28	1.51
May	5.85	4.77	5.35	5.13	5.51	4.26	5.07	4.38	4.39	5.39	4.75	1.32
June	5.77	5.02	5.15	5.09	5.06	4.38	5.19	4.23	4.74	5.74	5.15	1.53
July	5.67	5.20	5.18	5.16	4.94	4.23	5.10	4.20	4.73	5.70	5.00	1.48
August	5.56	5.24	5.27	4.92	4.66	4.59	4.99	4.25	4.78	5.39	4.63	1.31
September	5.10	5.52	5.32	4.92	4.46	4.69	4.89	4.16	4.74	5.13	4.23	1.12
October	4.93	5.70	5.15	4.76	4.57	4.89	4.73	4.31	4.85	5.07	3.76	1.06
November	4.87	5.16	5.06	4.58	4.59	5.04	4.66	4.33	4.84	4.70	2.86	1.00
December	4.49	5.24	4.88	4.88	4.52	4.94	4.50	4.27	4.93	4.60	2.26	0.93
20 Year Conventional Rate KORR												
January	6.04	4.36	4.91	4.52	4.81	4.46	4.73	4.55	4.05	4.77	4.54	3.72
February	5.98	4.47	4.80	4.58	4.83	4.37	4.80	4.58	4.13	4.80	4.68	3.85
March	5.90	4.64	4.64	4.56	5.12	4.51	4.69	4.79	4.28	4.73	4.54	3.48
April	5.73	4.58	4.71	4.84	5.14	4.64	4.91	4.63	4.38	4.95	4.77	3.48
May	5.79	4.83	4.77	4.98	5.45	4.44	5.03	4.43	4.59	5.08	4.95	3.63
June	5.59	4.92	4.68	5.10	5.03	4.38	5.07	4.30	4.60	5.32	5.22	3.79
July	5.63	4.88	4.70	5.05	4.92	4.59	4.99	4.33	4.60	5.28	5.09	3.77
August	5.43	4.82	4.79	4.83	4.65	4.67	4.88	4.34	4.58	5.04	4.62	3.76
September	5.02	4.97	4.90	4.94	4.46	4.74	4.83	4.24	4.49	4.89	4.67	3.79
October	4.92	4.97	4.84	4.80	4.59	4.85	4.73	4.37	4.53	4.92	4.65	3.68
November	4.79	4.46	4.64	4.55	4.65	4.93	4.64	4.31	4.48	4.73	4.33	3.83
December	4.49	4.56	4.51	4.75	4.61	4.80	4.53	4.22	4.41	4.71	3.70	3.95
10 Year Index-Linked Rate KORS												
January	3.01	2.00	2.11	2.21	2.61	2.07	1.88	1.73	1.48	2.24	1.60	1.77
February	2.94	1.94	2.16	2.30	2.53	1.81	1.90	1.81	1.54	2.27	1.29	1.18
March	2.89	1.90	2.06	2.34	2.55	1.88	1.76	1.99	1.65	2.18	0.76	0.83
April	2.80	1.74	2.08	2.55	2.45	1.90	1.94	1.83	1.65	2.61	1.12	0.79
May	2.83	1.96	2.15	2.61	2.58	1.74	2.10	1.71	1.96	2.59	1.48	0.47
June	2.81	1.93	2.13	2.56	2.35	1.59	2.17	1.67	1.94	2.73	1.77	0.53
July	2.67	1.93	2.14	2.57	2.46	1.67	2.12	1.66	1.92	2.68	1.61	0.13
August	2.55	2.20	2.25	2.45	2.37	1.89	2.04	1.63	1.80	2.37	1.64	0.01
September	2.59	2.32	2.29	2.56	2.24	1.99	1.95	1.49	1.76	2.01	1.69	–
October	2.66	2.26	2.33	2.55	2.42	2.08	1.83	1.89	1.89	1.99	2.38	–
November	2.39	2.03	2.32	2.42	2.39	2.16	1.85	1.64	1.87	1.70	3.44	−0.72
December	2.11	1.99	2.20	2.65	2.30	1.97	1.74	1.27	1.96	1.80	3.59	−1.26
20 Year Index-Linked rate KORT												
January	3.01	2.06	2.01	1.96	2.35	2.10	1.95	1.68	1.17	1.63	1.25	1.57
February	3.01	1.97	1.98	1.99	2.36	1.99	1.94	1.72	1.22	1.65	1.30	1.33
March	2.92	1.93	1.83	2.09	2.39	2.07	1.80	1.89	1.34	1.57	1.04	1.27
April	2.80	1.81	1.90	2.35	2.32	2.10	1.91	1.77	1.38	1.77	1.24	1.18
May	2.79	1.99	1.97	2.41	2.43	2.00	1.99	1.67	1.56	1.91	1.38	1.20
June	2.61	1.97	1.94	2.38	2.23	1.93	2.01	1.63	1.61	2.07	1.34	1.78
July	2.56	1.97	1.96	2.36	2.30	2.05	1.99	1.63	1.55	2.07	1.27	1.26
August	2.51	2.12	2.03	2.25	2.21	2.09	1.93	1.58	1.45	1.83	1.14	1.23
September	2.51	2.23	2.04	2.39	2.12	2.13	1.89	1.48	1.37	1.67	1.26	1.10
October	2.58	2.18	2.08	2.38	2.29	2.17	1.84	1.51	1.44	1.65	1.99	0.74
November	2.35	1.91	2.02	2.19	2.31	2.16	1.80	1.45	1.34	1.41	2.47	0.82
December	2.12	1.88	1.94	2.33	2.26	2.04	1.69	1.38	1.43	1.41	2.14	0.87

1 Working day average.
2 Discontinued from 6 December 2006.

Source: Bank of England: 020 7601 4444

23.13 Building societies[1,2]
United Kingdom

		1999[3]	2000[4]	2001	2002	2003	2004	2005	2006	2007	2008[5]
Number and balance sheets											
Societies on register (numbers)	KRNA	72	68	65	65	63	63	63	60	59	59
Share investors (thousands)	KRNB	21 774	22 237	20 311	20 724	20 901	20 734	22 090	22 396	23 038	..
Depositors (thousands)	KRNC	642	660	501	440	452	446	370	391	387	..
Borrowers (thousands)	KRND	2 868	2 925	2 579	2 520	2 520	2 570	2 617	2 626	2 642	..
Assets and liabilities (£ million)											
Liabilities:											
Shares	KRNE	109 137.7	119 298.5	119 815.2	132 372.9	142 477.1	153 844.0	171 935.0	188 943.0	206 782.5	224 424.0
Deposits and wholesale	KRNF	34 746.6	44 262.4	37 358.9	37 933.0	49 552.6	64 025.2	70 845.1	75 443.0	92 097.6	100 633.2
Taxation and other	KRNG	1 665.4	1 664.0	1 244.9	1 088.4	1 179.0	1 394.9	2 619.4	6 838.5	10 703.3	9 583.3
General reserves	KRNH	8 301.5	8 987.1	8 511.2	9 043.4	9 489.8	10 123.9	10 677.4	10 845.3	12 080.3	11 620.7
Other Capital	KRNI	1 529.2	1 861.0	1 416.1	1 709.2	2 534.7	3 599.1	4 566.5	5 510.9	6 073.8	..
Assets:											
Mortgages	KRNK	123 183.4	137 072.3	130 229.6	140 839.7	159 938.2	184 191.0	207 621.4	231 198.9	265 338.1	269 313.4
Investments and cash	KHVZ	29 917.8	36 574.2	35 925.9	38 952.7	43 067.9	46 234.1	49 240.3	52 349.4	57 843.5	72 477.7
Other	KRNN	2 279.2	2 426.6	2 190.7	2 354.4	2 226.9	2 562.0	3 781.7	4 032.3	4 555.9	8 100.4
Total	KRNJ	155 380.4	176 073.0	168 346.2	182 146.8	205 233.1	232 987.1	260 643.3	287 580.6	327 737.5	349 891.5
Current transactions (£ million)											
Mortgage advances	KRNU	23 997.9	28 233.6	29 320.0	33 077.0	43 392.4	51 089.0	50 059.4	52 327.5	61 678.8	47 215.6
Management expenses	KRNX	1 573.8	1 640.7	1 528.0	1 623.6	1 746.4	1 844.2	1 939.9	2 116.2	2 241.5	2 255.1

1 See chapter text.

2 The figures for each year relate to accounting years ending on dates between 1 February of that year and 31 January of the following year.

3 The societies which have converted to the banking sector, namely Cheltenham & Gloucester (August 1995), National & Provincial (August 1996), Alliance & Leicester (April 1997), Halifax (June 1997), Woolwich (July 1997), Bristol & West (July 1997), Northern Rock (October 1997), and Birmingham Midshires (April 1999) have been included in flow figures (using flows up to the date of conversion), but have been excluded from the end of year balances.

4 Bradford & Bingley, which converted to the banking sector in December 2000, is included within flow figures and the end of year balances.

5 2008 Reporting requirement changes - data is now sourced from QFS1 rather than AFS1. Mortgages Advances taken from MLAR (Mortgage Lenders and Administrators return)

Source: Financial Services Authority: 020 7066 1000

23.14 Consumer credit
United Kingdom

£ million

		2000	2001	2002	2003	2004	2005	2006	2007	2008	2009
Total amount outstanding	VZRD	135 168	150 802	169 209	180 649	198 856	211 038	212 835	221 687	233 164	226 827
Total net lending	VZQC	15 965	19 673	23 443	22 401	25 337	19 666	13 054	13 471	10 866	−713
of which											
Credit cards	VZQS	6 686	6 229	7 579	8 710	9 998	6 166	1 951	2 251	4 092	2 326
Other	VZQT	9 280	13 445	15 867	13 692	15 340	13 499	11 102	11 221	6 774	−3 039
Banks	AIKN	13 217	16 055	17 452	15 269	19 370	11 317	9 346	6 075	3 529	−1 622
Building societies' class 3 loans	ALPY	112	63	180	177	172	238	217	260	132	7
Other consumer credit lenders	BM59	2 640	3 554	5 811	6 954	5 796	8 112	3 489	7 135	7 205	901
Total gross lending	VZQG	160 744	177 452	196 451	207 255	221 318	217 467	207 460	204 632	193 149	170 513

As from Dec 2006 the Bank of England has ceased to update the separate data on consumer credit provided by other specialist lenders, retailers and insurance companies previously contained in these tables. These categories have been merged into 'other consumer credit lenders'.

Source: Office for National Statistics: 01633 456635

23.15 End-year assets and liabilities of investment trust companies, unit trusts[1] and property unit trusts[2]
United Kingdom

£ million

		1999	2000	2001	2002	2003	2004	2005	2006	2007	2008
Investment trust companies											
Short-term assets and liabilities (net):	CBPL	71	423	161	–	73	866	921	–155	1 194	1 351
Cash and UK bank deposits	AHAG	1 227	2 202	2 513	1 821	1 346	1 756	1 483	1 785	1 731	2 017
Other short-term assets	CBPN	1 097	1 082	656	805	1 189	1 344	1 549	353	1 572	1 380
Short-term liabilities	-CBPS	–2 253	–2 861	–3 008	–2 626	–2 462	–2 234	–2 111	–2 293	–2 109	–2 046
Medium and long-term liabilities and capital:	-CBPO	–57 616	–60 412	–54 630	–38 054	–48 076	–48 627	–55 076	–51 426	–57 508	–41 270
Issued share and loan capital	-CBPQ	–8 565	–8 934	–8 796	–8 711	–9 873	–8 210	–7 155	–5 492	–5 659	–3 834
Foreign currency borrowing	-CBPR	–880	–994	–933	–780	–682	–607	–839	–1 043	–1 118	–1 407
Other borrowing	-CBQA	–1 716	–2 503	–3 251	–2 246	–2 181	–1 728	–1 420	–1 447	–1 377	–1 245
Reserves and provisions, etc	-AHBC	–46 455	–47 981	–41 650	–26 317	–35 340	–38 082	–38 082	–43 444	–49 354	–34 784
Investments:	CBPM	56 491	59 948	54 822	37 748	48 035	47 212	53 265	50 052	55 608	39 079
British government securities	AHBF	1 217	821	645	471	303	466	769	533	715	628
UK company securities:											
Loan capital and preference shares	CBGZ	1 425	1 654	1 516	946	1 079	1 270	673	1 071	1 259	813
Ordinary and deferred shares	CBGY	28 010	33 456	30 338	19 475	23 292	23 941	25 037	22 870	23 034	14 366
Overseas company securities:											
Loan capital and preference shares	CBHA	979	963	1 143	458	603	682	937	741	1 038	623
Ordinary and deferred shares	AHCC	23 330	21 355	19 476	14 453	20 294	18 967	23 065	21 659	25 795	18 385
Other investments	CBPT	1 530	1 699	1 704	1 945	2 464	1 886	2 784	3 178	3 767	4 264
Unit trusts											
Short-term assets and liabilities:	CBPU	5 894	8 340	7 979	8 041	10 256	10 229	13 944	18 023	22 247	26 526
Cash and UK bank deposits	AGYE	4 797	6 969	5 748	5 321	5 243	6 302	7 740	12 336	16 443	16 257
Other short-term assets	CBPW	1 545	2 319	2 763	3 072	5 990	4 390	7 420	6 990	9 036	15 699
Short-term liabilities	-CBPX	–448	–948	–532	–352	–977	–463	–1 216	–1 303	–3 232	–5 430
Foreign currency borrowing	-AGYK	–	–	–	–	–	–	–	–	–	–
Investments:	CBPZ	213 553	222 844	204 899	210 002	245 516	269 064	351 645	420 153	457 729	388 282
British government securities	CBHT	3 627	4 693	4 690	7 077	9 125	9 768	25 181	31 603	32 120	33 466
UK company securities:											
Loan capital and preference shares	CBHU	13 322	14 654	16 318	21 152	23 972	22 467	29 293	29 876	30 626	30 174
Ordinary and deferred shares	RLIB	119 496	116 808	103 704	82 851	116 407	130 230	157 149	185 637	195 009	143 550
Overseas company securities:											
Loan capital and preference shares	CBHV	3 032	3 212	4 113	5 916	9 840	13 142	16 057	25 617	30 029	30 442
Ordinary and deferred shares	RLIC	70 256	79 601	71 329	63 152	75 074	81 034	105 443	127 409	142 211	113 667
Other assets	CBQE	3 820	3 876	4 800	9 997	11 098	12 801	18 522	20 011	27 734	36 983
Property unit trusts											
Short-term assets and liabilities (net)	AGVC	205	285	247	242	459	466	686	1 258	785	592
Property	CBQG	2 722	3 488	2 078	4 026	5 125	5 909	9 623	12 781	12 480	8 518
Other assets	AGVL	436	380	151	677	373	1 366	1 864	2 713	1 648	1 040
Long-term borrowing	-AGVM	–75	–391	–90	–75	–76	–63	–250	–90	–158	–177

Note: Assets are shown as positive: liabilities as negative.
1 Including open ended investment companies (OEICs).
2 Investments are at market value.

Source: Office for National Statistics: 01633 456635

23.16 Self-administered pension funds: market value of assets
United Kingdom
End year

£ million

		1996	1997	1998	1999	2000	2001	2002	2003	2004	2005	2006	2007	2008
Total pension funds[1]														
Total net assets	AHVA	543 879	656 874	699 191	812 228	765 199	711 572	610 441	692 694	761 066	914 955	1 010 794	1 023 979	864 606
Short-term assets	RYIQ	31 521	35 368	39 005	32 703	36 638	31 337	30 700	46 091	57 476	73 649	98 691	99 681	96 546
British government securities	AHVK	57 783	80 533	91 084	98 882	92 458	83 754	84 461	88 803	87 579	94 325	104 910	113 617	98 577
UK local authority long-term debt	AHVO	89	156	183	133	177	125	42	8	4	4	2	5	–
Overseas government securities	AHVT	11 800	13 079	15 493	16 684	19 206	20 383	16 031	16 340	15 075	19 037	21 776	22 434	21 527
UK company securities														
Ordinary shares	AHVP	276 001	339 687	334 648	357 230	299 318	260 696	186 437	186 426	180 561	199 199	208 473	152 048	110 571
Other	AHVQ	6 180	5 618	8 168	9 258	16 978	22 301	30 450	37 082	43 027	48 065	54 902	57 541	56 516
Overseas company securities														
Ordinary shares	AHVR	84 163	104 187	108 884	148 335	135 514	127 893	104 392	125 740	140 282	183 060	192 978	169 598	127 525
Other	AHVS	4 909	3 851	3 842	5 099	12 736	11 781	11 386	12 475	15 996	20 502	31 536	45 470	48 222
UK loans and mortgages	RLDQ	83	160	22	14	7	3	–	35	44	6	6	12	–
UK land, property and ground rent	AHWA	21 637	24 176	24 355	31 107	32 945	30 617	31 658	30 619	30 552	31 613	34 394	30 304	22 816
Authorised unit trust units	AHVU	21 767	21 979	30 596	33 731	34 587	38 083	36 530	62 029	67 482	86 660	94 638	134 176	102 685
Property unit trusts	AHVW	2 666	3 219	3 211	5 498	4 835	5 280	5 869	6 761	10 444	16 687	20 689	16 757	11 504
Other assets	RKPL	30 628	32 978	47 136	82 273	90 841	90 139	82 490	107 229	152 170	197 468	224 907	251 028	231 234
Total liabilities	GQFX	5 347	8 118	7 436	8 719	11 041	10 819	10 005	26 944	39 626	55 320	77 108	68 692	63 117

1 These figures cover funded schemes only and therefore exclude the main superannuation arrangements in the central government sector.

Source: Office for National Statistics: 01633 456635

23.17 Insurance companies: balance sheet market values
United Kingdom
End year

£ million

		1999	2000	2001	2002	2003	2004	2005	2006	2007	2008
Long-term insurance companies											
Assets											
Total current assets (gross)	RYEW	56 360	62 937	63 855	58 122	58 518	63 407	72 754	77 748	101 780	97 943
Agents' and reinsurance balances (net)	AHNY	508	384	..	6 373	4 720	..	..	..	984	−7 820
Other debtors[1]	RKPN	18 613	21 045	..	34 391	35 414	..	..	..	60 063	46 598
British government securities	AHNJ	126 223	116 734	119 513	131 305	142 920	157 019	161 906	161 641	158 694	166 879
UK local authority securities etc	AHNN	1 456	1 170	1 407	1 427	1 547	2 044	1 840	1 614	998	776
UK company securities[2]	RKPO	539 834	557 293	..	443 535	468 910	..	..	..	664 717	525 780
Overseas company securities	RKPP	120 665	107 439	..	110 738	110 193	..	..	..	234 388	219 957
Overseas government securities	AHNS	18 494	18 004	21 285	19 762	20 561	20 161	16 065	21 078	25 787	29 053
Loans and mortgages	RKPQ	10 914	9 687	..	10 994	12 107	..	..	..	13 655	21 926
UK land, property and ground rent	AHNX	50 387	49 705	53 726	52 658	57 174	60 502	61 037	58 918	66 169	46 484
Overseas land, property and ground rent	RGCP	206	1 975	498	158	184	94	27	61	–	
Other investments	RKPR	8 334	8 385	..	9 513	17 985	..	..	..	31 401	18 713
Total	RFXN	951 994	954 760	938 609	878 979	930 233	994 015	1 143 934	1 259 956	1 358 636	1 166 289
Net value of direct investment in:											
Non-insurance subsidiaries and associate companies in the United Kingdom	RYET	3 045	6 133	4 486	4 577	4 191	3 971	8 390	13 016	9 186	11 484
UK associate and subsidiary insurance companies and insurance holding companies	RYEU	2 245	3 586	4 206	4 569	5 054	3 473	2 528	6 114	7 578	7 890
Overseas subsidiaries and associates	RYEV	3 638	4 002	5 581	5 463	6 330	2 181	4 455	3 341	3 832	5 011
Total assets	RKBI	960 922	968 481	952 882	893 588	945 808	1 003 640	1 159 307	1 282 427	1 379 232	1 190 674
Liabilities											
Borrowing:											
Borrowing from UK banks	RGDF	6 064	8 272	8 790	4 958	4 164	5 358	5 037	2 862	3 795	5 083
Other UK borrowing	RGDE	3 070	2 823	5 350	7 406	10 923	8 385	9 036	9 542	6 705	4 838
Borrowing from overseas	RGDD	159	38	81	800	530	793	1 151	1 965	1 926	2 546
Long-term business:											
Funds	RKDC	800 184	838 485	831 051	794 177	824 766	873 071	1 037 658	1 125 221	1 205 183	1 069 993
Claims admitted but not paid	RKBM	2 032	2 249	2 547	3 234	3 699	3 579	3 481	3 513	3 848	3 426
Provision for taxation net of amounts receivable:											
UK authorities	RYPI	6 344	5 381	3 951	2 803	4 055	4 881	8 225	7 908	7 457	54
Overseas authorities	RYPJ	314	67	45	−20	2	−13	−2	199	5	−3
Provision for recommended dividends	RYPK	201	183	87	32	27	93	22	13	27	9
Other creditors and liabilities	RYPL	17 042	19 031	18 468	23 261	15 870	16 738	16 907	33 192	39 527	52 849
Excess of assets over above liabilities:											
Excess of value of assets over liabilities in respect of long-term funds	RKBR	116 951	79 173	63 337	36 517	62 546	65 641	59 132	71 017	75 066	16 131
Minority interests in UK subsidiary companies	RKTI	25	–	–	–	1	267	–	–	192	–
Shareholders' capital and reserves in respect of general business	RKBS	6 139	10 287	17 044	18 629	15 698	20 719	18 717	27 315	35 855	28 443
Other reserves including profit and loss account balances	RKBT	2 396	2 492	2 130	1 791	3 527	4 129	−57	−320	−354	7 305
Total liabilities	RKBI	960 922	968 481	952 882	893 588	945 808	1 003 640	1 159 307	1 282 427	1 379 232	1 190 674

23.17

Insurance companies: balance sheet market values
United Kingdom

continued   End year

£ million

		1998	1999	2000	2001	2002	2003	2004	2005	2006	2007	2008
Other than long-term insurance companies												
Assets												
Total current assets (gross)	RYME	8 524	10 468	8 772	12 264	17 671	20 036	29 258	26 561	24 942	25 810	27 563
Agents' and reinsurance balances (net)	AHMX	10 528	12 177	8 362	..	9 492	9 890	..	..	..	9 932	10 706
Other debtors[1]	RKPS	6 277	7 059	7 179	..	14 437	13 255	..	..	..	20 351	18 297
British government securities	AHMJ	16 409	15 938	14 561	15 064	18 390	19 645	19 662	19 818	19 296	16 026	18 441
UK local authority securities etc	AHMN	14	10	8	6	10	10	49	44	–	3	–
UK company securities[2]	RKPT	18 440	18 800	18 585	..	15 362	15 153	..	..	..	23 812	24 204
Overseas company securities	RKPU	8 676	6 284	8 190	..	7 394	7 124	..	..	..	14 773	20 258
Overseas government securities	AHMS	10 459	7 980	6 849	7 134	7 156	5 720	6 662	7 341	8 035	4 869	8 505
Loans and mortgages	RKPV	1 335	1 070	1 429	..	1 063	1 400	..	..	..	3 684	3 971
UK land, property and ground rent	AHMW	1 146	1 085	1 069	860	805	859	893	1 470	1 569	1 870	1 950
Overseas land, property and ground rent	RYNK	107	83	45	4	1	4	5	13	137	116	87
Other investments	RKPW	2 366	2 638	2 294	..	2 182	1 408	..	..	..	1 882	2 562
Total	RKAL	84 281	84 027	77 343	78 789	93 965	94 504	115 356	116 200	128 590	123 128	136 544
Net value of direct investment in:												
Non-insurance subsidiaries and associate companies in the United Kingdom	RYNR	5 553	7 074	7 038	10 456	11 706	13 408	19 028	20 530	20 111	21 954	21 259
UK associate and subsidiary insurance companies and insurance holding companies	RYNS	6 424	5 617	5 400	8 837	7 190	2 918	2 280	6 071	4 745	6 936	7 669
Overseas subsidiaries and associates	RYNT	14 239	17 775	15 993	14 260	9 014	5 718	5 507	6 446	9 657	9 445	10 815
Total assets	RKBY	110 497	114 493	105 774	112 342	121 875	116 548	142 171	149 247	163 103	161 463	176 287
Liabilities												
Borrowing:												
Borrowing from UK banks	RYMB	1 825	1 392	783	481	1 384	2 046	4 519	893	3 148	675	343
Other UK borrowing	RYMC	1 551	3 186	4 239	10 621	10 472	9 342	10 261	11 080	10 445	10 885	13 179
Borrowing from overseas	RYMD	1 600	3 045	1 867	1 964	2 916	2 918	2 476	2 817	5 459	7 037	6 692
General business technical reserves	RKCT	60 775	59 455	60 236	60 995	62 776	63 463	67 241	71 710	77 221	71 146	76 980
Long-term business:												
Funds	RKTF	–	–	–	–	▪	–	–	–	–	–	–
Claims admitted but not paid	RKTK	–	–	–	–	–	–	–	–	–	–	–
Provision for taxation net of amounts receivable:												
UK authorities	RYPO	1 197	939	874	594	941	834	1 094	1 796	2 376	2 259	809
Overseas authorities	RYPP	11	11	11	7	5	84	24	5	10	5	1
Provision for recommended dividends	RYPQ	1 318	1 817	2 682	1 957	958	1 082	1 311	5	270	222	48
Other creditors and liabilities	RYPR	3 793	4 981	6 293	6 410	8 025	9 567	10 817	10 718	16 226	22 069	21 149
Excess of assets over above liabilities:												
Excess of value of assets over liabilities in respect of long-term funds	RKCG	–	–	–	–	–	–	–	–	–	–	–
Minority interests In UK subsidiary companies	RKCH	68	29	33	276	4	6	6	–	–	599	1 902
Shareholders' capital and reserves in respect of general business	RKCI	34 397	35 372	24 699	26 190	31 982	25 153	39 695	43 264	42 186	38 145	47 225
Other reserves including profit and loss account balances	RKCJ	4 215	4 265	4 056	2 847	2 411	2 053	4 727	6 959	5 762	8 421	7 959
Total liabilities	RKBY	110 497	114 493	105 774	112 342	121 875	116 548	142 171	149 247	163 103	161 463	176 287

1 Including outstanding interest, dividends and rents (net).
2 Including authorised unit trust units.

Source: Office for National Statistics: 01633 456626

23.18 Individual insolvencies
United Kingdom

Numbers

		1999	2000	2001	2002	2003	2004	2005	2006	2007	2008	2009[7]
England and Wales												
Bankruptcies[1]	AIHW	21 611	21 550	23 477	24 292	28 021	35 898	47 291	62 956	64 480	67 428	74 670
Individual voluntary arrangements[2,3]	AIHI	7 195	7 978	6 298	6 295	7 583	10 752	20 293	44 332	42 165	39 116	47 641
Total	AIHK	28 806	29 528	29 775	30 587	35 604	46 651	67 584	107 288	106 645	106 544	134 142
Scotland												
Sequestrations[4]	KRHA	3 195	2 965	3 048	3 215	3 328	3 297	4 965	5 430	6 219	12 370	14 356
Protected Trust Deeds	GJ2I	2 144	2 801	3 779	5 174	5 452	6 024	6 881	8 208	7 595	7 542	9 126
Total	GJ2J	5 339	5 766	6 827	8 389	8 780	9 321	11 846	13 638	13 814	19 912	23 482
Northern Ireland												
Bankruptcies[5]	KRHB	401	349	292	334	517	666	821	1 035	898	1 079	1 237
Individual voluntary arrangements[3,6]	KJRK	172	267	176	207	318	449	633	774	440	559	722
Total	KRHD	573	616	468	541	835	1 115	1 454	1 809	1 338	1 638	1 959

1 Comprises receiving and administration orders under the Bankruptcy Act 1914 and bankruptcy orders under the Insolvency Act 1986. Orders later consolidated or rescinded are included in these figures.
2 Introduced under the Insolvency Act 1986.
3 For statistical purposes deeds of arrangement are now included with individual voluntary arrangements.
4 Sequestrations awarded but not brought into operation are included in these figures.

5 Comprises bankruptcy adjudication orders, arrangement protection orders and orders for the administration of estates of deceased insolvents. Orders later set aside or dismissed are included in these figures.
6 Introduced under the Insolvency Northern Ireland order 1989.
7 Provisional

Source: Insolvency Service: 020 7637 6504/6443

23.19 Company insolvencies
United Kingdom

Numbers

		1999	2000	2001	2002	2003	2004	2005	2006	2007	2008	2009[2]
England and Wales												
Compulsory liquidations	AIHR	5 209	4 925	4 675	6 231	5 234	4 584	5 233	5 418	5 165	5 494	5 643
Creditors' voluntary liquidations	AIHS	9 071	9 392	10 297	10 075	8 950	7 608	7 660	7 719	7 342	10 041	13 434
Total	AIHQ	14 280	14 317	14 972	16 306	14 184	12 192	12 893	13 137	12 507	15 535	19 077
Scotland												
Compulsory liquidations	KRGA	364	344	378	556	436	431	420	416	439	437	432
Creditors' voluntary liquidations	KRGB	208	239	224	232	195	190	149	133	100	87	152
Total	KRGC	572	583	602	788	631	621	569	549	539	524	584
Northern Ireland[1]												
Compulsory liquidations	KRGD	..	..	..	49	95	76	85	78	122	158	164
Creditors' voluntary liquidations	KRGE	..	..	..	53	47	45	53	50	42	51	83
Total	KRGF	..	..	..	102	142	121	138	128	164	209	247

1 Prior to 2002, the quality of the statistics on company liquidations in Northern Ireland are not robust enough and have been removed from this table.
2 Provisional.

Source: Insolvency Service: 020 7637 6504/6443

23.20 Selected financial statistics[1]

£ million

	Building societies		Unit trusts[3]	Net equity of households in life assurance and pension funds' reserves
	Advances[2]			
	Not seasonally adjusted	Seasonally adjusted		
Amount outstanding as at 31 Dec	AHIF		AGXB	
2009	..		480 601	
Transactions	AAMN	AHHU	AGXE	NBYD
2006	27 057	27 147	20 678	59 318
2007	24 975	24 861	3 870	65 070
2008	..	..	−2 151	19 930
2009	..	..	29 548	..
2008 Q4	..	..	88	−5 687
2009 Q1	..	..	5 627	1 027
Q2	..	..	7 741	12 164
Q3	..	..	8 892	2 301
2008 Dec	..	..	1 940	..
2009 Jan	..	..	1 928	..
Feb	..	..	2 325	..
Mar	..	..	1 374	..
Apr	..	..	1 883	..
May	..	..	3 863	..
Jun	..	..	1 995	..
Jul	..	..	2 448	..
Aug	..	..	2 693	..
Sep	..	..	3 751	..
Oct	..	..	1 964	..
Nov	..	..	2 800	..

	Banks[4]				Consumer credit[5]		of which Credit cards[5]	
	UK private sector deposits		Lending to the private sector					
	Sterling (Not seasonally adjusted)	Other currencies	Sterling (Not seasonally adjusted)	Other currencies	Not seasonally adjusted	Seasonally adjusted	Not seasonally adjusted	Seasonally adjusted
Amount outstanding as at 31 Dec	AEAS	AGAK	AECE	AECK	VZRD	VZRI	VZRE	VZRJ
2009	1 800 588	438 366	2 188 537	525 005	226 827	226 765	55 631	54 585
Transactions					Net lending	Net lending	Net lending	Net lending
	AEAT	AEAZ	AECF		VZQC	RLMH	VZQS	VZQX
2006	150 070	58 434	191 019		13 054	13 288	1 951	2 081
2007	162 298	71 345	213 349		13 471	13 012	2 251	2 031
2008	219 067	−37 030	234 087		10 866	11 218	4 092	4 229
2009	143 201	3 141	150 157		−713	−699	2 326	2 288
2009 Q2	−5 425	41 817	13 825		1 552	499	943	559
Q3	35 628	−12 883	45 929		−1 275	−736	520	422
Q4	42 701	−9 921	34 042		−313	−241	1 667	669
2010 Q1	..	..	..		531	1 278	−928	768
2009 Apr	−6 967	45 101	−13 240		746	222	453	250
May	3 342	−1 887	25 212		289	203	65	149
Jun	−1 800	−1 397	1 853		517	74	425	160
Jul	14 522	−10 302	11 606		−930	−272	−102	108
Aug	−2 654	11 281	3 330		−901	−305	424	200
Sep	23 760	−13 862	30 993		556	−159	197	115
Oct	55 414	−3 633	41 536		−784	−354	−115	176
Nov	2 608	10 092	−6 133		179	−212	771	262
Dec	−15 321	−16 380	−1 361		292	324	1 010	231
2010 Jan	−750	−3 367	2 963		105	376	−748	207
Feb	−257	17 657	−19 073		103	578	42	371
Mar	..	..	..		323	325	−222	190

1 For further details see *Financial Statistics*, Tables 1.2E, 3.2B, 4.2A, 4.3A, 4.3B, 5.2D, 6.2A, 10.5D.
2 Total administered by the Department for National Savings.
3 Including open ended investment companies (OEICs).
4 Monthly figures relate to calendar months.

5 Data have been revised back to February 2003 due to the inclusion of some additional other specialist lenders and the removal of some non-resident based securitisation vehicles.

Sources: Office for National Statistics;
Department for National Savings;
Building Societies Commission;
Association of Unit Trusts and Investment Funds;
Bank of England;
Department for Business, Enterprise and Regulatory Reform

23.21 Selected interest rates, exchange rates and security prices

	Selected retail banks' base rate	Average discount rate for 91 day Treasury bills	Inter bank 3 months bid rate	Inter bank 3 months offer rate	British government securities 20 years yield[1]	Exchange rate US spot
	ZCMG	AJNB	HSAJ	HSAK	AJLX	LUSS
2006 Feb	4.50	4.39	4.51	4.53	3.96	1.7511
Mar	4.50	4.41	4.54	4.56	4.15	1.7345
Apr	4.50	4.45	4.60	4.63	4.32	1.8179
May	4.50	4.51	4.66	4.68	4.43	1.8712
Jun	4.50	4.54	4.71	4.73	4.46	1.8494
Jul	4.50	4.58	4.73	4.74	4.45	1.8671
Aug	4.75	4.77	4.94	4.95	4.42	1.9018
Sep	4.75	4.87	5.02	5.05	4.29	1.8682
Oct	4.75	4.98	5.14	5.16	4.35	1.9073
Nov	5.00	5.04	5.20	5.22	4.27	1.9670
Dec	5.00	5.11	5.26	5.29	4.33	1.9570
2007 Jan	5.25	5.37	5.54	5.55	4.51	1.9574
Feb	5.25	5.31	5.48	5.50	4.59	1.9600
Mar	5.25	5.38	5.56	5.58	4.52	1.9613
Apr	5.25	5.47	5.66	5.70	4.72	1.9997
May	5.50	5.59	5.76	5.78	..	1.9782
Jun	5.50	5.77	5.93	5.98	..	2.0064
Jul	5.75	5.75	6.00	6.02	..	2.0322
Aug	5.75	5.77	6.55	6.65	4.80	2.0171
Sep	5.75	5.61	6.18	6.28	4.74	2.0374
Oct	5.75	5.57	6.17	6.25	4.74	2.0774
Nov	5.75	5.44	6.53	6.58	4.59	2.0561
Dec	5.50	5.24	5.95	5.95	4.59	1.9909
2008 Jan	5.50	5.01	5.50	5.58	4.46	1.9882
Feb	5.25	4.98	5.68	5.72	4.62	1.9892
Mar	5.25	4.77	5.95	6.02	4.54	1.9875
Apr	5.00	4.90	5.76	5.84	4.73	1.9803
May	5.00	5.04	5.80	5.87	4.85	1.9762
Jun	5.00	5.10	5.88	5.94	5.03	1.9901
Jul	5.00	5.09	5.75	5.79	4.94	1.9810
Aug	5.00	4.94	5.70	5.75	4.74	1.8237
Sep	5.00	4.51	6.15	6.30	4.66	1.7821
Oct	4.50	3.54	5.85	6.00	4.76	1.6158
Nov	3.00	1.68	3.85	4.10	4.69	1.5345
Dec	2.00	1.24	2.75	2.90	4.15	1.4376
2009 Jan	1.50	0.91	2.00	2.25	4.28	1.4416
Feb	..	0.66	1.95	2.15	4.34	1.4255
Mar	..	0.62	1.60	1.70	4.01	1.4331
Apr	..	0.57	1.30	1.45	4.24	1.4820
May	..	0.52	1.15	1.30	4.38	1.6125
Jun	..	0.49	1.15	1.20	4.47	1.6468
Jul	..	0.43	0.90	0.90	4.46	1.6579
Aug	..	0.37	0.70	0.70	4.22	1.6311
Sep	..	0.39	0.55	0.60	4.07	1.5993
Oct	..	0.46	0.50	0.70	4.05	1.6478
Nov	..	0.46	0.50	0.70	4.22	1.6411
Dec	..	0.49	0.55	0.70	4.33	1.6148
2010 Jan	..	0.49	0.50	0.70	4.42	1.6020
Feb	..	0.49	0.50	0.70	4.52	1.5224
Mar	..	0.51	0.50	0.70	4.57	1.5167

1 Average of working days.

Source: Bank of England

23.22 Mergers and acquisitions in the UK by UK companies: category of expenditure

£ million

	Number of companies acquired	Total[1]	Cash Independent companies	Cash Subsidiaries	Issues of ordinary shares[2]	Issues of fixed interest securities[2]
	AIHA	DUCM	DWVW	DWVX	AIHD	AIHE
1999	493	26 163	12 605	3 615	9 592	351
2000	587	106 916	33 906	6 168	65 570	1 272
2001	492	28 994	8 489	6 704	12 356	1 445
2002	430	25 236	9 574	7 991	6 780	891
2003	558	18 679	8 956	7 183	1 667	873
2004	741	31 408	12 080	7 822	10 338	1 168
2005	769	25 134	13 425	8 510	2 768	431
2006	779	28 511	..	8 131	..	335
2007	869	26 778	13 671	6 507	4 909	1 691
2008	558	36 469	31 333	2 851	1 910	375
1999 Q4	104	3 737	2 795	580	250	112
2000 Q1	139	33 739	17 483	1 136	14 960	160
Q2	133	21 469	4 224	1 881	15 045	319
Q3	163	16 852	6 934	2 237	7 367	314
Q4	152	34 856	5 265	914	28 198	479
2001 Q1	131	6 181	2 606	2 255	982	338
Q2	108	4 890	1 679	2 214	555	442
Q3	129	16 079	3 457	1 526	10 649	447
Q4	124	1 844	747	709	170	218
2002 Q1	83	3 853	2 201	1 298	104	250
Q2	120	4 228	801	3 179	78	170
Q3	88	6 333	4 695	1 426	184	28
Q4	139	10 822	1 877	2 088	6 414	443
2003 Q1	107	3 857	1 003	1 892	609	353
Q2	122	3 753	1 437	1 713	258	345
Q3	153	4 700	2 495	1 919	153	133
Q4	176	6 369	4 021	1 659	647	42
2004 Q1	151	12 639	2 819	655	8 807	358
Q2	169	5 359	2 555	1 682	822	300
Q3	211	8 109	3 469	4 026	240	374
Q4	210	5 301	3 237	1 459	469	136
2005 Q1	166	3 516	1 334	1 918	166	98
Q2	215	8 983	4 869	2 715	1 285	114
Q3	211	7 287	4 106	1 878	1 207	96
Q4	177	5 348	3 116	1 999	110	123
2006 Q1	207	6 969	4 069	2 427	431	42
Q2	208	4 222	3 298	527	384	13
Q3	163	11 376	..	4 580	..	216
Q4	201	5 944	4 690	597	593	64
2007 Q1	191	5 649	2 824	276	2 407	142
Q2	212	10 122	3 605	4 361	1 874	282
Q3	258	7 846	5 545	833	358	1 110
Q4	208	3 161	1 697	1 037	270	157
2008 Q1	172	4 545	2 578	913	786	268
Q2	183	9 593	8 845	520	187	41
Q3	104	4 133	3 408	328	341	56
Q4	99	18 198	16 502	1 090	596	10
2009 Q1	87	8 152	281	128	7 699	44
Q2	52	791	239	103	437	12
Q3	49	1 742	1 368	171	..	..

Missing data for any series have been suppressed to avoid the disclosure of information relating to individual enterprises.
1 Includes deferred payments.
2 Issued to the vendor as payment.

Source: Office for National Statistics

Service industry

Chapter 24

Service industry

Annual Business Inquiry

(Tables 24.1, 24.3 and 24.4)

For details of the Annual Business Inquiry, see the text accompanying **Table 22.1**.

Retail trade: index numbers of value and volume

(Table 24.2)

The main purpose of the Retail Sales Inquiry (RSI) is to provide up-to-date information on short period movements in the level of retail sales. In principle, the RSI covers the retail activity of every business classified in the retail sector (Division 52 of the 2003 Standard Industrial Classification (SIC(2003)) in Great Britain. A business will be classified to the retail sector if its main activity is one of the individual 4 digit SIC categories within Division 52. The retail activity of a business is then defined by its retail turnover, that is the sale of all retail goods (note that petrol, for example, is not a retail good).

The RSI is compiled from the information returned to the statutory inquiries into the distribution and services sector. The inquiry is addressed to a stratified sample of 5,000 businesses classified to the retail sector, the stratification being by 'type of store' (the individual 4 digit SIC categories within Division 52) and by size. The sample structure is designed to ensure that the inquiry estimates are as accurate as possible. In terms of the selection, this means that:

- each of the individual 4 digit SIC categories are represented – their coverage depending upon the relative size of the category and the variability of the data

- within each 4 digit SIC category the larger retailers tend to be fully enumerated with decreasing proportions of medium and smaller retailers

The structure of the inquiry is updated periodically by reference to the more comprehensive results of the Annual Business Inquiry (ABI). The monthly inquiry also incorporates a rotation element for the smallest retailers. This helps to spread the burden more fairly, as well as improving the representativeness between successive benchmarks.

During 2003 the RSI was rebased using detailed information from the 2000 ABI. The reference year is currently set at

2005=100 A review of the RSI was published in October 2008. The findings are available at: www.statistics.gov.uk/StatBase/Product.asp?vlnk=13527

The latest summary statistics are published each month by First Release. More disaggregated indices (not seasonally adjusted) are published each month in the Business Monitor SDM28. See: www.statistics.gov.uk/rsi

24.1 Retail businesses[1]
United Kingdom

		2003	2004	2005	2006	2007
Number of businesses	ZABE	202 604	200 606	201 419	200 004	198 644
Total turnover[2]	ZABL	278 373	288 716	295 952	309 668	319 216
Value Added Tax in total turnover	ZABM	28 505	29 420	29 923	31 239	31 888
Retail turnover[2]	ZABN	250 849	258 903	264 427	277 145	285 313
Non-retail turnover[2]	ZABO	27 524	29 812	31 525	32 524	33 903
Other income						
Value of commercial insurance claims received	ZABP	65	40	76	77	65
Subsidies received from UK government sources and the EC	ZAEN	5	10	16	10	12
Employment costs[3]	ZABQ	31 367	32 806	34 729	35 896	37 468
Gross wages and salaries	ZABR	28 294	29 481	30 938	32 080	33 486
Redundancy and severance payments	ZABS	134	158	251	170	150
Employers' National Insurance contributions	ZABT	1 991	2 142	2 282	2 385	2 482
Contributions to pension funds	ZABU	948	1 026	1 258	1 261	1 349
Stocks						
Increase during year	ZABV	978	957	726	1 178	1 753
Value at end of year	ZABW	23 024	23 527	24 211	25 150	25 837
Total turnover[3] divided by end-year stocks (Quotient)	ZABX	10.9	11.0	11.0	11.0	11.0
Purchases of goods, materials and services[3]	ZABY	194 169	199 773	205 399	214 698	221 531
Goods bought for resale without processing	ZABZ	161 304	165 667	169 676	176 219	180 725
Energy and water products for own consumption	ZACA	2 048	2 191	2 522	3 048	3 178
Goods and materials	ZACB	3 917	4 166	4 271	4 374	4 315
Hiring, leasing or renting of plant, machinery and vehicles	ZACC	946	727	576	600	625
Commercial insurance premiums	ZACD	1 001	1 061	1 034	931	948
Road transport services	ZACE	2 545	2 557	2 737	2 616	2 802
Telecommunication services	ZACF	624	626	607	574	634
Computer and related services	ZACG	765	915	816	824	954
Advertising and marketing services	ZACH	3 378	3 298	3 540	3 703	4 152
Other services	ZACI	17 642	18 565	19 620	21 809	23 197
Taxes, duties and levies	ZACJ	4 715	4 896	5 990	6 342	6 388
National non-domestic (business) rates	ZACK	3 859	3 937	4 336	4 693	5 017
Other amounts paid for taxes, duties and levies	ZACL	855	958	1 654	1 649	1 372
Capital expenditure						
Cost of acquisitions	ZACM	8 776	9 936	10 138	10 026	11 018
Proceeds from disposals	ZACN	1 328	1 590	1 516	1 688	1 968
Net capital expenditure	ZACO	7 448	8 346	8 622	8 338	9 050
Amount included in acquisitions for assets under finance leasing arrangements	ZACP	304	332	303	439	475
Work of a capital nature carried out by own staff (included in acquisitions)	ZACQ	142	149	176	188	122
Gross margin						
Amount	ZACR	88 904	93 830	95 667	102 001	107 174
As a percentage of adjusted turnover[4]	ZACS	*35.6*	*36.2*	*36.0*	*37.0*	*37.0*
Approximate gross value added at basic prices	ZACT	56 104	59 764	60 020	63 599	66 434

24.1 Retail businesses[1]
United Kingdom
continued

£ million

		2003	2004	2005	2006	2007
Total turnover	ZABL	278 373	288 716	295 952	309 668	319 216
Retail turnover	ZABN	250 849	258 903	264 427	277 145	285 313
1 Fruit (including fresh, chilled, dried, frozen, canned and processed)	DSSX	4 507	4 499	4 657	5 278	5 812
2 Vegetables (including fresh, chilled, dried, frozen, canned and processed)	DSSY	8 354	8 470	9 205	9 075	9 582
3 Meat (including fresh, chilled, smoked, frozen, canned and processed)	DSSZ	13 505	13 727	13 520	14 870	15 674
4 Fish, crustaceans and molluscs (including fresh, chilled, frozen, canned and processed)	DSTA	2 549	2 671	2 866	2 857	2 893
5 Bakery products and cereals (including rice and pasta products)	DSTC	12 314	11 880	12 967	14 154	14 608
6 Sugar, jam, honey, chocolate and confectionery (including ice-cream)	DSTD	6 446	6 534	6 406	7 533	7 807
7 Alcoholic drink	DSTE	12 297	12 931	13 099	14 028	14 433
8 Non-alcoholic beverages (including tea, coffee, fruit drinks and vegetable drinks)	DSTF	6 713	7 386	7 514	7 074	7 386
9 Tobacco (excluding smokers requisites, eg pipes, lighters, etc)	DSTG	9 204	9 020	8 960	9 143	9 233
10 Milk, cheese and eggs (including yoghurts and cream)	DSTH	7 390	7 995	8 356	8 947	9 479
11 Oils and fats (including butter and margarine)	DSTI	1 162	1 287	1 329	1 295	1 317
12 Food products not elsewhere classified (including sauces, herbs, spices and soups)	DSTJ	4 112	4 399	4 327	4 572	4 431
13 Pharmaceutical products	DSTK	2 963	2 987	3 090	3 384	3 520
14 National Health Receipts	DSTL	8 647	9 006	9 673	10 000	10 343
15 Other medical products and therapeutic appliances and equipment	DSTN	3 122	3 388	3 387	3 752	3 851
16 Other appliances, articles and products for personal care	DSTO	10 698	11 111	11 405	12 402	12 983
17 Other articles of clothing, accessories for making clothing	DSTP	1 955	2 089	2 452	2 805	3 040
18 Garments	DSTQ	29 691	30 375	31 294	31 772	32 698
19 Footwear (excluding sports shoes)	DSTR	5 622	5 904	6 037	6 600	6 526
20 Travel goods and other personal effects not elsewhere classified	DSTT	1 175	1 120	1 124	1 337	1 299
21 Household textiles (including furnishing fabrics, curtains, etc)	DSTV	3 799	3 890	3 700	3 846	4 431
22 Household and personal appliances whether electric or not	DSUA	6 776	6 798	6 957	6 901	6 456
23 Glassware, tableware and household utensils (including non-electric)	DSUB	2 843	2 743	3 124	3 022	2 909
24 Furniture and furnishings	DSUC	13 285	13 493	13 620	13 964	14 373
25 Audio and visual equipment (including radios, televisions and video recorders)	DSUE	4 818	5 130	5 646	6 180	6 384
26 Recording material for pictures and sound (including audio and video tapes, blank and pre-recorded records, etc)	DSUG	3 788	4 488	4 366	4 039	3 564
27 Information processing equipment (including printers, software, calculators and typewriters)	DSUL	3 077	3 743	3 600	3 703	4 091
28 Decorating and DIY supplies	DSUM	6 631	7 427	6 928	5 646	5 410
29 Tools and equipment for house and garden	DSUN	3 452	2 838	2 983	3 185	3 513
30 Books	DSUP	2 748	3 004	2 646	3 103	2 688
31 Newspapers and periodicals	DSUQ	4 067	4 053	4 048	4 246	3 979
32 Stationery and drawing materials and miscellaneous printed matter	DSUW	3 824	3 989	4 201	4 576	4 540
33 Carpets and other floor coverings (excluding bathroom mats, rush and door mats)	DSUX	3 757	3 386	3 526	3 481	4 169
34 Photographic and cinematographic equipment and optical instruments	DSUZ	1 670	1 842	2 052	2 064	1 630
35 Telephone and telefax equipment (including mobile phones)	DSVA	2 293	3 272	3 476	3 476	3 458
36 Jewellery, silverware and plate; watches and clocks	DSVB	4 312	4 681	4 697	5 329	4 950
37 Works of art and antiques (including furniture, floor coverings and jewellery)	DSVF	1 493	1 619	1 720	1 428	1 860
38 Equipment and accessories for sport, camping, recreation and musical instruments	DSVH	3 803	3 732	3 612	4 448	4 299
39 Spare part and accessories for all types of vehicle and sales of bicycles	DSVI	572	610	556	768	684
40 Games, toys, hobbies (including video game software, video game computers that plug into the tv, video-games cassettes and CD-ROMs)	DSVM	5 962	5 920	5 745	5 943	7 460
41 Other goods not elsewhere classified (including sale of new postage stamps and sales of liquid and solid fuels)	DSVN	3 134	2 884	2 623	3 912	4 415
42 Non-durable household goods (including household cleaning, maintenance products) and paper products and other non-durable household goods	DSVO	5 017	5 429	5 291	4 802	4 894
43 Natural or artificial plants and flowers	DSVQ	3 745	3 117	3 253	3 811	3 663
44 Pets and related products (including pet food)	DSVR	2 681	3 012	3 228	3 309	3 630
45 Repair of household and personal items	DSVS	875	1 021	1 161	1 084	947

1 See chapter text.
2 Inclusive of VAT.
3 Exclusive of VAT.
4 Turnover is adjusted to take out VAT.

Source: Office for National Statistics: 01633 456592

24.2 Retail trade: index numbers of value and volume of sales[1]
Great Britain

Not seasonally adjusted

		Sales in 2005 £ million	1999	2000	2001	2002	2003	2004	2005	2006	2007	2008	2009
Value													
All retailing	J5AH	311 836	80.5	84.4	88.0	91.6	94.1	98.6	100.0	103.8	107.9	111.0	110.9
Large	J5AI	244 990	75.4	79.8	84.4	88.7	93.2	98.0	100.0	104.7	109.7	115.0	116.8
Small	J5AJ	66 846	95.7	98.1	99.1	100.6	97.1	100.5	100.0	101.3	102.5	99.1	93.1
All retailing excluding automotive fuel	J43S	285 210	81.3	83.9	88.4	92.5	94.5	98.9	100.0	102.5	106.2	109.5	111.8
Predominantly food stores	EAFS	133 599	79.4	81.7	86.2	89.8	93.2	96.9	100.0	103.6	108.0	114.2	120.4
Predominantly non-food stores	EAFT	137 373	81.4	84.2	89.4	94.3	95.9	100.5	100.0	101.5	104.6	105.1	103.7
Non specialised predominantly non-food stores	EAGE	24 048	84.8	88.8	93.6	96.2	98.3	100.3	100.0	102.9	106.8	103.9	106.0
Textiles, clothing, footwear and leather	EAFU	38 492	76.2	79.8	86.1	91.0	94.3	99.1	100.0	104.6	107.5	107.2	108.5
Household goods stores	EAFV	32 295	85.8	88.7	95.3	99.8	99.5	103.3	100.0	100.7	104.2	102.1	97.6
Other specialised non-food stores	EAFW	42 538	80.6	82.2	85.5	91.9	93.3	99.6	100.0	98.9	101.2	106.3	103.1
Non-store retailing	J596	14 236	96.7	101.3	97.4	99.5	90.8	100.2	100.0	102.1	106.4	113.6	119.8
Automotive fuel	J43H	26 626	73.3	88.7	84.3	82.7	91.0	96.1	100.0	117.0	125.3	126.1	102.8
Volume													
All retailing	J5DD	311 836	77.6	80.8	84.4	89.4	92.6	97.9	100.0	103.9	107.8	109.0	109.7
All retailing excluding automotive fuel	J448	285 210	76.4	79.4	83.2	88.7	91.6	97.4	100.0	103.2	107.0	109.7	111.8
Predominantly food stores	EAGW	133 599	83.7	85.5	88.0	91.3	94.1	97.7	100.0	101.7	102.8	102.7	104.1
Predominantly non-food stores	EAGX	137 373	70.4	73.9	79.3	86.3	90.1	97.1	100.0	104.3	110.1	114.4	116.4
Non specialised predominantly non-food stores	EAHI	24 048	73.2	78.2	83.6	88.3	92.6	97.3	100.0	105.6	112.2	113.0	117.6
Textiles, clothing, footwear and leather	EAGY	38 492	60.4	64.9	73.3	82.0	87.4	95.3	100.0	107.8	113.8	119.2	128.3
Household goods stores	EAGZ	32 295	74.2	78.4	83.0	89.3	92.6	99.4	100.0	104.2	111.0	112.3	108.5
Other specialised non-food stores	EAHA	42 538	75.2	76.4	79.3	86.8	89.1	96.8	100.0	100.4	105.2	112.5	111.3
Non-store retailing	J5CL	14 236	83.4	88.8	86.8	91.4	85.5	97.0	100.0	104.8	112.4	124.1	134.7
Automotive fuel	J43V	26 626	90.5	96.9	97.0	97.7	103.8	104.0	100.0	111.0	115.3	101.6	88.9

1 See chapter text.

Source: Office for National Statistics

24.3 Motor trades[1]
United Kingdom

£ million and percentages

		Sale, maintenance and repair of,motor vehicles and motorcycles; retail sale of automotive fuel (SIC 2003 50.00)					Sale of motor vehicles (SIC 2003 50.10)			
		2004	2005	2006	2007		2004	2005	2006	2007
Number of businesses	MKEQ	70 265	70 994	71 201	71 183	MKER	24 199	23 924	23 614	23 175
Total turnover	CMRH	153 447	158 018	156 784	166 269	EWRI	103 594	107 586	106 338	112 098
Motor trades turnover	CMRI	147 850	152 554	151 800	160 636	FDFZ	102 579	105 909	104 463	110 362
Retail sales of:										
New cars	CMRJ	30 645	30 699	30 346	32 653	FDGA	28 427	28 744	28 115	30 288
Other new motor vehicles and motorcycles	CMRK	5 223	5 099	4 651	6 289	FDGB	4 358	4 152	3 694	5 309
Sales to other dealers of:										
New cars	CMRL	23 209	23 770	24 066	22 411	FDGC	22 790	23 451	23 677	22 017
Other new motor vehicles and motorcycles	CMRM	3 692	3 520	3 959	3 503	FDGD	3 074	2 913	2 768	2 538
Gross sales of used motor vehicles and motorcycles	CMRN	32 951	34 968	35 269	39 167	FDGE	30 560	32 890	31 703	34 848
Turnover from sales of petrol, diesel, oil and other petroleum products	CMRO	17 998	18 014	17 415	17 434	FDGF	806	702	693	1 042
Other motor trades sales and receipts (including parts and accessories, workshop receipts)	CMRP	34 131	36 483	36 094	39 180	FDGG	12 564	13 058	13 813	14 320
Non-motor trades turnover	CMRQ	5 598	5 464	4 984	5 633	FDHJ	1 015	1 677	1 875	1 737
Purchases of goods, materials and services										
Total purchases	CMNR	131 600	135 467	132 950	141 367	FDGH	91 714	94 598	92 902	98 411
Energy, water and materials	CMRS	1 696	2 017	2 166	2 489	FDGI	704	835	804	1 009
Used motor vehicles and motorcycles	COBU	29 352	30 698	31 717	34 919	FDGJ	27 397	28 946	28 728	31 272
Parts used solely in repair and servicing activities	CMRT	7 079	7 544	7 024	7 259	FDGK	2 682	2 975	3 536	3 684
Other goods for resale	CMRU	84 679	86 139	83 454	87 997	FDGL	55 864	56 738	54 814	57 450
Hiring, leasing and renting of plant, machinery and vehicles	CMRV	369	307	239	278	FDGM	84	84	69	84
Commercial insurance premiums	CMRW	561	609	542	575	FDGN	215	245	245	226
Road transport services	CMRX	753	715	633	579	FDGO	415	317	258	257
Telecommunication services	CMRY	295	307	276	298	FDGP	128	145	130	132
Computer and related services	CMRZ	388	352	411	383	FDGQ	187	201	245	216
Advertising and marketing services	CMSA	2 267	2 405	2 538	2 344	FDGR	1 897	1 964	2 105	1 920
Other services	CMSB	4 161	4 374	3 949	4 247	FDGS	2 140	2 147	1 968	2 159
Taxes, duties and levies										
Total taxes and levies	CMSC	972	1 077	1 060	1 100	FDGT	516	625	606	604
National (non-domestic business) rates	CMSD	613	660	659	693	FDGU	280	343	331	350
Other amounts paid for taxes, duties and levies	CMSE	359	417	401	407	FDGV	236	281	275	253
Capital expenditure										
Cost of acquisitions	CMSF	2 346	2 499	2 602	2 678	FDGW	1 425	1 610	1 794	1 599
Cost of disposals	CMSG	987	1 015	1 445	1 309	FDGX	671	736	1 166	1 023
Net capital expenditure	CMSH	1 359	1 484	1 157	1 370	FDGY	755	874	629	577
Work of a capital nature carried out by own staff (included in acquisitions)	CMSI	5	10	52	45	FDGZ	5	10	41	34
Stocks										
Increase during year	CMSJ	1 344	550	245	1 154	FDHA	1 138	403	219	907
Value at end of year	CMSK	14 923	15 621	15 812	16 863	FDHB	11 104	11 469	11 299	12 420
Total turnover divided by end-year stocks (Quotient)	CMSL	10.3	10.1	9.9	9.8	FDHC	9.3	9.4	9.4	9.0
Employment costs										
Total employment costs	CMSM	10 238	10 716	11 115	11 914	FDHD	5 327	5 608	5 511	6 033
Gross wages and salaries paid	COBP	9 062	9 382	9 714	10 411	FDHE	4 701	4 851	4 782	5 296
National insurance and pension contributions	COBQ	1 175	1 334	1 401	1 503	FDHF	625	757	730	737
Gross margin										
Amount	COBR	33 580	34 042	34 728	37 154	FDHG	18 770	19 283	19 434	20 585
As a percentage of adjusted turnover	COBS	*21.9*	*21.5*	*22.0*	*22.0*	FDHH	*18.1*	*17.9*	*18.0*	*18.0*
Approximate gross value added at basic prices	COBT	23 125	22 979	24 010	25 997	FDHI	13 011	13 363	13 639	14 605

24.3

Motor trades[1]
United Kingdom
continued

		Maintenance and repair of motor vehicles (SIC 2003 50.20)					Sale of motor vehicle parts and accessories (SIC 2003 50.30)			
		2004	2005	2006	2007		2004	2005	2006	2007
Number of businesses	MKES	30 050	30 973	31 666	32 631	MKET	7 952	8 067	8 096	8 067
Total turnover	FDHK	13 337	14 445	14 321	14 948	FDIW	13 694	13 659	14 427	15 826
Motor trades turnover	FDHL	13 023	14 082	14 041	14 538	FDIX	12 702	12 722	13 425	14 978
Retail sales of:										
New cars	FDHM	939	1 000	1 153	1 253	FDIY	1 241	880	904	930
Other new motor vehicles and motorcycles	FDHN	213	164	223	308	FDIZ	172	233	206	265
Sales to other dealers of:										
New cars	FDHO	..	23	38	46	FDJA	..	294	322	347
Other new motor vehicles and motorcycles	FDHP	..	..	429	307	FDJB	..	75	51	33
Gross sales of used motor vehicles and motorcycles	FDHQ	1 380	1 276	1 965	2 298	FDJC	374	251	493	499
Turnover from sales of petrol, diesel, oil and other petroleum products	FDHR	100	119	337	295	FDJD	86	1	4	1
Other motor trades sales and receipts (including parts and accessories, workshop receipts)	FDHS	10 386	11 500	9 896	10 031	FDJE	10 362	10 987	11 446	12 904
Non-motor trades turnover	FDHT	314	363	281	410	FDJF	992	936	1 002	848
Purchases of goods, materials and services										
Total purchases	FDHU	8 795	9 406	9 150	9 284	FDJG	10 958	11 223	11 737	12 587
Energy, water and materials	FDHV	652	735	758	727	FDJH	227	329	439	468
Used motor vehicles and motorcycles	FDHW	1 041	1 046	1 586	1 771	FDJI	371	272	387	566
Parts used solely in repair and servicing activities	FDHX	3 980	4 184	3 199	2 888	FDJJ	183	208	158	278
Other goods for resale	FDHY	1 453	1 739	2 284	2 472	FDJK	9 000	8 976	9 269	9 858
Hiring, leasing and renting of plant, machinery and vehicles	FDHZ	111	120	91	101	FDJL	136	62	53	49
Commercial insurance premiums	FDIA	227	242	174	156	FDJM	78	84	82	75
Road transport services	FDIB	104	79	40	28	FDJN	126	207	237	202
Telecommunication services	FDIC	103	97	76	80	FDJO	45	45	44	49
Computer and related services	FDID	72	39	43	43	FDJP	107	96	104	108
Advertising and marketing services	FDIE	125	111	84	103	FDJQ	208	290	274	263
Other services	FDIF	926	1 015	817	915	FDJR	478	655	691	672
Taxes, duties and levies										
Total taxes and levies	FDIG	215	218	217	234	FDJS	116	128	135	147
National (non-domestic business) rates	FDIH	152	146	156	159	FDJT	89	96	106	118
Other amounts paid for taxes, duties and levies	FDII	63	72	61	74	FDJU	27	32	29	29
Capital expenditure										
Cost of acquisitions	FDIJ	442	441	338	460	FDJV	199	194	210	306
Cost of disposals	FDIK	98	109	88	118	FDJW	54	76	97	122
Net capital expenditure	FDIL	345	332	250	342	FDJX	144	118	113	184
Work of a capital nature carried out by own staff (included in acquisitions)	FDIM	..	..	..	1	FDJY	..	..	6	10
Stocks										
Increase during year	FDIN	36	..	8	98	FDJZ	81	134	92	184
Value at end of year	FDIO	835	958	1 133	1 064	FDKA	1 807	1 818	2 069	2 126
Total turnover divided by end-year stocks (Quotient)	FDIP	16.0	15.1	13.0	14.0	FDKB	7.6	7.5	7.0	7.0
Employment costs										
Total employment costs	FDIQ	2 581	2 697	2 951	3 032	FDKC	1 565	1 618	1 773	1 919
Gross wages and salaries paid	FDIR	2 315	2 429	2 643	2 693	FDKD	1 391	1 423	1 556	1 675
National insurance and pension contributions	FDIS	266	268	308	339	FDKE	174	195	217	245
Gross margin										
Amount	FDIT	6 857	7 415	7 235	7 888	FDKF	4 199	4 313	4 691	5 298
As a percentage of adjusted turnover	FDIU	*51.4*	*51.3*	*51.0*	*53.0*	FDKG	*30.7*	*31.6*	*33.0*	*33.0*
Approximate gross value added at basic prices	FDIV	4 548	4 980	5 156	5 738	FDKH	2 796	2 547	2 772	3 420

24.3 Motor trades[1]
United Kingdom
continued

£ million and percentages

		Sale, maintenance and repair of motorcycles and related parts and accessories (SIC 2003 50.40)					Retail sale of automotive fuel (SIC 2003 50.50)			
		2004	2005	2006	2007		2004	2005	2006	2007
Number of businesses	MKEU	2 948	3 157	3 161	3 178	MKEV	5 116	4 873	4 664	4 132
Total turnover	FDKI	2 116	2 211	2 182	2 473	FDLV	20 708	20 118	19 517	20 924
Motor trades turnover	FDKJ	2 102	2 200	2 172	2 470	FDLW	17 444	17 641	17 700	18 289
Retail sales of:										
New cars	FDKK	..	35	54	99	FDLX	38	39	120	82
Other new motor vehicles and motorcycles	FDKL	479	550	465	403	FDLY	..	..	63	4
Sales to other dealers of:										
New cars	FDKM	–	–	–	–	FDLZ	1	2	29	1
Other new motor vehicles and motorcycles	FDKN	564	532	711	625	FDMA	–	–	–	–
Gross sales of used motor vehicles and motorcycles	FDKO	499	472	378	615	FDMB	138	80	730	907
Turnover from sales of petrol, diesel, oil and other petroleum products	FDKP	–	–	–	1	FDMC	17 006	17 192	16 381	16 097
Other motor trades sales and receipts (including parts and accessories, workshop receipts)	FDKQ	558	611	564	727	FDMD	261	328	375	1 198
Non-motor trades turnover	FDKR	14	11	10	3	FDME	3 263	2 476	1 817	2 634
Purchases of goods, materials and services										
Total purchases	FDKT	1 705	1 890	1 760	1 938	FDMF	18 428	18 350	17 400	19 147
Energy, water and materials	FDKU	13	21	23	29	FDMG	100	96	141	256
Used motor vehicles and motorcycles	FDKV	409	383	336	511	FDMH	134	51	680	798
Parts used solely in repair and servicing activities	FDKW	163	69	61	87	FDMI	71	108	70	322
Other goods for resale	FDKX	1 016	1 291	1 175	1 153	FDMJ	17 346	17 395	15 913	17 064
Hiring, leasing and renting of plant, machinery and vehicles	FDKY	1	2	1	–	FDMK	37	38	25	43
Commercial insurance premiums	FDKZ	8	13	9	11	FDML	32	25	32	107
Road transport services	FDLA	21	18	31	30	COBV	86	95	67	61
Telecommunication services	FDLB	5	6	6	5	COBW	14	14	21	31
Computer and related services	FDLC	3	5	5	3	COBX	19	11	15	12
Advertising and marketing services	FDLD	22	29	48	32	COBY	14	11	27	27
Other services	FDLE	42	52	64	76	COBZ	574	506	409	424
Taxes, duties and levies										
Total taxes and levies	FDLF	32	33	30	33	COCA	92	74	73	83
National (non-domestic business) rates	FDLG	..	..	11	13	COCB	..	..	55	52
Other amounts paid for taxes, duties and levies	FDLH	..	..	19	19	COCC	..	..	18	31
Capital expenditure										
Cost of acquisitions	FDLI	65	28	54	34	COCD	215	225	205	279
Cost of disposals	FDLJ	20	9	10	13	COCE	144	84	85	34
Net capital expenditure	FDLK	45	19	44	21	COCF	71	141	120	245
Work of a capital nature carried out by own staff (included in acquisitions)	FDLL	–	–	–	–	COCG	–	–	4	–
Stocks										
Increase during year	FDLM	−1	−29	−65	8	COCH	90	55	−8	−43
Value at end of year	FDLN	391	434	390	414	COCI	786	942	921	839
Total turnover divided by end-year stocks (Quotient)	FDLO	5.4	5.1	6.0	6.0	COCJ	26.3	21.3	21.0	25.0
Employment costs										
Total employment costs	FDLP	155	165	191	224	COCK	610	628	688	705
Gross wages and salaries paid	FDLQ	136	148	170	199	COCL	519	530	563	548
National insurance and pension contributions	FDLR	19	17	21	25	COCM	91	97	125	157
Gross margin										
Amount	FDLS	517	427	531	717	COCN	3 238	2 604	2 836	2 666
As a percentage of adjusted turnover	FDLT	*24.4*	*19.3*	*24.0*	*29.0*	CMQN	*15.6*	*12.9*	*15.0*	*14.0*
Approximate gross value added at basic prices	FDLU	400	281	343	529	CMQO	2 370	1 808	2 100	1 705

1 See chapter text. Figures are exclusive of VAT.

Source: Office for National Statistics: 01633 456592

24.4 Catering and allied trades[1]
United Kingdom

		Total catering and allied trades (SIC 2003 55.00)					Hotels and motels (SIC 2003 55.11 and 55.12)			
		2004	2005	2006	2007		2004	2005	2006	2007
Number of businesses	MKEK	126 706	130 180	132 563	134 651	MKEL	10 417	10 253	10 139	10 037
Total turnover[2]	CMKX	70 199	71 836	74 101	75 635	CMLW	13 009	13 438	14 742	15 441
Taxes and levies[3]										
Total taxes and levies	CMLM	1 848	1 949	1 996	1 994	CMML	427	461	502	491
National (non-domestic business) rates	CMLJ	1 673	1 749	1 849	1 827	CMMI	400	442	488	460
Other amounts paid for taxes, duties and levies	CMLL	175	200	147	167	CMMK	27	20	15	31
Capital expenditure[3]										
Capital acquisitions	CMLP	4 122	4 530	4 682	5 352	CMMO	934	1 110	1 326	1 600
Capital disposals	CMLQ	612	1 151	1 100	1 179	CMMP	150	336	176	249
Net capital expenditure	CMLK	3 510	3 379	3 582	4 172	CMMJ	783	773	1 150	1 352
Work of a capital nature carried out by your own staff (included in acquisitions)	CMLR	12	31	42	10	CMMQ	4	5	19	1
Stocks[3]										
Increase during year	CMLN	75	54	83	99	CMMM	2	2	1	12
Value at end of year	CMLO	1 253	1 267	1 283	1 343	CMMN	168	154	172	149
Purchases of goods and services[3]										
Total purchases	CMLI	31 813	33 358	33 990	34 379	CMMH	4 838	5 140	5 468	5 680
Energy, water and materials	CMKZ	13 374	12 839	12 762	13 364	CMLY	2 043	2 075	2 126	2 129
Goods for resale	CMLA	9 555	11 475	11 903	10 972	CMLZ	583	733	808	723
Hiring, leasing of plant, machinery etc.	CMLB	303	262	256	299	CMMA	66	49	46	53
Commercial insurance premiums	CMLC	545	525	523	504	CMMB	135	132	140	137
Road transport services	CMLD	103	146	135	155	CMMC	8	10	16	26
Telecommunication services	CMLE	265	253	229	225	CMMD	68	60	62	54
Computer and related services	CMLF	169	197	164	198	CMME	45	72	69	77
Advertising and marketing services	CMLG	713	727	768	928	CMMF	203	202	242	260
Other services	CMLH	6 786	6 934	7 250	7 736	CMMG	1 687	1 806	1 959	2 222
Employment costs[3]										
Total employment costs	CMKY	15 287	16 541	16 639	18 109	CMLX	3 270	3 660	3 821	4 241
Gross wages and salaries paid	CMKV	14 075	15 134	15 324	16 661	CMLU	2 993	3 295	3 472	3 880
National insurance and pension contributions	CMKW	1 212	1 406	1 314	1 448	CMLV	277	364	350	362
Gross margin[4]										
Amount	CMQP	51 047	50 616	52 234	54 543	CMQS	10 525	10 726	11 861	12 556
As a percentage of turnover	CMQQ	*84.1*	*81.4*	*81.0*	*83.0*	CMQT	*94.6*	*93.5*	*94.0*	*94.0*
Value added at basic prices[4]	CMQR	28 833	28 757	30 185	31 166	CMQU	6 272	6 327	7 203	7 605
Accommodation										
Number of establishments	CMLS	28 332	83 134	..	..	CMMR	14 190	24 367	..	..
Letting bedplaces	CMLT	2 676 991	2 441 159	..	..	CMMS	964 733	1 589 498	..	..

24.4 Catering and allied trades[1]
United Kingdom
continued

£ million and percentages

		Camping sites and other provision of short-stay accommodation (SIC 2003 55.21 to 55.23)					Restaurants or cafes, take-away food shops (SIC 2003 55.30)			
		2004	2005	2006	2007		2004	2005	2006	2007
Number of businesses	MKEM	4 703	5 027	5 225	5 460	MKEN	57 674	60 539	62 063	63 689
Total turnover[2]	CMMV	3 620	3 699	3 926	3 874	CMNU	21 731	22 601	23 027	24 909
Taxes and levies[3]										
Total taxes and levies	CMNK	90	91	93	94	CMOJ	556	627	647	663
National (non-domestic business) rates	CMNH	81	83	91	92	CMOG	483	544	582	605
Other amounts paid for taxes, duties and levies	CMNJ	8	7	2	3	CMOI	73	83	65	58
Capital expenditure[3]										
Capital acquisitions	CMNN	336	345	450	478	CMOM	1 153	1 339	1 415	1 492
Capital disposals	CMNO	55	47	155	76	CMON	130	253	285	260
Net capital expenditure	CMNI	281	298	294	402	CMOH	1 023	1 086	1 130	1 231
Work of a capital nature carried out by your own staff (included in acquisitions)	CMNP	–	17	4	1	CMOO	4	8	9	2
Stocks[3]										
Increase during year	CMNL	10	19	17	19	CMOK	12	13	43	30
Value at end of year	CMNM	137	194	192	198	CMOL	326	338	379	377
Purchases of goods and services[3]										
Total purchases	CMNG	1 747	1 763	1 852	1 735	CMOF	10 056	10 614	10 727	11 497
Energy, water and materials	CMMX	449	444	395	486	CMNW	5 080	4 810	4 835	5 119
Goods for resale	CMMY	594	592	720	567	CMNX	2 399	3 125	3 254	3 354
Hiring, leasing of plant, machinery etc.	CMMZ	14	10	9	8	CMNY	47	38	30	75
Commercial insurance premiums	CMNA	59	48	51	57	CMNZ	140	138	118	136
Road transport services	CMNB	11	17	16	11	CMOA	51	55	45	58
Telecommunication services	CMNC	17	18	17	16	CMOB	72	71	60	65
Computer and related services	CMND	13	15	14	17	CMOC	41	46	25	39
Advertising and marketing services	CMNE	111	101	117	107	CMOD	251	268	256	393
Other services	CMNF	480	517	515	465	CMOE	1 975	2 063	2 105	2 258
Employment costs[3]										
Total employment costs	CMMW	578	683	707	749	CMNV	4 642	5 131	5 069	5 846
Gross wages and salaries paid	CMMT	523	618	643	686	CMNS	4 305	4 725	4 702	5 392
National insurance and pension contributions	CMMU	55	65	64	64	CMNT	337	406	366	454
Gross margin[4]										
Amount	CMQV	2 586	2 734	2 770	2 910	CMQY	16 289	16 343	16 684	18 267
As a percentage of turnover	CMQW	*81.4*	*82.9*	*80.0*	*84.0*	CMQZ	*86.9*	*83.7*	*84.0*	*84.0*
Value added at basic prices[4]	CMQX	1 435	1 565	1 640	1 743	CMRA	8 660	8 863	9 217	10 129
Accommodation										
Number of establishments	CMNQ	6 255	43 033	..	..	CMOP	1 604	4 195	..	..
Letting bedplaces	CMRR	1 533 656	674 684	..	..	CMOQ	42 383	65 339	..	..

426

24.4 Catering and allied trades[1]
United Kingdom
continued

£ million and percentages

		Licensed clubs with entertainment, independent, tenanted, managed public houses or wine bars (SIC 2003 55.40)[5]					Canteen operator, catering contractor (SIC 2003 55.51 and 55.52)			
		2004	2005	2006	2007		2004	2005	2006	2007
Number of businesses	MKEO	48 147	48 400	49 001	49 112	MKEP	5 765	5 961	6 135	6 353
Total turnover[2]	CMOT	24 455	23 830	24 876	23 496	CMPS	7 383	8 268	7 531	7 915
Taxes and levies[3]										
Total taxes and levies	CMPI	748	725	724	699	CMQH	28	46	30	47
National (non-domestic business) rates	CMPF	688	652	666	628	CMQE	21	28	23	42
Other amounts paid for taxes, duties and levies	CMPH	59	73	58	71	CMQG	8	17	7	4
Capital expenditure[3]										
Capital acquisitions	CMPL	1 489	1 588	1 404	1 668	CMQK	211	148	88	113
Capital disposals	CMPM	260	490	450	567	CMQL	17	25	34	27
Net capital expenditure	CMPG	1 229	1 098	954	1 101	CMQF	194	123	54	86
Work of a capital nature carried out by your own staff (included in acquisitions)	CMPN	4	1	10	6	CMQM	–	–	–	..
Stocks[3]										
Increase during year	CMPJ	41	5	19	24	CMQI	9	15	3	13
Value at end of year	CMPK	512	443	415	466	CMQJ	109	138	124	153
Purchases of goods and services[3]										
Total purchases	CMPE	11 844	12 002	12 476	11 752	CMQD	3 328	3 839	3 467	3 715
Energy, water and materials	CMOV	3 458	3 007	3 186	3 467	CMPU	2 344	2 503	2 220	2 162
Goods for resale	CMOW	5 522	6 434	6 609	5 787	CMPV	457	590	512	542
Hiring, leasing of plant, machinery etc.	CMOX	138	120	109	84	CMPW	38	45	62	80
Commercial insurance premiums	CMOY	182	170	176	144	CMPX	30	36	38	30
Road transport services	CMOZ	17	44	43	41	CMPY	15	20	16	19
Telecommunication services	CMPA	86	77	66	65	CMPZ	23	28	24	24
Computer and related services	CMPB	48	38	38	44	CMQA	22	26	19	20
Advertising and marketing services	CMPC	129	121	131	133	CMQB	19	35	23	34
Other services	CMPD	2 264	1 992	2 118	1 987	CMQC	380	557	553	804
Employment costs[3]										
Total employment costs	CMOU	4 294	4 376	4 390	4 532	CMPT	2 503	2 691	2 652	2 740
Gross wages and salaries paid	CMOR	3 974	4 037	4 082	4 196	CMPQ	2 281	2 459	2 425	2 508
National insurance and pension contributions	CMOS	320	339	308	337	CMPR	222	232	227	232
Gross margin[4]										
Amount	CMRB	15 408	13 931	14 717	14 314	CMRE	6 238	6 882	6 201	6 495
As a percentage of turnover	CMRC	*73.6*	*68.2*	*69.0*	*71.0*	CMRF	*93.2*	*92.3*	*92.0*	*92.0*
Value added at basic prices[4]	CMRD	9 098	8 368	8 878	8 366	CMRG	3 368	3 633	3 248	3 322
Accommodation										
Number of establishments	CMPO	6 046	11 288	..	..					
Letting bedplaces	CMPP	110 130	84 174	..	..					

1 See chapter text.
2 Inclusive of VAT.
3 Exclusive of VAT.

4 The total turnover figure used to calculate these data excludes VAT.
5 Includes figures for managed public houses owned by breweries.

Source: Office for National Statistics: 01633 456592

Sources

This index of sources gives the titles of official publications or other sources containing statistics allied to those in the tables of this *Annual Abstract*. These publications provide more detailed analyses than are shown in the *Annual Abstract*. This index includes publications to which reference should be made for short–term (monthly or quarterly) series. Further advice on published statistical sources is available from the ONS Customer Contact Centre on the numbers provided on page ii.

Table number in Abstract	Government department or other organisation	Official publication or other source
Chapter 1: Area		
1.1	Ordnance Survey	
	Ordnance Survey of Northern Ireland	
	Office for National Statistics	Regional Trends (annual, Palgrave Macmillan)
Chapter 2: Parliamentary elections		
2.1	University of Plymouth for the Electoral Commission	British Electoral Facts 1832–2006 (Ashgate) Dod's Parliamentary Companion (annual)
2.2	University of Plymouth for the Electoral Commission	Vachers Parliamentary Companion (quarterly) Social Trends (annual, Palgrave Macmillan)
2.2 to 2.4	University of Plymouth for the Electoral Commission	British Electoral Facts 1832–2006 (Ashgate) Social Trends (annual, Palgrave Macmillan)
Chapter 3: International development		
3.1 to 3.2	Department for International Development	Statistics on International Development 2002/03–2007/08, Tables 1, 2, 3, 14 and 18
Chapter 4: Defence		
4.1 to 4.11	Ministry of Defence/DASA	UK Defence Statistics 2008 (The Stationery Office (TSO))
Chapter 5: Population		
Population		**Census**
5.1 to 5.3, 5.5	Office for National Statistics	*England and Wales*: Census reports 1911, 1921, 1931, 1951, 1961, 1971, 1981, 1991 and 2001 Key Population and Vital Statistics; Great Britain, Digest of Welsh Statistics (annual, National Assembly for Wales)
	General Register Office Scotland	*Scotland*: Census reports 1951, 1961, 1971, 1981, 1991 and 2001

Table number in Abstract	Government department or other organisation	Official publication or other source
	Northern Ireland Statistics and Research Agency	*Northern Ireland*: Census of population 1951, 1961, 1966, 1971, 1981, 1991 and 2001
		Resident population: mid–year estimates
5.1 to 5.3 and 5.5	Office for National Statistics	*England and Wales*: Series FM (Family statistics), DH (Death), MB (Morbidity), PP (Population estimates and projections), MN (Migration) and VS (Key population and vital statistics) Series PP1, Population estimates: The Registrar General's estimates of the population of regions and local government areas of England and Wales Population Trends (quarterly) Health Statistics Quarterly
	General Register Office Scotland	*Scotland*: Annual report of the Registrar General for Scotland Annual estimate of the population of Scotland
	Northern Ireland Statistics and Research Agency	*Northern Ireland*: Annual report of the Registrar General
5.6	Office for National Statistics	

Projections

| 5.1 to 5.3 | Office for National Statistics Government Actuary's Department | Series PP2, Population projections – national figures |

Migration

| 5.7 to 5.9 | Office for National Statistics | International Migration – statistical bulletin of 2007 estimates Series MN (International migration) Population Trends (quarterly) |
| 5.10 | Home Office | Control of immigration statistics United Kingdom (annual) Asylum Statistics United Kingdom (annual) |

Vital statistics

5.4 and 5.12 to 5.21	Office for National Statistics	*England and Wales*: Series FM (Births, marriages and divorce statistics) DH (Deaths), MB (Morbidity), PP (Population estimates and projections), MN (International migration) and VS (Key population and vital statistics)
	General Register Office Scotland	*Scotland*: Annual report of the Registrar General for Scotland Quarterly return of births, deaths and marriages
	Northern Ireland Statistics and Research Agency	*Northern Ireland*: Annual report of the Registrar General Quarterly return of births, deaths and marriages
5.14	Northern Ireland Court Service	Northern Ireland Judicial Statistics (annual)
5.18	Scottish Government Department of Health	

Sources

Table number in Abstract	Government department or other organisation	Official publication or other source
5.22	Office for National Statistics	*England and Wales*: Interim Life Table *Scotland*: Interim Life Table *Northern Ireland*: Annual Report of the Registrar General
5.23	Office for National Statistics General Register Office (Scotland) Northern Ireland Statistics and Research Agency	

Chapter 6: Education

6.1 to 6.11	Department for Children, Schools and Families (DCSF) (now Department for Education)	Education and Training Statistics for United Kingdom (Internet only) (annual, DCSF)
	Department For Innovation, Universities And Skills (DIUS)	United Kingdom higher education statistics (annual and ad–hoc, DIUS/Higher Education Statistics Agency (HESA))
	Welsh Assembly Government (WAG)	*Wales*: Statistics of education and training in Wales (annual and ad–hoc)
	Scottish Government (SG)	*Scotland*: Scottish educational statistics (annual and ad–hoc)
	Northern Ireland Department of Education (DENI)	*Northern Ireland*: Northern Ireland education statistics (annual and ad–hoc)
	Northern Ireland Department for Employment and Learning (DELNI)	Northern Ireland further and higher education statistics (annual and ad–hoc)

Chapter 7: Labour market

Labour force survey

7.1 to 7.3, 7.6, 7.9, 7.10, 7.11, 7.13, 7.16 to 7.18	Office for National Statistics	Economic and Labour Market Review (monthly, Palgrave Macmillan)
7.4, 7.5	Office for National Statistics	
7.7	Office for National Statistics	Labour Market Statistics
7.8	Office for National Statistics	Civil Service Statistics Monthly Digest of Statistics (Palgrave Macmillan)
7.9	Office for National Statistics	Economic and Labour Market Review (monthly, Palgrave Macmillan)
	Scottish Government	

Claimant count

7.12, 7.14, 7.15 and 7.25	Office for National Statistics	Economic and Labour Market Review (monthly, Palgrave Macmillan)

Table number in Abstract	Government department or other organisation	Official publication or other source
7.19	Office for National Statistics	Economic and Labour Market Review Monthly Digest of Statistics (Palgrave Macmillan)

Annual Survey of Hours and Earnings

7.20, 7.21, 7.24 and 7.25	Office for National Statistics	Annual Survey of Hours and Earnings (annual)

Average Earnings Index

7.22 and 7.23	Office for National Statistics	Economic and Labour Market Review Monthly Digest of Statistics (Palgrave Macmillan)
7.26	Certification Office	Certification Officers Annual Report

Chapter 8: Personal income, expenditure and wealth

8.1	Board of HMRC	http://www.hmrc.gov.uk/stats/income_distribution/menu.htm http://www.statistics.gov.uk/cci/article.asp?ID=2022
8.2	Office for National Statistics	(http://www.statistics.gov.uk/cci/article.asp?ID=2022)
8.3 to 8.5	Office for National Statistics	Expenditure and Food Survey, (annual) (1990 onwards edition–Family Spending) (annual, Palgrave Macmillan)

Chapter 9: Health

National Health Service

9.1	The NHS Information Centre for health and social care Welsh Assembly Government The Scottish Government, ISD Scotland part of NHS National Services Scotland Department of Health, Social Services and Public Safety (Northern Ireland)	 Summary of Health and Personal Social Services (Northern Ireland) Accounts (annual) Hospital Statistics (annual)
9.2	The Scottish Government, ISD Scotland part of NHS National Services Scotland	
9.3	Department of Health, Social Services and Public Safety (Northern Ireland)	Summary of Health and Personal Social Services (Northern Ireland) Accounts (annual) Hospital Statistics (annual)
9.4	The NHS Information Centre for health and social care	*England*: Health and Personal Social Services Statistics for England (annual) NHS Hospital and Community Health Services (HCHS):

Table number in Abstract	Government department or other organisation	Official publication or other source
9.5	Welsh Assembly Government	*Wales*: Health Statistics Wales (annual)

Public Health

9.6	Office for National Statistics	*England and Wales*: Death registrations series DH2
	General Register Office Scotland	*Scotland*: Annual Report of the Registrar General for Scotland
	Northern Ireland Statistics and Research Agency	*Northern Ireland*: Annual Report of the Registrar General for Research Agency Northern Ireland
9.7	HPA Centre for Infections	*England and Wales*: Communicable Disease Statistics (annual) Annual Review of Communicable Diseases
	NHS in Scotland NHS National Services Scotland	*Scotland*: Scottish Health Statistics (annual)
	Communicable Disease Surveillance Centre (NI)	*Northern Ireland*: Annual report of the Registrar General Northern Ireland
9.8 to 9.10	Health and Safety Executive	Health and Safety Statistics (annual)

Chapter 10: Social protection

Social security pensions, benefits and allowances

10.1	Department for Work and Pensions HM Revenue and Customs Department of Health, Social Services and Public Safety (Northern Ireland)	National Insurance Fund Account (annual)
10.2	Department for Work and Pensions	
10.3	HM Revenue and Customs	
10.4 and 10.5	Department for Work and Pensions (Information and Analysis Directorate) Ministry of Defence/DASA (Pay and Pensions)	Work and Pensions Longitudinal Study (WPLS, 100% sample)
	HM Revenue and Customs	
10.6 to 10.8, 10.12 to 10.19	Department for Work and Pensions (Information and Analysis Directorate)	Work and Pensions Longitudinal Study (WPLS, 100% sample)
10.9 and 10.11	HM Revenue and Customs	
10.15	Ministry of Defence/DASA (Health Information)	

Table number in Abstract	Government department or other organisation	Official publication or other source
Working Family Tax Credit		
10.10	Working Family Tax Credit Department for Work and Pensions (Information and Analysis Directorate)	Quarterly Enquiry United Kingdom
Social services		
10.20 to 10.24	Office for National Statistics Department for Education and Skills	Appropriation (annual) Northern Ireland Annual Abstract of Statistics
10.20	HM Treasury	HM Treasury Expenditure Statistical Analyses
Housing and community amenities		
10.25	Office for National Statistics	

Chapter 11: Crime and justice

11.1	Home Office	*England and Wales*: Police Service Strength England and Wales 2008 Home Office Statistical Bulletin 03/09
	Scottish Government Justice Analytical Services	
	The Police Service of Northern Ireland	*Northern Ireland*: The Chief Constable's Annual Report
11.3	Home Office	Crime in England and Wales 2007/08 (Home Office Statistical Bulletin 07/08)
11.4 to 11.9	Office for Criminal Justice Reform	Criminal Statistics, England and Wales (annual) (TSO) Offender Management Caseload Statistics 2008 (annual) Digest of Welsh Statistics (annual, Welsh Office)
11.2, 11.10 and 11.11	Ministry of Justice	Sentencing Statistics 2007 England & Wales Offender Management Caseload Statistics 2007
11.12	Ministry of Justice	HM Prison Service Annual Report and Accounts April 2007 – March 2008
11.13	Scottish Government Justice Analytical Services	Recorded Crime in Scotland, 2007/08
11.14 to 11.17	Scottish Government Justice Analytical Services	Criminal Proceedings in Scottish Courts, 2007/08
11.18 and 11.19	Scottish Government Justice Department	Prison Statistics Scotland, 2007/08 Scottish Prison Service Annual Report and Accounts

Table number in Abstract	Government department or other organisation	Official publication or other source
11.20	The Police Service of Northern Ireland	Northern Ireland: The Chief Constable's Annual Report 2008/09
11.21 to 11.24	Northern Ireland Office	A Commentary on Northern Ireland Crime Statistics 2004 'Court Prosecutions and Sentencing 2006' NIO Research and Statistical Bulletin 11/2008 Court Prosecutions and Sentencing for 10 to 17 year olds 2006' NIO Research and Statistical Bulletin 12/2008 The Northern Ireland Prison Population in 2007

Chapter 12: Lifestyles

12.1	Department for Culture, Media and Sports	
12.2	Department for Culture, Media and Sports	
12.3	Department for Culture, Media and Sports	
12.4	CAA/Nielsen EDI	
12.5 and 12.6	UK Film Council, CAA/Nielsen	08 Statistical Yearbook http://www.ukfilmcouncil.org.uk
12.7 and 12.10	Visit Britain	United Kingdom Tourism Survey
12.8 and 12.9	Office for National Statistics	International Passenger Survey Overseas Travel & Tourism MQ6 Overseas Travel & Tourism Statistical bulletin Travel Trends
12.11	Target Group Index, BMRB International	
12.12	Department for Culture, Media and Sports Gaming Commission National Lottery Commission	http://www.gamblingcommission.gov.uk/ http://www.natlotcomm.gov.uk/

Chapter 13: Environment

13.1, 13.2, 13.4, 13.8, 13.18 and 13.22	Office for National Statistics	Environmental Accounts Autumn 2008 http://www.statistics.gov.uk/downloads/theme_environment/ EADec2008.pdf
13.3, 13.6, 13.7, and 13.16	Department for Environment Food and Rural Affairs	e–Digest of Environmental Statistics (annual) www.defra.gov.uk/environment/statistics/index.htm The Environment in your Pocket (annual)

Table number in Abstract	Government department or other organisation	Official publication or other source
13.9 and 13.13	Centre for Ecology and Hydrology, Wallingford	www.ceh-nerc.ac.uk/data/NWA.htm
13.10	The Met Office	www.met-office.gov.uk
13.11 and 13.17	Environment Agency	www.environment-agency.gov.uk
13.12	Scottish Environment Protection agency	http://www.sepa.org.uk/water/monitoring_and_classification/scottish_monitoring_strategy.aspx
13.14	Water Services Regulation Authority (OFWAT)	Financial performance and expenditure of the water companies 2007–08 (annual) http://www.ofwat.gov.uk/regulating/reporting/rpt_fpr_2007-08.pdf
13.15	Environment Agency	*England and Wales*: www.environment-agency.gov.uk
	Scottish Environment Protection agency	*Scotland*: www.sepa.org.uk
	Environment & Heritage Services Northern Ireland	*Northern Ireland*: www.ehsni.gov.uk
13.19 and 13.20	Department for Environment Food and Rural Affairs	*England*: www.defra.gov.uk/environment/statistics/index.htm
	Welsh Assembly Government	*Wales*: www.wales.gov.uk/statistics
	Scottish Environment Protection agency	*Scotland*: www.sepa.org.uk
	Environment & Heritage Services Northern Ireland	*Northern Ireland*: www.ehsni.gov.uk
13.21	The Chartered Institute of Environmental Health	
	The Royal Environmental Health Institute of Scotland	

Chapter 14: Housing

14.1	Communities and Local Government	
	Welsh Assembly Government	
	Scottish Government	
	Department for Social Development, Northern Ireland	
14.2	Office for National Statistics	General Household Survey

Sources

Table number in Abstract	Government department or other organisation	Official publication or other source
14.3	Communities and Local Government	
	Welsh Assembly Government	*Wales*: Welsh Housing Statistics (annual)
	Scottish Government	*Scotland*: Statistical Bulletins on Housing (SG)
	Department for Social Development, Northern Ireland	*Northern Ireland*: Northern Ireland Housing Statistics (annual)
14.4	Communities and Local Government	
14.5	Communities and Local Government	
	Welsh Assembly Government	
14.6	HM Court Service Northern Ireland Court Service	
14.7	Council of Mortgage Lenders	
14.8	Communities and Local Government	
	Welsh Assembly Government	
	Scottish Government	
14.9	Communities and Local Government	Statutory Homelessness Statistical Release (quarterly) http://www.communities.gov.uk/index.asp?id=1156302

Chapter 15: Transport and communications

General

15.1, 15.2 and 15.4	Department for Transport	
15.3	Office for National Statistics	

Road Transport

15.5 to 15.12	Department for Transport	Vehicle Licensing Statistics (annual, TSO) Road Casualties Great Britain (annual, TSO) Road accidents Wales (annual, Welsh Assembly Government) Office for National Statistics: Department for Transport
15.11		Driving Standards Agency
15.13 and 15.14	Department for Regional Development, Northern Ireland	Publication: Transport Statistics NI Source: Driver and Vehicle Development, Agency

Rail Transport

15.20 and 15.21	Department for Transport	Office for National Statistics Health and Safety Executive: Industry and Services (annual) Bulletin of Rail Statistics (quarterly)
15.22 and 15.23	Department for Regional Development, Northern Ireland	Translink

Table number in Abstract	Government department or other organisation	Official publication or other source
Air Transport		
15.24 to 15.27	Civil Aviation Authority	Civil Aviation Authority; Annual Statements of Movements, Passengers and Cargo Civil Aviation Authority; Monthly Statements of Movements, Passengers and Cargo
Communications		
15.28 and 15.29	Ofcom	
	Office for National Statistics	
15.30	Royal Mail Parcel Force Capita Business Services Ltd Post Office Counters Ltd.	Monthly Digest of Statistics (Palgrave Macmillan) Post Office report and accounts (annual)

Chapter 16: National accounts

16.1 to 16.22	Office for National Statistics	United Kingdom National Accounts (annual, Palgrave Macmillan) Monthly Digest of Statistics (Palgrave Macmillan)

Chapter 17: Prices

Table number in Abstract	Government department or other organisation	Official publication or other source
Producer Prices		
17.1 and 17.2	Office for National Statistics	Producer Price Index Press Notice (monthly) Business Monitor MM22, Producer Price Indices Monthly Digest of Statistics (Palgrave Macmillan)
Consumer Prices		
17.3 to 17.6	Office for National Statistics	Economic and Labour Market Review (monthly, Palgrave Macmillan) Focus on Consumer Price Indices (monthly, National Statistics website)
17.7, 17.8	Department for Environment, Food and Rural Affairs	Agriculture in the UK (annual) Agricultural Price Indices, Statistical notice (monthly)
17.9	Office for National Statistics Eurostat	Economic and Labour Market Review (monthly)

Chapter 18: Government finance

Table number in Abstract	Government department or other organisation	Official publication or other source
Central Government		
18.1 to 18.3	Office for National Statistics	Financial Statistics (monthly, Palgrave Macmillan)
18.4 to 18.5 and 18.7	HM Treasury Office for National Statistics	Consolidated Fund and National Loans Fund Accounts Financial Statistics (monthly, Palgrave Macmillan)
18.5	HM Treasury Office for National Statistics	United Kingdom National Accounts (annual, Palgrave Macmillan)

Sources

Table number in Abstract	Government department or other organisation	Official publication or other source
18.6	Office for National Statistics	United Kingdom National Accounts (annual, Palgrave Macmillan)
18.8 and 18.9	HM Revenue & Customs	www.hmrc.gov.uk
18.10	Office for National Statistics	
Tax rates		
18.11 and 18.12	HM Revenue & Customs	www.hmrc.gov.uk
Rateable values		
18.13	HM Revenue & Customs	www.hmrc.gov.uk
Local Authorities		
18.14	Communities and Local Government Welsh Assembly Government Public Works Loan Board Scottish Executive Statistical Support for Local Government Department of Finance and Personnel for Northern Ireland Department of the Environment for Northern Ireland Chartered Institute of Public Finance and Accountancy	Local government financial statistics (England) (annual) Welsh local government financial statistics (annual) Annual report of the Public Works Loan Board Local Financial Returns (Scotland) (annual)
18.15 to 18.19	Communities and Local Government Welsh Assembly Government	Local government financial statistics (England) (annual) Welsh local government financial statistics (annual)
18.20 to 18.22	Scottish Government Statistical Support for Local Government	Local financial returns (Scotland) (annual) Capital Returns (Scotland) (annual)
18.23	Department of the Environment for Northern Ireland	District Council – Summary of Statement of Accounts (annual)

Chapter 19: External trade and investment

19.1 to 19.8	HM Revenue & Customs	OTS1 – Overseas Trade Statistics – Extra EC, (formerly MM20) (monthly) OTS2 – Overseas Trade Statistics – Intra EC and World (formerly MM20A) (monthly) OTSQ – Overseas Trade Statistics – Intra EC, (formerly MQ20) (quarterly) OTSA – Overseas Trade Statistics – Extra and Intra EC (formerly MA20) (annual)
		Business Monitor MM24, Monthly Review of External Trade Statistics (monthly, Palgrave Macmillan) Overseas Trade Analysed in Terms of Industries MQ10 (quarterly, Palgrave Macmillan)
	Office for National Statistics	Monthly Digest of Statistics (monthly, Palgrave Macmillan)

Table number in Abstract	Government department or other organisation	Official publication or other source
19.9 to 19.18	Office for National Statistics Bank of England	United Kingdom Balance of Payments (annual, Palgrave Macmillan) UK Economic Accounts (quarterly, Palgrave Macmillan) Financial Statistics (monthly, Palgrave Macmillan) Business Monitor Foreign Direct Investment MA4 (annual)

Chapter 20: Research and development

20.1 to 20.5	Office for National Statistics	Business Monitor MA14, Research and Development in UK Business (annual)

Chapter 21: Agriculture, fisheries and food

Agriculture

21.1 to 21.3	Department for Environment Food and Rural Affairs	Agriculture in the United Kingdom 2007 (annual)
21.6	Forestry Commission Department of agriculture and Rural Development (Northern Ireland)	Forestry Statistics (annual) Northern Ireland Annual Abstract of statistics

Fisheries

21.14 and 21.15	Department for Environment Food and Rural Affairs Scottish Government Agricultural Departments	

Family food

21.16	Department for Environment Food and Rural Affairs	Expenditure and Food Survey (annual) (1990 onwards edition–Family Spending) (annual, Palgrave Macmillan)

Chapter 22: Production

Production and construction

22.1	Office for National Statistics	Annual Business Inquiry (www.statistics.gov.uk/abi)

Manufacturers sales

22.2	Office for National Statistics	ProdCom: Product Sales and Trade Annual Reports – PRA series (annual, ONS) Product Sales and Trade Quarterly Reports – PRQ series (quarterly, ONS)
22.3	Office for National Statistics	UK Business: Activity, Size and Location (www.statistics.gov.uk/ukbusiness)

Sources

Table number in Abstract	Government department or other organisation	Official publication or other source
Energy		
22.4 to 22.13	Department of Energy and Climate Change	Digest of United Kingdom Energy Statistics (annual) Energy Trends (monthly and quarterly) Annual Business Inquiry (www.statistics.gov.uk/abi)
Iron and steel		
22.14 to 22.16	Iron and Steel Statistics Bureau	Iron and steel industry: annual statistics published by the Iron and Steel Statistics Bureau Corporation Regional Trends (annual, Palgrave Macmillan)
Industrial materials		
22.17	World Bureau of Metal Statistics Aluminium Federation	World Metal Statistics (monthly) Annual Business Inquiry (www.statistics.gov.uk/abi)
22.18	Agricultural Industries Confederation	Annual Business Inquiry (www.statistics.gov.uk/abi)
Minerals		
22.19	Communities and Local Government	Minerals (Business Monitor PA 1007) (annual)
	Department for Business, Enterprise and Regulatory Reform	Natural Environment Research Council: United Kingdom
	Department of Economic Development (Northern Ireland)	Minerals Yearbook Northern Ireland Annual Abstract of Statistics
Building materials		
22.20	Department for Business, Enterprise and Regulatory Reform	Monthly Statistics of Building Materials and Components (BERR) Monthly Digest of Statistics (Palgrave Macmillan)
Construction		
22.21 and 22.22	Office for National Statistics	Monthly Digest of Statistics (Palgrave Macmillan)
Engineering		
22.23 and 22.24	Office for National Statistics	Annual Business Inquiry (www.statistics.gov.uk/abi) UK Business: Activity, Size and Location (www.statistics.gov.uk/Ukbusiness)
Motor vehicle production		
22.25	Office for National Statistics	Monthly Digest of Statistics (Palgrave Macmillan)
Drink and tobacco		
22.26 and 22.27	HM Revenue & Customs	Annual report of the Commissioners of HM Revenue and Customs (www.hmrc.gov.uk/stats/tax_receipts/menu.htm) and HMRC Statistical Bulletins on UK Trade Information website (www.uktradeinfo.com/index.cfm?task=bulletins) Monthly Digest of Statistics (Palgrave Macmillan)

Table number in Abstract	Government department or other organisation	Official publication or other source

Chapter 23: Banking, insurance etc

Banking

23.1	Bank of England	Bank of England Annual Report and Accounts
23.2	Association for Payment Clearing Services	Yearbook of Payment Statistics 2008
23.3 to 23.7	Bank of England	Bank of England, Statistical Interactive Database
23.8	Bank of England	Bank of England Quarterly Bulletin
23.9 to 23.12	Bank of England	Financial Statistics (monthly, Palgrave Macmillan)

Other financial institutions

23.13	Financial Services Authority	Building Societies: Statistical Tables http://www.fsa.gov.uk/pages/Library/Other_publications/Miscellaneous/2007/bs_stats.shtml
23.14	Office for National Statistics	Business Monitor SDQ7, Assets and Liabilities of Finance Houses and Other Credit Companies (quarterly)
23.15	Office for National Statistics	Financial Statistics (monthly, Palgrave Macmillan) Monthly Digest of Statistics (Palgrave Macmillan) Business Monitor MQ5, Insurance Companies; Pension Funds and Trusts Investments (quarterly) Statistical bulletin
23.16 and 23.17	Office for National Statistics	Financial Statistics (monthly, Palgrave Macmillan) Business Monitor MQ5, Insurance Companies; Pension Funds and InsolvencyTrusts Investments (quarterly)
23.18 and 23.19	Insolvency service	

Chapter 24: Service industry

Retail trades

24.1	Office for National Statistics	Annual Business Inquiry (www.statistics.gov.uk/abi/2007-archive/default.asp)
24.2	Office for National Statistics	Business Monitor SDM 28, www.statistics.gov.uk/rsi

Motor trades

24.3	Office for National Statistics	Annual Business Inquiry (www.statistics.gov.uk/abi) (www.statistics.gov.uk/abi/2007-archive/default.asp)

Catering

24.4	Office for National Statistics	Annual Business Inquiry (www.statistics.gov.uk/abi) (www.statistics.gov.uk/abi/2007-archive/default.asp)

Sources

442

Index

Figures indicate table numbers

Index

Index

Index

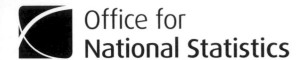
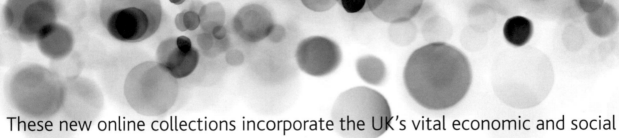